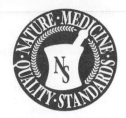

Natural Standard

MEDICAL CONDITIONS REFERENCE

An Integrative Approach

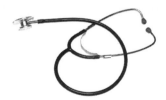 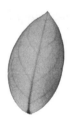

Natural Standard Research Collaboration

Somerville, Massachusetts, USA

www.naturalstandard.com

Chief Editor

Catherine Ulbricht, PharmD

Natural Standard Research Collaboration
Somerville, Massachusetts, USA
www.naturalstandard.com
Department of Pharmacy
Massachusetts General Hospital
Boston, Massachusetts, USA

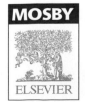

MOSBY

ELSEVIER

11830 Westline Industrial Drive
St. Louis, Missouri 63146

NATURAL STANDARD MEDICAL CONDITIONS
REFERENCE: AN INTEGRATIVE APPROACH   ISBN: 978-0-323-06405-7
Copyright © 2009 by Mosby, Inc., an affiliate of Elsevier Inc.

Notice

Knowledge and best practice in this field are constantly changing. As new research and experience broaden our knowledge, changes in practice, treatment and drug therapy may become necessary or appropriate. Readers are advised to check the most current information provided (i) on procedures featured or (ii) by the manufacturer of each product to be administered, to verify the recommended dose or formula, the method and duration of administration, and contraindications. It is the responsibility of the practitioner, relying on their own experience and knowledge of the patient, to make diagnoses, to determine dosages and the best treatment for each individual patient, and to take all appropriate safety precautions. To the fullest extent of the law, neither the Publisher nor the Editors assumes any liability for any injury and/or damage to persons or property arising out of or related to any use of the material contained in this book.

The Publisher

Library of Congress Cataloging-in-Publication Data
Natural Standard medical conditions reference : an integrative approach
/ edited by Catherine (Kate) Ulbricht. – 1st ed.
  p. ; cm.
 Includes bibliographical references and index.
 ISBN 978-0-323-06405-7 (pbk. : alk. paper) 1. Integrative
medicine–Handbooks, manuals, etc. I. Ulbricht, Catherine E. II.
Natural Standard (Firm) III. Title: Medical conditions reference.
 [DNLM: 1. Diagnostic Techniques and Procedures–Handbooks. 2. Signs
and Symptoms–Handbooks. WB 39 N2856 2009]
 R733.N3685 2009
 616.07'5–dc22

2008044244

Vice President and Publisher: Linda Duncan
Senior Editor: Kellie White
Senior Developmental Editor: Jennifer Watrous
Publishing Services Manager: Hemamalini Rajendrababu
Senior Project Manager: Mary Pohlman
Project Manager: Srikumar Narayanan
Senior Designer: Teresa McBryan

Printed in United States of America

Last digit is the print number: 9 8 7 6 5 4 3 2 1

PREFACE

Natural Standard Medical Conditions Reference: An Integrative Approach provides detailed information on over 120 common medical conditions along with prevention tips and conventional and integrative treatment options in 40 chapters. This trustworthy resource is compiled by the internationally renowned research collaboration that developed the subscription database www.naturalstandard.com, which is available to healthcare professionals and consumers. Finally, a subset of this epic work is available to the public in print format. Unlike other resources that aggregate and repurpose outdated information, Natural Standard has pioneered this intellectual property which further distinguishes this book from other typical conditions guides available on the market.

This evidence-based, unbiased resource compares drug therapies, surgical procedures, diet, exercise, nutrition, complementary/alternative modalities, and herb and supplement therapies, offering a whole body (integrative) approach to healthcare. Content has been reviewed by over 500 multidisciplinary healthcare providers and researchers from around the world to establish high quality, up-to-date consensus statements on the standard of care. Health is optimized by exploring all therapeutic options for medical conditions—not only prescription drugs.

WHO WILL BENEFIT FROM THIS BOOK?

This book is an all-inclusive reference tool for clinicians and their patients, providing the standard in evidence-based integrative patient care. Natural Standard facilitates understanding of common medical conditions, plus safety and efficacy of conventional and integrative therapies used to treat these conditions. Detailed prevention discussions help readers with strategies to reduce the risk of developing the condition or experiencing recurrences. Allied health professionals and educated consumers alike will benefit from this book.

WHY IS THIS BOOK IMPORTANT TO THE PROFESSION?

Integrative therapies have continued to gain popularity and constitute a multi-billion dollar commercial industry. As more patients adopt integrative approaches, it is increasingly important that healthcare providers and consumers have access to evidence-based information on these therapies for educated and safe decision making. This book serves as an information clearinghouse that fosters open dialogue amongst caregivers and the receivers of care to ensure teamwork and proper monitoring of all therapies.

Some herbs, supplements, and other complementary and alternative therapies are commonly used to treat medical conditions, despite a lack of evidence-based data supporting their use; this is an area of controversy. For example, many widely marketed dietary supplements are popularly used for weight loss, but proposed product effects may be primarily based on anecdotal or traditional evidence, rather than scientific data. Adequate safety information is often not readily available. For each herb, supplement, and integrative therapy in this book, Natural Standard consolidates the level of available evidence for a one stop look-up versus having to read multiple books and collating their results.

Although integrative therapies may be beneficial or more cost effective for many conditions, they may pose similar health risks as conventional therapies. For instance, herbs and supplements contain pharmacologically active constituents and may interact or potentiate the effects of other herbs or supplements, or drugs, foods, or laboratory assays. Despite these risks, many commercially available software programs, relied on in pharmacies as educational resources, do not recognize these interactions. This reference book aggregates the available safety data and concisely states the contraindications of each therapy so that pros and cons can be weighed before initiating a new healthcare regimen.

ORGANIZATION AND DISTINCTIVE FEATURES

Chapters are organized alphabetically by main medical condition, and cross-indexed by medical specialty on the inside back cover. Each chapter is divided into the following sections.

- **Background:** In the background section, the medical condition and related conditions are clearly defined. This section provides a concise and easy to understand summary of the disease.
- **Risk factors:** Here, risk factors are discussed, such as family history of the disease, age, or gender, that may predispose certain individuals to developing the condition.
- **Causes:** The causes section discusses the disease pathology. If the cause is unknown, theoretical etiology is described.

- **Signs and symptoms:** The defining signs and symptoms of the condition as well as its onset are discussed here. Additionally, uncommon and rare signs and symptoms are mentioned.
- **Diagnosis:** The diagnosis section explains which exam parameters and tests are used to diagnose and monitor a specific condition.
- **Complications:** Medical disorders associated with the main condition are discussed. When possible, this section states the prevalence of each complication, as well its severity and patient prognosis.
- **Treatment:** In the treatment section, it is clearly stated whether the disease has a known cure. Then, conventional medical treatment is thoroughly explained. Pharmacological (prescription and over-the-counter [OTC]) treatment methods, as well as non-pharmacological treatments, including lifestyle changes, are listed. Lastly, physical or occupational therapy treatment options, or surgical procedures are discussed.
- **Integrative therapies:** In each monograph, integrative therapies are categorized according to the available level of evidence. This text uses Natural Standard's validated, reproducible grading system to rate effectiveness. Therapies are categorized by strong scientific evidence, good scientific evidence, unclear or conflicting evidence (poor quality or confusing study results), fair negative scientific evidence (evidence suggests possible ineffectiveness) or strong negative scientific evidence (evidence suggests likely ineffectiveness). Safety concerns such as precautions and contraindications are also described so that readers are armed with data to make informed healthcare decisions based on all therapeutic options.
- **Prevention:** Prevention strategies are discussed. Even if a particular disorder is hereditary or not preventable, clinical suggestions are offered to help reduce symptoms, prevent complications, or reduce the risk of recurrences.

Given that many patients self-prescribe herbs and supplements regardless of potential safety risks, the information in these monographs is a necessary evidence-based guide for clinicians, investigators, and educated consumers to rely upon. Integrative care discussion promotes open communication between healthcare providers and patients. The sum of the information on each specific medical condition, treatment safety and efficacy, plus lifestyle suggestions and prevention measures make this text a complete resource for those interested in fully integrated medical practice.

OTHER RESOURCES

This volume is a welcome addition to the Natural Standard series of books including the *Natural Standard Herb & Supplement Reference: Evidence-based Clinical Reviews* and the *Natural Standard Herb & Supplement Handbook: The Clinical Bottom Line.* Coming soon—*Natural Standard Herbal Pharmacotherapy: An Integrative Approach.*

NOTE TO STUDENTS

As integrative therapies continue to gain popularity, it is increasingly necessary for students to have readily available access to evidence-based information regarding these therapies. Questions about these therapies appear on licensing exams, and integrative therapy products line the shelves of all retail stores. For the newly practicing clinician or student in residency, reliable safety and efficacy information on controversial and emerging therapies is critical to help minimize liability/malpractice risk. Students will be able to refer to this book as a trusted decision support tool and will be able to learn to counsel patients with more reliability and confidence in the area of integrative therapy.

ACKNOWLEDGMENTS

We are grateful for the on going contributions of Natural Standard's authors, peer reviewers, and editors since the founding of our international research collaboration (*see About Us on www.naturalstandard.com*). The hard work and dedication of the following content team members deserve special recognition for helping make this particular book available:

Dawn Costa, Shaina Tanguay-Colucci, Wendy Weissner, and Jen Woods. Additionally, we thank our operational, outreach, member services, and technical support teams, along with our Board of Directors for their ongoing support of evidence-based integrative medicine research.

CONTENTS

CONDITIONS: Addictions, Substance Abuse, Gambling Addiction

BACKGROUND

Addiction occurs when an individual becomes physically or psychologically dependent on something, such as alcohol, drugs (legal or illegal), or gambling. Individuals may become addicted to or have compulsive behaviors in regard to almost anything, including sex, food, exercise, shopping/spending money, work, and the Internet. The principles and consequences of addictions are generally the same, even if the particular addiction is different.

Substance Abuse (Drug Addiction): Substance abuse occurs when individuals use drugs (which may or may not be illegal) for recreational purposes. Commonly abused drugs include alcohol, central nervous system stimulants (such as nicotine, caffeine, and methamphetamine), cocaine, heroin, and marijuana. Drugs can be taken by mouth, injected into a vein, snorted through the nose, inhaled, or smoked.

When individuals abuse drugs, they are at risk of becoming physically and/or emotionally addicted. Over time, individuals begin to develop a tolerance for the drugs. As a result, they may start to use larger amounts of the drug more frequently. However, individuals can become addicted to substances without abusing them. Drug addictions cause compulsive drug cravings. Severe addictions may cause individuals to seek drugs, even at the expense of their jobs, families, and other important parts of their lives.

Drug addiction is considered a treatable disease if individuals want treatment and have the motivation and will power to stay sober. For many people, drug addiction is chronic, and it may last for years before they are willing and able to get help. Some individuals (not all) experience relapses after completing treatment programs.

Gambling Addiction: Gambling addiction, also called compulsive gambling, occurs when individuals are unable to control their gambling behaviors. Some individuals are constantly trying to win back lost money, and they may go to extremes to hide their gambling. Others compulsively gamble for the thrill and excitement of it, rather than for the actual winnings. Some individuals who are addicted to gambling may go to extreme lengths to perpetuate their addiction when money is scarce. In serious cases, this may include lying, stealing, cheating, or fraud.

Patients with gambling problems may develop associated conditions, such as alcohol dependence or drug addictions.

Stopping substance abuse or gambling addictions is often difficult. Fortunately, rehabilitation programs and support groups are available to help patients overcome their addictions. However, many patients relapse one or more times, even after long periods of abstinence from the drug or gambling. Support groups and social networks are available to help individuals overcome their addictions.

CAUSES

General: Most experts agree that a combination of biological, psychological, and environmental factors may predispose certain individuals to developing addictions.

It has also been suggested, but not scientifically proven, that individuals who are addicted to drugs or gambling may have addictive personalities. Supporters of this theory believe that this psychological trait may predispose someone to developing an addiction. However, this idea is the subject of much debate in the research community.

Substance Abuse: Initially, individuals may abuse drugs to get high. This desire to get high may stem from underlying causes, such as depression, bipolar disorder, stress, or low self-esteem. Others may try drugs out of curiosity or peer pressure. Once a person becomes addicted to a substance, it causes chemical changes in the brain that lead to intense drug cravings.

Recent studies suggest that trauma, substance abuse, and sexual risk behaviors are all interrelated. For instance, women who were sexually abused (as a child or as an adult) may have a hard time refusing unwanted sex and may use drugs as a coping mechanism.

Some research suggests that genetics may play a role in certain types of drug addictions. For instance, people with family histories of alcoholism are more likely to begin drinking before the age of 20 and to become alcoholics.

Individuals who experiment with illegal drugs and alcohol before the age of 16 have an increased risk of becoming drug addicts.

It has also been suggested that tobacco, alcohol, and marijuana are gateway drugs that may lead to experimentation with more serious drugs, such as heroin or cocaine. However, this theory has not been proven, and it is considered controversial.

Gambling Addiction: The exact cause of gambling addiction remains unknown. It has been suggested that chemicals in the brain, called serotonin, norepinephrine (noradrenaline), and dopamine, may be involved. These chemicals, also called neurotransmitters, allow nerve cells in the body to communicate. Serotonin helps regulate mood and behavior, norepinephrine helps the body handle stress, and dopamine causes the sensation of pleasure. It has been suggested that all three of these neurotransmitters may be involved in compulsive gambling.

SIGNS AND SYMPTOMS

General: Because individuals with addictions often deny they have problems, it is important for friends, family, coworkers, and others to watch for warning signs of addiction. When people are aware that a friend or loved one has a drug or gambling problem, they should try to persuade the person to undergo screening for drug or gambling addiction. If the person is still unable to recognize and seek help for his or her addiction, a group intervention may be planned to help the patient overcome the addiction.

Many patients who have substance abuse or gambling addictions share many of the same behavioral signs and symptoms. For instance, they may lie about their behaviors, deny they have problems, or use drugs or gamble in secret.

Substance Abuse: Individuals who are addicted to drugs typically experience compulsive drug cravings. In serious cases, these cravings may cause individuals to continue to seek drugs, even if it means risking their jobs, families, or other important parts of their lives. Specific symptoms of drug addiction depend on the substances that are being abused. Most substances cause a change in the patient's consciousness, usually a decrease in responsiveness. Other signs and symptoms may include the inability to relax while sober, mood swings and change in attitude, statements that do not make sense, and sudden changes in performance at school or work. Individuals may spend less time with friends and family members and/or stop participating in activities that they used to enjoy.

When individuals stop using drugs they are addicted to, withdrawal symptoms often develop. In general, symptoms of withdrawal may include irritability, headaches, nausea, vomiting, and mood swings. The severity of withdrawal symptoms varies, depending on the specific drug. For instance, individuals who are psychologically addicted to marijuana may experience symptoms of irritability, anxiety, and decreased appetite when they stop using the drug. In contrast, individuals who abuse methamphetamines experience much more severe withdrawal symptoms that may even be life threatening. Examples of these symptoms

include intense cravings for the drug, psychotic reactions, anxiety, moderate to severe depression, intense hunger, irritability, fatigue, mental confusion, and insomnia.

Gambling Addiction: Signs and symptoms of a gambling problem typically include being preoccupied with gambling, taking time away from work or loved ones to gamble, hiding gambling behaviors from friends and loved ones, feeling guilty or remorseful after gambling, borrowing or stealing money to use for gambling, and failing to limit or stop gambling behaviors.

COMPLICATIONS

General: Many complications associated with addictions, including drug addictions and gambling addictions, are the same. For instance, drug and gambling addictions may lead to social or interpersonal problems. Serious addictions may cause some patients to do things they normally would not (such as lie or steal) to fulfill their addictions. If this occurs, the person may have strained relationships with friends, family members, and loved ones.

Substance Abuse: Studies have shown that individuals who use illegal drugs (such as heroin or cocaine) typically engage in riskier behaviors than non–drug users. For instance, users may trade sex for drugs or money, or they may engage in behaviors that put them at risk for contracting infectious diseases (such as HIV or hepatitis) while under the influence of drugs. However, this is not true of all drug users.

Substance abuse during pregnancy may lead to serious birth defects or even prenatal death or stillbirth. If a woman uses drugs during pregnancy, the baby may be born with a drug addiction and go into withdrawal.

Individuals who are addicted to substances may have difficulty caring for loved ones, such as children or elderly parents.

Sharing intravenous needles with others increases the risk of transmitting or acquiring infectious diseases, including HIV, hepatitis B, and hepatitis C.

Drugs that are being abused may interact with other medications, herbs, or supplements and have serious medical consequences. For example, diabetics should not consume alcohol because it can affect blood sugar levels.

Amphetamines and cocaine have been shown to cause impotence in men.

Long-term abuse of stimulants changes the way the brain functions and may lead to severe mental disorders and memory loss. Long-term abuse of alcohol may lead to cirrhosis of the liver or liver failure.

Some drugs, including alcohol, heroin, cocaine, and methamphetamines, can be fatal if they are taken in high doses. Signs of an overdose include loss of consciousness, slowed or faint heartbeat, decreased blood pressure, slowed breathing, and chest pain. Individuals who experience any of these symptoms after using drugs should be taken to the nearest hospital immediately.

Gambling Addiction: Gambling may lead to drug abuse or alcohol dependence. This is because alcohol and drugs, like gambling, are often used to escape from problems.

DIAGNOSIS

Substance Abuse: Drug addiction is typically diagnosed after an evaluation by a psychiatrist, psychologist, or a professional addiction counselor. If drug addiction is suspected, the healthcare professional will ask many questions related to drug use. For instance, if the patient has felt like he/she uses drugs too frequently or if he/she has ever felt guilty about using drugs, this may suggest a drug addiction. Also, if friends or family members have criticized the patient's drug use, or the patient has used drugs first thing in the morning, this may also indicate a drug problem.

Drug screening tests are available for most substances. These tests can help a healthcare provider determine if drugs are present in the patient's body. These tests are especially helpful when drug use is suspected, but the patient denies it. However, the presence of a drug does not necessarily indicate a drug addiction. A doctor may take a sample of blood, urine, or hair from the patient. This sample is then analyzed in a laboratory for certain drugs. Over-the-counter (OTC) drug kits are available at most local pharmacies for home testing. Some drugs stay in the body for longer periods of time than others, regardless of how frequently the drugs are taken. For instance, marijuana can be detected in the blood for up to one month, while alcohol may be present in the blood for one to 12 hours.

Gambling Addiction: For compulsive gambling to be diagnosed, at least five of the following signs and symptoms must be present. 1) The patient is preoccupied with gambling. For instance, the individual may be constantly thinking about ways or places to gamble. 2) The patient has tried to stop or limit his/her gambling behaviors without success. 3) The patient needs more and more money to become excited about gambling. 4) The patient continues gambling in an effort to win back lost money. 5) When the patient tries to limit his/her gambling, he/she feels irritable. 6) Gambling is used as a way to escape or temporarily forget problems. 7) The patient lies to friends, family members, and/or loved ones about his/her gambling problem. 8) The patient commits crimes, such as theft or fraud, to get more gambling money. 9) The patient asks others for financial help when he/she runs out of money. 10) The patient risks an important relationship or career or educational career because of a gambling addiction.

PLANNING AN INTERVENTION

General: An intervention is a process that helps a drug addict recognize the seriousness of his/her problem. This technique is typically used when a patient does not realize the extent of his/her problem and has been unwilling to receive help up to this point. An intervention allows the individual to evaluate his/her own behavior through the eyes of others. During an intervention, friends and loved ones provide objective and non-judgmental feedback of the patient's behavior.

A group of friends and family members who plan to organize and conduct an intervention should receive guidance and counseling from a professional who is experienced with interventions. Friends and family members can also hire a qualified interventionist to moderate the intervention. This helps ensure that the intervention is safe. The interventionist also serves as an unbiased third party for the patient.

Form a Group: A group of the patient's closest friends and family members get together to plan an intervention. A leader should be chosen if an interventionist is not hired as a moderator. This person will serve as the moderator during the intervention.

Research: Individuals involved in the intervention should do as much research as possible before the intervention to learn about addiction, potential treatment options, and rehabilitation programs.

Make a Plan: The group that plans to do the intervention usually meets several times before the intervention takes place. The members share what they plan to say to the patient. They also choose a date and safe and comfortable location (usually a friend or family member's home) for the intervention.

Element of Surprise: The element of surprise is essential for an intervention. If the individual knows that an intervention will take place, he/she is unlikely to attend, especially if he/she does not believe he/she has a problem.

How to Approach the Addict: Each person involved in the intervention has a chance to speak with the addict. It is generally recommended that each person starts off by telling the addict how much he/she is cared for, followed by how his/her actions have affected the lives of others. Next, state the consequences. Experts recommend telling the addict that unless he/she gets help, there will be consequences to face. These consequences are not to punish the addict, but to protect the friend or family member from the harmful behavior of the abuser. For instance, a friend may say he/she will no longer give the addict any money unless the addict agrees to receive help.

Listen: After each person talks, the addict should have an opportunity to speak. The addict may have questions about treatment options. It is important that the interventionist, friends, and family members are prepared to provide the addict with information about professionals to contact for help.

If the person is still unwilling to accept help after the intervention, friends and family members should follow through with the consequences they discussed earlier. The person has to want help in order to be effectively treated.

TREATMENT

General: Substance abuse is typically treated with rehabilitation programs and support groups. Gambling additions are typically treated with psychotherapy, medications, and support groups. Risk reduction programs may also be beneficial for addicts.

Even with treatment, individuals may experiences relapses. It is estimated that about 33% of compulsive gamblers relapse within three months of initial treatment. Relapse statistics for drug addicts vary significantly depending on the specific drug used. Whenever possible, friends, family members, and loved ones should be included in therapy and treatment to provide support and help prevent relapses.

Rehabilitation Programs: Rehabilitation treatment programs are available to help patients recover from addiction. Treatment may include group therapy, motivational interviewing, family therapy, and one-on-one counseling. The duration of most rehabilitation programs is one to several months. Programs are tailored to specific individuals.

In addition to receiving treatment for the drug addiction, patients also receive treatment for the underlying cause. There are treatment centers that are specialized to help addicts with associated problems. For instance, some centers help drug addicts that have been sexually abused. Patients may receive psychotherapy and family counseling during rehab. Other centers specialize in drug addicts with psychological illnesses, such as bipolar

disorder or depression. These rehab centers may include psychotherapy and drug therapy to manage symptoms of psychological disorders.

During rehabilitation, medications called narcotic antagonists have been found useful in treating substance abuse specifically. In addition, medications such as buprenorphine may be prescribed to overcome withdrawal symptoms of opiate addictions.

Support Groups: Self-help and support groups are often beneficial for both substance abusers and gambling addicts. These groups provide support to individuals who are in the recovery process. National programs, such as Alcoholics Anonymous, Narcotics Anonymous, and Gamblers Anonymous, are some of the more widely known support groups that are available. However, many other programs are also available. Some support groups may include aspects of spirituality or religion. Others may be more specialized to meet the needs of addicts who also have psychological disorders or have been abused.

Support groups may also be beneficial for the friends and family members who are trying to rebuild relationships with the addict.

Not all support groups require face-to-face meetings. There are also many online support groups, which include chat rooms and message boards. They allow individuals to talk with others who share the same challenges.

Risk Reduction Programs: Risk reduction programs may also be beneficial for drug addicts and compulsive gamblers. These programs have trained counselors and advisors who teach skills to help individuals avoid unwanted consequences related to drugs or gambling. Drug risk reduction programs may also help prevent individuals who are predisposed to addictions from becoming dependent on drugs or gambling.

Psychotherapy: A form of psychotherapy, called cognitive behavior therapy, is often used to treat patients with compulsive gambling problems. During therapy, the patient meets with a qualified mental health professional to replace unhealthy and irrational beliefs and behaviors with positive ones. Counselors may also help patients learn how to manage stress, improve self-esteem, and deal with other factors that can potentially trigger relapses.

Group therapy also may be helpful. During group therapy sessions, the patient talks with other people who share the same challenges. This provides the patient with feedback and support from others.

Patients with drug addictions may also undergo various forms of psychotherapy during and after rehabilitation.

Medications: Patients with gambling addictions may benefit from some types of medications. For instance, antidepressants and mood stabilizers are often used to treat compulsive gambling. These medications may also help treat underlying psychological problems, such as depression or bipolar disorder. Also, medications called narcotic antagonists may help treat compulsive gambling.

INTEGRATIVE THERAPIES

Good Scientific Evidence

Thiamin: Thiamin (also spelled "thiamine") is a water-soluble B-complex vitamin. It is also known as vitamin B_1 or aneurine. Patients who suffer from chronic alcoholism or alcohol withdrawal are at risk of thiamin deficiency and its associated complications. Supplemental thiamin can help prevent deficiencies in these patients.

Thiamin is generally considered safe and relatively nontoxic, even at high doses. Avoid if allergic or hypersensitive to thiamin. Thiamin appears safe if pregnant or breastfeeding when taken in the recommended dosages.

Unclear or Conflicting Scientific Evidence

5-Hydroxy-L-Tryptophan (5-HTP): 5-HTP is the precursor for serotonin. Serotonin is the brain chemical associated with sleep, mood, movement, feeding, and nervousness. Early study suggests that 5-HTP may lessen alcohol withdrawal symptoms. Further research is needed to confirm these results.

Avoid if allergic to 5-HTP. Avoid with eosinophilia, Down's syndrome, or mitochondrial encephalomyopathy. Avoid if taking monoamine oxidase inhibitors. Use cautiously with gastrointestinal and kidney disorders. Use cautiously if taking antidepressants, carbidopa, phenobarbital, pindolol, reserpine, tramadol, or zolpidem. Avoid if pregnant or breastfeeding.

Acupressure, Shiatsu: During acupressure, finger pressure is applied to specific acupoints on the body. Acupressure is used around the world for relaxation, wellness promotion, and the treatment of many health problems. Preliminary evidence suggests that acupressure may be a helpful adjunct therapy to assist with the prevention of relapse, withdrawal, or dependence on drugs. Further research is necessary to confirm these findings before a firm conclusion can be reached.

With proper training, acupressure appears to be safe if self-administered or administered by an experienced therapist. No serious long-term complications have been reported, according to

scientific data. Hand nerve injury and herpes zoster ("shingles") cases have been reported after shiatsu massage. Forceful acupressure may cause bruising.

Acupuncture: Acupuncture is commonly used throughout the world. According to Chinese medicine theory, the human body contains a network of energy pathways through which vital energy, called "chi," circulates. These pathways contain specific points that function like gates, allowing chi to flow through the body. Needles are inserted into these points to regulate the flow of chi. Studies that evaluated the effectiveness of acupuncture in alcoholism have produced mixed results. More studies are needed to evaluate the use of acupuncture in this application.

More studies are needed before a recommendation can be made for or against the use of acupuncture in cocaine/opiate addictions.

Needles must be sterile in order to avoid disease transmission. Avoid with valvular heart disease, medical conditions of unknown origins, or infections. Acupuncture should not be applied to the chest in patients with lung diseases or on any area that may rely on muscle tone to provide stability. Avoid use in infants, young children, or in patients with needle phobias. Use cautiously with bleeding disorders, neurological disorders, seizure disorders, or diabetes. Use cautiously in elderly or medically compromised patients. Use cautiously in patients who will drive or operate heavy machinery after acupuncture. Use cautiously if taking anticoagulants. Avoid if pregnant.

Colon Therapy/Colonic Irrigation: Colon therapy is the use of herbs or water to clean out the colon or large intestine to treat certain health conditions. One small study of unclear methodology suggested that colonic irrigation employing Chinese herbs may augment dihydroetorphine and methadone therapy in heroin addicts going through withdrawal, possibly resulting in more rapid detoxification. However, the data provided are insufficient for making any definitive conclusions. More studies are needed.

Excessive treatments may allow the body to absorb too much water, which may cause electrolyte imbalances, nausea, vomiting, heart failure, fluid in the lungs, abnormal heart rhythms, or coma. Infections have been reported, possibly due to contaminated equipment or as a result of clearing out normal colon bacteria that destroys infectious bacteria. There is a risk of the bowel wall breaking, which is a serious complication that can lead to septic shock and death. Avoid with diverticulitis, ulcerative colitis, Crohn's disease, severe or internal hemorrhoids, rectal/colon tumors, or if recovering from bowel surgery. Avoid frequent treatments with heart or kidney disease. Colonic equipment must be sterile. Colonic irrigation should not be used as the only treatment for serious conditions. Avoid if pregnant or breastfeeding due to a lack of scientific data.

Dehydroepiandrosterone (DHEA): DHEA is a hormone that is produced by the adrenal glands. Preliminary study shows that DHEA is not beneficial in treating cocaine dependence, but further study is needed before a firm conclusion can be drawn.

Avoid if allergic to DHEA. Use cautiously with adrenal or thyroid disorders, depression, panic disorder, bipolar disorder, psychotic disorders, heart disorders, polycystic ovary syndrome, anovulatory infertility, steroid 21-hydroxylase deficiency, gynecomastia, overactive thyroid, bacterial infections, or diabetes. Use cautiously if at risk for prostate cancer, liver cancer, breast cancer, or ovarian cancer. Use cautiously in HIV patients with Kaposi's sarcoma or in patients who have received flu shots. Use cautiously if taking alprazolam, amlodipine, anastrozole, benfluorex, beta-adrenergic antagonists, calcium channel blockers, canrenoate, danazol, diltiazem, growth hormone, methylphenidates, metopirone, nitrendipine, or hormones or dietary supplements with hormone-like effects (e.g., chromium picolinate). Avoid if pregnant or breastfeeding.

Hypnotherapy, Hypnosis: Hypnosis is a trancelike state in which a person becomes more aware and focused and is more open to suggestion. Hypnotherapy has been used to treat health conditions and to change behaviors. There is inconclusive evidence on the effectiveness of hypnotherapy to treat drug addictions, including alcohol dependence. Additional study is needed before a firm conclusion can be drawn.

Use cautiously with mental illnesses (e.g., psychosis/schizophrenia, manic depression, multiple personality disorder, or dissociative disorders) or seizure disorders.

Kudzu: Kudzu has been traditionally used in China to treat alcoholism, diabetes, gastroenteritis, and deafness. Although preliminary study indicates that kudzu may help treat alcoholism, additional human study is needed to make a firm recommendation.

Avoid if allergic to kudzu, its constituents, or members of the Fabaceae/Leguminosae family. Avoid if taking methotrexate. Use cautiously if taking anticoagulants, drugs that treat diabetes, benzodiazepines, bisphosphonates, mecamylamine, neurologic agents, drugs that have estrogenic activity, drugs that lower blood pressure, or drugs that are broken down by the liver. Avoid if pregnant or breastfeeding due to a lack of safety evidence.

L-Carnitine: The human body produces L-carnitine in the liver, kidney, and brain. L-carnitine, or acetyl-L-carnitine, may be of benefit to alcoholics. Additional study is needed to make a firm recommendation.

Avoid if allergic to L-carnitine. Use cautiously with peripheral vascular disease, hypertension (high blood pressure), alcohol-induced liver cirrhosis, and diabetes. Use cautiously in low birth weight infants and individuals on hemodialysis. Use cautiously if taking anticoagulants (blood thinners), beta-blockers, or calcium channel blockers. Avoid if pregnant or breastfeeding.

Massage: The main goal of massage is to help the body heal itself. Touch is fundamental to massage therapy and is used by therapists to locate painful or tense areas, to determine how much pressure to apply, and to establish a therapeutic relationship with clients. Massage shows promise as an adjunct to traditional medical detoxification for alcohol. Further research is needed to confirm these results.

Avoid with bleeding disorders, low platelet counts, or if taking blood thinners. Areas should not be massaged where there are fractures, weakened bones from osteoporosis or cancer, open/healing skin wounds, skin infections, recent surgery, or blood clots. Use cautiously with a history of physical abuse or if pregnant or breastfeeding. Massage should not be used as a substitute for more proven therapies for medical conditions. Massage should not cause pain to the client.

Melatonin: Melatonin is a neurohormone produced in the brain. Levels of melatonin in the blood are highest before bedtime. A small amount of research has examined the use of melatonin to assist with tapering or cessation of benzodiazepines such as diazepam (Valium) or lorazepam (Ativan). Although preliminary results are promising, further study is necessary before a firm conclusion can be reached.

There are rare reports of allergic skin reactions after taking melatonin by mouth. Avoid with bleeding disorders or if taking blood thinners. Use cautiously with seizures disorders, major depression, psychotic disorders, diabetes, low blood sugar levels, glaucoma, high cholesterol, atherosclerosis, or if at risk of heart disease. Use cautiously if driving or operating heavy machinery.

Prayer: Prayer can be defined as a "reverent petition," the act of asking for something while aiming to connect with God or another object of worship. Initial research reports no effects of intercessory prayer on alcohol or drug dependency. Better research is necessary before a firm conclusion can be drawn.

Prayer is not recommended as the sole treatment approach for potentially serious medical conditions, and it should not delay the time it takes to consult with a healthcare professional or receive established therapies. Sometimes religious beliefs come into conflict with standard medical approaches and require an open dialog between patients and caregivers.

Psychotherapy: Psychotherapy is an interactive process between a person and a qualified mental health professional. The patient explores thoughts, feelings, and behaviors to help with problem solving. Psychotherapy or a combination of psychotherapy and prescription medication may help alcohol abuse patients prevent relapse, overcome withdrawal symptoms, and deal with underlying problems (such as depression or anxiety).

Psychotherapy, especially cognitive behavioral therapy, may help patients stop drug use and reduce relapses. Combination treatment of psychotherapy and certain medications is sometimes more effective than psychotherapy alone. Group therapy may be more effective than individual therapy.

Psychotherapy cannot always fix mental or emotional conditions. Psychiatric drugs are sometimes needed. In some cases, symptoms may worsen if the proper medication is not taken. Not all therapists are qualified to work with all problems. Use cautiously with serious mental illnesses or some medical conditions because some forms of psychotherapy may stir up strong emotional feelings and expressions.

Qi Gong: Qi gong is a type of traditional Chinese medicine that is thought to be at least 4,000 years old. It is traditionally used for spiritual enlightenment, medical care, and self-defense. A recent study looked at the effectiveness of qi gong therapy vs. medical and nonmedical treatment in the detoxification of heroin addicts. Results showed that qi gong may be beneficial in heroin detoxification without side effects, although the possibility of the placebo effect cannot be completely eliminated. Other treatments have been better studied for heroin detoxification and are recommended at this time. Qi gong may be used as an adjunct therapy.

Qi gong is generally considered to be safe in most people when learned from a qualified instructor. Use cautiously with psychiatric disorders. In cases of potentially serious conditions, qi gong should not be used as the only treatment instead of more proven therapies, and it should not delay the time it takes to see an appropriate healthcare provider.

Yoga: Yoga is an ancient system of relaxation, exercise, and healing with origins in Indian philosophy. Preliminary research suggests that yoga may be beneficial when added to standard therapies for the treatment of heroin or alcohol abuse. Additional studies are needed before a recommendation can be made.

Yoga is generally considered to be safe in healthy individuals when practiced appropriately. Avoid some inverted poses with disk disease of the spine, fragile or atherosclerotic neck arteries, extremely high or low blood pressure, glaucoma, detachment of the retina, ear problems, severe osteoporosis, cervical spondylitis, or risk for blood clots. Certain yoga breathing techniques should be avoided with heart or lung disease. Use cautiously with a history of psychotic disorders. Yoga techniques are believed to be safe during pregnancy and breastfeeding when practiced under the guidance of expert instruction. However, poses that put pressure on the uterus, such as abdominal twists, should be avoided in pregnancy.

Fair Negative Scientific Evidence

Ginkgo biloba: *Ginkgo biloba* has been used medicinally for thousands of years. One small study reports no benefit of ginkgo for cocaine dependence.

Avoid if allergic or hypersensitive to members of the Ginkgoaceae family. If allergic to mango rind, sumac, poison ivy or oak, or cashews, then allergy to ginkgo is possible. Avoid if taking anticoagulants due to an increased risk of bleeding. Ginkgo should be stopped two to three weeks before surgical procedures. Use cautiously with seizures or in children. Ginkgo seeds are dangerous and should be avoided. Skin irritation and itching may also occur due to ginkgo allergies. Do not use ginkgo in supplemental doses if pregnant or breastfeeding.

Traditional or Theoretical Uses Lacking Sufficient Evidence

Aromatherapy: Aromatherapy refers to many different therapies that use essential oils. The oils are sprayed in the air, inhaled, or applied to the skin. Essential oils are usually mixed with a carrier oil (usually a vegetable oil) or alcohol. Theoretically, aromatherapy may help treat patients with addictions. However, scientific studies have not evaluated the safety and efficacy of this particular use. Further research is warranted.

Essential oils should be administered in a carrier oil to avoid toxicity. Avoid with a history of allergic dermatitis. Use cautiously if driving or operating heavy machinery. Avoid consuming essential oils. Avoid direct contact of undiluted oils with mucous membranes. Use cautiously if pregnant. Sage, rosemary, and juniper oils should be avoided if pregnant or breastfeeding.

Detoxification Therapy: Detoxification is a broad concept that encompasses many different modalities and substances used in cleansing the body's systems and organs. Detoxification therapy has been historically used to treat alcoholism and drug addictions. However, scientific evidence is lacking. Until research is conducted in this area, a firm conclusion cannot be reached.

In cases of illness, the various forms of detoxification should be used under professional guidance. See specific monographs for precautions and warnings associated with modalities of detoxification.

Relaxation Therapy: Relaxation techniques include behavioral therapeutic approaches that differ widely in philosophy, methodology, and practice. The primary goal is usually non-directed relaxation. Relaxation therapy has been suggested as a possible treatment for drug addictions, including alcohol dependence. However, a firm conclusion cannot be made until scientific studies evaluate the safety and efficacy of this therapy.

Avoid with psychiatric disorders, such as schizophrenia/psychosis. Jacobson relaxation (flexing specific muscles, holding that position, and then relaxing the muscles) should be used cautiously with illnesses, such as heart disease, high blood pressure, or musculoskeletal injury. Relaxation therapy is not recommended as the sole treatment approach for potentially serious medical conditions, and it should not delay the time to diagnosis or treatment with more proven techniques.

PREVENTION

General: Risk reduction programs may help prevent individuals who are predisposed to addictions from becoming dependent on drugs or gambling. These programs have trained counselors and advisors who teach skills to help individuals avoid unwanted consequences related to drugs or gambling.

Substance Abuse: Having knowledge about drug abuse is the key to preventing drug addictions.

Individuals who feel depressed, suffer from psychological disorders, or were abused should seek help. Treating such conditions promptly reduces the chances that the patient will self-medicate with drugs.

Individuals who are recovering from drug addictions should avoid the temptation to use drugs. Individuals should not spend time with others who are using drugs or expose themselves to environments where drugs are present.

Individuals who use intravenous drugs (such as heroin) should not share needles with others. Sharing needles increases the risk of transmitting or acquiring infectious diseases, including HIV and hepatitis.

Gambling Addiction: There is currently no known method to prevent gambling addictions. However, individuals may decrease their risks of developing gambling problems by limiting the amount of time they spend gambling.

It is also important to seek help as soon as a problem is identified. This may help prevent the addiction from worsening.

Individuals who have gambling addictions should avoid temptations to gamble. Recovering compulsive gamblers who suddenly feel the urge to gamble should talk to their healthcare providers to prevent a relapse from occurring.

ALLERGIES

CONDITIONS: Allergies, Pollen Allergy, Food Allergy, Dust/Mold/Dander Allergy

BACKGROUND

An allergy, or hypersensitivity reaction, occurs when the body's immune system overreacts to a substance that is normally harmless (allergen), such as mold, pollen, animal dander, or dust mites. The white blood cells of an allergic individual produce an antibody called immunoglobulin E (IgE), which attaches to the allergen. This triggers the release of histamine and other inflammatory chemicals that cause allergic symptoms, such as runny nose, watery eyes, and hives.

If the allergen is airborne, the allergic reaction will primarily affect the eyes, nose, and lungs. If the allergen is ingested, the allergic reaction will primarily affect the mouth, stomach, and intestines. If enough inflammatory chemicals are released, a reaction such as hives or rash could occur throughout the body. The most severe allergic reaction, known as anaphylaxis, can lead to low blood pressure, breathing difficulties, shock, and loss of consciousness, all of which can be fatal.

Allergies are extremely common, affecting more than 20% of Americans. The most common allergy triggers include pollen, dust mites, molds, animal dander, latex, foods, and insect venom.

Allergy treatment depends on the type of allergy and severity of symptoms. Commonly used allergy medications include antihistamines, nasal sprays, decongestants, leukotriene inhibitors. and allergen immunotherapy (allergy shots).

TYPES OF ALLERGIC REACTIONS

Allergic reactions can be classified into four immuno-pathological categories using various classification systems. The Gell and Coombs allergic classification system is based on the immune system's response to the allergen, not on the severity of the reaction.

Type I: Type I allergic reactions involve IgE, which is specific for a particular drug, antigen, or other allergen that triggers the allergic reaction. The allergen binds to the immunoglobulin on specific immune cells called basophils and mast cells. This binding results in the release of chemicals that cause inflammation in the body (such as histamine, serotonin, proteases, bradykinin generating factor, chemotactic factors from immune cells, leukotrienes, prostaglandins, and thromboxanes) within 30 minutes of exposure. These chemical mediators cause allergy symptoms, such as urticaria (hives), runny nose, watery eyes, sneezing, wheezing, and itching. This type of allergic reaction is often seen with penicillin, latex, blood products, and vaccines.

Type II: This classification is called a cytotoxic reaction because it involves the destruction of the host cells. An antigen associated with a specific cell initiates cytolysis (breakdown of the cell) by an antigen-specific antibody, such as IgG or IgM. This reaction often involves blood elements, such as red blood cells, white blood cells, or platelets. It often occurs within five to 12 hours of exposure to the allergen, which may include penicillin, quinidine, phenylbutazone, thiouracils, sulfonamides, or methyldopa.

Type III: This category involves the formation of an antigen-antibody immune complex, which deposits on blood vessel walls and activates cell components called complements. This causes a serum sickness–like syndrome involving fever, swelling, skin rash, and enlarged lymph nodes in about three to eight hours. It may be caused by a variety of allergens, including penicillins, sulfonamides, intravenous contrast media, and hydantoins.

Type IV: This classification involves delayed cell-mediated reactions. Antigens on the allergen release inflammatory mediators within 24 to 48 hours of exposure. This type of reaction is seen with graft rejection, latex, contact dermatitis, and tuberculin reaction.

CAUSES

Most allergies are inherited, which means they are passed on to children by their parents. Although people inherit a tendency to be allergic, they may not inherit an allergy to the same allergen. When one parent is allergic, the child has a 50% chance of having allergies. That risk jumps to 75% if both parents have allergies.

Typically, an allergic response is not triggered the first time the body encounters the allergen. After the body is exposed to an allergen, the immune system becomes sensitized and prepares to react to the next encounter with the allergen. Once sensitized, the immune system can quickly detect the drug in the body and produce IgE. These antibodies trigger the release of chemical mediators, including histamine, which may cause allergic symptoms up to and including anaphylaxis.

Common allergy triggers include pollen, dust mites, molds, animal dander, latex, foods, and insect venom.

COMMON TRIGGERS

Pollen: Each spring, summer, and fall, plants release tiny particles called pollen into the air in order to reproduce. Pollen from plants, such as ragweed, can trigger allergy symptoms.

Dust: Dust mites are microscopic organisms that live in dust and in the fibers of household objects like pillows, mattresses, and carpets. Dust mites prefer warm, humid areas. Household dust is a combination of potentially allergenic materials, including fibers from different fabrics, animal dander, bacteria, mold, fungus spores, food particles, bits of plants, or other allergens.

Molds: Molds are parasitic, microscopic fungi (like *Penicillium*) that have spores that float in the air like pollen. Mold is a common trigger for allergies, and it is usually found in damp areas such as the basement or bathroom as well as outside in grass, leaf piles, hay, or mulch. In some people, symptoms of mold allergy may be triggered or worsened after eating certain foods, such as cheese processed with fungi. Mold spores peak during hot, humid weather.

Animal Dander: Animals secrete oily fluids that contain allergens from their skin. These fluids collect on fur, feathers, and other surfaces inside the home. Proteins in the animal's saliva also cause allergic reactions. The allergens are capable of triggering reactions for several months. Allergies to animals can take two or more years to develop, and symptoms may not subside until months after discontinuing contact with the animal.

Latex: Latex, a substance found in products like rubber gloves and condoms, can also trigger allergic reactions in sensitive people. A component of the latex substance itself is an allergen. In addition, the latex glove powder residue is an airborne allergen that causes upper airway allergic reactions in some people. Latex reactions may cause a potentially life-threatening allergic reaction called anaphylaxis. According to the American Academy of Allergy Asthma & Immunology (AAAAI) about 220 cases of anaphylaxis and three deaths per year are attributed to latex allergies.

Foods: Food allergens are those parts of foods, usually proteins, that lead to allergic reactions. Most allergens can still cause allergic reactions even after they are cooked or have been digested. However, some allergens (usually from fruit and vegetables) only cause allergic reaction if eaten raw. These reactions are usually limited to the mouth and throat. According to the AAAAI, six foods, including milk, peanuts, soy, eggs, wheat, and tree nuts (like pecans and walnuts), cause 90% of food allergies in children. Children usually outgrow allergies to milk, eggs, and soy, but peanut, tree nut, fish, and shellfish allergies continue throughout adulthood.

Insect Venom: The honeybee, yellowjacket, paper wasp, white-faced hornet (bald-faced hornet), and fire ant are among the most common insects that trigger insect sting or bite allergies. Since the stinger is a modified egg-laying apparatus, only females can sting.

SIGNS AND SYMPTOMS

Common allergy symptoms include runny nose, tearing eyes, burning or itching eyes, red or swollen eyes, coughing, wheezing, difficulty breathing, hives, skin rash, stomach cramps, vomiting, diarrhea, headache, itchy nose, postnasal drip, and impaired smell as well as itchy mouth, throat, or skin.

COMPLICATIONS

Anaphylaxis is a rapid, immune-mediated (allergic), systemic reaction to allergens to which the individual has previously been exposed. Anaphylaxis is a medical emergency that requires immediate medical treatment as well as follow-up care with an allergist or immunologist. Symptoms of anaphylaxis can vary from mild to severe and may be potentially life threatening. The most dangerous symptoms are low blood pressure, breathing difficulties, shock, and loss of consciousness, all of which can be fatal. Epinephrine is a medication used to treat anaphylaxis. Administering the epinephrine as soon as possible improves the chances of survival and a quick recovery.

Individuals who have a history of anaphylaxis should carry an autoinjectable epinephrine device (EpiPen) with them at all times. If symptoms of anaphylaxis appear after exposure to an allergen or medication, the patient uses the device to inject the epinephrine into his/her thigh. A trained family member or friend may help the patient administer the epinephrine, if necessary.

DIAGNOSIS

Skin Test: A skin test is used to determine whether a patient is allergic to certain substances, such as mold, dust mites, or animal dander. During the test, the skin is exposed to different allergy-causing substances (allergens) and then observed for an allergic reaction. Some tests, like the percutaneous (puncture, prick, or scratch) test, detect immediate allergic reactions, which develop within minutes of exposure to an allergen. Other tests, like the epicutaneous (patch) test, detect delayed allergic reactions that develop over the course of several days. If an allergen triggers an allergic reaction to a test, the patient will develop reddening, swelling, or a raised, itchy red wheal (bump) that looks similar to a mosquito bite. The healthcare provider will measure the size of the wheal and record the results. The larger the wheal, the more severe the allergy.

Radioallergosorbent Test (RAST): An allergen-specific IgE test, commonly referred to as RAST, is a type of blood test that can help determine if a patient who experiences allergy symptoms, such as runny nose, watery eyes, and hives, is allergic to particular substances called allergens.

The in vitro test (performed outside of the body in a laboratory setting) exposes a blood sample to suspected allergens (like dust mites, pollen, or animal dander) to determine whether the patient has developed allergen-specific IgE antibodies. Antibodies are proteins that recognize and bind to specific antigens.

During the procedure, a sample of blood is taken from the patient. The blood is then sent to a laboratory that performs specific IgE blood tests. An allergen-antigen complex is bound to an allergosorbent paper disk and the patient's blood is added. If the blood contains antibodies to the specific antigen, it will bind to the "tagged" immunoglobulins.

RAST is less accurate than a skin test. However, if the patient has a severe skin disease (like eczema or psoriasis) that is present on large areas of skin on the arms or back, a skin test may not be possible. This is because the skin test may only be performed on the arms and back, and there may not be enough unaffected skin to perform a conclusive test. For these patients, an allergen-specific IgE test is the preferred diagnostic method.

TREATMENT

General: Allergy treatment depends on the type of allergy and severity of symptoms. Commonly used allergy medications include antihistamines, nasal sprays, decongestants, leukotriene inhibitors, and immunotherapy (allergy shots).

Short-Acting Antihistamines: Short-acting antihistamines like diphenhydramine (Benadryl) have been used to relieve mild to moderate allergy symptoms. Most short-acting antihistamines are available over the counter. These medications often cause drowsiness, and they have shown to blunt learning in children (even in the absence of drowsiness). However, loratadine (Claritin), an over-the-counter

medication, does not cause drowsiness or affect learning in children. Patients should consult their healthcare providers to determine whether these medications are safe for children.

Longer Acting Antihistamines: Longer acting antihistamines like fexofenadine (Allegra) or cetirizine (Zyrtec) are available by prescription for mild to moderate allergy symptoms. They cause less drowsiness than short-acting antihistamines, and they are equally effective. These medications do not usually interfere with learning. Patients should consult their healthcare providers to determine whether these medications are safe for children.

Nasal Corticosteroid Sprays: Nasal corticosteroid sprays can effectively relieve allergy symptoms in patients who are not responding to antihistamines. Commonly prescribed corticosteroid sprays include fluticasone (Flonase), mometasone (Nasonex), and triamcinolone (Nasacort AQ).

Decongestants: Decongestants may help relieve symptoms such as nasal congestion (stuffy nose). These drugs shrink the tissues and blood vessels in the eyes and nose that swell in response to contact with an allergen. Nasal decongestant sprays like oxymetazoline (Afrin) should not be used more than twice daily for three consecutive days because rebound nasal congestion may result. Decongestants in pill form do not cause this effect.

Cromolyn Sodium: Cromolyn sodium is available as a nasal spray (Nasalcrom) for treating hay fever. Eye drop versions of cromolyn sodium are also available for itchy, bloodshot eyes.

Leukotriene Inhibitors: Leukotriene inhibitors like montelukast (Singulair) have been used to control allergic asthma and to help relieve seasonal allergy symptoms.

Immunotherapy (Allergy Shots): Allergen immunotherapy, also known as allergy shots, is often used to treat patients who suffer from severe allergies or those who experience allergy symptoms more than three months a year. Allergen immunotherapy involves injecting increasing amounts of an allergen to a patient over several months.

INTEGRATIVE THERAPIES
Good Scientific Evidence

Bromelain: Bromelain may be a useful addition to other therapies used for sinusitis (such as antibiotics) due to its ability to reduce inflammation/swelling. Studies report mixed results, although overall bromelain appears to be beneficial for reducing swelling and improving breathing. Better studies are needed before a firm conclusion can be made.

Avoid if allergic to bromelain, pineapple, honeybee, venom, latex, birch pollen, carrots, celery, fennel, cypress pollen, grass pollen, papain, rye flour, wheat flour, or other members of the Bromeliaceae family. Use cautiously with history of bleeding disorders, stomach ulcers, heart disease, liver disease, or kidney disease. Use cautiously before dental or surgical procedures or while driving or operating machinery. Avoid if pregnant or breastfeeding.

Butterbur: Good scientific evidence suggests that butterbur may effectively prevent allergic rhinitis in susceptible individuals. Comparisons of butterbur to prescription drugs, such as fexofenadine (Allegra) and cetirizine (Zyrtec), have reported similar efficacy. Additional studies are warranted before a firm conclusion can be made.

Avoid if allergic or hypersensitive to *Petasites hybridus* or other plants from the Asteraceae/Compositae family (like ragweed, marigolds, daisies, and chrysanthemums). Raw, unprocessed butterbur plant should not be eaten due to the risk of liver or kidney damage or cancer. Avoid if pregnant or breastfeeding.

Nasal Irrigation: Good scientific evidence suggests that nasal irrigation can effectively treat allergic rhinitis. A well-conducted, randomized controlled trial that fully reports the data would make the case for allergic rhinitis stronger.

There is also good scientific evidence that nasal irrigation may effectively treat chronic sinusitis. A large, randomized, double-blind study would lend strong support to the usage of nasal irrigation for the treatment of chronic sinusitis.

Nasal irrigation is generally well tolerated. Use cautiously with history of frequent nosebleeds. If the irrigation liquid is hot, the nose may become irritated.

Probiotics: Use of probiotic *Enterococcus faecalis* bacteria in hypertrophic sinusitis (sinus inflammation) may reduce frequency of relapses and the need for antibiotic therapy.

Probiotics are generally considered safe and well tolerated. Avoid if allergic or hypersensitive to probiotics. Use cautiously if lactose intolerant.

Unclear or Conflicting Scientific Evidence

Acupuncture: More well-designed studies are needed to determine whether or not acupuncture offers benefit in chronic sinusitis patients.

Preliminary research suggests that acupuncture may effectively treat hives. However, further research is needed to confirm these results.

Applied Kinesiology: Applied kinesiology is commonly used to diagnose food allergies. However,

there is conflicting scientific evidence as to whether applied kinesiology is an effective diagnostic tool. Further research is warranted before a firm conclusion can be drawn.

Aromatherapy: Despite widespread use in over-the-counter agents and vapors, there is not enough scientific evidence to recommend use of eucalyptus oil as a decongestant-expectorant (by mouth or inhaled form). The available studies are of poor quality and have used combination therapies or 1,8-cineole (eucalyptol), which is a component of eucalyptus. Further studies are needed before a firm conclusion can be made.

Cat's Claw: It has been suggested that cat's claw may help treat allergic respiratory diseases. However, there is limited scientific evidence to support this claim. More well-designed trials are needed to determine whether cat's claw is a beneficial treatment.

Choline: Oral tricholine citrate effectively relieved allergic rhinitis symptoms in one study. However, further research is needed before a firm conclusion can be made.

Ephedra: A preliminary study suggests that ephedrine nasal spray, a chemical in ephedra, may help treat symptoms of nasal allergies. Additional research is needed before a firm conclusion can be made.

Honey: Currently there is insufficient human evidence to recommend honey for the treatment of rhinoconjunctivitis. One poor-quality trial reported no benefit of the use of honey for the treatment of rhinoconjunctivitis. Further research is necessary before a firm conclusion can be made.

Hypnotherapy, Hypnosis: It has been suggested that hypnotherapy may help treat hay fever. However, further research is necessary to determine whether it is an effective treatment.

Lactobacillus Acidophilus: A small study was conducted to evaluate the effects of *Lactobacillus acidophilus* strain L-92 on the symptoms of Japanese cedar pollen allergy with positive results. Further research is needed before a decision can be made.

Perilla: Preliminary evidence suggests some benefit of perilla extract for seasonal allergies. Further clinical trials are required before a firm conclusion can be made.

Probiotics: Only a few types and combinations of probiotics have been studied as a possible treatment for allergies. They have been studied mostly in children, teenagers, and young adults. Further research is necessary before a firm conclusion can be made.

Sorrel: There is no reliable human evidence evaluating sorrel monotherapy as a treatment for bronchitis. However, it is an ingredient in the combination herbal product Sinupret, which also contains cowslip flower, European elderflower, gentian root, and verbena. This proprietary formula has been used historically in Europe for the treatment of acute bronchitis and sinusitis. Although no studies have been conducted comparing the combination product to placebo, there is initial evidence from a comparison trial of various expectorants vs. Sinupret in the treatment of acute bronchitis. Additional evidence is necessary before a firm conclusion can be drawn regarding the use of sorrel or Sinupret in the management of bronchitis.

Stinging Nettle: For many years, a freeze-dried preparation of *Urtica dioica* has been prescribed by physicians and sold over the counter to treat allergic rhinitis. Clinical trials demonstrating statistical significance over placebo, and/or equivalence with other available treatments, are needed before a firm conclusion can be made.

Vitamin E: Although thought to aid in reducing the nasal symptoms of allergies, vitamin E intake may not be effective. However, current evidence is limited, and more studies are needed before a firm conclusion can be drawn.

PREVENTION

Avoid substances that trigger allergic reactions. Patients who are allergic to pollen should remain indoors in the morning and evening, when outdoor pollen levels are highest.

Keep windows closed and use the air conditioner, if possible, in the house and car.

Do not dry clothes outside.

Avoid unnecessary exposure to other environmental irritants such as insect sprays, tobacco smoke, air pollution, and fresh tar or paint.

Regularly wash the hands and face to remove pollen.

A humidifier may help remove some of the allergens out of the air.

Children who have been breastfed are less likely to develop allergies. In addition, a mother who avoids cow's milk, eggs, nuts, and peanuts while breastfeeding may help prevent allergy-related conditions, such as eczema, in some children.

There is evidence that infants who are exposed to airborne allergens like dust mites and animal dander may be less likely to develop related allergies.

Individuals with a history of anaphylaxis should carry an autoinjectable epinephrine device (EpiPen) with them at all times.

ALZHEIMER'S DISEASE

CONDITION: Alzheimer's Disease

BACKGROUND

Alzheimer's disease (AD) is an irreversible, progressive disorder in which neurons (brain cells) deteriorate, resulting in the loss of cognitive (thought) functions, primarily memory, judgment, reasoning, movement coordination, and pattern recognition. In advanced stages of the disease, all memory and mental functioning may be lost.

AD may cause death; it is the eighth leading cause of death in the United States. However, an individual with AD often dies from an additional illness like pneumonia.

AD is the most common form of dementia. Dementia is a group of disorders that impairs mental functioning. Dementia means loss of the ability to think. Alzheimer's is progressive and irreversible. Abnormal changes in the brain worsen over time, eventually interfering with many aspects of brain function. Memory loss is one of the earliest symptoms, along with a gradual decline of other intellectual and thinking abilities, called cognitive functions, and changes in personality or behavior. Other forms of dementia include vascular dementia (due to a lack of blood flow to the brain), mixed dementia (presence of both AD and vascular dementia), and Creutzfeldt-Jakob disease (rapidly declining memory and cognition due to consumption of cattle with "mad cow" disease).

AD advances in stages, progressing from mild forgetfulness and cognitive impairment to widespread loss of mental abilities. In advanced AD, people become dependent on others for every aspect of their care. The time course of the disease varies by individual, ranging from five to 20 years. The most common cause of death is infection.

Age is the most important risk factor for AD. The number of people with the disease doubles every five years beyond age 65.

It is estimated that about five million Americans suffer from AD, and about 360,000 people are newly diagnosed every year. Alzheimer's affects about 10% of people ages 65 and up, and the number doubles roughly every ten years after age 65. Half of the population ages 85 and up may have AD.

There are an estimated 24 million people with general dementia worldwide. Every 72 seconds in the United States someone develops AD. By 2050, the estimated range of AD prevalence will be 11.3 million to 16 million Americans, with a middle estimate of 13.2 million unless a cure or prevention is found. Medicare and other healthcare insurance help offset the costs for individuals.

It has been reported that the direct and indirect costs of AD and other dementias amount to more than $148 billion annually in the United States alone. The financial cost of caring for someone with AD can be overwhelming and is estimated to be about $50,000 per year in direct medical expenses.

There is no known cure for AD, although researchers have made progress on determining the causes of AD.

RISK FACTORS

Age: The risk for AD increases with each decade of adult life. AD usually affects people older than 65, but it may rarely affect those younger than 40. Less than 5% of people between 65-74 years old have AD. For people 85 and older, that number jumps to nearly 50%.

Heredity: The risk of developing AD appears to be slightly higher if a first-degree relative (a parent, sister, or brother) has the disease. Although the genetic link of AD among families remains largely unexplained, researchers have identified a few genetic mutations that greatly increase risk in some families. A clear inherited pattern of AD exists in less than 10% of cases. In addition, one form of the apolipoprotein E (ApoE) gene increases the chances of developing late-onset AD. Nearly all individuals with Down's syndrome who live into their 40s develop the disease. Down's syndrome is a condition in which extra genetic material causes delays in the way a child develops and often leads to mental retardation. It affects one in every 800 babies born. Three genetic mutations in DNA are known to cause early-onset AD.

Sex: It is thought that gender plays a role because several clinical studies suggest that women are afflicted with AD more often than men. This was explained by the life span of women being usually longer than men. However, the evidence is inconsistent and some studies report that the disease is more common in men. Therefore, more research is needed to obtain conclusive evidence regarding prevalence in gender.

Lifestyle: The same factors that put an individual at risk of heart disease, including hypertension (high blood pressure) and hypercholesterolemia (high cholesterol), may also increase the likelihood that the person will develop AD. Poorly controlled diabetes is another risk factor. Exercise and diet are very important to prevent and control AD. Some clinical studies have suggested that remaining mentally active throughout life, especially in the later years, reduces the risk of AD. Mental activity can be doing crossword puzzles daily, reading the newspaper or books, and increasing social activities.

Education Levels: Clinical studies have found an association between less education and the risk of developing AD. Some researchers theorize that the more an individual uses his/her brain, the more synapses are created, which provide a greater reserve as an individual ages. It remains unclear, however, whether less education and less mental activity create a risk of AD or if it is simply harder to detect AD in individuals who exercise their minds frequently or who have more education. Reading, working, puzzles, and social activities help exercise the mind.

Toxicity: Another theory is that overexposure to metals (such as lead, mercury, and aluminum) or chemicals may cause AD. For a time, aluminum was thought to increase the likelihood of developing AD. This was due to the findings that more individuals with AD have deposits of aluminum in their brains. After many years of studies, however, no true link to developing AD has been found with aluminum exposure. A study found that workers exposed to aluminum experienced neurotoxicity (nerve damage) and symptoms of early AD, such as decreased cognitive performance. More studies need to be performed to link heavy metals to AD.

Head Injury: The observation that some ex-boxers eventually develop dementia suggests that serious traumatic injury to the head (for example, a concussion with a prolonged loss of consciousness) may be a risk factor for AD. Findings are mixed and more research is needed.

Hormone Replacement Therapy: The exact role hormone replacement therapy may play in the development of dementia and AD is not yet clear. Early evidence seemed to report that estrogen supplements given after menopause could reduce the risk of dementia and AD. But results from the large-scale Women's Health Initiative Memory Study indicated an increased risk of AD for women taking estrogen after age 65. The verdict is not yet in on whether estrogen affects the risk of dementia and AD if given at an earlier age. More research is needed.

CAUSES

Genetic Factors: Genetic factors are known to play a role in some cases of AD. A gene, called the amyloid beta precursor protein (APP) gene, has been linked to the occurrence of AD in Down's syndrome

patients who survive beyond 40 years. Some families with a history of early-onset AD also have a mutation on the APP gene. The ApoE gene also has been implicated in the disease. ApoE is a protein found with beta amyloid (a protein found in the brains of AD patients) in neuritic (inflamed nerve) plaques. Together, these genetic mutations account for less than 10% of all AD cases.

Plaques and Tangles: The causes of AD are poorly understood, but its effect on brain tissue has been demonstrated clearly. AD damages and kills brain cells. A healthy brain has billions of nerve cells called neurons. Neurons generate electrical and chemical signals that are relayed from neuron to neuron to help an individual think, remember, and feel (physically and emotionally). Brain chemicals called neurotransmitters help these signals flow seamlessly between neurons. Initially in people with AD, neurons in certain locations of the brain begin to die. When they die, lower levels of neurotransmitters are produced, creating signaling problems in the brain. One neurotransmitter, known as acetylcholine, has been found to be deficient in the brains of those with AD. Medication treatment is based around increasing the amount of acetylcholine in the brain.

Plaques and tangles in brain tissue are considered hallmarks of AD. Studies of plaques and tangles from the brains of people who have died of AD suggest several possible roles these structures might play in the disease.

Plaques are made up of beta-amyloid, a normally harmless protein. Although the ultimate cause of neuron death in AD is not known, mounting evidence suggests that a form of beta-amyloid protein may be the cause. The plaque is responsible for memory deterioration in individuals with AD.

The internal support structure for brain neurons depends on the normal functioning of a protein called tau. In people with AD, threads of tau protein undergo alterations that cause them to become twisted or tangled. Many researchers believe that this may seriously damage neurons, causing them to die.

Inflammation: Researchers have observed inflammation in the brains of some people with AD. Inflammation is the body's response to injury or infection and a natural part of the healing process. Even as beta-amyloid plaques develop in the spaces between neurons, immune cells are at work getting rid of dead cells and other waste products in the brain. Although research has found that the inflammation occurs before plaques have fully formed, it is not known how this development relates to the disease process. There is also debate about whether inflammation has a damaging effect on neurons or whether it is beneficial in clearing away plaques.

SIGNS AND SYMPTOMS

Because early symptoms of AD progress slowly, diagnosis is difficult and often delayed. The disease's course varies from person to person. Eight years is the average length of time from diagnosis of AD to death. Survival begins to decline three years after diagnosis, but some people live more than a decade with the disease.

Stages of AD: In individuals with AD, changes in the brain may begin 10–20 years before any visible signs or symptoms appear. Some regions of the brain may begin to shrink (found during brain imaging such as positron emission tomography), resulting in memory loss and the first visible sign of AD. Over time, AD progresses through three main stages: mild (early), moderate, and severe.

Mild Symptoms: Individuals with mild symptoms of AD often seem healthy, but mental deterioration, such as memory impairment and confusion, are occurring. Symptoms and early signs of AD may include difficulty learning and remembering new information, difficulty with daily tasks (such as managing finances, planning meals, and taking medication on schedule), and depression symptoms (sadness, decreased interest in usual activities, loss of energy). The individual is usually still able to do most activities such as driving a car but may get lost going to familiar places. People with early and mild symptoms of AD may exhibit mood swings. They may express distrust in others, show increased stubbornness, and withdraw socially. This may be a response to the frustration they feel as they notice uncontrollable changes in their memory. Restlessness also is a common sign. As the disease progresses, people with AD may become anxious or aggressive and behave inappropriately.

Moderate Symptoms: In individuals with moderate symptoms of AD, the damaging processes occurring in the brain worsen and spread to other areas that control language, reasoning, sensory processing, and thought. In this stage, symptoms and signs of AD become more severe and behavioral problems may become more obvious. Signs and symptoms of moderate AD may include forgetting old facts, continually repeating stories, and/or asking the same questions over and over. The individual may make up stories to fill memory gaps. They have difficulty performing tasks such as keeping a checkbook, shopping for groceries, or following written notes. The individual may not shower or go to the toilet as they did previously, and help with these tasks is needed. They become agitated and restless easily. Repetitive movements, such as rocking to and fro or rubbing the hands, are seen. The individual may wander off and needs to be watched closely. Paranoia, delusions, and hallucinations may occur. Deficiencies in intellect and reasoning, along with a lack of concern for appearance, hygiene, and sleep, become more noticeable.

Severe Symptoms: In the advanced stage of AD, damage to the brain's nerve cells is widespread. At this point, full-time care is typically required. The patient is generally bedridden. For friends, family, and caregivers, this can be the most difficult stage. Individuals with severe AD may have difficulty walking, and they often suffer complications from other illnesses such as pneumonia. Signs of severe AD may include groaning, screaming, mumbling, or speaking gibberish. They refuse to eat and may inappropriately cry out. Individuals with severe or advanced symptoms fail to recognize the faces of family members or caregivers. Apraxia (inability to perform physical tasks such as dressing, eating) and aphasia (loss of ability in comprehension of spoken or written language) are seen. They have great difficulty with all essential activities of daily life.

DIAGNOSIS

There is no one test to diagnose AD. Typically, doctors start the diagnostic process by ruling out other diseases and conditions that may also cause memory loss. Small, undetected strokes, which are caused by a lack of oxygen to the brain resulting in neurological damage, can cause dementia. Individuals with Parkinson's disease, a degenerative nerve disorder, also may develop dementia. Depression can also cause lapses in memory. In addition, many older adults are on multiple medications that may decrease their ability to think clearly.

Medical History: Questions regarding general health and current medications will be asked. Past medical problems, including diseases and surgeries, will be discussed. Family members will usually be involved in the medical history process.

Blood Tests: Blood tests to determine basic health will be used. A complete blood count will determine thyroid problems, electrolyte (such as sodium and potassium) balances, vitamin deficiencies, and immune health.

Mental Status Evaluation: A Mental Status Evaluation screens memory, problem-solving abilities, attention span, counting skills, and language skills. Questions such as "What day is it today?" or "Who is the president of the United States?" may be asked. Recall tests are another example. Doctors may list familiar objects and then ask a person to repeat them immediately and again five minutes later. The Clock Drawing Test, the Mini-Mental State Examination, and the Functional Assessment Staging are commonly used mental status evaluation tools for determining if AD is present. On the tests, the final score helps confirm a diagnosis of AD.

Sometimes doctors will more extensively assess memory, problem-solving abilities, attention span, counting skills, and language. This is especially helpful in trying to detect AD and other dementias at an early stage. Doctors use formal psychological tests to determine if an individual's mental abilities are as expected for his or her age and education. The patterns of any mental deficits observed during neuropsychological testing can help doctors sort out possible causes of dementia.

Brain Scans: Doctors may want to take a picture of the brain using a brain scan. Several types of brain scans are available, including computerized tomography (CT) scan, magnetic resonance imaging (MRI) scan, and positron emission tomography (PET) scan. Doctors can pinpoint visible abnormalities in the brain using these imaging techniques. A CT scan uses x-rays to take many pictures of the brain and then combines the pictures by computer that provides a detailed picture. A CT scan can often show changes in brain structure. MRI's for AD diagnosis display a cross-section of the brain using radio waves and strong magnets instead of radiation. A contrast dye may be injected, although it is used less often with MRI. PET scans involve the injection of radioactivity into the blood that goes to the brain. Images can then be analyzed for changes in function and structure of the brain. They may take longer than CT scans, and the patient is placed inside a confining tube. CT, MRI, and PET are performed at a clinic or hospital. Some individuals will be sedated with mild sedatives (such as alprazolam [Xanax] or midazolam [Versed]). These medications may cause drowsiness and it is not recommended that the individuals drive. The individual should bring a friend or family member to the clinic or hospital.

Genetic Testing: Due to the discovery of genes that are associated with developing AD, genetic testing may be used in the future as a routine diagnostic tool for determining the chances of developing AD. Genetic testing is not approved by the U.S. Food and Drug Administration (FDA) for use in AD diagnosis.

COMPLICATIONS

Mental Illness: Depression is common in patients with AD, especially during the earlier stages when they may be aware of losing mental functions.

Falls and Their Complications: Individuals with AD may become disoriented, increasing their risk of falls. Falls can lead to bone fractures that require hospitalization, medications, and surgery. Falls may also lead to an increase in the severity of AD symptoms, such as confusion and agitation. In addition, falls are a common cause of serious head injuries, such as brain hemorrhage (bleeding in the brain). Long-term immobilization after surgery and hospitalization may also increase the risk of a pulmonary embolism (blood clot in the lungs), which can be life threatening.

Infections: In advanced AD, people may lose all ability to care for themselves. This can make them more prone to additional health problems such as pneumonia (a bacterial infection of the lungs and respiratory system). They may have difficulty swallowing food and liquids, which may cause individuals with AD to inhale some of what they eat and drink into their airways and lungs, which may then lead to pneumonia.

Urinary Incontinence: Urinary incontinence, or the loss of bladder control causing urine leakage, may require the placement of a urinary catheter, which increases the risk of urinary tract infections (UTIs). UTIs can lead to more serious, life-threatening infections.

TREATMENT

The primary symptoms of AD include memory loss, disorientation, confusion, and problems with reasoning and thinking. These symptoms worsen as brain cells die and the connections between cells are lost. Progressive loss of brain cells usually occurs. Although current drugs cannot alter the progressive loss of cells, they may help minimize or stabilize symptoms. These medications may also delay the need for nursing home care.

Cholinesterase Inhibitors: The FDA has approved two classes of drugs to treat cognitive symptoms of AD. The first to be approved were cholinesterase inhibitors, which increase the amount of the brain chemical acetylcholine. Three of these drugs that are commonly prescribed include donepezil (Aricept), rivastigmine (Exelon), and galantamine (Razadyne). Tacrine (Cognex), the first cholinesterase inhibitor, was approved in 1993 but is rarely prescribed today because of associated side effects, including possible liver damage. About half of the people who take cholinesterase inhibitors experience a modest improvement in cognitive symptoms, such as memory. Side effects include diarrhea, vertigo (dizziness), drowsiness, fatigue (extreme tiredness), nausea, and vomiting. Individuals with liver disease, peptic ulcer disease, chronic obstructive pulmonary disease, and slow heart rate should not take these drugs.

Memantine: Memantine (Namenda) is a drug approved by the FDA for treatment of moderate to severe AD. Memantine is the first AD drug of this type approved in the United States. It appears to work by regulating the activity of glutamate, one of the brain's specialized messenger chemicals involved in information processing, storage, and retrieval. Glutamate plays an essential role in learning and memory. Excess glutamate, on the other hand, may lead to disruption and death of brain cells. Memantine may protect cells against excess glutamate by partially blocking NMDA receptors. Side effects include headache, constipation, confusion, and dizziness.

Other Medications: Medications may be needed to treat the symptoms associated with AD. These symptoms interfere with normal daily activities and sleeping. Depression that occurs during the early stages is commonly treated with antidepressant medications, such as selective serotonin reuptake inhibitors, including fluoxetine (Prozac) and sertraline (Zoloft), and the tricyclic antidepressants (TCAs), including amitriptyline (Elavil). Side effects include drowsiness, fatigue, and sedation. TCAs may increase mental confusion. Agitation may be treated with antipsychotic medication, such as haloperidol (Haldol), risperidone (Risperdal), olanzapine (Zyprexa), and quetiapine (Seroquel). Antipsychotics are not FDA approved to treat symptoms of AD and may increase the risk for death in elderly dementia patients. Side effects include sedation, confusion, and tardive dyskinesia (an irreversible movement disorder characterized by lip smacking, facial grimacing, and unsteady walking).

Prognosis: Patients may survive eight to 10 years with AD. Some have been known to live 25 years with the disease. Death usually occurs from infections (including pneumonia), heart disease, or malnutrition.

INTEGRATIVE THERAPIES
Strong Scientific Evidence

Ginkgo: *Ginkgo biloba* has been used medicinally for thousands of years. The scientific literature overall does suggest that ginkgo benefits people with early-stage AD and multi-infarct dementia and may be as helpful as acetylcholinesterase inhibitor drugs such as donepezil (Aricept). Well-designed research comparing ginkgo to prescription drug therapies is needed. Ginkgo may cause bleeding, especially in sensitive individuals such as those taking medications for bleeding disorders (including warfarin [Coumadin]).

Good Scientific Evidence

Aromatherapy: Aromatherapy is the use of essential oils from plants for healing purposes. There is suggestive preliminary evidence that aromatherapy using essential oil of lemon balm (*Melissa officinalis*) can effectively reduce agitation in people with severe dementia when applied to the face and arms twice daily. Other research reports that steam inhalation of lavender aromatherapy may have similar effects. However, there is a conflicting study that reports no benefits of aromatherapy using lemon balm, *Lavender officinalis,* sweet orange (*Citrus aurantium*), or tea tree oil (*Melaleuca alternifolia*). Overall, the evidence does suggest potential benefits. It is not clear if this is because of anxiety-reducing qualities of these therapies. Additional study is necessary. There is also preliminary research suggesting that aromatherapy used with massage may help to calm people with dementia who are agitated. However, it is not clear if this approach is any better than massage used alone.

Bacopa: *Bacopa monnieri* leaf extract is called brahmi in Ayurvedic medicine (medicine practiced in India) and is widely used in India for memory enhancement and pain relief and treating epilepsy. Although bacopa is traditionally used in Ayurvedic medicine to enhance cognition, high-quality clinical trials are lacking. Two methodologically weak studies found some evidence that bacopa improves cognition. However, more high-quality and independent research is needed before bacopa can be recommended for enhancing brain function in adults or children. Bacopa may interact with medications such as calcium channel blockers (used for arrhythmias and high blood pressure), thyroid medications, phenytoin (Dilantin), and drugs metabolized by the liver.

Ginseng: Several clinical studies report that ginseng (*Panax ginseng*) can modestly improve thinking or learning. Mental performance has been assessed using standardized measurements of reaction time, concentration, learning, math, and logic. Benefits have been seen both in healthy young people and in older ill patients. Effects have also been reported for the combination use of ginseng with *Ginkgo biloba*. However, some negative results have also been reported. Therefore, although the sum total of available scientific evidence does suggest some effectiveness of short-term use of ginseng in this area, better research is necessary before a strong recommendation can be made.

Music Therapy: Music is used to influence physical, emotional, cognitive, and social well-being and improve quality of life for healthy people as well as those who are disabled or ill. It may involve either listening to or performing music, with or without the presence of a music therapist. In people with AD and other mental disorders in older adults, music therapy has been found to reduce aggressive or agitated behavior, improve mood, and improve cooperation with daily tasks such as bathing. Music therapy may also be beneficial for dementia-associated neuropsychiatric symptoms such as depression and aggressive behavior.

Unclear or Conflicting Scientific Evidence

Acupuncture: Acupuncture has been reported to help improve memory and cognitive performance in the elderly. However, there is insufficient available evidence for the use of acupuncture in cognitive and communication disorders. More research is necessary.

Art Therapy: Art therapy enables the expression of inner thoughts or feelings when verbalization is difficult or not possible. The aesthetic aspect of the creation of art is thought to lift one's mood, boost self-awareness, and improve self-esteem. Art therapy also allows the opportunity to exercise the eyes and hands, improve eye-hand coordination, and stimulate neurological pathways from the brain to the hands. Art therapy may be an effective means of improving quality of life in the elderly. There is evidence that the nondirected use of visual art (pictures) as a means of encouraging communication among elderly nursing home residents may increase well-being. It may also reduce blood pressure and improve medical health status with regard to reported dizziness, fatigue, pain, and use of laxatives.

Boron: Boron is a mineral that is essential for health. Preliminary human studies report better performance on tasks of eye-hand coordination, attention, perception, short-term memory, and long-term memory with the use of boron. Although boron has not been studied in AD, it may be beneficial in improving memory.

Coenzyme Q10: Coenzyme Q10 (CoQ10) is produced by the human body and is necessary for the basic functioning of cells. Promising preliminary evidence suggests that CoQ10 supplements may slow, but not cure, dementia in people with AD. Additional well-designed studies are needed to confirm these results before a firm conclusion can be made.

Copper: Copper is a mineral that occurs naturally in many foods, including vegetables, legumes, nuts, grains, and fruits as well as shellfish, avocado, and beef (organs such as liver). Conflicting study results report that copper intake may either increase or decrease the risk of developing AD. Additional research is needed.

Cranberry: Preliminary study results show that cranberry juice may increase overall ability to remember. Further well-designed clinical trials are needed to confirm these results. It is best not to use sweetened cranberry juice or cranberry juice cocktail due to the high sugar content. The use of 100% cranberry juice products are recommended by healthcare providers.

Melatonin: Melatonin is a naturally occurring hormone that helps regulate the sleep/wake cycles (circadian rhythm). There is limited study of melatonin for improving sleep disorders associated with AD (including nighttime agitation or poor sleep quality in patients with dementia). It has been reported that natural melatonin levels are altered in people with AD, although it remains unclear if supplementation with melatonin is beneficial. Further research is needed in this area before a firm conclusion can be reached.

Dehydroepiandrosterone (DHEA): DHEA is an endogenous hormone (made in the human body) secreted by the adrenal gland. DHEA serves as precursor to male and female sex hormones (androgens and estrogens). DHEA levels in the body begin to decrease after age 30 and may need to be taken as supplements.

Folic Acid: Folate and folic acid are forms of a water-soluble B vitamin. Folate occurs naturally in food; folic acid is the synthetic form of this vitamin. Preliminary evidence indicates that low folate concentrations might be related to AD. Well-designed clinical trials of folate supplementation are needed before a conclusion can be drawn.

Guided Imagery: The term guided imagery may be used to refer to a number of techniques, including metaphor, story telling, fantasy, game playing, dream interpretation, drawing, visualization, active imagination, or direct suggestion using imagery. Early research suggests that guided imagery of short duration may improve working memory performance. Further research is needed before a firm conclusion can be drawn.

Kundalini Yoga: Kundalini yoga is one of many traditions of yoga that share common roots in ancient Indian philosophy. It is comprehensive in that it combines physical poses with breath control exercises, chanting (mantras), meditations, prayer, visualizations, and guided relaxation. Breathing exercises are an important part of Kundalini yoga. There is some evidence from studies with healthy volunteers that use of certain breathing techniques (such as breathing solely through one nostril or the other) may improve different aspects of cognitive functioning. More studies are needed to determine if these techniques can reliably be used to improve cognitive performance and possibly aid in treating cognitive and nervous system disorders.

Lemon Balm: Clinical data suggest that the use of standardized lemon balm (*Melissa officinalis*) extract has some effect on particular self-reported measures of mood and cognition. More rigorous studies need to be conducted using patient-relevant outcomes to better assess the validity of these results as they apply to patient care.

Massage: Massage with or without essential oils has been used in patients with dementia in long-term care facilities to assess effects on behavior. There is compelling early evidence that aromatherapy with essential oils may reduce agitation in patients with dementia, although the effects of massage itself are not clear.

Pet Therapy: In the institutionalized elderly, there is evidence that pet therapy may reduce depression, blood pressure, irritability, and agitation and increase social interaction. In AD, there is evidence that the presence of a companion animal may increase social behaviors such as smiles, laughs, looks, leans, touches, verbalizations, or name-calling.

Riboflavin: Adequate nutrient supplementation with riboflavin (vitamin B_2) may be required for the maintenance of adequate cognitive function. Treatment with B vitamins, including riboflavin, has been reported to improve scores of depression and cognitive function in patients taking TCAs. This may be related to tricyclic-caused depletion of riboflavin levels.

Vitamin B_1: Because thiamin (vitamin B_1) deficiency can result in a form of dementia (Wernicke-Korsakoff syndrome, a neurological condition), its relationship to AD and other forms of dementia has been investigated. Whether thiamin supplementation is of benefit in AD remains controversial. Further evidence is necessary before a firm conclusion can be reached.

Vitamin B_{12}: Some patients diagnosed with AD have been found to have abnormally low vitamin B_{12} (cyanocobalamin) levels in their blood. However, vitamin B_{12} deficiency itself often causes disorientation and confusion and thus mimics some of the prominent symptoms of AD. Well-designed clinical trials are needed.

Vitamin E: Vitamin E has been proposed and evaluated for the prevention or slowing of dementia (including Alzheimer's type) based on antioxidant properties and findings of low vitamin E levels in some individuals with dementia. There is some evidence that all-rac-alpha-tocopherol (synthetic vitamin E) is similar in effects to a commonly used drug for AD, selegiline (Eldepryl), in slowing cognitive function decline in patients with moderately severe AD. No additive effect was observed when used in combination with selegiline. Retrospective data suggest that long-term combination therapy with donepezil (Aricept) may help slow cognitive decline in patients with AD. Overall, the evidence remains inconclusive in this area. Other research suggests that vitamin E from dietary sources or supplements does not affect the risk of developing AD or vascular dementia. Vitamin E may cause bleeding, especially in sensitive individuals such as those taking medications for bleeding disorders (including warfarin [Coumadin]).

Other supplements that have unclear or conflicting scientific evidence include black and green tea (*Camellia sinensis*), iodine, iron, omega-3 fatty acids (fish oils), policosanol (sugar cane wax), soy (*Glycine max*), and yoga.

Historical or Theoretical Uses Lacking Sufficient Evidence

Integrative therapies used in AD treatment that have historical or theoretical uses but lack sufficient clinical evidence include: 5-hydroxytryptophan, ashwagandha (*Withania somnifera*), astaxanthin, cat's claw (*Uncaria tomentosa*), cordyceps (*Cordyceps sinensis*), garlic (*Allium sativum*), gotu kola (*Centella asiatica*), hypnosis, muira puama (*Ptychopetalum olacoides*), rosemary (*Rosmarinus officinalis*), taurine, turmeric (*Curcuma longa*), and zinc.

PREVENTION

Healthy Aging: Some of the most recent research indicates that taking steps to improve cardiovascular (heart) health, such as losing weight, exercising, and controlling hypertension (high blood pressure) and high cholesterol, may also help prevent AD.

Nonsteroidal Antiinflammatory Drugs (NSAIDs): Several clinical studies have reported that the NSAIDs ibuprofen (Advil, Motrin), naproxen sodium (Aleve), and indomethacin (Indocin) may reduce the risk of developing AD. This may be because inflammation appears to play a role in AD. Because NSAIDs can cause stomach and intestinal bleeding and kidney problems, clinical trials need to be completed before it is clear whether individuals should take NSAIDs solely to prevent AD.

Statins: Statin drugs are used to lower cholesterol levels. They include atorvastatin (Lipitor) and simvastatin (Zocor). Recent studies have reported that statin drugs may reduce the risk of AD. More studies are being done to determine exactly what role, if any, statins may have in AD prevention. Researchers believe that statins help improve blood flow to the brain by decreasing particles in the blood such as cholesterol and triglycerides.

Selective Estrogen Receptor Molecules: Drugs called selective estrogen receptor molecules, including raloxifene (Evista), are used to protect against the bone loss associated with osteoporosis. These drugs also appear to lower the risk of developing mild cognitive impairment, a memory disorder that often precedes AD. The mechanism is not known.

Mental Fitness: Maintaining mental fitness may delay onset of dementia. Some researchers believe that lifelong mental exercise and learning may promote the growth of additional synapses, the connections between neurons, and delay the onset of dementia. Other researchers argue that advanced education gives a person more experience with the types of memory and thinking tests used to measure dementia. Doing crossword puzzles, reading books, and increasing social activities are recommended by healthcare providers.

CONDITIONS: Anxiety, Generalized Anxiety Disorder (GAD), Panic Attacks/Panic Disorder, Phobias, Posttraumatic Stress Disorder (PTSD), Obsessive-Compulsive Disorder (OCD)

BACKGROUND

Anxiety is an unpleasant complex combination of emotions often accompanied by physical sensations such as heart palpitations (irregular heartbeat), nausea, angina (chest pain), shortness of breath, tension headache, and nervousness.

Anxiety disorders affect about 40 million American adults age 18 years and older (about 18%) in a given year. Only about one-third of those suffering from an anxiety disorder receive treatment. Anxiety disorders are reported to cost the United States more than $42 billion a year.

Unlike the relatively mild, brief anxiety that can be caused by a stressful event (such as testing, a job interview, the death of a loved one, or public performance/speaking), anxiety disorders last at least six months and can become worse if not treated. Anxiety disorders can commonly occur along with other mental or physical illnesses, including alcohol or substance abuse, depression, or bipolar illness, which may mask anxiety symptoms or make them worse.

Individuals with an anxiety disorder are three to five times more likely to go to the doctor and six times more likely to be hospitalized for psychiatric disorders than nonsufferers.

TYPES OF ANXIETY

Generalized Anxiety Disorder (GAD): Most people experience anxiety at some point in their lives and some nervousness in anticipation of a real situation. However, if a person cannot shake unwarranted worries, or if the feelings are jarring to the point of causing avoidance of everyday activities, he or she most likely has an anxiety disorder. GAD is characterized by excessive, unrealistic worry that lasts six months or more. In adults, the anxiety may focus on issues such as health, money, or career. Physical symptoms may also appear such as nervousness or heart palpitations. GAD affects about 5% of Americans in the course of their lives and is more common in women than in men. Some experts believe that it is underdiagnosed and more common than any other anxiety disorder. GAD usually begins in childhood and often becomes a chronic ailment, particularly when left untreated. Depression in adolescence may be a strong predictor of GAD in adulthood. Depression commonly accompanies this anxiety disorder.

Obsessive-Compulsive Disorder (OCD): In OCD, individuals are plagued by persistent, recurring thoughts (obsessions) that reflect exaggerated anxiety or fears. Typical obsessions include worrying about being contaminated with germs or fears of behaving improperly or acting violently. The obsessions may lead an individual to perform a ritual or routine (compulsions) such as washing hands, repeating phrases, or hoarding. OCD occurs equally in men and women, and it affects about 2-3% of people over a lifespan. About 80% of people who develop OCD show signs of the disorder in childhood, although the disorder usually develops fully in adulthood.

Panic Attacks and Panic Disorder: Panic disorder is characterized by repeated, unexpected panic attacks. These panic attacks strike without warning and usually last a terrifying 15-30 minutes. Panic disorder may also be accompanied by agoraphobia, which is a fear of being in places where escape or help would be difficult in the event of a panic attack. Agoraphobia is characterized by individuals likely to avoid public places such as shopping malls or confined spaces such as an airplane. Studies indicate that the prevalence of panic disorder among adults is 1.6-2% and is much higher in adolescence (3.5-9%). In one study, 18% of adult patients with panic disorder reported the onset of the disorder before 10 years of age. In general, however, panic disorder tends to begin in late adolescence and peaks at around 25 years of age.

Posttraumatic Stress Disorder (PTSD): PTSD can follow an exposure to a traumatic event such as a sexual or physical assault, witnessing a death, the unexpected death of a loved one, or natural disaster. There are three main symptoms associated with PTSD: "reliving" of the traumatic event (such as flashbacks and nightmares); avoidance behaviors (such as avoiding places related to the trauma) and emotional numbing (detachment from others); and physiological arousal such as difficulty sleeping, irritability, or poor concentration. Researchers now know that anyone, even children, can develop PTSD if they have experienced, witnessed, or participated in a traumatic occurrence—especially if the event was life threatening. Studies estimate a lifetime risk for PTSD in the United States of up to 8%. People exposed to traumatic events, of course, are at highest risk, but many people can go through such events and not experience PTSD. Studies also estimate that 6-30% or more of trauma survivors develop PTSD, with children and young people being among those at the high end of the range. Women have twice the risk of PTSD as men. PTSD can also occur in people not directly involved with a traumatic event.

Phobias: A phobia is an unrealistic or exaggerated fear of a specific object, activity, or situation that in reality presents little to no danger. Common phobias include fear of animals such as snakes and spiders, fear of flying, and fear of heights. In the case of a severe phobia, one might go to extreme lengths to avoid the thing feared.

Separation Anxiety: Separation anxiety is a normal part of child development. It consists of crying and distress when a child is separated from a parent or away from home. If separation anxiety persists beyond a certain age or interferes with daily activities, it may be a sign of separation anxiety disorder.

Social Anxiety Disorder (SAD)/Social Phobia: SAD is characterized by extreme anxiety about being judged by others or behaving in a way that might cause embarrassment or ridicule. This intense anxiety may lead to avoidance behavior. Physical symptoms associated with this disorder include heart palpitations, faintness, blushing, and profuse sweating. Performance anxiety (better known as stage fright) is the most common type of social phobia. Social phobia is currently estimated to be the third most common psychiatric disorder in the United States. Studies have reported a prevalence of 7-12% in Western nations.

RISK FACTORS

Gender: With the exception of OCD and possibly social anxiety, women have twice the risk for most anxiety disorders as men. A number of factors may increase the reported risk in women, including hormonal factors, cultural pressures to meet everyone else's needs except their own, and fewer self-restrictions on reporting anxiety to doctors. Pregnant women and women experiencing menopause may be more susceptible to symptoms of anxiety. Also, women have about twice the risk for panic disorder as men.

Age: In general, phobias, OCD and separation anxiety show up early in childhood, while social phobia and panic disorder are often diagnosed during the teen years. Reports have estimated that approximately 3-5% of children and adolescents have some type of anxiety disorder. This number may be low, particularly since symptoms in children may differ from those in adults. Reports indicate that if such children could be identified as early as two

years of age they possibly could be treated to avoid later anxiety disorders.

Environmental Factors: A person's environment can play a huge role in the development of anxiety disorders. Difficulties such as poverty, early separation from the mother, family conflict, critical and strict parents, parents who are fearful and anxious themselves, and the lack of a strong support system can all lead to chronic anxiety. Studies report that anxiety in new mothers can affect their infants. One study reported a higher rate of crying and an impaired ability to adapt to new situations in infants of mothers who had been stressed and anxious during pregnancy. In another, infants of mothers with panic disorder had higher levels of stress hormones and more sleep disturbances than other children.

Personality Traits: Personality differences can affect whether or not an anxiety disorder develops. People with anxiety disorders often are very self-conscious, have poor coping skills, and have low self-esteem. Children's personalities may indicate higher or lower risk for future anxiety disorders, such as extremely shy children and those likely to be the target of bullies, who are at a higher risk for developing anxiety disorders later in life.

Heredity: Anxiety disorders tend to run in families. People with anxiety disorders often have a family history of anxiety disorders, mood disorders, or substance abuse.

CAUSES

Brain Chemistry: Studies suggest that an imbalance of the brain's neurotransmitters (chemical messengers) such as serotonin, gamma-aminobutyric acid, epinephrine, and norepinephrine may contribute to anxiety disorders. Abnormalities in the stress hormone cortisol, produced by the adrenal glands, have also been found. Most medications prescribed for anxiety disorders aim to readjust the brain's chemical balance.

Trauma: An anxiety disorder may develop in response to a traumatic event, such as a car accident or a marital separation. Anxiety may also have its roots in early life abuse or developmental trauma. Trauma in infancy and early childhood can be particularly damaging, leaving a pervasive and lasting sense of helplessness that can develop into anxiety or depression in later life.

Medications: Some prescription and nonprescription medications may cause symptoms of anxiety, including caffeine and other stimulants; drugs such as heroin, cocaine, and amphetamines; over-the-counter medications such as decongestants;

steroids such as cortisone and prednisone; inhalers and other respiratory medications; some herbal supplements such as ephedra (no longer available on the U.S. market), *Citrus aurantium,* yerba mate tea, and guarana; weight loss products; high blood pressure medications; withdrawal from alcohol; medications for attention deficit–hyperactivity disorder (Ritalin, Adderall, Dexedrine) withdrawal from benzodiazepines (Xanax, Valium); and hormones such as birth control pills and thyroid medications.

Medical Conditions: Many medical conditions can cause or mimic symptoms of anxiety disorders. They include thyroid disorders, diabetes, hypoglycemia (low blood sugar), asthma, sleep disorders, adrenal disorders, epilepsy (seizures), heart conditions including arrhythmias (irregular heartbeat), migraine headaches, and certain psychiatric illnesses such as bipolar disorder (characterized by mania and depression) and depression.

Nutritional Deficiencies: Nutritional deficiencies stemming from poor diet and/or digestion can also contribute to anxiety. Depleted levels of minerals, especially magnesium and zinc, have been linked to the presence of anxiety. A deficiency of B vitamins, especially vitamin B_{12}, can be a significant contributing factor to the development of anxiety disorders.

SIGNS AND SYMPTOMS

The primary symptoms of anxiety disorders are fear and worry. However, anxiety disorders are also characterized by additional emotional and physical symptoms.

Physical: Physical symptoms include heart palpitations (irregular heartbeat), angina (chest pain), hot flashes or chills, cold and clammy hands, stomach upset or queasiness, frequent urination, diarrhea, shortness of breath, sweating, vertigo (dizziness), tremors, muscle tension or aches, fatigue (tiredness), and insomnia (inability to sleep).

Emotional/Psychological: Emotional or psychological symptoms can include apprehension, uneasiness, dread, impaired concentration or selective attention, feeling restless or on edge, avoidance, nightmares, irritability, confusion, behavioral problems (especially in children and adolescents), nervousness, jumpiness, self-consciousness, insecurity, fear of dying or going crazy, and a strong desire to escape.

GAD: Specific symptoms for GAD can include chronic exaggerated worry, tension, and irritability that appear to have no cause or are more intense than the situation warrants. Physical signs, such as restlessness, trouble falling or staying asleep, headaches,

trembling, twitching, muscle tension, or sweating, often accompany these psychological symptoms.

Panic Disorder: Panic disorder symptoms include heart palpitations (irregular heartbeat), angina (chest pain), lightheadedness or dizziness, nausea, shortness of breath, feelings of imminent danger, shaking or trembling, choking, fear of dying, sweating, feelings of unreality, numbness or tingling, hot flashes or chills, and a feeling of going crazy. Since many of the symptoms of panic disorder mimic those found in illnesses like heart disease, thyroid problems, and breathing disorders, people with panic disorder often make multiple visits to emergency rooms or doctors' offices, convinced they have a life-threatening illness (hypochondria).

SAD: Specific symptoms for SAD include blushing, sweating, trembling, nausea, rapid heartbeat, dizziness, and headaches. Some people may have an intense fear of a single social or performance circumstance such as giving a speech, talking to a salesperson, or making a phone call but be perfectly comfortable in other social settings. Others may have a more generalized form of SAD, ranging from such behaviors as becoming anxious in a variety of routines to clinging behavior and throwing tantrums.

PTSD: People with PTSD typically avoid situations that remind them of the traumatic event because they provoke intense distress or even panic attacks. PTSD is characterized by three main types of symptoms, including re-experiencing the trauma through intrusive distressing recollections of the event, flashbacks, and nightmares; emotional numbness and avoidance of places, people, and activities that are reminders of the trauma; and increased arousal, including difficulty sleeping and concentrating, feeling jumpy, and becoming easily irritated and angered.

OCD: Common obsessions include constant, irrational worry about dirt, germs, or contamination; nagging feelings that something bad will happen if certain items aren't in an exact place, position, or order; fear that one's negative or blasphemous thoughts or images will cause personal harm or harm to a loved one; preoccupation with losing or throwing away objects with little or no value; and rumination about accidentally or purposefully injuring another person. Common compulsions include repeatedly washing one's hands, bathing, or cleaning household items, often for hours at a time; checking and re-checking, several to hundreds of times per day, that the doors are locked, stove is turned off, hairdryer is unplugged, etc.; inability to stop repeating a name, phrase, or tune; an excessive, methodical, and painstakingly slow approach to daily activities; and hoarding, such as saving useless items like old newspapers or magazines, bottle caps, or rubber bands.

Obsessions and rituals can substantially interfere with a person's normal routine, schoolwork, job, or family or social activities. Many hours of each day may be spent focusing on obsessive thoughts and performing rituals, and normal concentration and the performing of daily functions becomes very difficult.

Children can also suffer from OCD, but unlike adults, children with OCD do not realize that their obsessions and compulsions are excessive and ritualistic.

Phobias: Specific phobias are characterized by strong, irrational, involuntary fear reactions to a particular object, place, or situation. The reactions to these fears lead the individual to dread confronting common, everyday situations or avoid them altogether, even though they logically know there isn't any threat of danger. Symptoms of phobias include heights, flying in airplanes, insects, snakes and other animals, dental procedures, thunder, public transportation, and elevators. The fear doesn't make any sense, but nothing seems to be able to stop it. When confronted with the feared situation, someone with a phobia may even have a panic attack.

DIAGNOSIS

GAD: GAD is diagnosed when an individual spends at least six months worried excessively about everyday problems. However, incapacitating or troublesome symptoms warranting treatment may exist for shorter periods of time.

Panic Disorder: Panic disorder (or panic attack) is diagnosed by either four attacks within four weeks or one or more attacks followed by at least a month of persistent fear of having another attack. Also, a minimum of four of the symptoms listed for panic disorders developed during at least one of the attacks. Most panic attacks last only a few minutes and up to an hour in rare cases. They can occur at any time, even during sleep.

Phobias: Phobia present with extreme anxiety with exposure to the object or situation. The individual recognizes that his or her fear is excessive or unreasonable and finds that normal routines, social activities, or relationships are significantly impaired as a result of these fears.

OCD: A mental health professional will diagnose OCD after a thorough evaluation. Criteria are based upon the Diagnostic and Statistical Manual of Mental Disorders (DSM-IV-TR), a clinical book of mental illness diagnoses. OCD diagnosis is based upon recurrent and persistent thoughts, impulses,

or images that are intrusive and cause distress; thoughts that aren't simply excessive worries about real problems; an attempt to ignore or suppress these thoughts, images, or impulses; and the recognition that these thoughts, images, and impulses are a product of the mind.

Compulsions must meet specific criteria— including repetitive behaviors, such as handwashing, or repetitive mental acts, such as counting silently— that the individual feels driven to perform. These behaviors or mental acts are meant to prevent or reduce distress about unrealistic obsessions.

PTSD: Although many of the symptoms of PTSD may be an appropriate initial response to a traumatic event, they are considered part of a disorder when they persist beyond three months.

COMPLICATIONS

Anxiety can also worsen many preexisting medical conditions, such as ulcers, hypertension (high blood pressure), asthma, and chronic obstructive pulmonary disease. Anxiety may also be associated with mitral valve prolapse (condition where the mitral valve does not close properly), chronic fatigue syndrome, sleep apnea, irritable bowel syndrome, and chronic tension headaches.

Depression: Anxiety and depression usually go hand in hand in both the young and old. The combination of depression and anxiety may increase both substance abuse and suicide.

The lifetime risk for depression in people with anxiety disorders may be higher than 70%. Most patients with GAD will experience at least one episode of significant depression and many develop recurrent episodes. In patients with both disorders, GAD usually precedes the onset of depression. Social anxiety during adolescence or young adulthood has been associated with a higher risk for depression, and the presence of both increases the chances for severe depression. People with PTSD are four to seven times as likely to be depressed as are people without PTSD.

Bipolar Disorder: Symptoms of panic disorder are very common in people with bipolar disorder (manic depression). In fact, people with bipolar disorder have 26 times the rate of panic disorder as in the general population. To complicate matters, anxiety can worsen bipolar disorder.

Suicide: Anxiety disorders may also contribute to an increased risk for suicide, developing alcoholism and other forms of substance abuse, and overeating; may have very negative effects on work, school, and relationships; and decrease the individual's overall health.

Physical Injury: Individuals with OCD may experience physical injury such as skin problems from excessive washing, injuries from repetitive physical acts, and hair loss from repeated hair pulling (trichotillomania). Studies have reported that PTSD may be associated with shrinkage in the brain associated with memory and learning, possibly due to the continued release of the stress hormone cortisol.

Physical Effects of Anxiety on Children: Anxiety may be associated with a higher risk for sleep disorders in children, such as frequent nightmares, restless legs syndrome, and bruxism (grinding and gnashing of the teeth during sleep).

TREATMENT

Psychotherapy Techniques

Generally, anxiety disorders are treated with medications, specific types of psychotherapy, or both. Treatment choices depend on the symptoms and the preference of the doctor and patient.

Psychotherapy: Psychotherapy involves talking with a trained mental health professional, such as a psychiatrist, psychologist, social worker, or counselor, to discover what causes an anxiety disorder and how to deal with its symptoms.

Cognitive-Behavior Therapy: Many therapists use a combination of cognitive and behavior therapies (CBT). CBT is based on the scientific fact that thoughts cause feelings and behaviors—not external things, like people, situations, and events. The benefit of this fact is that an individual can change the way he/she thinks to feel and act better even if the situation causing the problem does not change.

Relaxation Techniques: Relaxation techniques help individuals develop the ability to more effectively cope with the stresses that contribute to anxiety as well as with some of the physical symptoms of anxiety. The techniques taught include breathing re-training and exercise.

Antianxiety Medications

Benzodiazepines: Benzodiazepines are fast-acting sedatives that typically relieve anxiety symptoms within 30 minutes to one hour. The rapid relief when using benzodiazepines makes them very effective when taken during a panic attack or another overwhelming anxiety episode.

Unfortunately, benzodiazepines can be addictive. If taken regularly for more than a couple of weeks, physical and psychological addiction is likely to occur. Benzodiazepines may create tolerance, with larger doses needed to achieve the same effect, and serious withdrawal symptoms can occur when going off the medication, including increased anxiety, depression, and insomnia. Some benzodiazepines, including diazepam (Valium) have a longer half-life in the body, meaning they stay in the body longer. The addictive potential is why benzodiazepines are usually recommended only for short-term use. To minimize the withdrawal reaction, it is important to slowly taper off these medications.

Some examples of benzodiazepines include alprazolam (Xanax), chlordiazepoxide (Librium), clonazepam (Klonopin), clorazepate (Tranxene), lorazepam (Ativan), oxazepam (Serax), and diazepam (Valium). Clonazepam is commonly used for social phobia and GAD, lorazepam is used for panic disorder, and alprazolam is useful for both panic disorder and GAD.

Most common side effects include drowsiness, impaired coordination, fatigue, confusion and disorientation, dizziness, decreased concentration, short-term memory problems, dry mouth, blurred vision, and irregular heartbeat.

Azapirones: Azapirones were developed more recently than benzodiazepines and are antianxiety drugs prescribed for GAD and OCD. Compared to benzodiazepines, the azapirones are slow acting, taking from two to four weeks to provide anxiety symptom relief. Advantages of these drugs over benzodiazepines include less sedation and effects on coordination and less memory impairment. Withdrawal effects with azapirones are minimal compared to benzodiazepines. Buspirone (Buspar) is the only azapirone approved for medical use.

Side effects may include nausea, headaches, dizziness, drowsiness, upset stomach, constipation, diarrhea, and dry mouth. Azapirones are not to be taken with monoamine oxidase inhibitors (a type of antidepressant) due to the increase risk of life-threatening high blood pressure.

Antidepressant Medications

Selective Serotonin Reuptake Inhibitors (SSRIs): SSRIs are antidepressants that alter the levels of the neurotransmitter serotonin in the brain. SSRIs have been used to treat panic disorder, OCD, and GAD. They are often prescribed because they have less severe side effects than the older antidepressants.

Some SSRIs used in anxiety disorders include fluoxetine (Prozac), sertraline (Zoloft), escitalopram (Lexapro), paroxetine (Paxil), and citalopram (Celexa), which are commonly prescribed for panic disorder, OCD, PTSD, and social phobia. SSRIs are also used to treat panic disorder when it occurs in combination with OCD, social phobia, or depression. SSRIs generally are started at low doses and gradually increased until they have a beneficial effect.

Tricyclic Antidepressants (TCAs): TCAs are older antidepressants that may be prescribed for panic disorder, OCD, and GAD. TCAs can also be prescribed for anxiety disorders co-occurring with depression. TCAs typically take around two weeks to provide symptom relief.

TCAs include imipramine (Tofranil), which is prescribed for panic disorder and GAD, and clomipramine (Anafranil), which is the only tricyclic antidepressant useful for treating OCD.

Monoamine Oxidase Inhibitors (MAOIs): MAOIs are the oldest class of antidepressant medications.

The MAOIs most commonly prescribed for anxiety disorders are phenelzine (Nardil), followed by tranylcypromine (Parnate), and isocarboxazid (Marplan), which are useful in treating panic disorder and social phobia.

Atypical Antidepressants

There are several newer atypical antidepressants that target other neurotransmitters either alone or in addition to serotonin. Some of the brain chemicals they affect include norepinephrine and dopamine. Venlafaxine (Effexor), an atypical antidepressant, is used to treat GAD.

Antidepressants take up to four to six weeks to begin relieving symptoms, so they aren't helpful if first taken during a panic attack. Antidepressants are often prescribed instead of benzodiazepines because the risk for dependency and abuse is less. Antidepressants can cause loss of sexual desire, nausea, insomnia, sweating, nervousness, dizziness, weight gain or weight loss, dry mouth, constipation, and blurred vision. MAOIs also have severe interactions with certain foods, drinks, and medications. When an individual takes an MAOI, he or she must carefully monitor what is eaten and what drugs are taken. Items that are restricted include many cheeses, chocolate, wine, and beer.

Beta-Blockers

Beta-blockers are a type of drug used to treat high blood pressure and heart problems. In anxiety, beta-blockers can help control physical symptoms such as nervousness, rapid heart rate, trembling voice, sweating, dizziness, and shaky hands. Beta-blockers are prescribed off-label for anxiety.

Because they don't affect the emotional symptoms of anxiety such as worry, beta-blockers are most helpful for phobias, particularly social phobia and performance anxiety (such as a speech or being in front of an audience). Examples of beta-blockers include propranolol (Inderal), metoprolol (Lopressor), and atenolol (Tenormin).

Side effects include lightheadedness, sleepiness, short-term memory loss, unusually slow pulse, fatigue, insomnia, diarrhea, cold hands and feet, and sexual side effects.

INTEGRATIVE THERAPIES

Strong Scientific Evidence

Kava: Kava kava (*Piper methysticum*) is a shrub from the South Pacific islands that has been used for centuries to produce calming effects in humans. Studies have found moderate benefit of kava in the treatment of anxiety, and preliminary evidence suggests that kava may be equivalent to benzodiazepine drugs such as diazepam (Valium). In one human study, kava's effects were reported to be similar to the prescription drug buspirone (Buspar) used for GAD. However, a recent study found no effect in GAD. The kava supplement should be standardized for best results.

There is concern regarding kava's potential toxicity, based on multiple reports of liver damage in Europe and a number of cases in the United States, including hepatitis, cirrhosis, and liver failure. The U.S. Food and Drug Administration has issued warnings to consumers and physicians. Kava should not be used in individuals with preexisting liver conditions or a history of alcohol or drug abuse. Caution is advised when taking kava as numerous adverse effects, including sedation and drug interactions, are possible. Kava should not be used if pregnant or breastfeeding.

Music Therapy: Music is an ancient tool of healing. Many different forms of music intervention have been used to reduce anxiety in a variety of medical conditions and medical procedures. Most studies have positive findings, although not all do. There is evidence that music interventions help reduce anxiety related to cataract surgery, sigmoidoscopy, bronchoscopy, breast biopsy, cesarean delivery, colonoscopy, esophagogastroduodenoscopy, cardiac catheterization, hospitalized asthmatic patients, psychotherapy, general medical procedures, radiation therapy, treatment for acute myocardial infarction, preparation for surgery, total knee arthroplasty, ventilator dependence, and transurethral resection of the prostate. Many of these studies have found reduced blood pressure and heart rate as well. A minority of studies found no benefit, including studies related to mammogram, ischemic heart disease, pediatric outpatient surgery, and cardiac catheterization. The choice of music may be a factor in outcomes: listening to music of one's preference has been found to be an important consideration. Overall, the evidence favors use of music interventions for anxiety, although more studies are needed to determine what forms work best.

Good Scientific Evidence

Aromatherapy: Fragrant oils have been used for thousands of years. Aromatherapy is a technique in which essential oils from plants are used with the intention of preventing or treating illness, reducing stress, or enhancing well-being. Several small studies report that lavender essential oil aromatherapy is able to cause reductions in anxiety levels. Additionally, rosemary (*Rosmarinus officinalis*) essential oil is frequently used in aromatherapy for treatment of a variety of conditions, including anxiety. Early study has shown benefit in reducing stress levels and increasing alertness. More study is needed to draw a firm recommendation. The use of aromatherapy for anxiety disorders needs more research.

Art Therapy: Art therapy may enable the expression of inner thoughts or feelings when verbalization is difficult or not possible. Some evidence suggests that creative expression programs in schools involving art therapy may help alleviate problems of self-esteem and can improve social functioning in school-age children. However, there is some evidence suggesting that art therapy may not benefit children with PTSD symptoms. Limited evidence suggests that art therapy, in the context of group psychotherapy, may contribute to reduction of symptoms of emotional distress in military personnel receiving mental health treatment.

Hypnosis: Hypnosis is associated with a deep state of relaxation. Several studies support the use of hypnosis to reduce anxiety, particularly prior to dental or medical procedures, or in the management of phobias. Early evidence suggests that these effects may last for up to three years with benefits reported in children and adults.

Psychotherapy: Psychotherapy is an interactive process between a person and a qualified mental health professional (psychiatrist, psychologist, clinical social worker, licensed counselor, or other trained practitioner). Psychotherapy, especially CBT, may help decrease the symptoms of anxiety disorders when used along with medications, including GAD, OCD, panic disorder, and PTSD.

Relaxation Therapy: Clinical studies suggest that relaxation techniques may be beneficial in patients with anxiety, although these approaches do not appear to be as effective as psychotherapy. Numerous human studies report that relaxation techniques (for example, using audiotapes or group therapy) may moderately reduce anxiety, particularly in individuals without significant mental illness. Relaxation may be beneficial for phobias such as agoraphobia (fear of crowds); panic disorder; work-related stress; and anxiety due to serious illnesses, prior to medical procedures, or during pregnancy. However, there are many types of relaxation techniques used in studies, and many trials do not clearly describe design or results.

Yoga: Yoga is an ancient system of relaxation, exercise, and healing with origins in Indian philosophy. Yoga may reduce daily stress and anxiety in healthy people when practiced several times weekly. Several human studies support the use of yoga therapy in the treatment of clinical anxiety disorders, including GAD and OCD. Available data remain inconclusive, yet thousands of years of effectiveness in India for stress and anxiety must be appreciated.

Unclear or Conflicting Scientific Evidence

Acupressure: Acupressure, or shiatsu, has been used in China for thousands of years for health and healing. Preliminary clinical trials suggest that acupressure may significantly reduce GAD and preoperative anxiety. However, these studies have been small and poorly designed, warranting better-quality research.

Acupuncture: Acupuncture, or the use of needles to manipulate the "chi," or body energy, originated in China over 5,000 years ago. Several studies have reported benefits in anxiety disorders, but the studies have been small and poorly designed, leaving the scientific evidence on acupuncture use in anxiety inconclusive.

Bacopa: Bacopa (*Bacopa monnieri*) is commonly called "brahmi" and is used in the Ayurvedic system of medicine in India. Although bacopa is traditionally used for anxiety, high-quality clinical trials are lacking. One weak study found some evidence that bacopa reduces clinical anxiety. However, more independent research is needed. Caution is advised when taking bacopa supplements as numerous adverse effects, including heart palpitations, are possible.

Gotu Kola: In the traditional Indian system of Ayurvedic medicine, gotu kola is said to develop the crown chakra, the energy center at the top of the head, and to balance the right and left hemispheres of the brain. It has traditionally been used by yogis as a food for meditation. Animal research has demonstrated anxiolytic (anxiety reducing) properties of gotu kola, but human studies are lacking. A single randomized trial assessing the effects of gotu kola on startle responses in healthy (nonanxious) individuals has reported some benefits. These preliminary findings are promising, although further research should be performed. Gotu kola is not related to the cola nut and does not contain caffeine. Gotu kola is generally reported as safe when used in humans for short-term use.

Guided Imagery: Guided imagery may include a number of techniques, such as metaphor, story telling, fantasy, game playing, dream interpretation, drawing, visualization, active imagination, or direct suggestion using imagery. Therapeutic guided imagery may be used to help patients relax and focus on images associated with personal issues they are confronting. Initial evidence suggests that guided imagery relaxation audiotapes may reduce anxiety after surgeries and may improve healing. More studies are needed.

Healing Touch: Preliminary data from an uncontrolled trial suggests healing touch may help reduce symptoms of PTSD in women. More studies are needed.

Lemon Balm: Preliminary human evidence has been published that supports the use of lemon balm (*Melissa officinalis*) for anxiety. In a large case series that included 1,599 patients with symptoms of anxiety, a combination of lemon balm and valerian (*Valeriana officinalis*) was found to improve symptoms of anxiety, including nervousness, fatigue, and sleep disturbances, in over 90% of the patients. Although only mild side effects were reported, caution is advised when taking lemon balm supplements as numerous adverse effects, including drowsiness and drug interactions, are possible.

Massage: Various forms of therapeutic superficial tissue manipulation have been practiced for thousands of years across cultures. Several human trials have assessed the effects of massage in patients with anxiety, including those with cancer, chronic illnesses, preoperative anxiety (anxious about themselves or for family members having surgery), dementia, multiple sclerosis, premenstrual syndrome, or fibromyalgia; in patients before/during medical procedures; those who are hospitalized for psychiatric disorders; depressed adolescent mothers; and elderly institutionalized patients. Additional research is necessary in order to form a scientifically based recommendation.

Meditation: Various forms of meditation, including mindfulness, transcendental meditation, and "meditation-based stress reduction programs" have been studied for their effects on anxiety. Better studies are needed.

Qi Gong: Qi gong is a type of traditional Chinese medicine that is thought to be at least 4,000 years old. Preliminary study shows that qi gong may be beneficial for relieving stress. Available data remain inconclusive, yet thousands of years of effectiveness in China for stress and anxiety must be appreciated.

Reflexology: Reflexology involves the application of manual pressure to specific points or areas of the feet that are believed to correspond to other parts of the body. There is preliminary evidence that reflexology may be useful for relaxation and to decrease anxiety. However, it is not clear that reflexology is equivalent or superior to massage or other types of physical manipulation. Better research is needed in this area.

Therapeutic Touch: Results of different studies do not agree with each other, and therefore it is currently unclear if therapeutic touch is a useful anxiety treatment. Some trials report benefits, while others find no effects. Also, there is early evidence that therapeutic touch may reduce anxiety in children with life-threatening illnesses, reduce stress in teenagers with psychiatric disease, and help relax premature infants. Most studies have not been well designed, and better research is necessary in order to draw firm conclusions.

Valerian: Valerian (*Valeriana officinalis*) has traditionally been used for sleep improvement and for stress and anxiety. Studies have generally been of poor methodological quality, and several have used valerian in combination with other herbs, such as passion flower (*Passiflora incarnata*), lemon balm (*Melissa officinalis*), and St. John's wort (*Hypericum perforatum*). Studies report that valerian is generally well tolerated for up to four to six weeks in recommended doses. Caution is advised when taking valerian supplements as numerous adverse effects, including drowsiness, sedation, and drug interactions, are possible. Do not use valerian if pregnant or breastfeeding.

ARTHRITIS

CONDITIONS: Arthritis, Periarthritis, Rheumatoid Arthritis, Osteoarthritis

BACKGROUND

The term arthritis literally means joint inflammation or swelling. More than 100 different diseases fall under the general category of arthritis. Arthritis conditions affect the joints, the tissues surrounding the affected joints, and other connective tissues. Common forms of arthritis include rheumatoid arthritis, osteoarthritis, and periarthritis.

Osteoarthritis, also called degenerative joint disease or osteoarthrosis, occurs when the cartilage in the joints starts to break down. The cartilage serves as a cushion between bones, allowing the joint to move without pain. Therefore, patients with osteoarthritis experience pain and reduced mobility in their joints. Osteoarthritis may affect any joint in the body. Osteoarthritis occurs most often in individuals older than 45 years, but it may develop at any age. Females are more likely to develop the disorder than males, suggesting that heredity may play a role in the development of the condition. Individuals who are obese, have weak muscles, have cartilage disorders, and/or have malformed joints have an increased risk of developing osteoarthritis.

Rheumatoid arthritis is an autoimmune disorder that occurs when the body's immune system, which normally fights against disease and infection, attacks itself. Unlike osteoarthritis, which only affects the bones and cartilage, rheumatoid arthritis may also cause swelling in other areas of the body. Women are two to three times more likely to develop rheumatoid arthritis than men. Most cases of rheumatoid arthritis occur in individuals who are 20-50 years old. However, rheumatoid arthritis may also develop in young children and older adults. Although there is currently no cure for osteoarthritis or rheumatoid arthritis, treatment can help reduce pain and help individuals remain active.

Periarthritis is a chronic inflammatory disease of a joint and the tissues surrounding it. The condition primarily affects patients who are 50 years old or older. Periarthritis most commonly affects the shoulder. Periarthritis of the shoulder is also called adhesive capsulitis or frozen shoulder. Patients typically receive cortisol injections, antiinflammatories, and physical therapy. Without aggressive treatment, periarthritis of the shoulder can be permanent.

CAUSES

Osteoarthritis: The exact cause of osteoarthritis remains unknown. Most researchers believe that several factors, including obesity, age, joint injury or stress, genetics, and muscle weakness, may contribute to the development of osteoarthritis.

Some researchers believe that cartilage damage may occur when cartilage releases too many enzymes that allow for the natural breakdown and regeneration of cartilage. If the body releases too many of these enzymes, the cartilage will be destroyed faster than it can be regenerated. However, it is unknown exactly what causes an imbalance of the cartilage enzyme.

When individuals have osteoarthritis, their bodies try to repair the cartilage damage. However, the body cannot regenerate enough cartilage. Instead, new bone grows alongside the existing bone, causing small lumps to form. Although these lumps cause minimal if any pain, they may be disfiguring and limit the joint's mobility.

Rheumatoid Arthritis: The exact cause of rheumatoid arthritis remains unknown. Rheumatoid arthritis is considered an autoimmune disorder because the immune system does not function properly. Normally, the immune system helps the body fight against harmful foreign invaders, such as bacteria, that may cause disease and infection. However, in rheumatoid arthritis patients, the immune system attacks body cells because they are mistaken for harmful invaders.

Patients with rheumatoid arthritis have high levels of white blood cells in the synovial membrane, which lines the body's joints. As a result, the joints became painful and swollen. The inflammation causes proteins to be released over months or years, which then results in the thickening of the synovial membranes. This may also lead to damaged bones, cartilage, tendons, and ligaments.

Some researchers believe that this autoimmune process is triggered by an infection with a virus or bacterium. Heredity may also play a role in the development of rheumatoid arthritis.

Periarthritis: Periarthritis typically occurs after the joint becomes injured, which causes scarring, thickening, and shrinkage of the joint. It may also occur after exposure to cold temperatures. Periarthritis typically affects the shoulder.

Individuals who have other types of long-term arthritis that affect the shoulders have an increased risk of developing periarthritis of the shoulder, also called adhesive capsulitis or frozen shoulder.

SIGNS AND SYMPTOMS

Osteoarthritis: Because osteoarthritis develops slowly, many patients do not experience symptoms right away. Once symptoms develop, they are generally the worst during the first year of the disease. Common symptoms include joint pain, swelling and/or stiffness in a joint (especially after use), joint discomfort before or during a change in the weather, bony lumps on the fingers, and loss of joint flexibility. The joints that are most often affected by osteoarthritis include the fingers, spine, and weight-bearing joints, such as the hips, ankles, feet, and knees.

If patients overuse the affected joints and do not receive treatment, the cartilage in the joints may wear down completely. When this happens, the bone may rub against bone, causing severe pain.

Rheumatoid Arthritis: Rheumatoid arthritis often affects many joints at the same time. The severity of symptoms varies among patients. Symptoms, which may come and go, typically include pain and swelling in the joints (especially in the hands and feet), generalized aching or stiffness of the joints and muscles (especially after periods of rest), loss of motion of the affected joints, weakness in the muscles near the affected joints, low-grade fever, and general feeling of discomfort. In general, both sides of the body are affected equally. For instance, if arthritis is in the hands, both hands will be equally affected. Early in the disease, the joints in the hands, wrists, feet, and knees are most frequently affected. Over time, arthritis may develop in the shoulders, elbows, jaw, hips, and neck.

Over time, the joints may become deformed. Small lumps, called rheumatoid nodules, may develop under the skin at pressure points. These lumps, which range from the size of a pea to a quarter, may be visible near the elbows, hands, feet, Achilles tendon, back of the scalp, knee, or lungs. Rheumatoid nodules are not painful. However, bone deformities or swelling may reduce the flexibility of the joints.

In addition to the joints, other areas of the body may also be affected. Rheumatoid arthritis may cause swelling in other parts of the body, including the tear ducts, salivary glands, the lining of the heart, the lungs and, occasionally, blood vessels.

Periarthritis: Periarthritis causes swelling and pain in the joint. Most patients develop periarthritis of the shoulder. When the shoulder is affected, the joint's mobility is significantly or completely reduced, aggressive treatment is started.

COMPLICATIONS

Cosmetic Concerns: Arthritis may cause small bumps, called nodules, to form on bones. These bumps can occur on any joint, but they are most common in the hands. These nodules may be disfiguring.

Depression: Some arthritis patients may suffer from depression. This may happen if the arthritis interferes significantly with the patient's lifestyle. Patients should consult their healthcare providers if they experience feelings of sadness, low self-esteem, loss of pleasure, apathy, and possibly difficulty functioning for two weeks or longer with no known underlying cause. These may be signs of depression.

Joint Damage: In some cases, arthritis can lead to severe joint damage. In such cases, surgery, such as a joint replacement, may be necessary. Patients should regularly visit their healthcare providers to monitor their conditions.

Limited Mobility: Patients with arthritis may have limited mobility in their joints. Joint mobility decreases as the joint becomes more damaged. Patients with periarthritis of the shoulder, also called frozen shoulder, may be completely unable to move their joints without aggressive treatment. If arthritis is not properly managed with nonsteroidal antiinflammatories, arthritis may interfere with a patient's daily life.

Pain: Arthritis may cause severe pain. Patients should stay in close contact with their healthcare providers to ensure that their medications are properly managing the pain. In some cases, the medication or dosage may need to be changed.

DIAGNOSIS

General: Once patients are diagnosed with arthritis, they should visit their healthcare providers regularly, at least once a year. Patients should stay in close contact with their physicians to ensure that their symptoms are managed and to monitor joint damage.

Osteoarthritis: X-rays are often the first test performed if a patient has symptoms of osteoarthritis. If the patient has osteoarthritis, the x-ray images will often show loss of cartilage in the affected joints, narrowing of the space between bones, and bumps called nodules.

A procedure called arthrocentesis may also be performed at a healthcare provider's office. During the procedure, a needle is inserted into the affected joint and a small sample of fluid is removed. The fluid is then analyzed to rule out other conditions, such as gout or infection. This test may also temporarily relieve some pain and inflammation in the joint.

A surgical procedure called arthroscopy may also be performed. During the surgery, a small incision is made into the affected joint. Then a tube called an arthroscope is inserted into the joint. This tube has a small light and camera, which allow the healthcare provider to see the inside of the joint. If abnormalities such as cartilage or ligament damage are seen, the patient is diagnosed with osteoarthritis.

Rheumatoid Arthritis: A blood test may be performed to determine if an antibody called the rheumatoid factor is present. Most patients with rheumatoid arthritis eventually have this abnormal protein in their blood. However, it may not present when symptoms first develop. If rheumatoid factor is present, a positive diagnosis is made. If patients test negative but rheumatoid arthritis is suspected, a healthcare provider may recommend treatment to reduce symptoms. Another test may be performed in the future to confirm a diagnosis.

Periarthritis: Periarthritis is usually diagnosed after a healthcare provider takes a detailed medical history and performs a physical examination. The affected joint will have very limited mobility. In some cases, an x-ray may be needed to confirm a diagnosis. During the procedure, a contrast dye is injected into the affected joint and x-rays are taken. If the patient has periarthritis, the joint will appear shrunken and scarred.

TREATMENT

General: Osteoarthritis, rheumatoid arthritis, and periarthritis are managed with medications that reduce pain and inflammation. Patients with rheumatoid arthritis may also require treatment with medications that weaken the immune system, such as corticosteroids or immunosuppressants. In severe cases, surgery may be necessary to repair damage.

In order to properly manage pain and prevent joint damage, patients should take their medications exactly as prescribed by their healthcare providers. Patients should also tell their healthcare providers if they are taking any other drugs (prescription or over-the-counter) because they may interfere with treatment.

Abatacept (Orencia): Batacept (Orencia) is a type of drug called a costimulation modulator. Abatacept reduces inflammation and joint damaged caused by rheumatoid arthritis. The drug prevents white blood cells, called T cells, from attacking the joints. Patients receive a monthly injection through a vein in the arm.

Side effects may include headache, nausea, and mild infections, such as upper respiratory tract infections. Serious infections, such as pneumonia, may develop.

Antidepressants: Some patients with arthritis may also suffer from depression. Commonly prescribed antidepressants for arthritis patients include amitriptyline, nortriptyline (Aventyl, Pamelor), and trazodone (Desyrel).

Arthroscopic Lavage and/or Debridement: In some cases, patients with osteoarthritis may suffer from severe joint damage. In such cases, surgical procedures called arthroscopic lavage and/or arthroscopic debridement may be recommended. During the surgery, a small incision is made near the joint. A small tubular instrument called an arthroscope is then inserted. The arthroscope has a small light and camera attached to it, allowing the surgeon to see inside the joint. During arthroscopic lavage, the surgeon squirts saline into the joint to remove any blood, fluid, or loose debris inside the joint. During arthroscopic debridement, loose fragments of bone or cartilage are removed from the joint. In some cases, built-up scar tissue may also be removed.

Both of these procedures may provide temporary pain relief and improved joint function. However, recent studies suggest that they may not be effective in some patients with osteoarthritis. Therefore, patients should discuss the potential risks and health benefits of the procedure with their healthcare providers.

Corticosteroids: Corticosteroids, such as prednisone (e.g., Deltasone) and methylprednisolone (Medrol), have been used to reduce inflammation and pain and slow joint damage caused by rheumatoid arthritis. These drugs are generally very effective when used short term. However, if these drugs are used for many months to years, they may become less effective and serious side effects may develop. Side effects may include easy bruising, thinning of bones, cataracts, weight gain, a round face, and diabetes.

Occasionally, corticosteroids are used to treat patients with severe osteoarthritis. The medication is injected into the affected joints to reduce pain and inflammation. Patients with periarthritis typically receive corticosteroid injections into affected joints to reduce pain and inflammation. Corticosteroids are usually prescribed for a certain amount of time and then the patient is gradually tapered off the medication. Patients should not stop taking corticosteroids suddenly or change their dosages without first consulting their healthcare providers.

Cool Compress or Ice Pack: Applying a cool compress or ice pack to the affected joint during a flare-up may help reduce swelling and pain.

Disease-Modifying Antirheumatic Drugs (DMARDs): During the early stages of rheumatoid arthritis, patients typically receive DMARDs to limit the amount of permanent joint damage. These drugs may take weeks to months before they begin to take effect. Therefore, they are often used in combination with nonsteroidal antiinflammatory drugs (NSAIDs) or corticosteroids. Commonly prescribed DMARDs include the gold compound auranofin (Ridaura), hydroxychloroquine (Plaquenil), minocycline (Dynacin, Minocin), sulfasalazine (Azulfidine), and methotrexate (Rheumatrex).

Heat: Applying a hot pack to affected joints may help reduce pain, relax muscles, and increase blood flow to the joint. It may also be an effective treatment before exercise. Alternatively, patients may take a hot shower or bath before exercise to help reduce pain.

Immunosuppressants: Patients with rheumatoid arthritis may take prescription drugs called immunosuppressants. These medications weaken the body's immune system, which limits the amount of joint damage. Commonly prescribed immunosuppressants include leflunomide (Arava), azathioprine (Imuran), cyclosporine (Neoral, Sandimmune), and cyclophosphamide (Cytoxan).

These medications may have serious side effects, including increased risk of infections, kidney problems, high blood pressure, and decreased levels of red blood cells. Other side effects may include increased hair growth, loss of appetite, vomiting, and upset stomach.

Fusing Bones: If there is serious joint damage, the bones of a joint, such as the ankle, may be surgically fused to together in a procedure called arthrodesis. This surgery helps increase stability and reduces pain. However, the joint no longer has any flexibility and cannot bend or move.

Joint Replacement Surgery: In some cases, patients with osteoarthritis or rheumatoid arthritis suffer from permanent joint damage. In such instances, joint replacement surgery may be necessary. During the procedure, the damaged joint is surgically removed and it is replaced with a plastic or metal device called a prosthesis. The most commonly replaced joints are the hip and knee, but other joints, including the elbow, shoulder, finger, or ankle joints, can be replaced.

Joint replacement surgeries are generally most successful for large joints, such as the hip or knee. Researchers estimate that hip or knee replacements last at least 20 years in 80% of patients. After a successful surgery and several months of rehabilitation, patients are able to use their new joints without pain.

As with any major surgery, there are risks associated with joint replacements. Patients should discuss the potential health risks and benefits of surgery with their healthcare providers.

Lifestyle: Many lifestyle changes, including regular exercise, weight management, and healthy diet may help reduce symptoms of osteoarthritis. A healthcare provider may recommend a physical therapist or nutritionist to help a patient determine the best treatment plan for him/her.

Individuals with osteoarthritis or rheumatoid arthritis should wear comfortable footwear that properly supports their weight. This may reduce the amount of strain put on the joints during walking.

Patients with osteoarthritis or rheumatoid arthritis may require canes, walkers, or other devices to help them get around. If the hands are severely affected, braces may be beneficial. Patients should talk to their healthcare providers about assistive devices that are available.

Individuals with osteoarthritis or rheumatoid arthritis should maintain good posture. This allows the body's weight to be evenly distributed among joints.

Nonselective Nonsteroidal Anti-inflammatory drugs (NSAIDs): NSAIDs have been used to relieve pain and inflammation caused by osteoarthritis, rheumatoid arthritis, and periarthritis. Commonly used over-the-counter NSAIDs include ibuprofen (Advil, Motrin) and naproxen sodium (Aleve). Higher doses of these drugs are also available by prescription. Commonly prescribed NSAIDs include diclofenac (Cataflam, Voltaren), nabumetone (Relafen), and ketoprofen (Orudis). NSAIDs may be taken by mouth, injected into a vein, or applied to the skin. These medications are generally taken long term to manage symptoms.

The frequency and severity of side effects vary. The most common side effects include nausea, vomiting, diarrhea, constipation, decreased appetite, rash, dizziness, headache, and drowsiness. The most serious side effects include kidney failure, liver failure, ulcers, heart-related problems, and prolonged bleeding after an injury or surgery. About 15% of patients who receive long-term NSAID treatment develop ulcers in the stomach or duodenum.

Pain Relievers: Prescription pain relievers, including tramadol (Ultram), have been used to reduce pain caused by osteoarthritis or rheumatoid arthritis. Although this drug, which is available by prescription, does not reduce swelling, it has fewer side effects than NSAIDs. Tramadol is generally taken as a short-term treatment to reduce symptoms of flare-ups.

Narcotic pain relievers, such as acetaminophen/codeine (Tylenol with codeine), hydrocodone/acetaminophen (Lorcet, Lortab, Vicodin), or oxycodone (OxyContin, Roxicodone), may be prescribed to treat severe arthritis pain. However, they do not reduce swelling. These medications are only used short term to treat flare-ups. Common side effects include constipation, drowsiness, dry mouth, and difficulty urinating. Narcotic pain relievers should be used cautiously because patients may become addicted to them.

Rituximab (Rituxan): A medication called rituximab (Rituxan) has been used to treat patients with rheumatoid arthritis. This medication, which is injected into the patient's vein, reduces the number of B cells in the body. This medication helps reduce swelling because the B cells are involved in inflammation.

Side effects may include flulike symptoms, such as fever, chills, and nausea. Some people experience extreme reactions to the infusion, such as difficulty breathing and heart problems.

Selective Cyclooxygenase-2 (COX-2) Inhibitors: Celecoxib (Celebrex) has been taken by mouth to reduce pain and inflammation caused by osteoarthritis, rheumatoid arthritis, or periarthritis. Celecoxib is currently the only COX-2 inhibitor that is approved by the U.S. Food and Drug Administration. Celecoxib is generally taken long term to manage symptoms.

COX-2 inhibitors have been linked to an increased risk of serious heart-related side effects, including heart attack and stroke. Selective COX-2 inhibitors have also been shown to increase the risk of stomach bleeding, fluid retention, kidney problems, and liver damage. Less serious side effects may include headache, indigestion, upper respiratory tract infection, diarrhea, sinus inflammation, stomach pain, and nausea.

Topical Pain Relievers: Topical pain relievers are creams, ointments, gels, and sprays that are applied to the skin. Many over-the-counter pain relievers may temporarily help reduce the pain caused by osteoarthritis. Products such as Aspercreme, Sportscreme, Icy Hot, and Ben-Gay may help reduce arthritis pain. Capsaicin cream, which is made from the seeds of hot peppers, may reduce pain in joints that are close to the skin surface, such as the fingers, knees, and elbows.

INTEGRATIVE THERAPIES

Strong Scientific Evidence

Glucosamine: Glucosamine is a natural compound that is found in healthy cartilage. Based on human research, there is good evidence to support the use of glucosamine sulfate in the treatment of mild-to-moderate knee osteoarthritis. Most studies have used glucosamine sulfate supplied by one European manufacturer (Rottapharm, Monza, Italy), and it is not known if glucosamine preparations made by other manufacturers are equally effective. Although some studies of glucosamine have not found benefits, these

have either included patients with severe osteoarthritis or used products other than glucosamine sulfate. The evidence for the effect of glycosaminoglycan polysulfate is conflicting and merits further investigation. More well-designed clinical trials are needed to confirm safety and effectiveness and to test different formulations of glucosamine.

Avoid if allergic or hypersensitive to shellfish or iodine. Some reports suggest a link between glucosamine/chondroitin products and asthma. Use cautiously with diabetes or with a history of bleeding disorders. Avoid if pregnant or breastfeeding.

Willow Bark: Willow bark that contains salicin has been used to treat many different kinds of pain. Willow bark is a traditional analgesic (pain relieving) therapy for osteoarthritis. Several studied have confirmed this finding. Additional study comparing willow bark to conventional medicinal agents for safety and effectiveness is warranted.

Avoid if allergic/hypersensitive to aspirin, willow bark (*Salix* spp.), or any of its constituents, including salicylates. Use cautiously with gastrointestinal problems (e.g., ulcers), liver disorders, diabetes, gout (foot inflammation), high blood pressure, or high cholesterol. Use cautiously with a history of allergy, asthma, or leukemia. Use cautiously if taking protein-bound medications, antihyperlipidemia agents, alcohol, leukemia medications, beta-blockers, diuretics, phenytoin (Dilantin), probenecid, spironolactone, sulfonylureas, valproic acid, or methotrexate. Use cautiously if predisposed to headaches. Use cautiously in tannin-containing herbs or supplements. Avoid operating heavy machinery. Avoid in children with chickenpox and any other viral infections. Avoid with blood and renal disorders. Avoid if taking other NSAIDs, acetazolamide, or other carbonic anhydrase inhibitors. Avoid with elevated serum cadmium levels. Avoid if pregnant or breastfeeding.

Good Scientific Evidence

Borage Seed Oil: Borage (*Borago officinalis*) is an herb native to Syria that has spread throughout the Middle East and Mediterranean. Borage flowers and leaves may be eaten, and borage seeds are often pressed to produce oil that is very high in gamma-linolenic acid (GLA). GLA has known antiinflammatory effects that may make it beneficial in treating rheumatoid arthritis. A few human studies have generally found positive results and no side effects were reported. However, more research is needed to determine the optimal dose and administration.

Avoid if allergic or hypersensitive to borage, its constituents, or members of the Boraginaceae family. Avoid with a weakened immune system. Use cautiously with bleeding disorders, epilepsy, or if taking drugs used to treat these disorders. Avoid if pregnant or breastfeeding.

Glucosamine: Glucosamine is a natural compound that is found in healthy cartilage. Several human studies and animal experiments report benefits of glucosamine in treating osteoarthritis of various joints of the body. However, the evidence is less plentiful than that for knee osteoarthritis. Some of these benefits include pain relief (possibly due to an antiinflammatory effect of glucosamine) and improved joint function. Overall, these studies have not been well designed. Although there is some promising research, more study is needed in this area before a firm conclusion can be made.

Avoid if allergic or hypersensitive to shellfish or iodine. Some reports suggest a link between glucosamine/chondroitin products and asthma. Use cautiously with diabetes or with a history of bleeding disorders. Avoid if pregnant or breastfeeding.

Omega-3 Fatty Acid: Multiple studies report improvements in morning stiffness and joint tenderness with the regular intake of fish oil supplements for up to three months. Benefits have been reported as additive with antiinflammatory medications, such as NSAIDs (e.g., ibuprofen). However, because of weaknesses in study designs and reporting, better research is necessary before a strong favorable recommendation can be made. Effects beyond three months of treatment have not been well evaluated.

Avoid if allergic or hypersensitive to fish, omega-3 fatty acid products that come from fish, nuts, linolenic acid, or omega-3 fatty acid products that come from nuts. Avoid during active bleeding. Use cautiously with bleeding disorders, diabetes, low blood pressure, or if taking drugs, herbs, or supplements that treat any such conditions. Use cautiously before surgery. The Environmental Protection Agency recommends that fish intake be limited in pregnant/nursing women to a single six-ounce meal per week and in young children to less than two ounces per week. For farm-raised, imported, or marine fish, the U.S. Food and Drug Administration recommends that pregnant/nursing women and young children avoid eating types with higher levels of methyl mercury and less than 12 ounces per week of other fish types. Women who might become pregnant are advised to eat seven ounces or less per week of fish with higher levels of methyl mercury or up to 14 ounces per week of fish types with about 0.5 parts per million (such as marlin, orange roughy, red snapper, or fresh tuna).

Physical Therapy: The goal of physical therapy is to improve mobility, restore function, reduce pain, and prevent further injuries. Several techniques, including exercises, stretches, traction, electrical stimulation, and massage, are used. Physical therapy for osteoarthritis of the knee may provide short-term benefits, but long-term benefits do not appear better than standard treatments. Physical therapy, either as an individually delivered treatment or in a small group format, appears effective. Only one available study compared physical therapy to a sham group (subtherapeutic ultrasound) and found that a combination of manual physical therapy and supervised exercise was beneficial for patients with osteoarthritis of the knee. One method of physical therapy, infrared short-wave diathermy-pulsed patterns and interferential therapy, showed more effectiveness than intra-articular hyaluronan drugs in two studies. More research using consistent treatment protocols and outcomes measures would be helpful in this area.

Not all physical therapy programs are suited for everyone, and patients should discuss their medical history with their qualified healthcare professionals before beginning any treatments. Based on the available literature, physical therapy appears generally safe when practiced by a qualified physical therapist. Physical therapy may aggravate preexisting conditions. Persistent pain and fractures of unknown origin have been reported. Physical therapy may increase the duration of pain or cause limitation of motion. Pain and anxiety may occur during the rehabilitation of patients with burns. Both morning stiffness and bone erosion have been reported in the physical therapy literature, although causality is unclear. Erectile dysfunction has also been reported. All therapies during pregnancy and breastfeeding should be discussed with a licensed obstetrician/gynecologist before initiation.

Psychotherapy: Psychotherapy is an interactive process between a person and a qualified mental health professional. The patient explores thoughts, feelings, and behavior to help with problem solving. Although group therapy may somewhat decrease pain in people with rheumatoid arthritis and depression, individual therapy coupled with antidepressants may be more effective.

Psychotherapy cannot always fix mental or emotional conditions. Psychiatric drugs are sometimes needed. In some cases, symptoms may get worse if the proper medication is not taken. Not all therapists are qualified to work with all problems. Use cautiously with serious mental illness or some medical conditions because some forms of psychotherapy may stir up strong emotional feelings and expression.

Acupuncture: Acupuncture is commonly used throughout the world. According to Chinese medicine theory, the human body contains a network of energy pathways through which vital energy, called chi, circulates. These pathways contain specific "points" that function like gates, allowing chi to flow through the body. Needles are inserted into these points to regulate the flow of chi. According to early research, acupuncture for the treatment of periarthritis of the shoulder shows promising results. Further research is needed before a firm conclusion can be made.

Some studies of weak design have reported that acupuncture may relieve pain associated with rheumatoid arthritis. However, a well-designed trial was unable to confirm this. More evidence is needed to clarify if or when acupuncture is beneficial in rheumatoid arthritis.

Needles must be sterile in order to avoid disease transmission. Avoid with valvular heart disease, infections, bleeding disorders, medical conditions of unknown origin, or neurological disorders. Avoid on areas that have received radiation therapy and during pregnancy. Avoid if taking drugs that increase the risk of bleeding (anticoagulants). Use cautiously with pulmonary disease (such as asthma or emphysema). Use cautiously in medically compromised patients, diabetics, or the elderly. Use cautiously with a history of seizures. Avoid electroacupuncture with arrhythmia (irregular heartbeat) or in patients with pacemakers.

Astaxanthin: Astaxanthin is found in microalgae, yeast, salmon, trout, krill, shrimp, crayfish, crustaceans, and the feathers of some birds. Astaxanthin has been suggested as a possible treatment for rheumatoid arthritis. However, further research is warranted.

Avoid if allergic or hypersensitive to astaxanthin or related carotenoids, including canthaxanthin or an astaxanthin algal source. Use cautiously if taking 5-alpha-reductase inhibitors, hypertensive agents, asthma medications, drugs that are broken down by the liver, menopause agents, birth control pills, or *Helicobacter pylori* agents. Use cautiously with high blood pressure, parathyroid disorders, or osteoporosis. Avoid with hormone-sensitive conditions, immune disorders, or if taking immunosuppressive therapies. Avoid with previous experience of visual changes while taking astaxanthin and with low eosinophil levels. Avoid if pregnant or breastfeeding.

Ayurveda: Ayurveda is a form of natural medicine that originated in ancient India more than 5,000 years ago. Ayurveda is an integrated system of techniques that uses diet, herbs, exercise, meditation, yoga, and massage or bodywork to achieve optimal health on all levels (physical, psychological, and spiritual). There is some evidence that a traditional Ayurvedic herbal formula RA-1 may reduce joint swelling but not other symptoms in rheumatoid arthritis. RA-1 contains *Withania somnifera* (ashwagandha), *Boswellia serrata* (gugulla), *Zingiberis officinale* (ginger), and *Curcuma longa* (turmeric). A resin that is extracted from Boswellia serrata (H15, indish incense) is regarded in Ayurvedic medicine as having antiinflammatory properties. However, evidence from one study showed no benefit in patients with rheumatoid arthritis. More studies are needed to determine efficacy of these treatments in rheumatoid arthritis.

Ayurvedic herbs should be used cautiously because they are potent and some constituents can be potentially toxic if taken in large amounts or for a long time. Some herbs imported from India have been reported to contain high levels of toxic metals. Ayurvedic herbs may interact with other herbs, foods, or drugs. A qualified healthcare professional should be consulted before taking. Avoid Ayurveda with traumatic injuries, acute pain, advanced disease stages, or medical conditions that require surgery.

Beta-Sitosterol: Beta-sitosterol is found in plant-based foods, such as fruits, vegetables, soybeans, breads, peanuts, and peanut products. It is also found in bourbon and oils, such as olive oil, flaxseed, and tuna. Beta-sitosterol has been shown to reduce inflammation and it has therefore been suggested as a possible treatment for rheumatoid arthritis. Further research is needed to confirm these claims.

Avoid if allergic or hypersensitive to beta-sitosterol, beta-sitosterol glucoside, or pine. Use cautiously with asthma or breathing disorders, diabetes, primary biliary cirrhosis (destruction of the small bile duct in the liver), ileostomy, neurodegenerative disorders (such as Parkinson's disease or Alzheimer's disease), bulging of the colon, short-bowel syndrome, celiac disease, or sitosterolemia. Use cautiously with a history of gallstones. Avoid if pregnant or breastfeeding.

Black Cohosh: Black cohosh is a popular alternative for menopausal hormonal symptoms, such as hot flashes, migraine headache, mood changes, sleep changes, sweating, fast heartbeat, and vaginal dryness. The exact action of black cohosh is unclear. Although it has been suggested that black cohosh may help relieve joint pain associated with rheumatoid arthritis and osteoarthritis, further research is needed.

Use cautiously if allergic to members of the Ranunculaceae family, such as buttercups or crowfoot. Avoid with hormone conditions (e.g., breast cancer, ovarian cancer, uterine cancer, endometriosis). Avoid if allergic to aspirin products, NSAIDs (such as ibuprofen), or blood thinners (such as warfarin). Avoid with a history of blood clots, stroke, seizures, or liver disease. Stop use two weeks before and immediately after surgery/dental/diagnostic procedures with bleeding risks.

Black Currant: The black currant shrub grows naturally in Europe and parts of Asia. Traditionally, black currant fruit has been cultivated mainly for dietary and confectionary purposes. Black currant may help reduce inflammation and morning stiffness associated with arthritis. However, additional research is needed before a firm conclusion can be made.

Avoid if allergic or hypersensitive to black currant, its constituents, or plants in the Saxifragaceae family. Avoid with bleeding disorders or if taking blood thinners unless otherwise recommended by a qualified healthcare provider. Use cautiously with venous disorders or gastrointestinal disorders. Use cautiously if taking antidepressants or vitamin C supplements. Avoid if pregnant or breastfeeding.

Boswellia: Boswellia (*Boswellia serrata*) is an herb that has been shown to have antiinflammatory properties. Therefore, boswellia has been suggested as a potential treatment for rheumatoid arthritis and osteoarthritis. However, data are conflicting and sometimes combination products have been used. Therefore, there is currently insufficient evidence to recommend for or against the use of boswellia for arthritis.

Avoid if allergic or hypersensitive to boswellia. Avoid with a history of stomach ulcers or stomach acid reflux disease. Avoid if pregnant or breastfeeding.

Bromelain: Bromelain is an herb that contains a digestive enzyme that comes from the stem and the fruit of the pineapple plant. When taken with meals, bromelain may aid in the digestion of proteins. When taken on an empty stomach, it acts as an antiinflammatory agent. In one study of a combination product ERC (enzyme-rutosid combination: rutosid, bromelain, trypsin), results showed that ERC may be considered as an effective and safe alternative to prescription antiinflammatory drugs (NSAIDs) such as diclofenac, in the treatment of painful episodes of osteoarthritis of the knee. Further well-designed clinical trials of bromelain alone are needed to confirm these results.

Bromelain has also been suggested as a possible treatment for rheumatoid arthritis. Further research is needed before a firm conclusion can be made.

Avoid if allergic to bromelain, pineapple, honeybee venom, latex, birch pollen, carrots, celery, fennel, cypress pollen, grass pollen, papain, rye flour, wheat flour, or other members of the Bromeliaceae family. Use cautiously with a history of bleeding disorders, stomach ulcers, heart disease, liver disease, or kidney disease. Use cautiously before dental or surgical procedures or while driving or operating machinery. Avoid if pregnant or breastfeeding.

Cat's Claw: Cat's claw is widely used in the United States and Europe, and it is one of the top herbal remedies sold despite a lack of high-quality human evidence. In Germany and Austria, cat's claw is only available by prescription. Several laboratory and animal studies suggest that cat's claw may reduce inflammation; this has led to research of cat's claw for inflammatory conditions such as arthritis. Early research also suggests that cat's claw may reduce pain from knee osteoarthritis. Large, high-quality human studies are needed comparing effects of cat's claw alone vs. placebo before a conclusion can be drawn.

Avoid if allergic to cat's claw, Uncaria plants, or plants in the Rubiaceae family (such as gardenia, coffee, or quinine). Avoid with a history of conditions affecting the immune system (such as AIDS, HIV, some types of cancer, multiple sclerosis, tuberculosis, or lupus). Use cautiously with bleeding disorders or with a history of stroke. Use cautiously if taking drugs that may increase the risk of bleeding. Stop use two weeks before and immediately after surgery/dental/diagnostic procedures with bleeding risk. Avoid if pregnant or breastfeeding. Cat's claw may be contaminated with other Uncaria species. Reports exist of the potentially toxic Texan grown plant *Acacia greggii* being substituted for cat's claw.

Chlorophyll: Chlorophyll is responsible for the green pigment in plants. It can be obtained from green leafy vegetables (broccoli, Brussels sprouts, cabbage, lettuce, and spinach), algae (*Chlorella* and *Spirulina*), wheat grass, and numerous herbs (alfalfa, damiana, nettle, and parsley). Diets high in chlorophyll have been hypothesized to modify intestinal flora, resulting in improved management of immune disorders, including rheumatoid arthritis. More evidence is needed to support the use of chlorophyll in autoimmune diseases.

Avoid if allergic or hypersensitive to chlorophyll or any of its metabolites. Use cautiously with photosensitivity, compromised liver function, diabetes, or gastrointestinal conditions or obstructions. Use cautiously if taking immunosuppressant agents or antidiabetes agents. Avoid if pregnant or breastfeeding.

Copper: Copper is a mineral that occurs naturally in many foods, including vegetables, legumes, nuts, grains, fruits, shellfish, avocado, beef, and animal organs, such as liver and kidney. The use of copper bracelets in the treatment of arthritis has a long history of traditional use, with many anecdotal reports of effectiveness. There are research reports suggesting that copper salicylate may reduce arthritis symptoms more effectively than either copper or aspirin alone. Further study is needed before a recommendation can be made.

Avoid if allergic/hypersensitive to copper. Avoid use of copper supplements during the early phase of recovery from diarrhea. Avoid with hypercupremia, which occasionally occurs in disease states, including cutaneous leishmaniasis, sickle-cell disease, unipolar depression, breast cancer, epilepsy, measles, Down syndrome, or controlled fibrocalculous pancreatic diabetes (a unique form of secondary diabetes mellitus). Avoid with genetic disorders affecting copper metabolism, such as Wilson's disease, Indian childhood cirrhosis, or idiopathic copper toxicosis. Avoid with HIV/AIDS. Use cautiously with water-containing copper concentrations greater than six milligrams per liter. Use cautiously with anemia, arthralgias, or myalgias. Use cautiously if taking oral contraceptives. Use cautiously if at risk for selenium deficiency. The recommended dietary allowance (RDA) is 1,000 micrograms for pregnant women. The RDA for nursing women is 1,300 micrograms.

Dehydroepiandrosterone (DHEA): DHEA is a hormone that is produced by the adrenal glands. Preliminary evidence from a case series suggests that DHEA likely offers no benefit to individuals with rheumatoid arthritis. Well-designed human studies are needed before firm conclusions can be made.

Avoid if allergic to DHEA. Avoid with a history of seizures. Use cautiously with adrenal or thyroid disorders. Use cautiously if taking anticoagulants or drugs, herbs, or supplements that treat diabetes, heart disease, seizure, or stroke. Stop use two weeks before and immediately after surgery/dental/diagnostic procedures with bleeding risks. Avoid if pregnant or breastfeeding.

Dimethyl Sulfoxide (DMSO): DMSO is naturally found in vegetables, fruits, grains, and animal products. DMSO is available for both nonmedicinal and medicinal uses. Applying DMSO to the skin may help treat symptoms of rheumatoid arthritis. More research is needed before a conclusion can be drawn.

Avoid if allergic or hypersensitive to DMSO. Use cautiously with urinary tract cancer, liver disorders, or kidney dysfunction. Avoid if pregnant or breastfeeding.

Dong Quai: Dong quai (*Angelica sinensis*), also known as Chinese angelica, has been used for thousands of years in traditional Chinese, Korean, and Japanese medicine. Dong quai is traditionally used to treat arthritis. However, there is insufficient reliable human evidence to recommend the use of dong quai alone or in combination with other herbs for osteoarthritis or rheumatoid arthritis.

Although dong quai is accepted as being safe as a food additive in the United States and Europe, its safety in medicinal doses is not known. There are no reliable long-term studies of side effects available. Avoid if allergic or hypersensitive to *Angelicae radix* or members of the Apiaceae/Umbelliferae family (such as anise, caraway, carrot, celery, dill, and parsley). Avoid prolonged exposure to sunlight or ultraviolet light. Use cautiously with bleeding disorders or if taking drugs that may increase the risk of bleeding. Use cautiously with diabetes, glucose intolerance, or hormone sensitive conditions (such as breast cancer, uterine cancer, or ovarian cancer). Do not use before dental or surgical procedures. Avoid if pregnant or breastfeeding.

Evening Primrose Oil: Evening primrose oil contains the omega-6 essential fatty acid GLA, which is believed to be the active ingredient. Benefits of evening primrose oil in the treatment of arthritis have not been clearly shown. More information is needed before a recommendation can be made.

Avoid if allergic to plants in the Onagraceae family (willow's herb, enchanter's nightshade) or GLA. Avoid with seizure disorders. Use cautiously if taking mental illness drugs. Stop use two weeks before surgery with anesthesia. Avoid if pregnant or breastfeeding.

Feverfew: Feverfew (*Tanacetum parthenium*) is an herb native to Asia Minor. It is unclear clear if feverfew is an effective treatment for rheumatoid arthritis symptoms, such as joint stiffness or pain.

Avoid if allergic to feverfew and other plants of the Compositae family (such as chrysanthemums, daisies, marigolds, and ragweed). Stop use before and immediately after surgery and dental or diagnostic procedures. Avoid with drugs that increase bleeding risk. Avoid stopping feverfew use all at once. Instead, slowly take less and less over several days. Avoid with a history of heart disease, anxiety, or bleeding disorders. Use cautiously with a history of mental illness, depression, or headaches. Avoid if pregnant or breastfeeding.

Gamma-Linolenic Acid (GLA): Gamma-linolenic acid (GLA) is a dietary fatty acid. It is found in many plant oil extracts. A limited amount of GLA is found naturally in human breast milk, cold-water fish, and organ meats, such as liver. GLA is commonly sold as a dietary supplement either in the form of capsules or oil.

Several human studies indicate significant therapeutic improvements in rheumatoid arthritis symptoms, including decreased joint tenderness, joint swelling, and pain. Some studies also suggest that GLA may be a more tolerable alternative to the standard pain-reduction therapies, such as COX-2 inhibitors and NSAIDs. However, there is some concern on dosage control and additional study is needed to make a strong recommendation in this area.

Use cautiously with drugs that increase the risk of bleeding, such as anticoagulants and antiplatelet drugs. Avoid if pregnant or breastfeeding.

Ginger: The underground stems called rhizomes and above-ground stems of ginger have been used in Chinese, Japanese, and Indian medicine for hundreds of years. It is unclear if ginger can improve joint and muscle pain caused by rheumatoid arthritis or osteoarthritis.

Avoid if allergic to ginger or other members of the Zingiberaceae family (such as red ginger, *Alpinia purpurata*, *Alpinia zerumbet* (shell ginger), green cardamom, and balsam of Peru). Use cautiously if driving or operating machinery. Stop two weeks before and immediately after surgery/dental/diagnostic procedures due to risk of bleeding. Avoid with a history of irregular heartbeat (arrhythmia). Use cautiously with a history of ulcers, acid reflux, heart conditions, inflammatory bowel disease, blocked intestines, or bleeding disorders. Use cautiously if pregnant or breastfeeding.

Glucosamine: Glucosamine is a natural compound that is found in healthy cartilage. Preliminary human research reports benefits of glucosamine in the treatment of joint pain and swelling in rheumatoid arthritis. However, this is early information and additional research is needed before a conclusion can be drawn. The treatment of rheumatoid arthritis can be complicated and a qualified healthcare provider should follow people with this disease.

Avoid if allergic or hypersensitive to shellfish or iodine. Some reports suggest a link between glucosamine/chondroitin products and asthma. Use cautiously with diabetes or with a history of bleeding disorders. Avoid if pregnant or breastfeeding.

Green Tea: Green tea is made from the dried leaves of *Camellia sinensis*, an evergreen shrub. Research indicates that green tea may benefit arthritis by reducing inflammation and slowing cartilage breakdown. Further studies are required before a recommendation can be made.

Avoid if allergic or hypersensitive to caffeine or tannin. Use cautiously with diabetes or liver disease.

Guggul: Guggul (gum guggul) is a resin produced by the mukul mirth tree. There is insufficient evidence to support the use of guggul or guggul derivatives for the management of rheumatoid arthritis.

Avoid if allergic to guggul. Avoid with a history of thyroid disorders, anorexia, bulimia, or bleeding disorders. Signs of allergy to guggul may include itching and shortness of breath. Avoid if pregnant or breastfeeding.

Guided Imagery: Guided imagery refers to a number of techniques, including metaphor, storytelling, fantasy, game playing, dream interpretation, drawing, visualization, active imagination, and direct suggestion, using imagery. Therapeutic guided imagery may be used to help patients relax and focus on images associated with personal issues they are confronting. Cognitive-behavioral interventions for pain may be an effective adjunct to standard pharmacological interventions for pain in patients with juvenile rheumatoid arthritis. Further research is needed to confirm these results.

Guided imagery is usually intended to supplement medical care, not to replace it, and guided imagery should not be relied on as the sole therapy for a medical problem. Contact a qualified healthcare provider if mental or physical health is unstable or fragile. Never use guided imagery techniques while driving or doing any other activity that requires strict attention. Use cautiously with physical symptoms that can be brought about by stress, anxiety, or emotional upset because imagery may trigger these symptoms.

Hydrotherapy: Hydrotherapy is broadly defined as the external application of water in any form or temperature (hot, cold, steam, liquid, ice) for healing purposes. It may include immersion in a bath or body of water (such as the ocean or a pool), use of water jets, douches, application of wet towels to the skin, or water birth. Historically, hydrotherapy has been used to treat symptoms related to rheumatoid arthritis and osteoarthritis. Multiple studies have been published, largely based on therapy given at Dead Sea spa sites in Israel. Although most studies report benefits in pain, range of motion, or muscle strength, due to design flaws there is not enough reliable evidence to draw a firm conclusion.

Avoid sudden or prolonged exposure to extreme temperatures in baths, wraps, saunas, or other forms of hydrotherapy, particularly with heart disease, lung disease, or if pregnant. Avoid with implanted medical devices, such as pacemakers, defibrillators, or hepatic (liver) infusion pumps. Vigorous use of water jets should be avoided with fractures, known blood clots, bleeding disorders, severe osteoporosis, open wounds, or during pregnancy. Use cautiously with Raynaud's disease, chilblains, acrocyanosis, erythrocyanosis, or impaired temperature sensitivity, such as neuropathy. Use cautiously if pregnant or breastfeeding. Hydrotherapy should not delay the time to diagnosis or replace treatment with more proven techniques or therapies. Hydrotherapy should not be used as the sole approach to illnesses. Patients with known illnesses should consult their physicians before starting hydrotherapy.

Hypnosis, Hypnotherapy: Hypnosis is a trancelike state in which a person becomes more aware and focused and is more open to suggestion. Hypnotherapy has been used to treat health conditions or to change behaviors. Although multiple trials report diminished pain levels or requirements for pain-relieving medications after hypnotherapy, there is limited research for rheumatoid arthritis pain specifically. Other signs of rheumatoid arthritis, such as joint mobility or blood tests for rheumatoid factor, have not been adequately assessed.

Use cautiously with mental illnesses like psychosis/schizophrenia, manic depression, multiple personality disorder, dissociative disorders, or seizure disorders.

Magnet Therapy: Magnetic fields play an important role in Western medicine. For instance, they are used for magnetic resonance imaging, pulsed electromagnetic fields, and experimental magnetic stimulatory techniques. Several studies have evaluated the use of magnetic field therapy applied to areas of osteoarthritis or degenerative joint disease. In particular, this research has focused on knee osteoarthritis. However, most studies have been small or poorly designed or reported. Efficacy remains unclear. Notably, one promising small study published in 2004 by Wolsko et al. reported some benefits. Larger and better quality studies are needed before a recommendation can be made in this area.

Initial evidence has failed to show improvements in knee pain with the use of magnet therapy. However, due to methodological weaknesses with this research, the conclusions cannot be considered definitive.

Avoid with implantable medical devices, such as heart pacemakers, defibrillators, insulin pumps, or hepatic artery infusion pumps. Avoid with myasthenia gravis or bleeding disorders. Avoid if pregnant or breastfeeding. Magnet therapy is not advised as the sole treatment for potentially serious medical conditions and should not delay the time to diagnosis a condition. It should not replace treatment with more proven methods. Patients are advised to discuss magnet therapy with their qualified healthcare providers before starting treatment.

Mistletoe: Once considered a sacred herb in Celtic tradition, mistletoe has been used for centuries for high blood pressure, epilepsy, exhaustion, anxiety, arthritis, vertigo (dizziness), and degenerative inflammation of the joints. According to one retrospective case study, mistletoe injections may help manage arthritis. Further research is needed before a firm conclusion can be made.

Avoid if allergic or hypersensitive to mistletoe or any of its constituents. A life-threatening allergic reaction called anaphylaxis has been described after injections of mistletoe. Avoid with acute highly febrile inflammatory disease, thyroid disorders, seizure disorders, or heart disease. Use cautiously with diabetes, glaucoma, or if taking cholinergics.

Moxibustion: Moxibustion is a therapeutic method used in traditional Chinese medicine, classical acupuncture, and Japanese acupuncture. During the therapy, an herb, usually mugwort, is burned above the skin or on the acupuncture points to introduce heat into an acupuncture point to relieve symptoms. There is preliminary evidence suggesting that patients suffering from rheumatoid arthritis may experience improved immune function as a result of acupuncture and moxibustion. However, evidence is insufficient at this time for making concrete recommendations.

Use cautiously over large blood vessels and thin or weak skin. Avoid with aneurysms, any kind of "heat syndrome," heart disease, convulsions, cramps, diabetic neuropathy, extreme fatigue and/or anemia, fever, or inflammatory conditions. Avoid using over allergic skin conditions, ulcerated sores, or skin adhesions. Avoid areas with an inflamed organ, contraindicated acupuncture points, face, genitals, head, inflamed areas in general, and nipples. Avoid in patients who have just finished exercising or taking a hot bath or shower. Avoid if pregnant or breastfeeding. Use cautiously with elderly people with large vessels. Not advisable to bathe or shower for up to 24 hours after a moxibustion treatment.

Pantothenic Acid (Vitamin B$_5$): Pantothenic acid is found in many foods, including meats, liver, kidney, fish/shellfish, chicken, vegetables, legumes, yeast, eggs, and milk. It has been reported that pantothenic acid levels are lower in the blood of patients with rheumatoid arthritis compared to healthy individuals. However, it is unclear if this is a cause, effect, or a beneficial adaptive reaction. There is currently insufficient scientific evidence in this area in order to form a clear conclusion.

Pantothenic acid has also been suggested as a possible treatment for osteoarthritis. However, further research is needed to determine whether or not this treatment is effective.

Avoid if allergic or hypersensitive to pantothenic acid or dexpanthenol. Avoid with gastrointestinal blockage. Pantothenic acid is generally considered safe in pregnant and breastfeeding women when taken at recommended doses.

Physical Therapy: The goal of physical therapy is to improve mobility, restore function, reduce pain, and prevent further injuries. Several techniques, including exercises, stretches, traction, electrical stimulation, and massage, are used. Physical therapy for osteoarthritis of the knee may provide short-term benefits, but long-term benefits do not appear better than standard treatments. Several studies have indicated that treatment of rheumatoid arthritis should be conducted by a specially trained physical therapist and that physical therapy may help improve morning stiffness and grip strength. Some researchers have suggested a long-term, high-intensity exercise program. Beneficial effects may last up to one year. Despite promising early evidence, better-designed studies are needed to draw a firm conclusion.

Not all physical therapy programs are suited for everyone and patients should discuss their medical history with their qualified healthcare professionals before beginning any treatments. Based on the available literature, physical therapy appears generally safe when practiced by a qualified physical therapist. Physical therapy may aggravate preexisting conditions. Persistent pain and fractures of unknown origin have been reported. Physical therapy may increase the duration of pain or cause limitation of motion. Pain and anxiety may occur during the rehabilitation of patients with burns. Both morning stiffness and bone erosion have been reported in the physical therapy literature, although causality is unclear. Erectile dysfunction has also been reported. All therapies during pregnancy and breastfeeding should be discussed with a licensed obstetrician/gynecologist before initiation.

Podophyllum: Podophyllum rhizomes have a long medicinal history among native North American tribes who used a rhizome powder as a laxative or to treat infections with worms or parasites. A topical poultice of the powder was also used to treat warts and tumorous growths on the skin. Preliminary research suggests that podophyllum may be helpful for rheumatoid arthritis. Research is limited due to the possible adverse effects like severe diarrhea associated with taking podophyllum by mouth. However, additional research is needed before a firm conclusion can be drawn.

Avoid if allergic/hypersensitive to podophyllum or the Berberidaceae family. Podophyllum, when applied topically, may be absorbed through the skin and cause irritation of the stomach and intestines. Podophyllum toxicity may cause heart palpitations and blood pressure changes, muscle paralysis, difficulty walking, confusion, and convulsions. Using podophyllum and laxatives may result in dehydration and electrolyte depletion. Use cautiously with arrhythmia, Crohn's disease, cardiovascular problems, gallbladder disease or gallstones, high blood pressure, irritable bowel syndrome, liver insufficiency, muscular disorders, neurological disorders, psychosis, and kidney insufficiency. Use cautiously if taking antimiotic agents (e.g., vincristine), antipsychotic agents, or laxatives. Avoid if pregnant or breastfeeding.

Prayer: Prayer can be defined as a "reverent petition," the act of asking for something while aiming to connect with God or another object of worship. Prayer on behalf of the ill or dying has played a prominent role throughout history and across cultures. Initial research suggests that praying for others in the presence of patients may reduce pain, fatigue, tenderness, swelling, and weakness when it is used in addition to standard care. Better-quality research is necessary before a firm conclusion can be drawn.

Prayer is not recommended as the sole treatment approach for potentially serious medical conditions, and it should not delay the time it takes to consult with a healthcare professional or receive established therapies. Sometimes religious beliefs come into conflict with standard medical approaches and require an open dialog between patients and caregivers.

Probiotics: Probiotics are beneficial bacteria that are sometimes called friendly germs. They help maintain a healthy intestine and aid in digestion. They also help keep harmful bacteria and yeasts in the gut under control. Most probiotics come from food sources, especially cultured milk products. Probiotics can be taken as capsules, tablets, beverages, powders, yogurts, and other foods. In a small study *Lactobacillus* GG was associated with improved subjective well-being and trends in reduced symptoms of rheumatoid arthritis. However, the results were not statistically significant. More studies on the effects of probiotics on rheumatoid arthritis are needed.

Probiotics are generally considered safe and well tolerated. Avoid if allergic or hypersensitive to probiotics. Use cautiously if lactose intolerant.

Propolis: Bees make propolis to form their hives. Propolis is made of the buds of conifer and poplar trees and it is combined with beeswax and other bee secretions. Based on antiinflammatory action observed in laboratory research, propolis has been proposed as a possible treatment for rheumatic and other inflammatory diseases. However, there is currently not enough scientific human study to make a clear recommendation.

Avoid if allergic or hypersensitive to propolis, black poplar (*Populus nigra*), poplar bud, bee stings, bee products, honey, or balsam of Peru. Severe allergic reactions have been reported. There has been one report of kidney failure with the ingestion of propolis that improved upon discontinuing therapy and deteriorated with re-exposure. Avoid if pregnant or breastfeeding because of the high alcohol content in some products.

Relaxation Therapy: Relaxation techniques include behavioral therapeutic approaches that differ widely in philosophy, methodology, and practice. The primary goal is usually nondirected relaxation. In a randomized study of patients with osteoarthritis pain, Jacobson relaxation was reported to lower the level of subjective pain over time. The study concluded that relaxation might be effective in reducing the amount of analgesic medication taken by participants. Further well-designed research is needed to confirm these results.

Limited preliminary research reports that muscle relaxation training may improve function and well being in patients with rheumatoid arthritis. Additional research is necessary before a conclusion can be reached.

Avoid with psychiatric disorders, such as schizophrenia or psychosis. Jacobson relaxation, which involves flexing and relaxing specific muscles, should be used cautiously with illnesses such as heart disease, high blood pressure, or musculoskeletal injury. Relaxation therapy is not recommended as the sole treatment approach for potentially serious medical conditions and it should not delay the time to diagnosis or treatment with more proven techniques.

Selenium: Selenium is a mineral found in soil, water, and some foods. Selenium supplementation has been studied in rheumatoid arthritis patients with mixed results. Additional research is necessary before a clear conclusion can be drawn.

Avoid if allergic or sensitive to products containing selenium. Avoid with a history of nonmelanoma skin cancer. Selenium is generally regarded as safe for pregnant or breastfeeding women. However, animal research reports that large doses of selenium may lead to birth defects.

Shark Cartilage: Shark cartilage is one of the most popular supplements in the United States, with more than 40 brand-name products sold. Shark cartilage has been suggested as a possible treatment for inflammatory conditions, including rheumatoid arthritis and osteoarthritis. However, additional research is needed to determine if this treatment is safe and effective in humans.

Avoid if allergic to shark cartilage or any of its ingredients (including chondroitin sulfate and glucosamine). Use cautiously with sulfur allergy. Avoid with a history of heart attack, vascular disease, heart rhythm abnormalities (arrhythmias), or heart disease. Use cautiously with a history of liver or kidney disorders, tendency to form kidney stones, breast cancer, prostate cancer, multiple myeloma, breathing disorders (such as asthma), cancers that raise calcium levels (such as breast, prostate, multiple myeloma, or squamous cell lung cancer), or diabetes. Avoid if pregnant or breastfeeding.

Stinging Nettle: Stinging nettle is found in Africa, Europe, the United States, and Canada. It is a perennial plant that has been used as a medical treatment since ancient times. Nettle is widely used as a folk remedy to treat arthritic and rheumatic conditions throughout Europe and in Australia. Preliminary evidence suggests that certain constituents in the nettle plant have antiinflammatory and/or immunomodulatory activity. More study is needed to confirm these findings.

Nettle has historically been used in several different forms to treat pain of varying origins, including arthritis. However, there is a lack of available scientific evidence to confirm this use and additional study is needed.

Avoid if allergic or hypersensitive to nettle, the Urticaceae family, or any ingredient of nettle products. Use cautiously with diabetes, bleeding disorders, or low sodium levels in the blood. Use cautiously with diuretics and antiinflammatory drugs. The elderly should also use nettle cautiously. Avoid if pregnant or breastfeeding.

Transcutaneous Electrical Nerve Stimulation (TENS): TENS is a noninvasive technique in which a low-voltage electrical current is delivered through wires from a small power unit to electrodes located on the skin. Electrodes are temporarily attached with paste in various patterns, depending on the specific condition and treatment goals. Preliminary studies of TENS in rheumatoid arthritis report improvements in joint function and pain. However, most research is not well designed or reported and better studies are necessary before a clear conclusion can be reached.

Avoid with implantable devices, such as defibrillators, pacemakers, intravenous infusion pumps, or hepatic artery infusion pumps. Use cautiously with decreased sensation (such as neuropathy) or with seizure disorders. Avoid if pregnant or breastfeeding due to a lack of safety evidence.

Thymus Extract: Thymus extracts for nutritional supplements are usually derived from young calves (bovine). Thymus extract is commonly used to treat primary immunodeficiencies, bone marrow failure, autoimmune disorders, chronic skin diseases, recurrent viral and bacterial infections, hepatitis, allergies, chemotherapy side effects, and cancer. Further research is needed to determine whether or not thymus extract can effectively treat symptoms of rheumatoid arthritis.

Avoid if allergic or hypersensitive to thymus extracts. Use bovine thymus extract supplements cautiously due to potential for exposure to the virus that causes "mad cow disease." Avoid use with an organ transplant or other forms of allografts or xenografts. Avoid with thymic tumors, myasthenia gravis (neuromuscular disorder), or untreated hypothyroidism. Avoid if taking immunosuppressants or hormonal therapy. Avoid if pregnant or breastfeeding. Thymic extract increases human sperm motility and progression.

Turmeric: Turmeric is a perennial plant native to India and Indonesia. It is often used as a spice in cooking. Laboratory and animal studies show antiinflammatory activity of turmeric and its constituent curcumin, which may be beneficial in people with osteoarthritis or rheumatoid arthritis. Reliable human research is lacking.

Avoid if allergic or hypersensitive to turmeric (curcumin), yellow food colorings, or plants belonging to the Curcuma and Zingiberaceae (ginger) families. Use cautiously with a history of bleeding disorders, immune system deficiencies, liver disease, or gallstones. Use cautiously if taking blood thinners, such as warfarin (Coumadin). Use cautiously if pregnant or breastfeeding.

Zinc: Zinc formulations have been used since ancient Egyptian times to enhance wound healing. The majority of trials do not show significant improvements in arthritis symptoms following zinc treatment. Interpretation of some data is difficult because patients in the studies were permitted to continue their previous arthritis medication and most studies used a small number of participants. Well-designed clinical trials are needed before a decision can be made.

Zinc is generally considered safe when taken at the recommended dosages. Avoid zinc chloride since studies have not been done on its safety or effectiveness. While zinc appears safe during pregnancy in amounts lower than the established upper intake level, caution should be used since studies cannot rule out the possibility of harm to the fetus.

Fair Negative Scientific Evidence

Willow Bark: Willow bark that contains salicin has been used to treat many different kinds of pain. There is good evidence that willow bark may be effective in treating chronic pain from osteoarthritis. However, willow bark extract did not show efficacy in treating rheumatoid arthritis. Additional study is needed to make a firm recommendation.

Avoid if allergic/hypersensitive to aspirin, willow bark (*Salix* spp.), or any of its constituents, including salicylates. Use cautiously with gastrointestinal problems such as ulcers, liver disorders, diabetes, gout (joint inflammation), high blood pressure, or high cholesterol. Use cautiously with a history of allergy, asthma, and leukemia. Use cautiously if taking protein-bound medications, antihyperlipidemia agents, alcohol, leukemia medications, beta-blockers, diuretics, Phenytoin (Dilantin), probenecid, spironolactone, sulfonylureas, valproic acid, or methotrexate. Use cautiously if predisposed to headaches. Use cautiously in tannin-containing herbs or supplements. Avoid operating heavy machinery. Avoid in children with chickenpox and any other viral infections. Avoid with blood and kidney disorders. Avoid if taking other NSAIDs, acetazolamide, or other carbonic anhydrase inhibitors. Avoid with elevated serum cadmium levels. Avoid if pregnant or breastfeeding.

PREVENTION

Rheumatoid Arthritis: Currently, there is no known method of prevention for rheumatoid arthritis.

Osteoarthritis: Individuals who maintain a healthy body weight have a decreased risk of developing osteoarthritis. Eating a healthy and well-balanced diet may help individuals control their weight. The U.S. government issued a revised food pyramid in 2005 in an effort to help Americans live healthier. The new pyramid provides 12 different models, which are based on daily calorie needs, ranging from the 1,000-calorie diets for toddlers to 3,200-calorie diets for teenage boys.

Regular exercise may also help patients control their weight. There are many ways for people to exercise including gardening, walking, sports activities, and dancing. Patients who are beginning an exercise program should choose activities that fit their levels of strength and endurance. The type of exercise is not as important as a consistent exercise schedule. Most experts today agree that burning calories should not be the goal of exercise. Exercise that causes extreme pain or discomfort is considered by many experts as unhealthy and may even cause permanent damage to the body.

Periarthritis: Patients can reduce their risks of developing periarthritis by avoiding injuries. In order to reduce the risk of injury, all workouts should begin with a warm-up routine and end with a cool-down segment that includes stretching exercises. Patients should talk to their healthcare providers before starting new exercise programs.

ASTHMA

BACKGROUND

Asthma is a chronic, inflammatory lung disease. The air passages within the lungs are constantly swollen, restricting the amount of air allowed to pass through the trachea. Asthmatics have recurrent breathing problems and a tendency to cough and wheeze. According to the American Lung Association, about 20 million Americans have asthma, which causes about 5,000 deaths each year. Asthma is incurable, but many medications and changes in behavior may help manage the condition.

Allergic asthma occurs when allergens cause the airway to become inflamed. When the airway becomes constricted during vigorous physical activity, the condition is known as exercise-induced asthma. Cough-variant asthma is a chronic, persistent cough without shortness of breath. Occupational asthma occurs as a result of a particular environment. Once the patient is out of the environment, symptoms gradually disappear.

CLASSIFICATIONS OF ASTHMA

Asthma is classified as either allergic or nonallergic. Both conditions cause airway obstruction and inflammation that is partly reversible by medication. They also produce the same symptoms. The main difference, however, is their cause.

Allergic (Extrinsic) Asthma: An allergic reaction triggers what is known as allergic asthma. Inhaled allergens like dust mites, mold spores, pollen and pet dander may trigger allergic asthma. It is the most common form of asthma, affecting more than 50% of asthma sufferers.

Nonallergic (Intrinsic) Asthma: Nonallergic asthma is not related to allergies and does not involve the immune system. Instead, factors like anxiety, stress, exercise, cold air, dry air, smoke, hyperventilation, viruses, and other irritants trigger the disease.

SYMPTOMS

Symptoms of asthma include: bronchospasm (abnormal contraction of the bronchi, resulting in airway obstruction), coughing (constantly or intermittently), wheezing or whistling sounds when exhaling, shortness of breath or rapid breathing, chest tightness or chest pain, and fatigue.

Infants may have trouble feeding and may grunt during suckling.

CHILDHOOD ASTHMA

Nine million U.S. children, from newborns to 18-year-olds, have been diagnosed with asthma, according to a 2002 National Health Interview Survey. Asthma rates in children younger than five years old have increased more than 160% from 1980 to 1994. One study found a strong correlation between obesity and asthma but no similar relationship between obesity and allergies. Researchers believe that asthma was the result of the increased physical exertion of the lungs in obese individuals.

Many children with asthma have what is known as allergic asthma. In such cases, exposure to allergens like dust mites, pollen, mold, and animal dander may irritate the airways, causing even more constriction, as well as causing the production of excess mucus and inflammation of the airway passages.

ADULT-ONSET ASTHMA

Asthma symptoms may appear at any time in life. Individuals who develop asthma as adults have what is known as adult-onset asthma. It is possible to develop asthma at the age of 50 or later.

Unlike children who usually experience intermittent symptoms, individuals with adult-onset asthma are more likely to experience persistent symptoms.

The cause of adult-onset asthma is unknown. However, some evidence suggests that allergy and asthma may be genetically inherited. In addition, obesity appears to significantly increase the risk of developing asthma as an adult.

PREGNANCY AND ASTHMA

Asthma is one of the most common, potentially serious medical problems that occur during pregnancy. According to some studies, asthma may complicate up to 7% of all pregnancies. Researchers estimate that about one-third of pregnant women with asthma will experience increased symptoms during the pregnancy; another third will experience the same symptoms, while the last third will experience a lessening of symptoms.

Pregnant women with asthma have an increased risk of delivering prematurely or giving birth to an infant with low birth weight. In addition, pregnant women with asthma are more likely to experience hypertension (high blood pressure) or a related condition called preeclampsia (swelling, high blood pressure, and kidney malfunction).

If asthma is not controlled, the mother has lower levels of oxygen in her blood. This may result in decreased oxygen in the fetal blood, which may also cause growth deficiencies or death in the fetus. However, proper treatment and management of asthma symptoms help reduce the risk of complications, according to research.

ASPIRIN-INDUCED ASTHMA

Aspirin and other nonsteroidal antiinflammatory drugs (NSAIDs) like ibuprofen (Advil, Motrin), may cause asthma symptoms, nasal congestion, watery eyes and, occasionally, facial flushing and swelling in about 10% of asthmatics. Since sensitization and immunoglobulin E production are not involved in aspirin-sensitive asthma, it is not considered an allergic reaction. In the body, these drugs inhibit the cyclooxygenase-1 enzyme, which produces inflammation and fever. Their ability to inhibit the enzyme allows NSAIDs to reduce pain, inflammation, and fever.

Inhibiting the enzyme also allows NSAIDs to clear the way for different enzymes that have adverse effects in some people. One of these enzymes triggers the release of chemicals that can cause the airways to swell and increase mucus production, leading to an asthma attack. The process is an unwanted side effect NSAIDs, not an immune-system reaction to NSAIDs.

Asthmatics, and especially asthmatics who also have nasal polyps, are vulnerable to asthma as a side effect of aspirin and aspirin-like drugs.

SEVERITY OF ASTHMA

Mild Intermittent: Symptoms occur twice a week or less. Exacerbations are short and the intensity varies. Nighttime symptoms occur twice a month or less.

Mild Persistent: Symptoms occur more than twice a week but less than once a day. Exacerbations may affect daily activities. Nighttime symptoms occur more than twice a month.

Moderate Persistent: Symptoms occur daily. Exacerbations occur twice a week or more. Nighttime symptoms occur more than once a week.

Severe Persistent: Symptoms are constant and limit the individual's physical activities. Frequent exacerbations disrupt daily activities, and nighttime symptoms occur more than twice a week.

PREDISPOSITION TO ASTHMA

Infants or young children who wheeze and suffer from viral upper respiratory infections.

Individuals with strong allergies.

Individuals with a family history of asthma and/or allergy.

Perinatal exposure to tobacco smoke and allergens.

DIAGNOSIS

Spirometry is a noninvasive way to evaluate the air capacity of the lungs. Physicians are able to measure the volume of air exhaled before and after a bronchodilator (inhaler) is used. During this procedure, the spirometer measures the airflow when the patient exhales, comparing lung capacity to the average capacity for the individual's age and racial group. Then the patient inhales medicine from a short-acting bronchodilator. The doctor once again measures the patient's lung capacity. If there is an increase in capacity it is likely that the asthma symptoms can be controlled.

In addition, the physician should have the patient perform some form of physical activity to increase the breathing rate and check for changes in lung capacity (both with and without a bronchodilator).

TREATMENT

Long Term

Combined Therapy Medicine: Combined therapy involves both a controller (long-acting bronchodilator) and reliever (corticosteroid) medicine. This therapy is used to manage asthma symptoms for the long term.

Cromolyn Sodium and Nedocromil Sodium: Cromolyn sodium (Intal) and nedocromil sodium (Tilade) are used to help prevent the airways from swelling when they are exposed to asthma triggers. These inhaled nonsteroids may also help prevent exercise-induced asthma attacks.

Immunotherapy: During immunotherapy (also known as allergy shots), the patient receives periodic injections, as determined by the allergist/immunologist, over the course of three to five years. The solutions in the injections contain the substances the individual is allergic to. The treatment helps the immune system tolerate the allergens and lessens the need for medications.

Peak Flow Meter: A peak flow meter is a portable device that measures airflow, or peak expiratory flow. When asthmatics blow into the device quickly and forcefully, the peak flow reading indicates how open the airways are. Patients should compare their daily peak flow recordings with their "personal best" recording. The device helps patients determine the severity of the asthma. It is enables patients to check their responses to treatment and monitor their treatment progress.

Inhaled Corticosteroids: Inhaled corticosteroids (Aerobid, Azmacort, Beclovent, Flovent, Pulmicort, Vanceril) are used to prevent and reduce airway swelling as well as decrease the amount of mucus in the lungs. These medications are generally considered safe when taken as directed.

Leukotriene Modifiers: Leukotriene modifiers (Accolate, Singulair) are a new type of long-term control medication. They help prevent airway inflammation and swelling as well as decrease the amount of mucus in the lungs.

Long-Acting Beta-Agonists: Long-acting beta-agonists, such as salmeterol (Serevent, which is inhaled) may be taken with or without antiinflammatories to help control persistent symptoms. Long-acting, inhaled beta-agonists should not be used as a substitute for antiinflammatories. This type of medicine may also prevent exercise-induced asthma. However, these medications cannot relieve symptoms quickly, and they should not be used to treat an acute attack. A short-acting, inhaled beta-agonist should be used to treat acute symptoms.

Oral Corticosteroids: Oral corticosteroids (Aristocort, Celestone, Decadron, Medrol, Prednisone, Sterapred) are available in pill/tablet format for adults. Liquid corticosteroids (Pediapred, Prelone) are available for children. These medications can be used short term for severe asthma episodes or as long-term therapy for individuals who have severe asthma.

Trigger Avoidance: Since asthma can be triggered by allergens, symptoms can be caused or aggravated by the environment. An allergist or immunologist can help patients recognize the allergens and irritants that trigger asthma attacks. Exposure to common irritants, including pollen, animal dander, mold spores, and dust mites, may trigger asthma.

Eliminate potential food allergens, including dairy (milk, cheese, and sour cream), eggs, nuts, shellfish, wheat (gluten), corn, preservatives, and food additives (like dyes and fillers). Food allergies can be a contributing factor in immune imbalance, triggering symptoms of asthma.

Short Term

Oral Beta-Agonists: Oral beta-agonists (Alupent, Brethine, Bricanyl, Proventil, Proventil Repetabs, Ventolin, Volmax) may be used to decrease acute symptoms that arise quickly. Oral beta-agonists are available in pill, syrup, and inhaled form.

Short-Acting Bronchodilators: Short-acting bronchodilators are also used for quick relief of asthma symptoms. They open airways by relaxing the muscles that tighten around airways during an asthma attack.

Short-Acting Beta-Agonists: Short-acting beta-agonists (Albuterol, Brethaire, Bronkosol, Isoetharine, Maxair, Medihaler-Iso, Metaprel, Proventil, Tornalate, Ventolin) may help relieve asthma symptoms quickly. These medications may also help prevent exercise-induced asthma. If these medications are taken daily, or if they are taken more than three times in a single day, the asthma may be worsening or the inhaler may not be used correctly.

Theophylline: Theophylline (Aerolate, Elixophyllin, Quibron-T, Resbid, Slo-bid, T-Phyl, Theolair, Theo-24, Theo-Dur, Theo-X, Uni-Dur, Uniphyl) may be used to treat persistent asthma symptoms and to prevent nighttime asthma. In order to be effective, theophylline must remain at a constant level in the bloodstream. If the level is too high, it can be potentially dangerous. A qualified healthcare provider will perform regular blood tests to ensure safety. Sustained-release theophylline is not the preferred primary long-term control treatment, but it has been shown to be effective when taken with antiinflammatories to control nighttime asthma attacks.

Pregnancy

General: Many asthma medications are considered safe for pregnant patients because the risk of adverse effects appears to be less than the risk of uncontrolled asthma. Medications that have been used in pregnant women include inhaled bronchodilators, cromolyn sodium, and beclomethasone, all of which have a local effect. Theophylline has also been used during pregnancy if the asthma is not adequately controlled by the other medications. Oral steroid medications, such as prednisone, should only be used when necessary for severe asthma during pregnancy. Consult a qualified healthcare professional before beginning any treatment.

TYPES OF INHALERS

Dry Powder Inhaler: Dry powder inhalers are the most common inhalers used today. This type of inhaler does not need a propellant. Instead, the individual inhales the medicine so it can reach the lung. Children, people with severe asthma, and people suffering from acute attacks may be unable to produce enough airflow to use these inhalers successfully.

Metered-Dose Inhaler (MDI): The most efficient way to get asthma medication into the airways is with an MDI. When used properly, about 12-14% of the medication is inhaled deep into the lungs with each puff of the MDI. They are especially important for delivering quick relief medication—short-acting beta-agonists—that relieve an acute asthma attack. MDIs are also used to deliver some long-term control medications, including antiinflammatories and long-acting bronchodilators, which are taken routinely to manage asthma symptoms. An MDI is especially recommended for use with inhaled steroids because it reduces the amount of drug dispersed into the mouth, which reduces the risk of side effects.

MDIs are designed to release a premeasured amount of medication into the lungs. There are several different types, but in general, they all have a chamber that holds the medication and a propellant that turns the medication into a fine mist. A button is pushed to force the medication out through the mouthpiece.

Medication that is inhaled acts more quickly than medication taken by mouth. It also causes few adverse effects because the medication goes directly to the lungs and not to other parts of the body.

If an MDI is not used correctly, symptoms may persist or worsen. Individuals who have trouble using the device correctly may use a spacer to help them get the medication they need. Spacers are attached to the mouthpiece, and they hold the discharged, premeasured medication in a chamber until the patient breathes in. Spacers are recommended for young children and older adults who have trouble coordinating breathing and activating the MDI.

Nebulizer: A nebulizer is an electrical device that sends medicine directly into the mouth by a tube (or mask in children). This method does not require hand-breath coordination. The patient puts the prescribed amount of medication into the tube and then places the tube in the mouth (or places the mask over the child's nose and mouth). Then the patient breathes normally until all of the medication is gone.

INTEGRATIVE THERAPIES

Good Scientific Evidence

Boswellia: Boswellia has been proposed as a potential chronic asthma therapy. Future studies are needed to assess the long-term efficacy and safety of boswellia and to compare the efficacy of boswellia to standard therapies. Boswellia should not be used for the relief of acute asthma exacerbations. Boswellia is generally believed to be safe when used as directed, although safety and toxicity have not been well studied in humans. Avoid if allergic to boswellia or similar herbs or if pregnant or breastfeeding.

Choline: Choline is possibly effective when taken orally for asthma. Choline supplements seem to decrease the severity of symptoms, number of symptomatic days, and the need to use bronchodi-

lators in asthma patients. There is some evidence that higher doses of 3 grams daily might be more effective than lower doses of 1.5 grams daily. Choline is generally regarded as safe and appears to be well tolerated. Pregnant or breastfeeding women should not take doses that exceed adequate intake levels.

Coleus: There is a lack of sufficient data to recommend for or against the use of coleus in the treatment of bronchial asthma. Preliminary data appear to be promising. However, larger, randomized, controlled trials are needed to confirm the safety and efficacy of coleus in bronchial asthma. Coleus is generally regarded as safe, as very few reports have documented adverse effects. However, only a few short-term trials have assessed its safety in a small sample size of patients. Avoid if allergic to *Coleus forskohlii* and related species or with bleeding disorders. Avoid if pregnant or breastfeeding.

Ephedra: Ephedra contains the chemicals ephedrine and pseudoephedrine, which are bronchodilators (expand the airways to assist in easier breathing). It has been used and studied to treat asthma and chronic obstructive pulmonary disease in both children and adults. Other treatments such as beta-agonist inhalers (for example, albuterol) are more commonly recommended due to safety concerns with ephedra or ephedrine. However, the U.S. Food and Drug Administration has collected thousands of reports of serious toxicity linked to ephedra (including over 100 deaths). Ephedra products are banned from dietary supplements because of serious health risks, including heart attack, heart damage, breathing difficulties, and fluid retention in the lungs. Avoid ephedra if pregnant or breastfeeding.

Psychotherapy: Family psychotherapy may slightly improve wheezing and thoracic gas volume for children with asthma, according to several studies.

Yoga: Multiple human studies report benefits of yoga (such as breathing exercises), when added to other treatments for mild-to-moderate asthma (such as standard drug therapy, diet, or massage). Better research is needed before a firm conclusion can be drawn.

Unclear or Conflicting Scientific Evidence

Acupressure: Preliminary research suggests that patients with chronic asthma who receive acupressure may experience improved quality of life. Further well-designed studies are needed before firm conclusions can be drawn.

Ayurveda: There is early evidence that daily supplementation with gum resin of *Boswellia serrata,* known in Ayurveda as salai guggal, may reduce dyspnea (shortness of breath), rhonchi, and the number of attacks in bronchial asthma.

Another herb, devadaru *(Cedrus deodara),* may have antispasmodic effects and reduce symptoms in bronchial asthma, particularly for patients with shorter histories of asthma and lower frequencies of attacks. Further research is needed in this area before a recommendation can be made.

Black Tea: Research has shown caffeine to cause improvements in airflow to the lungs (bronchodilation). However, it is not clear if caffeine or tea use has significant clinical benefits in people with asthma. Better research is needed in this area before a conclusion can be drawn.

Butterbur: Historically, butterbur has been used to treat asthma. Preclinical studies report antiinflammatory and leukotriene inhibitory properties, which may lead to clinical effects. Initial human research suggests possible benefits. However, controlled trials with adequate sample sizes are necessary in order to clarify whether there are true benefits in humans.

Chiropractic: Several studies report the effects of chiropractic spinal manipulative therapy on breathing indices and quality of life in children and adults with asthma. Results are variable, and in the studies with positive results, mostly subjective but not objective (lung function test) changes are reported. Due to methodological problems and variable results, no clear conclusions can be drawn in this area.

Green Tea: Research has shown caffeine to cause improvements in airflow to the lungs (bronchodilation). However, it is not clear if caffeine or tea use has significant benefits in people with asthma. Better research is needed in this area before a conclusion can be drawn.

Hypnotherapy, Hypnosis: Preliminary research for the use of hypnosis for the management of asthma symptoms does not provide clear answers. Anxiety associated with asthma may be relieved with hypnosis. Additional research is needed before a firm conclusion can be drawn.

Lactobacillus Acidophilus: *Lactobacillus acidophilus* has been suggested as a possible treatment for asthma. However, further research is necessary before a firm conclusion can be made.

Lycopene: Laboratory research suggests that lycopene, like other carotenoids, may have antioxidant properties. It has been suggested that antioxidants may be helpful in the prevention of asthma that is caused by exercise. There is limited, poor-quality research in this area, and further evidence is needed before a firm conclusion can be made.

Massage: Promising initial evidence suggests that massage therapy may improve lung function in children with asthma. Additional research is necessary before a firm conclusion can be drawn.

Meditation: Preliminary research of transcendental meditation for asthma reports benefits. However, due to unclear design or study description, these results cannot be considered definitive.

Sahaja yoga, which incorporates meditation techniques, may have some benefit in the management of moderate to severe asthma. Further studies of meditation alone are needed before any a firm conclusion can be drawn.

Melatonin: Based on preliminary research, melatonin may improve sleep in patients with asthma. Further studies that evaluate the long-term effects of melatonin on airway inflammation and bronchial hyperresponsiveness are needed before a firm conclusion can be made.

Omega-3 Fatty Acids, Fish Oil, Alpha-Linolenic Acid: Several studies in this area do not provide enough reliable evidence to form a clear conclusion, with some studies reporting no effects, and others finding benefits. Because most studies have been small without clear descriptions of design or results, the results cannot be considered conclusive.

Perilla: Preliminary evidence suggests some benefit of perilla oil for symptoms of asthma. Further clinical trials are required before a definitive conclusion can be reached.

Physical Therapy: Chest physical therapy and physiotherapy breathing retraining have been studied in both children and adults to improve quality of life and improve lung function in severe and acute asthma. Early evidence is mixed. Studies often include combination treatment with drug therapy or are not well designed, which make it difficult to assess the magnitude of benefit, if any, of physical therapy alone. More research is warranted.

Pycnogenol: Pycnogenol (Horphag Research, Berlin) may offer clinical benefit to both children and adults with asthma. Additional study is needed before a strong recommendation can be made.

Relaxation Therapy: Preliminary studies of relaxation techniques in individuals with asthma report a significant decrease in asthma symptoms, anxiety and depression, along with improvements in quality of life and measures of lung function. Further large trials in humans are needed to confirm these results.

Selenium: Preliminary research reports that selenium supplementation may help improve asthma symptoms. Further research is needed to confirm these results.

Tylophora: Methodologically weak trials make extrapolation to clinical practice difficult. Available studies of *Tylophora* for asthma show conflicting results. Therefore, efficacy remains unproven.

Vitamin B$_6$: Preliminary research suggests that children with severe asthma might have inadequate pyridoxine status. Theophylline, a prescription drug used to help manage asthma, seems to lower pyridoxine levels. Studies of pyridoxine supplementation in asthma patients taking theophylline yield conflicting results. Further research is needed before a conclusion can be drawn.

Vitamin C: It has been suggested that low levels of vitamin C (or other antioxidants) may increase the risk of developing asthma. The use of vitamin C for asthma has been studied since the 1980s (particularly exercise-induced asthma), although the evidence in this area remains inconclusive. Additional research is necessary before a clear conclusion can be drawn.

Fair Negative Scientific Evidence

Evening Primrose Oil: Small studies do not show evening primrose oil to be useful in the treatment of asthma. Further research is needed to confirm this conclusion.

Vitamin E: There is preliminary evidence that vitamin E does not provide benefits in individuals with asthma.

Strong Negative Scientific Evidence

L-Arginine: Although it has been suggested that arginine may be a treatment for asthma, studies in humans have actually found that arginine worsens inflammation in the lungs and contributes to asthma symptoms. Therefore, taking arginine by mouth or by inhalation is not recommended in people with asthma.

PREVENTION

Avoidance of Known Allergens: Asthma is strongly associated with allergies, and exposure to allergens can worsen asthma symptoms.

Avoidance of Secondhand Smoke: Children are especially susceptible to developing asthma or experience a worsening in symptoms if they are exposed to secondhand smoke. Children breathing secondhand smoke are more likely to suffer from bronchitis and pneumonia, ear infections, coughing and wheezing, and more frequent and severe asthma attacks.

ATTENTION DEFICIT–HYPERACTIVITY DISORDER (ADHD)

CONDITION: Attention Deficit–Hyperactivity Disorder (ADHD)

BACKGROUND

Attention deficit–hyperactivity disorder (ADHD) is classified as a psychiatric disorder characterized by a continual pattern of inattention, distractibility, impulsivity, and hyperactivity.

Beginning in childhood, ADHD is one of the most commonly diagnosed psychiatric disorders in children and adolescents. ADHD becomes apparent in some children in the preschool and early school years. ADHD is thought to affect about 9.2% of boys and 2.9% of girls who are of school age.

While it is estimated that about 4.4% of adults also suffer from ADHD, the condition often goes unrecognized in adults. It is believed that around 60% of children diagnosed with ADHD retain the disorder as adults. Adults with ADHD are diagnosed under the same criteria, including the stipulation that their symptoms must have been present prior to the age of seven.

ADHD is divided into three subtypes based on symptoms, including inattentive type, hyperactive-impulsive type, and combined type with both inattention and hyperactivity-impulsiveness. The most common ADHD subtype is the combined type; females are more likely to have the inattentive type.

RISK FACTORS

Heredity: ADHD tends to run in families. About one in four children with ADHD has at least one relative with the disorder, and when one identical twin has ADHD, the other twin almost always has it as well.

Diet: Recent studies have found that children with ADHD may have vitamin and mineral deficiencies. Decreases in zinc, essential fatty acids, iron, B vitamins, and glyconutrients have been reported in children with ADHD. Protein deficiencies may also contribute to the development of ADHD.

Food and Additive Allergies: Food allergies (including wheat, soy, corn, dairy, shellfish, and tree nuts, such as walnuts and peanuts) and food additives (such as dyes and preservatives) have been reported to aggravate the symptoms of ADHD.

Heavy Metal Toxicity and Other Environmental Toxins: Environmental toxins (chemicals) and heavy metal (including lead, mercury, and cadmium) exposure during pregnancy or in childhood may contribute to the development of ADHD. Smoking during pregnancy has been reported to increase the chances of developing ADHD.

Violence, Abuse, and Other Emotional Traumas: While no conclusive evidence has been offered that parenting methods can cause ADHD in otherwise normal children, some clinicians believe this is the case.

CAUSES

The exact cause of ADHD remains unknown. Most of the causes have been reported to be dysfunction in the brain and nervous system.

Altered Brain Function: Dopamine is a brain neurochemical necessary for proper function. Research has found that individuals with ADHD may have a deficiency of dopamine. Also, individuals with ADHD may have decreased blood flow to the brain.

Thyroid Disorders: Thyroid abnormalities have been associated with ADHD and other childhood psychiatric disorders.

Head Injuries: Head trauma in childhood may cause neurological problems leading to the development of ADHD.

Drug Induced: Hyperactivity may be caused by high or repeated doses of caffeine or stimulants.

SIGNS AND SYMPTOMS

Individuals with ADHD have many symptoms, including extreme inattentiveness and/or impulsiveness and hyperactivity. Many people with ADHD continue to have symptoms throughout life. The symptoms of ADHD fall into the following two broad categories.

Inattention: Symptoms of inattention include failure to pay close attention to details, trouble keeping focused during play or tasks, appearing not to listen when spoken to, failure to follow instructions or finish tasks, avoiding tasks that require a high amount of mental effort and organization such as school projects, frequently losing items required to facilitate tasks or activities such as school supplies, excessive distractibility, forgetfulness, procrastination, inability to begin an activity, difficulties with household activities (cleaning, paying bills, etc.), difficulty falling asleep, frequent emotional outbursts, easily frustrated, and easily distracted.

Hyperactivity-Impulsive Behavior: Hyperactive-impulsive symptoms include fidgeting with hands or feet or squirming in seat, leaving seat often even when inappropriate, running or climbing at inappropriate times, difficulty in quiet play, frequently feeling restless, excessive speech, answering a question before the speaker has finished, failure to wait one's turn, interrupting the activities of others at inappropriate times, and impulsive spending leading to financial difficulties.

A positive diagnosis is usually only made if the person has experienced six of the above signs and symptoms for at least three months. Symptoms must appear consistently in varied environments (not only at home or school) and interfere with general functioning.

Children who grow up with ADHD often continue to have signs and symptoms as they grow into adulthood. Adults living with ADHD may experience challenges in the areas of self-control, self-motivation, and decision making as well as depression, anxiety, and substance abuse. Adults may have more signs and symptoms of inattention and less of hyperactivity-impulsive behavior than children.

DIAGNOSIS

Diagnosis of ADHD is mainly based on observed symptoms and behavior.

Clinical Testing: The American Academy of Pediatrics Clinical Practice Guideline for children with ADHD states that a diagnosis should be based upon the following three criteria:

1. The use of explicit criteria for the diagnosis using the *Diagnostic and Statistical Manual of Mental Disorders* (the clinical reference for psychiatric illnesses). The Conners Rating Scale is commonly used.
2. The importance of obtaining information about the child's symptoms in more than one setting. This is completed by obtaining a personal medical and family history from parents, teachers, and the patient.
3. The search for coexisting conditions that may make the diagnosis more difficult or complicate treatment planning. This is done with psychological and intelligence testing.

Analytical Testing: Some clinicians use brain scan technology to determine if there is a problem with brain function or blood flow. These tests include magnetic resonance imaging, positron emission tomography, and single-photon emission computed tomography. Scientists have concluded, however,

that there is not enough evidence to use these methods to determine if an individual has ADHD.

Computerized Tests: These generally determine the attention span of the individual. However, due to a high rate of false negatives, this testing modality is not commonly used to determine if an individual has ADHD.

COMPLICATIONS

Individuals with ADHD struggle to function normally in daily life. Children often struggle in the classroom, which can lead to academic failure and ridicule from other children and adults.

Children with ADHD are much more likely to experience minor trauma, such as fractures and cuts, than are other children. Adults and teenagers are also more likely to become involved in car accidents and have other injuries. Individuals with ADHD may also be more likely to have trouble with following the law and commit crimes.

As many as one in three children with ADHD also have other psychological or developmental conditions.

Oppositional Defiant Disorder (ODD): Generally defined as a pattern of negative, defiant and hostile behavior toward authority figures, ODD tends to occur more frequently in children who are impulsive and hyperactive and is especially common in boys.

Conduct Disorder: A more serious condition than ODD, conduct disorder is marked by distinctly antisocial behavior such as stealing, fighting, destroying property, harming people and animals, and committing crimes. Children with conduct disorder need immediate help.

Depression: Depression may occur in both children and adults with ADHD. It's more likely to appear when there is a family history of depression.

Anxiety Disorders: Anxiety disorders tend to occur fairly often in children with ADHD and may cause overwhelming worry and nervousness as well as physical signs and symptoms, such as a rapid heartbeat, sweating, and dizziness. Although anxiety disorders can cause severe symptoms, most people can be helped with therapy or medication. Once anxiety is under control, children are better able to deal with the problems arising from ADHD.

Learning Disabilities: Children with both ADHD and learning disabilities are the children most in need of special education services.

Tourette's Syndrome: Many children with ADHD are at increased risk of Tourette's syndrome, a neurological disorder characterized by compulsive muscular or vocal tics.

Alcohol and Drug Abuse: Individuals with ADHD may be more likely to develop addiction problems with alcohol or drugs due to factors including altered brain function and the continued use of stimulants.

TREATMENT

Family Therapy: Family therapy can help parents and siblings deal with the stress of living with a child who has ADHD.

Behavioral Therapy (BT): BT helps individuals with ADHD develop more effective ways to work on immediate issues. Practical assistance may be offered, such as helping organize school tasks and studying for school or assisting the individual with powerful emotional issues. Anger control is an example of BT.

Psychotherapy: Psychotherapists work to help people with ADHD to live as functioning members of society, increasing self-esteem and dealing with other psychological issues. Psychotherapy alone, however, does not address the symptoms or underlying causes of the disorder. Upsetting thoughts and feelings are verbalized, along with exploration of self-defeating patterns of behavior. Individuals with ADHD can learn alternative ways to handle their emotions.

Social Skills Training: Social relationships are studied with a therapist to help the individual with ADHD develop and maintain social relationships, like waiting for a turn, sharing toys, asking for help, or responding to teasing. Social skills training helps the child to develop better ways to play and work with other children and provides the adult with better social skills.

Support Groups: Support groups help individuals with ADHD and parents to connect with other people who have similar problems and concerns. Meetings occur on a regular basis (usually weekly) to share frustrations and successes and to hear lectures from experts on ADHD and obtain referrals to qualified specialists and information about what works.

Parenting Skills Training: Parents face special obstacles when raising a child with ADHD and often feel frustrated and as if there is no help. Parenting skills training is offered by therapists or in special classes and can give parents tools and techniques for managing their child's behavior. Time outs, reward systems, and organization are just a few of the skills taught.

Stimulants: The most frequently prescribed medications for ADHD are stimulants, which work by stimulating the areas of the brain responsible for focus, attention, and impulse control. Stimulant drugs include methylphenidate (Ritalin, Metadate, Focalin, Concerta, and Daytrana, a topical methylphenidate patch), amphetamine, mixed salts (Adderall, Adderall XR), dextroamphetamine (Dexedrine), modafinil (Provigil), methamphetamine (Desoxyn), and the recently approved lisdexamfetamine (Vyvanse).

Nonstimulants: Atomoxetine (Strattera) is a norepinephrine reuptake inhibitor and helps regulate brain function. Atmoxetine is usually taken once or twice a day, depending on the individual, every day, and takes up to 6 weeks to begin working fully.

Amantadine (Symmetrel) is used to increase dopamine in the brain. Reports suggest that low-dose amantadine has been successfully used off label to treat ADHD.

Antidepressant medications may be used off label for ADHD, including serotonin reuptake inhibitors, monoamine oxidase inhibitors (including selegiline [Emsam]), and bupropion (Wellbutrin).

INTEGRATIVE THERAPIES

Good Scientific Evidence

Zinc: One study has shown a correlation between low serum free fatty acids and zinc serum levels in children with ADHD. Two other studies found that zinc supplements reduced hyperactive, impulsive, and impaired socialization symptoms but did not reduce attention deficiency symptoms. Zinc supplementation may be a more effective treatment for older children with higher body mass index scores.

Unclear or Conflicting Scientific Evidence

Flaxseed and Flaxseed Oil (*Linum Usitatissimum*): Preliminary evidence supports the idea that deficiencies or imbalances in certain highly unsaturated fatty acids may contribute to ADHD. Based on preliminary clinical evidence, alpha linolenic acid–rich nutritional supplementation in the form of flax oil may improve symptoms of ADHD. More research is needed to confirm these results.

Gamma-Linolenic Acid (GLA): Clinical trials investigating the effect of GLA on symptoms associated with ADHD are limited. There is no evidence of effectiveness of treatment with GLA, but more study is needed to confirm these results.

Glyconutrients: Glyconutrients are supplements that contain monosaccharides (sugar-type molecules), which are required for the synthesis of glycoproteins (help form hormones and immune system components). The effect of a glyconutritional product has been investigated in children with ADHD. A decrease in the number and severity of symptoms was noted.

Iron: Based on preliminary data, taking iron orally might improve symptoms of ADHD. A recent study found a three-year-old child with ADHD and low iron levels improved significantly on ADHD testing scores after an eight-month treatment with ferrous sulfate, 80 milligrams daily. Caution should be used when taking iron supplements as drug interactions are possible.

L-Carnitine: One study has reported positive effects of using L-carnitine (also called acetyl-L-carnitine) supplements in children (boys) with ADHD. Acetyl-L-carnitine is an antioxidant and may help blood flow as well as neurological function.

Massage: Preliminary research suggests massage therapy may improve mood and behavior in children with ADHD.

Melatonin: There is some research of the use of melatonin in children with ADHD both in the treatment of ADHD and insomnia in ADHD children. Melatonin is not used for extended periods of time. Interactions with drugs may occur.

Music Therapy: Music relaxes and may cause reduced heart rate, reduced blood pressure, reduced tension, and many other beneficial changes. Evidence that music therapy can lead to the relaxation response has been found in healthy individuals and individuals with health problems. More study is needed in the area of ADHD.

Pycnogenol: Pycnogenol (Horphag Research, Berlin) is a potent antioxidant that may be effective in decreasing neurological imbalances. Preliminary research comparing Pycnogenol vs. placebo in adults with ADHD reported improved concentration with both agents. In more recent studies in children, improvements in attention and various rating scales were noted with Pycnogenol supplementation. Pycnogenol is safe in recommended dosages. If pregnant or breastfeeding, consult a qualified health care provider.

S-Adenosylmethionine (SAMe): SAMe is formed in the body from the essential amino acid methionine and is used in depression and mood disorders. Preliminary evidence from an open trial suggests that SAMe may be of benefit for adults with ADHD. Caution should be used when taking SAMe supplements as drug interactions are possible.

Vitamin B$_6$ (Pyridoxine): Some research suggests that pyridoxine supplementation alone or in combination with high doses of other B vitamins might help ADHD. Vitamin B$_6$ may also be found in a multivitamin or a B-complex vitamin supplement.

Yoga: There is limited study in humans of yoga in the treatment of ADHD. Further research is needed before a recommendation can be made.

Traditional or Theoretical Uses Lacking Sufficient Evidence

Biofeedback: Ordinarily, this stress-reduction technique is used to help people learn to control certain body responses, such as heart rate and muscle tension. It has also been used with the intent of teaching adults and children with ADHD to change their brain wave patterns to more normal ones.

Omega-3 Fatty Acids: Essential fatty acids have many roles in the body, including proper nerve and brain function. Preliminary evidence supports the idea that deficiencies or imbalances in certain highly unsaturated fatty acids may contribute to ADHD. More research is needed in this area.

Fair Negative Scientific Evidence

Evening Primrose Oil (*Oenothera biennis L.*): Small human studies show no benefit from evening primrose oil in ADHD. Further research is needed to confirm this conclusion.

Psychotherapy: Psychotherapy is an interactive process between a person and a qualified mental health professional. Psychotherapy may not improve parenting, enhance academic achievement, or improve emotional adjustment for children ages seven to nine with ADHD. It is unclear whether psychotherapy will reduce the use of stimulants, such as methylphenidate, in these children. More studies are needed in this area.

PREVENTION

Nutritional changes along with the addition of supplements (vitamins, minerals, and herbs) may be effective in preventing ADHD and improving the symptoms.

Avoid caffeine and other stimulants, alcohol, and smoking.

Eliminate potential food allergens, including dairy (milk, cheese, and sour cream), eggs, nuts, shellfish, wheat (gluten), corn, preservatives, and food additives (such as dyes and fillers). Food allergies can be a contributing factor in mental imbalance.

Avoid refined foods such as white breads, pastas, and sugar. Doughnuts, pastries, bread, candy, soft drinks, and foods with high sugar content may all contribute to worsening symptoms of ADHD.

BACK PAIN

BACKGROUND

Back and neck pain are the most common chronic pain conditions. Back and neck pain can arise from soft tissues, bony parts of the back and neck, and joints holding the spine in alignment. It can arise directly or indirectly from the discs in the back or neck, and it can occur when nerves and nervous tissue, normally protected by the bones of the spine, are compressed by those bones.

Back pain can range from a dull, constant ache to a sudden, sharp pain that leaves the individual suffering and/or incapacitated. Back pain can be acute (immediate) or chronic (long term). Acute back pain usually gets better on its own without treatment. However, chronic back pain may require medication and/or surgery.

The back is an intricate structure of bones, ligaments, muscles, nerves, and tendons. The spine, or backbone, is made up of 33 bony segments called vertebrae. The vertebrae are arranged in a long vertical column and held together by ligaments that are attached to muscles by tendons. Between each vertebra lies a gel-like cushion called an intervertebral disc, consisting of a semifluid matter that is surrounded by a capsule of elastic fibers.

The spinal cord is an extension of the brain that runs through a long, hollow canal in the column of the vertebrae. The meninges (membranes that surround the brain and spinal cord), cerebrospinal fluid (fluid that circulates around the brain and spinal cord), fat, and a network of veins and arteries nourish and protect the spinal cord. Thirty-one pairs of nerve roots emerge from the spinal cord through spaces in each vertebra. The spinal cord and peripheral (outside the brain and spinal column) nerves perform essential sensory and motor activities of the body. The peripheral nervous system conveys sensory information from the body to the brain and conveys motor signals from the brain to the body.

Back problems are the most frequent cause of activity limitations in working-age adults. About 85% of Americans experience back pain by age 50. More than 26 million Americans between the ages of 20-64 experience frequent back pain. Two-thirds of American adults will have back pain during their lifetimes. Back pain is the leading cause of disability in Americans under 45 years old. Each year 13 million people go to the doctor for chronic back pain. It is estimated that the condition leaves 2.4 million Americans chronically disabled and another 2.4 million temporarily disabled. Back pain is the second most common reason why individuals in the United States seek medical care from their primary care physicians.

RISK FACTORS

Age: The first attack of low back pain typically occurs between the ages of 30-40. Back pain becomes more common with age. Aging produces wear and tear on the spine that may result in conditions (such as disc degeneration or spinal stenosis) that produce neck and back pain. Having a previous back injury puts the individual at risk for another injury and increased pain.

Diet: A diet high in calories and fat, especially trans fats found in fried foods, combined with an inactive lifestyle, can lead to obesity. Obesity has been found to be a major risk factor in the development of back pain due to increased stress on the back.

Heredity: Some causes of back pain, including disc disease, may be genetic or passed from one generation to the next through genes. More research is being performed in the area of back pain and heredity.

Race: Race can be a factor in back problems. African-American women, for example, are two to three times more likely than white women to develop spondylolisthesis, a condition in which a vertebra of the lower spine (lumbar spine) slips out of place.

Occupation: Physically demanding occupations, such as construction work and healthcare, which require repetitive bending and lifting, have a high incidence of back injury. Jobs that require long hours of standing without a break (such as hairdressing and fast food service) or sitting in a chair that does not support the back well (e.g., computer keyboard operation) also put a person at risk for neck and lower back injury.

Lifestyle: Back pain is more common among people who are not physically fit. Weak back and abdominal muscles may not properly support the spine. Clinical studies report that low-impact aerobic exercise is good for the discs that cushion the vertebrae.

Although smoking tobacco may not directly cause back pain, it increases the risk of developing low back pain and low back pain with sciatica. Sciatica is back pain that radiates to the hip and/or leg due to pressure on a nerve. Smoking has been reported to negatively affect bone mineral density, lumbar disc disease, the rate of hip fractures, and the rate and extent of bone and wound healing.

Poor posture, such as slouching in a chair, driving hunched over, standing incorrectly, and using poor body mechanics when lifting and carrying heavy loads, are risk factors. Sleeping on a soft or sagging mattress also can lead to back pain.

Sports that involve twisting the back, such as golf and basketball, can result in back injury and they also worsen existing lower back pain.

CAUSES

Movement Problems: A movement or mechanical problem is a problem with the way the spine moves or the way an individual feels when moving the spine in certain ways. Perhaps the most common mechanical cause of back pain is intervertebral disc degeneration. In this condition, the discs located between the vertebrae of the spine break down with age. As the vertebrae deteriorate, they lose their cushioning ability. This problem can lead to pain if the back is stressed. Other mechanical causes of back pain include spasms, muscle tension, and ruptured or herniated discs.

Injuries: Spinal injuries, such as sprains and fractures, can cause either acute (short-lived) or chronic (long-term) pain. Sprains or tears in the ligaments that support the spine can occur from twisting or lifting improperly. Fractured vertebrae are often the result of osteoporosis, a condition that causes weak, porous bones. Less commonly, back pain may be caused by more severe injuries that result from accidents and falls.

Whiplash is a nonmedical term used to describe neck pain following an injury to the soft tissues of the neck, specifically ligaments, tendons, and muscles. Whiplash is caused by an accidental motion or force applied to the neck that results in movement beyond the neck's normal range of motion. Whiplash occurs in motor vehicle accidents, sporting activities, accidental falls, and assault.

Conditions and Diseases: Many diseases can cause or contribute to back pain. These include various forms of arthritis, such as herniated disc (occurs when disc material presses on a nerve), osteoarthritis, rheumatoid arthritis, and ankylosing spondylitis, and cancers from elsewhere in the body that may spread to the spine. Scoliosis, which causes curvature of the spine, does not usually cause pain until mid-life. Spinal stenosis, or a narrowing of the spinal column that puts pressure on the spinal cord and nerves, also contributes to back pain. While osteoporosis itself is not painful, it can lead to painful fractures of the vertebrae. Other causes of back pain include pregnancy, kidney stones or infections, endometriosis

(the buildup of uterine tissue in places outside the uterus), and fibromyalgia (which causes fatigue and widespread muscle pain).

Infections and Tumors: Although they are not common causes of back pain, infections can cause pain when they involve the vertebrae. Osteomyelitis is an infection (typically caused by bacteria) of bone and bone marrow in which the resulting inflammation can lead to a reduction of blood supply to the bone. Diskitis is when the infection involves the discs that cushion the vertebrae. Tumors are relatively rare causes of back pain. Occasionally, tumors begin in the back, but more often they appear in the back as a result of cancer that has spread from elsewhere in the body.

Emotional Stress: Although the causes of back pain are usually physical, emotional stress may also play an important role in back pain and how severe and long it lasts. For example, stress may cause back muscles to become tense and painful.

SIGNS AND SYMPTOMS

Pain: Pain can be constant or intermittent (off and on). Intensity can vary from a dull ache to searing agony. The onset may be sudden or acute (short term), with or without apparent reason, or gradual and chronic (long term).

Most back pain resolves in a few days or weeks with or without treatment. However, some individuals have chronic pain that lasts months or years.

Severe pain lasting more than a few days without improvement may require medical attention. Individuals having difficulty passing urine; numbness in the back or genital area; numbness, pins and needles, or weakness in the legs; shooting pain down the leg; or unsteadiness when standing should see a doctor immediately.

Pain is often described as aching, tight, stiff, sore, burning, throbbing, or pulling. The pain may worsen while bending, sitting, walking, or standing too long in one position. It may also be more prevalent at different times of the day, such as when a person wakes up in the morning.

Pinched nerves produce numbness or tingling, warm or cold sensations, and burning or stabbing pain that begin in the back and radiate down the leg or the arm. Activities such as coughing, sneezing, or walking may increase pressure on the pinched nerve and aggravate the pain.

Compressed nerves may cause numbness and weakness in the muscle associated with the nerve. The muscle may atrophy (waste away) if the compression is not relieved.

DIAGNOSIS

Examination: Diagnosing the underlying cause of neck and back pain can be difficult. A medical history that includes age, weight, current and past medical problems, medications, and height is taken. Also, a complete physical examination, which may include a neurological exam, is performed.

X-Ray: X-rays show the alignment of the spine and may reveal degenerative joint diseases, fractures, or tumors.

Magnetic Resonance Imaging (MRI): MRI scans provide clear images of disc deterioration, pathologies of the spinal cord, spinal stenosis, herniated discs, spinal tumors, and abnormalities in nerves and ligaments. MRIs are conducted in a small, confined areas and some individuals may find this uncomfortable. Some individuals may have to be sedated using a mild sedative such as alprazolam (Xanax) or lorazepam (Ativan). If the individual is sedated, transportation should be organized with a family member or friend to bring and take the individual home due to drowsiness and decreased coordination.

Computerized Tomography (CT): A CT scan is an x-ray that uses computer technology and can be enhanced with the injection of a contrast dye. CT scans are used to show abnormalities in bones and soft tissue. CT scans can be used for individuals who are unable to tolerate MRIs.

Myelography: Myelography is used to examine the spinal canal and cord. Contrast dye is injected into the cerebrospinal fluid in the spine. This allows the doctor to outline the spinal cord and nerve roots, and abnormal disc conditions or bone spurs can then be visualized using an x-ray or CT scan.

Electromyogram (EMG): An EMG is the use of tiny electrodes inserted into muscle tissue to test for abnormal electrical signals. Abnormal electrical signals may indicate that a nerve root is pinched or irritated at the spine. An anesthetic, such as lidocaine (Xylocaine), is used to reduce the pain of electrode insertion into the skin.

Spinal Tap: Spinal tap involves drawing a sample of cerebrospinal fluid and analyzing it for elevated pressure, infection, bleeding, or tumor. Spinal tap may be painful and may require sedation.

Radioactive Bone Scan: Radioactive bone scans locate problems (such as a fracture or osteoporosis) in the vertebrae. A chemical called a radioactive tracer is injected into the patient and, after several hours, a gamma camera picture will reveal bone undergoing rapid changes where large amounts of tracer accumulate.

COMPLICATIONS

Complications of back pain include limited mobility, such as trouble walking up stairs, standing, or sitting; pain; lost work time; surgery; and disability.

TREATMENT

In many cases, it is not necessary to see a doctor for back pain because pain usually goes away without treatment. However, individuals should see a doctor if they experience numbness or tingling, severe pain, or pain that does not improve with medication and rest. Also, individuals should see a doctor if they have pain after a fall or an injury. It is also important to see a doctor if pain occurs along with any of the following problems: trouble urinating; weakness, pain, or numbness in the legs; fever; or unintentional weight loss. Such symptoms could signal a serious medical condition that requires treatment.

Applying ice as soon as possible during the 48 hours after straining a muscle can reduce pain. Ice slows inflammation and swelling, numbs soft tissue, and slows nerve impulses in the injured area. After spasms and acute pain subside, heat can be applied to loosen tight muscles. Over-the-counter pain-relieving medications, such as acetaminophen (Tylenol), ibuprofen (Advil), or naproxen (Aleve), may be used short term (less than two weeks). Two or three days of bed rest followed by a gradual return to normal activity is sometimes recommended.

Physical Therapy and Exercise: A physical therapist may apply a variety of treatments (such as heat, ice, ultrasound, electrical stimulation, and muscle release techniques) to the back muscles and soft tissues to reduce pain. As pain improves, the physical therapist can teach the individual specific exercises to increase flexibility, strengthen the back and abdominal muscles, and improve posture. Regular use of these techniques may help prevent pain from coming back. Exercise can correct current back problems, help prevent new ones, and relieve back pain, particularly after an injury. Exercise also strengthens bones and reduces the risk of falls and injuries.

Prescription Medications: A doctor may prescribe nonsteroidal antiinflammatory drugs (such as flurbi-profen [Ansaid] and celecoxib [Celebrex]), muscle relaxants (such as cyclobenzaprine [Flexeril]), and narcotic pain relievers (such as hydrocodone [Lortab]). A skin patch containing an opioid called transdermal fentanyl (Duragesic) may relieve chronic back pain more effectively than oral opioid drugs. Muscle relaxants, opiate agonists, and narcotic pain relievers may cause drowsiness. Narcotic pain relievers may also cause physical dependence and should be used with caution. Corticosteroid injections (steroids, such as dexamethasone [Decadron]) may be used if pain-relieving and antiinflammatory medications do not offer relief. The long-term use of steroid medications can cause complications such as weakened immune systems and swelling.

Tricyclic antidepressants, such as amitriptyline (Elavil) and nortriptyline (Pamelor), may be used for numbness, burning, aching, throbbing, or stabbing pains that shoot down the limbs. Side effects of these drugs include drowsiness, dry mouth, blurred vision, and constipation.

Surgery: Few individuals need surgery for back pain. Surgery is usually reserved for pain caused by a herniated disc. If the individual is experiencing unrelenting pain that is unable to be relieved by medications or progressive muscle weakness caused by nerve compression, surgery may be beneficial.

Disc Removal: There are three common types of surgeries that involve the removal of damaged or herniated discs in the spine, including laminotomy, laminectomy, and diskectomy. A laminotomy is the surgical removal of part of the lamina (bony arch) above and below an affected nerve. A laminectomy consists of the surgical removal of most of the lamina of a vertebra. A laminectomy is most often performed when back pain fails to improve with more conservative medical treatments such as pain medications and physical therapy. A diskectomy is the surgical removal or partial removal of a spinal disc.

Fusion Surgery: Fusion surgery involves joining two vertebrae to eliminate painful movement. Recovery following fusion surgery generally takes longer compared to other types of spinal surgery. Patients typically stay in the hospital for three or four days, but a longer stay after more extensive surgery is not uncommon. A short stay in a rehabilitation unit after release from the hospital is often recommended for patients who have had extensive surgery or for elderly or debilitated patients. Pain from surgery varies.

Intradiskal Electrothermal Therapy: In intradiskal electrothermal therapy, doctors insert a needle through a catheter into the damaged spinal disc. The needle is heated to a high temperature for up to 20 minutes. The heat thickens and seals the disc wall, reducing disc bulge and the related spinal nerve irritation. It is unclear whether this treatment is effective for back pain.

Implanted Pumps: Pumps may be implanted into the spinal area to deliver a constant flow of pain-relieving medications (such as opiates like morphine).

Surgically implanted spinal cord stimulators modulate the pain response so that the individual with a back condition experiences less pain. The implantation may put the individual at an increased risk for infection.

INTEGRATIVE THERAPIES

Good Scientific Evidence

Chiropractic: Chiropractic is a healthcare discipline that focuses on the relationship between musculoskeletal structure (primarily the spine) and body function (as coordinated by the nervous system) and how this relationship affects the preservation and restoration of health. The broad term "spinal manipulative therapy" incorporates all types of manual techniques, including chiropractic. Multiple clinical studies have examined the effects of spinal manipulation in patients with acute or chronic neck pain. Overall, the quality of studies has been poor, and reviews of this topic have been unable to form clear or convincing conclusions. Better-quality clinical research for the use of chiropractic for neck pain is necessary before a firm conclusion can be drawn. Although chiropractic helps many people with back pain (including lower back pain), there is not enough reliable scientific evidence to conclude whether chiropractic techniques are beneficial in the management of back pain when compared to conventional approaches, such as medication and surgery. Chiropractic has also been studied in lumbar disc herniation and whiplash injuries, with mixed results.

Devil's Claw: Devil's claw (*Harpagophytum procumbens*) has traditionally been used as an antiinflammatory and pain reliever for joint diseases, back pain, and headache. There are several human studies that support the use of devil's claw for the treatment of low back pain. However, most studies have been small with flaws in their designs, and many have been done by the same authors. Therefore, although these results can be considered promising early evidence, additional well-designed trials are necessary before a firm conclusion can be reached. It is not clear how devil's claw compares to other therapies for back pain. Devil's claw may lower blood sugar levels. A qualified healthcare provider should monitor patients taking drugs for diabetes by mouth or insulin closely. Medication adjustments may be necessary. Devil's claw may increase stomach acidity and therefore may interact with drugs used to decrease the amount of acid in the stomach, such as antacids, sucralfate, ranitidine (Zantac), and esomeprazole (Nexium).

Hydrotherapy: Hydrotherapy is broadly defined as the external application of water in any form or temperature (hot, cold, steam, liquid, ice) for healing

B

purposes. It may include immersion in a bath or body of water (such as the ocean or a pool), use of water jets, douches, application of wet towels to the skin, or water birth. Several small controlled clinical trials report that regular use of hot whirlpool baths with massaging jets decreases the duration and severity of back pain when added to standard therapy, compared to standard therapy alone. It is not clear if there is a reduced need for pain control drugs or if benefits are longstanding. Because these studies are small with flaws in design and reporting, better-quality research is necessary before a strong conclusion can be drawn.

White Willow: White willow (*Salix alba*) bark has been compared to cyclooxygenase-2 inhibitors (commonly used for back pain and arthritis), and many of the studies found willow bark to be as effective or superior to other methods. Cost-effectiveness studies have also been performed between white willow bark and conventional treatment; they found that willow bark was more cost effective. Additional study in humans is needed.

Unclear or Conflicting Scientific Evidence

Acupressure, Shiatsu: The practice of applying finger pressure to specific acupoints (energy points) throughout the body has been used in China since 2000 BC. Shiatsu technique can incorporate palm pressure, stretching, massaging, and other manual techniques. Shiatsu practitioners commonly treat musculoskeletal and psychological conditions, including neck/shoulder and lower back problems, arthritis, depression, and anxiety. One clinical study reported that acupressure was effective in reducing low back pain in terms of disability, pain scores, and functional status. The benefit was sustained for six months. More research is needed.

Acupuncture: Evidence is inconsistent regarding the effects of acupuncture in back pain. The research on acupuncture for neck pain and cervical myofascial pain also shows mixed results. Additionally, early study does not show that laser acupuncture is any more effective than sham laser acupuncture when used in combination with drugs and other mobilization therapies. Further human research is needed.

Alexander Technique: The Alexander technique is an educational program that teaches movement patterns and postures with an aim to improve coordination and balance, reduce tension, relieve pain, alleviate fatigue, improve various medical conditions, and promote well-being. There is limited evidence in this area, and no firm conclusion can be drawn based on scientific research.

Healing Touch: One poor-quality clinical study using 20 participants with chronic low back pain suggested that healing touch may significantly decrease pain, improve range of motion, and improve orthopedic measurements. However, more research using healing touch for back pain needs to be performed before a conclusion can be drawn.

Magnet Therapy: The use of permanent or harnessed bipolar magnets in the treatment of chronic back pain is controversial. Early evidence with stronger magnets (up to 2,000 gauss strength) reported benefits, while more recent study with lower strength (450 gauss strength) noted no effects. Additional research is necessary in this area before a firm conclusion can be drawn.

Massage: Several human trials report temporary improvements in low back pain with various massage methods. A clinical study reported slightly more efficacy for traditional therapy such as pain medications and surgery. However, the additional benefits of massage may contribute to its value for holistic nursing practice. Further research is necessary.

Meditation: Various forms of meditation have been practiced for thousands of years throughout the world, with many techniques originating in Eastern religious practices. Based on preliminary research, patients suffering from chronic low back pain may improve with breath therapy. Further clinical research is needed to confirm these results.

Transcutaneous Electrical Nerve Stimulation (TENS): TENS is a noninvasive technique in which a low-voltage electrical current is delivered through wires from a small power unit to electrodes located on the skin. Electrodes are temporarily attached with paste in various patterns, depending on the specific condition and treatment goals. The effects of TENS or acupuncture-like TENS on low back pain remain controversial, and multiple controlled trials have been published in this area. Studies have not been consistent in the type of TENS techniques used (location, intensity, frequency, duration) or in definitions of back pain, and most trials have not been well designed or reported. Published meta-analyses have grouped some of these studies together to try to determine whether this technique is effective but have also yielded inconsistent results, with some authors reporting overall benefits and others finding no clear advantage over placebo. Better-designed research is needed before a firm conclusion can be reached.

Trigger Point Therapy: Trigger points are discrete, focal, hyperirritable spots located in skeletal muscle. The spots may be painful on compression and associated with pain and tenderness, motor dysfunction, and autonomic nervous system phenomena. The goal of trigger point therapy for back pain is to eliminate the trigger points and thus lessen the pain. There have been few studies that addressed the therapeutic potential of this therapy. Overall, the evidence is positive and demonstrates that this therapy might be effective for the treatment of back pain. However, because back pain may be insidious and brought on by unrecognized causes, future studies should address trigger point therapy in various causes of back pain.

Yoga: Yoga is an ancient system of relaxation, exercise, and healing with origins in Indian (Hindu) philosophy. Preliminary research reports that yoga may improve chronic low back pain in humans. However, larger, better-designed studies are needed before a firm conclusion can be drawn.

Fair or Negative Scientific Evidence

Reflexology: Reflexology involves the application of manual pressure to specific points or areas of the feet that are believed to correspond to other parts of the body. Reflexology is often used with the intention to relieve stress or prevent/treat physical disorders. Pressure may also be applied to the hands or ears. A large trial comparing reflexology to relaxation or no therapy reports that reflexology is not effective for managing chronic lower back pain.

Historical or Theoretical Uses Lacking Sufficient Evidence

Integrative therapies used in back pain or related conditions that have historical or theoretical uses but lack sufficient clinical evidence include homeopathic aconite (*Aconitum napellus*), alizarin (1,2-dihydroxyathraquinones), homeopathic arnica (*Arnica montana*), aromatherapy, bacopa (*Bacopa monnieri*), black cohosh (*Actaea racemosa*), bromelain, chamomile (*Matricaria recutita, Chamaemelum nobile*), detoxification therapy (cleansing), dong quai (*Angelica sinensis*), glucosamine, homeopathic nux vomica (*Strychnos nux-vomica*), and spiritual healing.

PREVENTION

Proper Body Mechanics: Many options exist for individuals wishing to prevent back and neck pain. Learning proper body mechanics, such as bending, lifting, and twisting, is particularly important if the individual's occupation involves repetitive bending, lifting, and twisting, as is the case with athletes and construction workers.

Exercise: Regular exercise helps to keep back muscles strong and flexible. Regular low-impact aerobic activities do not strain or jolt the back and neck. Low-impact aerobic exercises may also increase strength and endurance in the back and allow the muscles to function better. Walking and swimming are also recommended by health professionals. Abdominal and back muscle exercises, also called core-strengthening exercises, help condition back muscles so that they function more efficiently and help protect the back from injury. Flexibility in the hips and upper legs aligns the pelvic bones to improve back comfort. A healthcare professional can help the individual choose the best exercise program.

Posture: Maintaining good posture, such as sitting straight in a chair and not slumping, can prevent and decrease back pain. Individuals with jobs that require long standing or sitting should take frequent breaks from standing or sitting positions to help prevent back pain.

Weight Control: Maintaining weight within an ideal range for the individual's body size is very important. Excess weight has been directly linked with the development and worsening of back pain.

Diet: Eating a healthy diet is important to prevent back pain. A healthy diet, including fresh fruits and vegetables, provides the body with essential nutrients for health.

Smoking Cessation: Smokers have diminished oxygen levels in their spinal tissues that can hinder the healing process. Clinical studies have found mixed results on whether cigarette smoking leads to back conditions, but there is evidence that smoking may increase the risk of developing sciatica or back pain that radiates to the hip and/or leg due to pressure on a nerve.

CANCER

BACKGROUND

Cancer, also called malignancy or neoplasm, develops when cells in a specific part of the body begin to grow out of control. Unlike normal cells, cancer cells do not stop reproducing after they have doubled 50-60 times. Normal body cells grow, divide, and die in an orderly, natural fashion. Normal cells divide more rapidly during the early years of an individual's life. After adulthood is reached, cells in most parts of the body divide only to replace worn-out or dying cells and to repair injuries. Cancer cells continue to grow and divide, forming new abnormal cells.

Cancer cells usually form a tumor. Some cancers, such as leukemia or cancer of the bone marrow and blood, do not form tumors. Instead, these cancer cells circulate through other tissues where they grow. Not all tumors are cancerous. Benign (noncancerous) tumors do not metastasize (spread) to other parts of the body and, with very rare exceptions, are not life threatening. Different types of cancer can grow at different rates and respond to different treatments. Malignant, or cancerous, tumors may metastasize and cause further damage to organs and tissues in the body.

Cancer cells develop because of damage to DNA (the material inside the nucleus of a cell that carries genetic information). DNA occurs in most cells of the body and is the blueprint for how the body grows, functions, and stays healthy. Usually, when DNA becomes damaged the body is able to repair it. In cancer cells, the damaged DNA is not able to be repaired. Individuals can inherit damaged DNA; such is the case with inherited cancers. More often, though, an individual's DNA becomes damaged by exposure to something in the environment, such as smoking or radiation from the sun.

The immune system, which is made up of special cells, proteins, tissues, and organs, defends individuals against invasion by pathogens (disease-causing agents) such as cancer cells, bacteria, and viruses. The differences between cancer cells and normal cells may not be as easily detected, and the immune system may not always recognize cancer cells as pathogens. Most healthy individuals have immune systems that can keep up with the pathogens, but sometimes problems with the immune system can lead to illness and infection.

Cancer cells sometimes travel through the blood or lymphatic system to other parts of the body. The cancerous cells begin to grow and replace normal tissue in a process called metastasis. Regardless of where cancer may spread, it is always named for the place it began. For instance, colon cancer that spreads to the liver is still called colon cancer, not liver cancer.

Symptoms and treatment depend on the cancer type and how advanced it is. Treatment plans may include surgery, radiation, and/or chemotherapy. The most common cancers are breast cancer, lung cancer, bowel or colon cancer, prostate cancer, bladder cancer, non-Hodgkin's lymphoma, stomach cancer, melanoma, esophageal cancer, pancreatic cancer, leukemia, and ovarian cancer.

Cancer is the leading cause of death among Americans under the age of 85. Half of all men and one third of all women in the United States will develop cancer during their lifetimes. Although cancer occurs in Americans of all racial and ethnic groups, the rate of cancer occurrence varies from group to group. Two-thirds of individuals diagnosed with cancer are over 65 years. In 2005, 7.6 million people died of cancer out of 58 million deaths worldwide. More than 70% of all cancer deaths worldwide occur in low- and middle-income countries, where resources available for prevention, diagnosis, and treatment of cancer are limited or nonexistent. Based on projections, cancer deaths will continue to rise; an estimated 9 million people will die from cancer in 2015, and 11.4 million may die in 2030.

Early diagnosis makes it more likely that cancer can be treated successfully. It is important that individuals are aware of possible symptoms and that individuals see a doctor for regular check-ups.

TYPES OF CANCER

There are over 100 types of cancer that can affect the human body. Each of the types of cancer has its own name, behavior, and course of treatment. All cancers involve the abnormal growth of cells. The most commonly found cancers in humans include carcinoma, sarcoma, leukemia, lymphoma, and adenoma.

Carcinoma: More than 85% of cancers are carcinomas. Carcinomas start in the cells that line and cover internal and external organs. The most common carcinomas are lung cancer, breast cancer, skin cancer, and bowel cancer.

Sarcoma: Sarcoma begins in supportive tissues of the body, such as muscle, bone, cartilage, blood vessels, fat, and connective tissue.

Leukemia: Leukemia is cancer of the blood cells that grows in the bone marrow.

Lymphoma: Lymphomas develop in the lymph nodes and tissues of the immune system.

Adenoma: An adenoma is a tumor (usually benign) that begins in glandular tissue, such as the adrenal, pituitary, or thyroid gland.

Risk Factors and Causes

Age: The chances of developing cancer increase with age. In the United States, more than 60% of cancers occur in people older than 65. The risk of developing cancer doubles every five years after the age of 25. The increased cancer rate is probably due to a combination of increased and prolonged exposure to carcinogens and weakening of the body's immune system.

Environmental Factors: The environment we live in can cause an individual to have an increased risk of developing various types of cancers. Studies have reported that individuals exposed to high amounts of benzene, which is commonly found in gasoline, cigarettes, and pollution, are at an increased risk for developing cancer.

Certain chemicals found in pesticide products, such as lawn and garden chemicals, may increase the risk of developing cancers such as lymphoma. Long-term use of hair products, including permanent hair dyes (especially dark colors) and hair-straightening chemicals doubles an individual's risk of developing lymphoma, particularly among women and persons who used hair dyes before 1980. These dyes contained more carcinogenic (cancer-causing) substances than the dyes used today due to changes in regulation by the U.S. Food and Drug Administration (FDA).

Studies have reported that exposure to chemicals and pesticides can significantly increase the chances of developing breast cancer. Being overweight increases the chances of developing many types of cancer, such as ovarian cancer. A high-fat diet may increase the chances of developing colon cancer. Exercising at least 30 minutes a day, five days a week may reduce the risk of developing cancer.

Diet and Lifestyle: Exposure to charred red meat has been reported to increase the risk of developing colon cancer. Diets low in fruits and vegetables are linked to an increased risk of cancers, including cervical cancer.

Heredity: Heredity or genetics plays a large role in cancer development. A family history of cancer, such as breast, ovarian, or colon cancer, increases the risk of the individual developing that type of cancer. When cancer is genetic, a mutated gene has been passed down. However, this does not always mean that the genetically predisposed individual will always develop cancer. Genetic tests are available for many cancers that are hereditary.

Personal History of Cancer: If an individual has had any type of cancer, there is an increased risk of developing that cancer again. Cancer can be in remission, or a period of time when the cancer is responding to treatment or is under control, and then return at a later time.

Preexisting Medical Conditions: Preexisting medical conditions can increase an individual's risk of developing various forms of cancer. Inflammatory bowel diseases such as ulcerative colitis and Crohn's disease increase the risk of colon cancer. Individuals with diabetes have as high as a 40% increased risk of developing colorectal cancer. A recent report found that men with testicular cancer had a higher rate of colorectal cancer. Men who receive radiation therapy for prostate cancer have also been reported to have a higher risk of rectal cancer.

Ethnicity: Some research suggests that ethnicity may play a role in the development of various types of cancer. However, it is important to note that the following statistics may be correlations that do no necessarily have to do with ethnicity/genetics, but may be influenced by social factors associated with people of certain ethnicities (such as diet, access to healthcare, and quality of healthcare). Caucasian families have about a 17% risk for developing lung cancer, while African-Americans have a much higher risk, around 25%. Jews of Eastern European descent (Ashkenazi Jews) have a higher incidence of developing colon cancer. Caucasian women are more likely to develop breast cancer than African-American or Latino women. In the United States, African-American men have a 60% higher incidence rate of developing prostate cancer as compared to Caucasian men.

Sun Exposure: Individuals who spend a considerable amount of time in the sun can develop skin cancer, especially if the skin is not protected by sunscreen or clothing. Ultraviolet (UV) rays from the sun can damage the DNA of skin cells and cause the mutation into cancerous cells. Tanning is the skin's injury response to excessive UV radiation and increases the risk of skin cancer. Every time an individual gets sunburned or is exposed to too much UV radiation, there is an increased risk of damaging skin cells and developing skin cancer. One or more severe, blistering sunburns can increase the risk of skin cancer as an adult.

Tobacco: Smoking cessation decreases the risk for developing various types of cancer. According to the National Cancer Institute, smoking causes

30% of all cancer deaths in the United States and is responsible for 87% of cases of lung cancer. Smoking affects the lungs and kidneys and has been reported to cause pancreatic, cervical, and stomach cancers and acute myeloid leukemia. Cancers of the mouth, larynx, bladder, cervix, and esophagus are also related to tobacco. A study found that exposure to secondhand smoke increases the risk of breast cancer in premenopausal women and lung cancer in the general population.

Weak Immune System: Individuals with a weakened immune system, including those living with human immunodeficiency virus (HIV) or acquired immunodeficiency syndrome (AIDS), leukemia, and those taking immunosuppressant drugs after an organ transplant, are at a greater risk for developing certain types of cancer, including skin cancer.

Viral Infections: Practicing unsafe sex can increase the risk of developing human papillomavirus (HPV). HPV is a group of over 100 viruses that increases the risk of developing cervical, anal, vulvar, and vaginal cancer. Hepatitis B virus can cause liver cancer. Some human retroviruses cause lymphomas and other cancers of the blood system. Some viruses produce cancer in certain countries but not in others. For instance, the Epstein-Barr virus causes Burkitt's lymphoma (a type of cancer) in Africa and cancers of the nose and pharynx in China.

SIGNS AND SYMPTOMS

There are over 100 different types of cancer. They are all unique with their own symptoms and characteristics. Each cancer affects the body in a different way. Although cancers differ greatly, there are a few cancer symptoms that are commonly experienced by most cancer patients. Symptoms can be general (also called nonspecific), such as pain or unexplained weight loss. Other symptoms are more specific, such as unusual bleeding in the vagina, common in vaginal cancer, or difficulty swallowing, common in esophageal cancer.

Nonspecific Symptoms

Depression: Cancer often results in depression. Depression can be related to the symptoms of the illness, a fear of dying, or a loss of independence. Additionally, some cancers may produce tumors that directly cause depression by affecting normal brain function.

Fatigue: Fatigue, or extreme tiredness, is one of the most commonly experienced symptoms of cancer. Fatigue may occur early in cancers that cause a chronic loss of blood, including colon or stomach cancers and leukemia. Fatigue is usually more common when the cancer is advanced but still occurs in the early stages.

Fever: Most cancer patients experience a fever at some point, particularly if the cancer or its treatment (including chemotherapy and radiation) affects the immune system and reduces resistance to infection. Less often, fever may be an early sign of cancer, such as with leukemia or lymphoma.

Neurological and Muscular Symptoms: Cancer can grow directly onto or compress nerves, causing any of several neurological and muscular symptoms, including a change in sensation (such as tingling sensations) or muscle weakness. When a cancer grows in the brain, symptoms may be hard to pinpoint but can include confusion, dizziness, headaches, nausea, changes in vision, and seizures.

Pain: Pain is normally present when cancer progresses. However, pain can be present early on in some cancers, such as bone or testicular cancers.

Respiratory Symptoms: Cancer can compress or block physical structures, such as the airways in the lungs or trachea, causing shortness of breath, cough, or pneumonia. Shortness of breath can also occur when the cancer causes a fluid or bleeding into the lungs or anemia (a lack of red blood cells, which carry oxygen to tissues).

Skin Changes: Skin changes such as jaundice, hyperpigmentation (darkening of the skin), abnormal hair growth, erythema (reddening), boils, and skin itchiness can indicate certain types of cancers.

Unintentional Weight Loss: Most individuals with cancer will lose weight at some time with their disease. Losing 10 or more pounds without dieting or intending to lose weight can be one of the first symptoms experienced with cancer, particularly cancers of the pancreas, stomach, esophagus, or lung.

Specific Symptoms

Bladder Cancer: Individuals with bladder cancer may have blood in the urine, pain or burning upon urination, frequent urination, or cloudy urine.

Bone Cancer: Individuals with bone cancer may often experience pain in the bone or swelling around the affected site, fractures in bones, weakness, fatigue, weight loss, repeated infections, nausea, vomiting, constipation, problems with urination, weakness or numbness in the legs, and/or bumps and bruises that do not heal easily.

Brain Cancer: Individuals with brain cancer often experience dizziness, drowsiness, abnormal eye movements or changes in vision, weakness, loss of feeling in arms or legs or difficulties in walking, fits or convulsions, changes in personality, changes in memory or speech, headaches that tend to be worse in the morning and ease during the day, and headaches that may be accompanied by nausea or vomiting.

Breast Cancer: Although most lumps are not cancerous, individuals with breast cancer may have a lump or thickening of the breast; the most common sign of breast cancer for both men and women is a lump or thickening in the breast. Often the lump is painless. Other symptoms of breast cancer may include a spontaneous clear or bloody discharge from the nipple often associated with a breast lump, retraction, or indentation of the nipple; a change in the size or contours of the breast; flattening or indentation of the skin over the breast; and redness or pitting of the skin over the breast (similar to the skin of an orange).

Colorectal Cancer: Individuals with colorectal cancer often experience rectal bleeding (red blood in stools or black stools), abdominal cramps, constipation alternating with diarrhea, weight loss, loss of appetite, weakness, changes in bowel habits, or pale complexion.

Kidney Cancer: Individuals with kidney cancer often experience blood in urine, dull ache or pain in the back or side, or a lump in the kidney area, sometimes accompanied by high blood pressure or abnormality in red blood cell count.

Leukemia: Individuals with leukemia often experience weakness; paleness; fever and flulike symptoms; bruising and prolonged bleeding; enlarged lymph nodes, spleen, or liver; pain in bones and joints; frequent infections; weight loss; or night sweats.

Lung Cancer: Individuals with lung cancer often experience a wheezing, persistent cough for months, blood-streaked sputum, persistent ache in chest, congestion in lungs, or enlarged lymph nodes in the neck.

Melanoma: Individuals with melanoma often experience a change in a mole or other bump on the skin, including bleeding or change in size, shape, color, or texture.

Non-Hodgkin's Lymphoma: Individuals with non-Hodgkin's lymphoma often experience painless swelling in the lymph nodes in the neck, underarm, or groin; persistent fever; feeling of fatigue; unexplained weight loss; itchy skin and rashes; small lumps in skin; bone pain; swelling in the abdomen; and liver or spleen enlargement.

Oral Cancer: Individuals with oral cancer often experience a lump in the mouth; ulceration of the lip, tongue, or inside of the mouth that does not heal within a couple of weeks; dentures that no longer fit well; or oral pain, bleeding, foul breath, loose teeth, and changes in speech.

Ovarian Cancer: Individuals with ovarian cancer often experience abdominal swelling, abnormal vaginal bleeding (in rare cases), and digestive discomfort.

Pancreatic Cancer: Individuals with pancreatic cancer often experience upper abdominal pain and unexplained weight loss; pain near the center of the back; inability to eat fatty foods without experiencing gas, bloating, nausea, or vomiting; yellowing of the skin; abdominal masses; and enlargement of liver and spleen.

Prostate Cancer: Individuals with prostate cancer often experience urination difficulties due to blockage of the urethra, urinary retention creating frequent feelings of urgency to urinate, especially at night, incomplete bladder emptying, burning or painful urination bloody urine, tenderness over the bladder, and dull ache in the pelvis or back.

Stomach Cancer: Individuals with stomach cancer often experience indigestion or heartburn, discomfort or pain in the abdomen, nausea and vomiting, diarrhea or constipation, bloating after meals, loss of appetite, weakness and fatigue, and bleeding such as vomiting blood or blood in the stool.

Uterine Cancer: Individuals with uterine cancer often experience abnormal vaginal bleeding, a watery bloody discharge in postmenopausal women, painful urination, pain during intercourse, and pain in the pelvic area.

Cancer Remission: Remission is a period of time when the cancer is responding to treatment or is under control. Cancer cells stop growing out of control. In a complete remission, all the signs and symptoms of the disease disappear. It is also possible for a patient to have a partial remission in which the cancer shrinks but does not completely disappear. Remissions can last anywhere from several weeks to many years. Complete remissions may continue for years and be considered cures. If the disease returns, another remission often can occur with further treatment. A cancer that has recurred may respond to a different type of therapy, including a different drug combination. Recurrence of cancer may not respond to the same medications and treatments as the cancer did before remission.

Spontaneous remission of cancer refers to exceptional and unexplained partial or complete disappearance of cancer without medical intervention.

DIAGNOSIS

Cancer is diagnosed based on an individual's symptoms, the results of a physical examination, and sometimes the results of screening tests. Confirmation that cancer is present requires diagnostic tests.

Screening

Screening tests serve to detect the possibility that a cancer is present before symptoms occur. Screening tests are an important prophylactic measure for detecting cancer early, and healthcare professionals recommend cancer screening. Screening tests usually are not perfect; results are confirmed or disproved with further examinations and tests. Diagnostic tests are performed once a doctor suspects that an individual has cancer.

Although screening tests can help save lives, they can be costly and can produce false-positive results or results that suggest a cancer is present when it actually is not. False-positive results can create undue psychological stress and can lead to other tests that are expensive and risky. Screening tests can also produce false-negative results, or results that show no presence of a cancer that is actually present. However, cancer screening is important for individuals with risk factors for cancer, including age, race, heredity, and lifestyle (such as smoking, lack of exercise, or being overweight). The American Cancer Society has cancer screening guidelines that are widely used by healthcare providers.

Recommendations for cancer screening are influenced by many factors, including age, race, previous medical history, and lifestyle. These screening recommendations are for individuals with no symptoms and with an average risk of cancer. For individuals with a higher risk, such as those with a strong family history of certain cancers or those who have had a previous cancer, screening may be recommended more frequently or to start at a younger age. Screening tests other than those listed here may also be recommended. An individual's physician will help decide when to begin screening and which tests should be used.

Breast Cancer: Breast self-examination is recommended monthly after age 20. A physical examination by a healthcare provider is recommended every three years between the ages of 20 and 39, then yearly. A mammography is recommended yearly starting at age 40.

Cervical Cancer: A Papanicolaou (Pap) test is recommended yearly for individuals younger than 30 years of age. Some women 65-70 years of age or older who have had three or more normal Pap tests in a row may choose to stop having cervical cancer screening. For women over 30, some doctors recommend testing every three years with a conventional Pap test plus the human papillomavirus DNA test.

Lung Cancer: Chest x-ray, sputum cytology (examining the sputum for changes in cells), and computed tomography (CT) are not recommended on a routine basis. If an individual presents with symptoms of lung cancer, such as persistent hoarseness or cough, these tests may be performed.

Prostate Cancer: A rectal examination is recommended yearly for men after age 50. A prostate-specific antigen blood test is also recommended yearly after age 50.

Rectal and Colon Cancer: A stool examination for occult (hidden) blood should be performed yearly after age 50. A sigmoidoscopic examination should be performed every five years beginning at age 50, or a colonoscopic examination every 10 years beginning at age 50. In a sigmoidoscopic exam, the doctor uses a flexible, slender, and lighted tube to examine the rectum and sigmoid colon (approximately the last two feet of the colon). The test is fast but can sometimes be uncomfortable. If a polyp or colon cancer is found during this exam, the doctor will recommend a colonoscopy to look at the entire colon and remove any polyps for further examination under a microscope.

Skin Cancer: A physical examination should be part of a routine checkup. More frequent examinations may be needed for individuals at high risk for developing skin cancer, such as those with fair skin or frequent sunburns. Whole-body photography is not routinely needed, although it may be helpful for those with multiple moles or in whom examination of the skin is difficult.

Diagnosis

Generally, when a doctor first suspects cancer, some type of imaging study, such as x-ray, ultrasonography, CT, or magnetic resonance imaging is performed. Although these tests can show the presence, location, and size of an abnormal mass, they usually cannot confirm that cancer is the cause. Cancer is confirmed by finding cancer cells on microscopic examination of samples from the suspected area. Usually, the sample must be a piece of tissue, although sometimes examination of the blood is enough (such as in leukemia). Obtaining a tissue sample is termed a biopsy. Biopsies can be performed by cutting out a small piece of tissue with a scalpel (surgical knife), but very commonly the sample is obtained using a hollow needle. Such tests are commonly done without the need for an overnight hospital stay and are called outpatient procedures. Doctors often use ultrasonography or a CT scan to guide the needle to the right location. Because biopsies can be painful, the individual is usually given a local anesthetic (such as lidocaine [Xylocaine]) to numb the area.

In cases with findings on examination or imaging tests that suggest cancer, measuring blood levels of tumor markers may provide additional evidence for or against the diagnosis of cancer. Tumor markers are substances produced by tumor cells or by other cells of the body in response to cancer or certain benign (noncancerous) conditions. Tumor markers can be found in the blood, the urine, the tumor tissue, or in other tissues. Different tumor markers are found in different types of cancer, and levels of the same tumor marker can be altered in more than one type of cancer. In addition, tumor marker levels are not altered in all people with cancer, especially if the cancer is early stage. Some tumor marker levels can also be altered in patients with noncancerous conditions. In individuals who have been diagnosed with certain types of cancer, tumor markers may be useful to monitor the effectiveness of treatment and to detect possible recurrence of the cancer. For some cancers, the level of a tumor marker drops following treatment and increases if the cancer recurs. Common cancer tumor markers include: alpha-fetoprotein, which may be raised in individuals with colon cancer; β_2-microglobulin, which may occur in individuals with multiple myeloma; carcinoembryonic antigen, which may be raised in individuals with colon cancer; prostate-specific antigen, which may be increased in individuals with prostate cancer; and carbohydrate antigen 27.29, which may be increased in individuals with breast cancer. Using tumor markers for cancer diagnosis is beneficial because of the ease of obtaining and measuring their presence; also, there is less discomfort for patients.

Staging

After cancer is diagnosed, it is staged. Staging is the process of finding out how far the cancer has spread. Staging the cancer is a vital step in determining the treatment choices, and it will also give the healthcare team a clearer idea of the outlook for recovery. There can be several different processes for staging each individual cancer, such as with brain cancer, lymphoma, or melanoma.

The TNM system is the most widely used staging. The "T" describes the size of the tumor, and whether the cancer has invaded nearby tissues and organs. The "N" describes how far the cancer has spread to nearby lymph nodes. The "M" shows whether the cancer has metastasized (spread) to other organs of the body. Once the TNM descriptions have been established, they can be grouped together into a simpler set of stages, stages 0 through stage IV (0-4). In general, the lower the number, the less the cancer has spread. A higher number, such as stage IV (4), means a more serious, widespread cancer. A T1N2M0 cancer would be a cancer with a T1 tumor, N2 involvement of the lymph nodes, and no metastases (no spreading through the body).

COMPLICATIONS

Metastasis: Metastasis (spreading) to other organs, such as the liver, pancreas, lungs, and lymph nodes, may occur, causing an increased chance of death. Metastasis allows cancerous cells to spread to other tissues in the body and more than one body system, causing damage.

Cardiac Tamponade: Cardiac tamponade occurs when fluid accumulates in the pericardium, the baglike structure surrounding the heart. This fluid puts pressure on the heart and interferes with its ability to pump blood. Fluid can accumulate when a cancer invades and irritates the pericardium.

Pleural Effusion: Pleural effusion occurs when fluid accumulates in the pleural cavity surrounding the lungs, causing shortness of breath.

Superior Vena Cava Syndrome: Superior vena cava syndrome occurs when cancer partially or completely blocks the superior vena cava, which is a vein that drains blood from the upper part of the body into the heart. Blockage of the superior vena cava causes the veins in the upper part of the chest and neck to swell, resulting in swelling of the face, neck, and upper part of the chest.

Spinal Cord Compression: Spinal cord compression occurs when cancer compresses the spinal cord or the spinal cord nerves, resulting in pain and loss of function (such as urinary or fecal incontinence). The longer the compression of the spinal cord or spinal cord nerves persists, the less likely normal nerve function will return when the compression is relieved.

Brain Dysfunction: Brain dysfunction occurs when the brain functions abnormally as a result of a cancer growing within the brain, either as a primary brain cancer or more commonly as a metastasis from a cancer elsewhere in the body. Tumors may develop and put pressure on sensitive nerves and blood vessels, causing symptoms such as confusion, drowsiness, agitation, headaches, abnormal vision, abnormal sensations, weakness, nausea, vomiting, and seizures.

Bleeding: At first, a cancer may bleed slightly because its cells are not well attached to each other and its blood vessels are fragile. Later, as the cancer enlarges and invades surrounding tissues, it may grow into a nearby blood vessel, causing bleeding. The bleeding may be slight and undetectable or detectable only with testing. Such is often the case in early-stage colon cancer. Or, particularly with advanced cancer, the bleeding may be more significant, even massive and life threatening. The site of the cancer determines the site of the bleeding. Cancer anywhere along the gastrointestinal tract can cause bleeding in the stool. Cancer anywhere along the urinary tract can cause bleeding in the urine. Other cancers can bleed into internal areas of the body. Bleeding into the lungs can cause the individual to cough up blood.

TREATMENT

The number of treatment choices an individual has will depend on the type of cancer, the stage of the cancer, and other individual factors such as age, health status, and personal preferences. Individuals should discuss all treatment options with their cancer team. It is important to ask questions and to understand all the cancer treatment options available.

The four major types of treatment for cancer are surgery, radiation, chemotherapy, and biological therapies. The specific cancer treatment will be based on the individual's needs. Certain types of cancer respond very differently to different types of treatment, so determining the type of cancer is a vital step toward knowing which treatments will be most effective. The cancer's stage (how widespread it is) will also determine the best course of treatment, since early-stage cancers respond to different therapies than later-stage ones. The individual's overall health, lifestyle, and personal preferences will also play a part in deciding which treatment options will be best.

It is important for individuals to understand the goals of treatment. The treatment can either be palliative, which helps control symptoms (such as pain), or curative, which may help cure the cancer and decrease the chances of it returning. The goal of cancer treatments and therapies is to increase the quality of life for the individual suffering from this condition.

Chemotherapy

While surgery and radiation therapy are used to treat localized cancers, chemotherapy is used to treat cancer cells that have metastasized (spread) to other parts of the body. Chemotherapy is also used in combination with surgery and/or radiation or to shrink tumors, which helps surgery be easier on the patient and safer. Depending on the type of cancer and its stage of development, chemotherapy can be used to cure cancer, to keep the cancer from spreading, to slow the cancer's growth, to kill cancer cells that may have spread to other parts of the body, or to relieve symptoms caused by cancer. Not all individuals will respond the same way to chemotherapy treatments, and some individuals will have more success than others.

Prior to Chemotherapy: The individual undergoing chemotherapy may be asked to take some medications prior to the procedure (called premedications), including steroids, such as prednisone (Deltasone) or hydrocortisone (Solu-Medrol); antihistamines (allergy medications), such as diphenhydramine (Benadryl); antinausea medications, such as ondansetron (Zofran); sedatives, such as alprazolam (Xanax); or antibiotics, such as levofloxacin (Levaquin).

During Chemotherapy: Individuals will be given the chemotherapy medication(s) by whichever route the doctor thinks best. Chemotherapy drugs can be given by mouth, injected through a syringe into a vein, artery, or muscle; given intravenously through a drip device; placed into a catheter (tube) that goes into the bladder, chest cavity, brain, spinal cord, liver, or abdomen; or, they can be applied to the skin. The decision on what route to use depends on several factors, mainly the type of tumor and the drug being used.

At the same time, individuals may be given other medications to fight the side effects of chemotherapy, including steroids, allergy medications (antihistamines), antinausea medications, sedatives, and antibiotics.

Chemotherapy Drugs: Almost all chemotherapy agents currently available kill cancer cells by affecting DNA synthesis or function, a process that occurs through the cell cycle. Each drug varies in the way this occurs within the cell cycle.

The major categories of chemotherapy agents are alkylating agents, antimetabolites, plant alkaloids, antitumor antibiotics, and steroid hormones. Each drug is categorized according to its effect on the cell cycle and cell chemistry.

Alkylating agents kill cells by directly attacking DNA. Alkylating agents may be used in the treatment of chronic leukemias; Hodgkin's disease; lymphomas; and certain carcinomas of the lungs, breasts, prostate, and ovaries. Cyclophosphamide (Cytoxan) is an example of a commonly used alkylating agent.

Nitrosoureas act similarly to alkylating agents and also inhibit changes necessary for DNA repair. These agents cross the blood-brain barrier and are therefore used to treat brain tumors, lymphomas, multiple myeloma, and malignant melanoma. Carmustine (BCNU, BiCNU) and lomustine (CCNU, CeeNU) are the major drugs in this category.

Antimetabolites are drugs that block cell growth by interfering with certain activities, usually DNA synthesis. Once ingested into the cell, they halt normal development and reproduction. Antimetabolites may be used in the treatment of acute and chronic leukemias; choriocarcinoma; and some tumors of the gastrointestinal tract, breast, and ovary. Examples of commonly used antimetabolites are 6-mercaptopurine (Purinethol) and 5-fluorouracil (5FU, Leucovorin).

Antitumor antibiotics are a diverse group of compounds. In general, they act by binding with DNA and preventing RNA synthesis. These agents are widely used in the treatment of a variety of cancers. The most commonly used drugs in this group are doxorubicin (Adriamycin), mitomycin-C (Mutamycin), and bleomycin (Blenoxane).

Plant (vinca) alkaloids are antitumor agents derived from the periwinkle plant (*Vinca* spp.). These drugs act specifically by blocking cell division during mitosis (a stage of division). They are commonly used in the treatment of acute lymphoblastic leukemia; Hodgkin's and non-Hodgkin's lymphomas; neuroblastomas; Wilms' tumor; and cancers of the lungs, breasts, and testes. Vincristine (Oncovin) and vinblastine (Velbe) are commonly used agents in this group.

Steroid hormones are useful in treating some types of tumors. This class includes adrenocorticosteroids, estrogens, antiestrogens, progesterones, and androgens. Although their specific mechanism of action is not clear, steroid hormones modify the growth of certain hormone-dependent cancers. Tamoxifen (Nolvadex) is an example used for estrogen-dependent breast cancer.

Platinum-based chemotherapy drugs contain the metal platinum. They are used to treat various types of cancers, including sarcomas, some carcinomas (e.g., small-cell lung cancer and ovarian cancer), lymphomas, and germ cell tumors. Examples include cisplatin (Platinol), carboplatin (Paraplatin), and oxaliplatin (Eloxatin).

Often, a combination of chemotherapy is used instead of a single drug. Chemotherapy is given in cycles, each followed by a recovery period. The total course of chemotherapy is often about six months, usually ranging from three to nine months. After a cancer is removed by surgery, chemotherapy can significantly reduce the risk of cancer returning. The chances of cancer returning and the potential benefit of chemotherapy depend on the type of cancer and other individual factors.

After Chemotherapy: After chemotherapy, individuals may be given any of the following medications: antinausea drugs, injections of immune-system boosting drugs (to increase white blood cells that fight potential infections) several days after the chemotherapy has been given, or other drugs, including steroids, antihistamines, antinausea medications, sedatives, and/or antibiotics.

Side Effects of Chemotherapy: A major concern with chemotherapy is the possibility of long-term side effects and complications, such as heart damage, lung damage, liver damage, and secondary cancers (including leukemia). Although these severe effects occur in only a small number of people, great effort is being put into finding equally effective regimens with less toxicity. Drug regimens have been developed that substantially diminish the likelihood of long-range,

life-threatening complications, including acute leukemia in people who have received multiple courses of chemotherapy and radiation therapy.

Side effects of chemotherapy depend on the type of drugs, the amounts taken, and the length of treatment. The most common are nausea and vomiting, temporary hair loss, increased chance of infections, and fatigue (extreme tiredness). Many of these side effects can be uncomfortable or emotionally upsetting. However, most side effects can be controlled with medicines, supportive care measures, or changing the treatment schedule.

Fatigue is one of the most common side effects of radiation and chemotherapy. Like most other side effects, fatigue will usually disappear once the treatment is complete. Individuals need to get plenty of rest, eat a well-balanced diet (less meat, dairy, and fat and more vegetables), and drink plenty of water.

Hair loss may occur with some types of chemotherapy. Some individuals experience hair loss during chemotherapy treatments (and sometimes with radiation treatment to the head) while others do not, even with the same drugs. If hair loss does occur, it usually begins within two weeks of the start of therapy and gets worse one to two months after the start of therapy. Hair growth often begins even before therapy is completed. Most people are able to find suitable ways of managing the hair loss until it grows back, with specially designed hats, scarves, and wigs.

Medications for Side Effects of Chemotherapy: Some individuals who experience certain side effects of chemotherapy may be prescribed medications to counteract these effects. Several drugs are now available for use alone or in combination to help reduce a few of the most common side effects, such as nausea, vomiting, and fatigue.

Dolasetron Mesylate (Anzemet): Dolasetron mesylate helps prevent and relieve nausea and vomiting from surgery or chemotherapy. Researchers believe that nausea and vomiting during chemotherapy is associated with the release of serotonin from special cells in the small intestine. Dolasetron mesylate blocks these nerve endings in the intestine and prevents signals to the central nervous system. Dolasetron mesylate is available in tablet form and by injection.

Prochlorperazine (Compazine): Prochlorperazine helps control nausea and vomiting after surgery or chemotherapy. Prochlorperazine is available in capsule, tablet, and liquid form and by suppository or injection. Prochlorperazine can cause drowsiness and may interact with other medications or alcohol.

Granisetron Hydrochloride (Kytril): Granisetron hydrochloride is an antinausea medication approved by the FDA for patients undergoing chemotherapy. Granisetron hydrochloride is typically given 60 minutes before chemotherapy. In some cases, a second dose is given about 12 hours after the first dose. Granisetron hydrochloride is available in tablet form and by injection.

Promethazine (Phenergan): Promethazine has sedative, antihistamine, and mild antinausea properties. It may be used to help prevent or treat nausea due to chemotherapy. Promethazine may be available in tablet form or as an oral syrup, suppository, or injection.

Epoetin Alfa (Procrit): Epoetin alfa helps the body produce more red blood cells, which helps relieve fatigue due to chemotherapy. Since chemotherapy affects both normal and cancerous cells, it can decrease the number of red blood cells, which leads to anemia (lack of red blood cells to carry oxygen) and a feeling of extreme tiredness.

Filgrastim (Neupogen): Filgrastim is the name for granulocyte colony stimulating factor. Filgrastim is a protein-based drug that stimulates the production of white blood cells. White blood cells are important for protecting the body from infection. Filgrastim is used to increase white blood cells and to decrease the risk of infection in conditions such as cancer. Filgrastim can be used subcutaneously or intravenously. Side effects may include nausea, bone pain, and swelling or redness at the injection site. Contacting a doctor immediately is recommended by healthcare providers if the individual develops a fever, chills, sore throat, congestion, or diarrhea or redness, pain, or swelling around a wound or sore while using filgrastim.

Ondansetron (Zofran): Ondansetron helps to relieve nausea and vomiting associated with chemotherapy. Ondansetron is available in pill form, as a liquid solution, and by injection. The first dose of ondansetron (tablet form) is usually administered 30 minutes before chemotherapy and then at regular intervals for one to two days after chemotherapy.

Myelodysplastic Syndromes: Myelodysplastic syndromes are diseases of the blood and bone marrow, often caused by chemotherapy. Blood cells, such as red blood cells that carry oxygen to tissues and white blood cells that help produce cells for immunity, are damaged by chemotherapy medicines. Symptoms of myelodysplastic syndrome include fatigue and chronic tiredness, shortness of breath, chilled sensation, chest pain (occasionally), an increased susceptibility to infection, and an increased

susceptibility to bleeding. Patients who experience low blood cells counts during chemotherapy may also be given medications to help raise blood cell or platelet counts. For example, patients who suffer from neutropenia, a decrease in the number of neutrophils (a type of white blood cell), may be given certain growth factors, such as the granulocyte-macrophage colony stimulating factor (sargramostim [Leukine]) or filgrastim.

Radiation Therapy

Radiation therapy uses high-energy rays to kill cancer cells. It is considered a local therapy, meaning that it should be used to target areas of the body invaded by tumor masses. A radiation oncologist will plan and supervise therapy. The area to be treated will be carefully mapped out and the treatment machine will be adjusted so that only the lymphoma cells are exposed to a full dose of radiotherapy. Because of the need to target the radiation at exactly the right area of the body, a mold is sometimes made that will help to hold that part of the body still and in position during the treatment sessions.

Normal cells surrounding the lymphoma are spared the full dose, and these cells are usually able to repair themselves more easily than lymphoma cells. Therefore, radiotherapy can often control or destroy lymphoma cells, while causing only temporary damage to normal cells.

Radiotherapy is usually given on an outpatient basis, with the patient visiting the hospital up to five times a week. Before each treatment, the patient is carefully positioned, usually lying on a treatment table. Parts of the body that are not being treated may be covered. It is important to remain completely still during the treatment. Each treatment usually lasts only a few minutes and causes no discomfort. Although the patient is left alone during the actual treatment, the radiotherapy technician watches from an observation room and it is possible to talk to the individual through a microphone. A course of radiotherapy typically lasts between two and six weeks, depending on the patient's individual circumstances. The length of radiation treatment varies depending on the stage of the disease. Radiation therapy may be used alone, but is commonly used in conjunction with chemotherapy.

Depending on how and where the radiation is administered, it may cause certain side effects such as fatigue (extreme tiredness), loss of appetite, nausea, diarrhea, and skin problems. Radiation of lymph node areas may result in suppression of the immune system to varying degrees. Irradiation of the underlying bone and the marrow within the bone may result in suppression of the blood count.

Surgery

Surgery is the treatment of choice for many types of cancer, such as colon or breast. Treatment depends on the stage of the disease and the overall health of the patient. Chemotherapy and radiation therapy may be used as adjuvant treatment or in addition to surgery.

Cryosurgery: During cryosurgery, a doctor uses very cold material, such as liquid nitrogen spray, or a cold probe to freeze and destroy cancer cells or cells that may become cancerous (such as irregular cells in the cervix that could become cervical cancer).

Electrosurgery: Electrosurgery is the application of high-frequency electrical currents by a doctor. These currents can kill cancer cells, such as in the mouth or on the skin.

Laser Surgery: Laser surgery is used to treat many types of cancer. Laser therapy uses high-intensity light to treat cancer and other illnesses. Lasers can be used to shrink or destroy tumors. Lasers are most commonly used to treat superficial cancers (cancers on the surface of the body or the lining of internal organs) such as basal cell skin cancer and the very early stages of some cancers, such as cervical, penile, vaginal, vulvar, and non–small-cell lung cancer.

Mohs' Surgery: Mohs' surgery is useful for removing cancer from sensitive areas such as near the eye. Mohs' surgery is also useful for assessing how deep a cancer is growing. Mohs' surgery is performed by carefully removing cancer layer by layer with a scalpel or knife. After removing a layer, the doctor will evaluate the cells under a microscope until all the abnormal cells have been removed and the surrounding tissue shows no evidence of cancer.

Laparoscopic Surgery: In laparoscopic surgery (or minimally invasive surgery), a surgeon uses a laparoscope to see inside the body without making large incisions. A laparoscope is a telescopic rod lens system that is usually connected to a video camera. Several small incisions are made and a tiny camera and surgical tools are inserted into the body. The surgeon watches a monitor that projects what the camera sees inside the body. The smaller incisions mean faster recovery and a reduced risk of complications. Laparoscopic surgery is used in cancer diagnosis, staging, treatment, and symptom relief.

Robotic Surgery: In robotic surgery, the surgeon sits away from the operating table and watches a screen that projects a three-dimensional image of the area being operated on. The surgeon uses hand controls that tell a robot how to maneuver surgical tools to perform the operation. Robotic surgery helps the surgeon operate in hard-to-reach areas. But robotic surgical systems are expensive and require specialized training, so robotic surgery is only available in specialized medical centers.

C

Clinical Trials

Human studies of promising new or experimental treatments are known as clinical trials. A clinical trial is only done when there is some reason to believe that the treatment being studied may be valuable to the patient. Treatments used in clinical trials are often found to have real benefits. Clinical trials are not commonly used as treatments for cancer, but are an option. A doctor will help get information on various clinical trials available for certain types of cancer. There is no guarantee of success in clinical trials for the patients, and some individuals will actually not receive medication (the placebo).

Types of Clinical Trials: There are three phases of clinical trials in which a treatment is studied before it can be approved by the FDA.

Phase I Clinical Trials: The purpose of a phase I study is to find the best way to give a new treatment and find out how much of it can be given safely. Doctors watch patients carefully for any harmful side effects. The treatment has been well tested in lab and animal studies, but the side effects in patients are not completely known. Doctors running the clinical trial start by giving very low doses of the drug to the first patients and increasing the dose for later groups of patients until side effects appear. Although doctors are hoping to help patients, the main purpose of a phase I study is to test the safety of the drug.

Phase II Clinical Trials: These studies are designed to see if the drug works. Patients are given the best dose of the drug (based on the results of the phase I study) and closely observed for an effect on the cancer. The doctors will also look for side effects.

Phase III Clinical Trials: Phase III studies are done to see if the new treatment is better than what is already available. They involve large numbers of patients. One group (the control group) receives the standard (most accepted) treatment. The other group receives the new treatment. All patients in phase III studies are closely watched. The study will be stopped if the side effects of the new treatment are too severe or if one group has had much better results than the others.

If an individual enrolls in a clinical trial, a team of experts will monitor their progress very carefully. The study is especially designed to pay close attention to the individual with cancer. However, there may be risks. Even with animal testing and laboratory studies, it is difficult to determine what side effects may occur in individuals undergoing clinical trials for cancer. It is important to discuss all potential risks and benefits carefully with a healthcare provider before making a decision to enroll in a clinical trial.

Other Therapies

Photodynamic Therapy (PDT): PDT is another type of cancer treatment that uses lasers. In PDT, a drug called a photosensitizer or photosensitizing agent is injected into a patient and absorbed by cells all over the individual's body. After a couple of days, the agent is found mostly in cancer cells. Laser light is then used to activate the agent and destroy cancer cells. Because the photosensitizer makes the skin and eyes sensitive to light for approximately six weeks, individuals undergoing PDT are advised to avoid direct sunlight and bright indoor light during that time.

Perillyl Alcohol: Perillyl alcohol is a naturally occurring chemical with anticancer activity. Perillyl alcohol is found in lavender, cherries, and mint. The use of perillyl alcohol for cancer treatments is in phase I clinical trials.

Laetrile: Laetrile is a substance derived from a chemical called amygdalin, which is found in the seeds of apricots, plums, and bitter almonds. Laetrile is publicized as an antineoplastic (prevents the development of a tumor or neoplasm) drug, although there is no supporting evidence.

Pain Control

Pain may be acute or chronic. Acute pain is severe and lasts a relatively short time. It is usually a signal that body tissue is being injured in some way, and the pain generally disappears when the injury heals. Chronic or persistent pain may range from mild to severe, and it is present to some degree for long periods of time. Some individuals with chronic pain that is controlled by medicine can have breakthrough pain. This occurs when moderate to severe pain "breaks through" or is felt for a short time. Breakthrough pain may occur several times a day, even when the proper dose of medicine is given for chronic and persistent pain.

Pain may be caused by the cancer itself. Whether the individual has pain and the amount of pain he or she has may depend on the type of cancer, the stage (extent) of the disease, and the individual's pain threshold (tolerance for pain). Most of the pain comes when a tumor presses on bones, nerves, or body organs. Pain can also be caused by the treatment or procedures for diagnosing cancer.

Cancer pain is usually treated with analgesic (pain relieving) drugs, both prescription and nonprescription, and with nondrug treatments such as relaxation techniques, biofeedback, imagery, and others. Healthcare providers recommend asking a doctor or pharmacist for advice before taking any medicine for pain.

Pain will generally be graded on a pain intensity scale. Using a pain scale is helpful in describing how much pain a patient is feeling. Using the pain intensity scale, individuals answer questions and assign a number from zero to 10 according to their pain level. No pain gets a zero, while a 10 is the highest level of pain imaginable. Questions can include the severity of pain, how pain changes with medication, and how bad the pain is during the day and night. If one medicine or treatment does not work for the pain, there is almost always another one that can be tried. Changes may also be made in the frequency and dosages to help increase the pain relief.

Medications for Pain: The type of medicine and the method by which the medicine is given depend on the type and cause of pain. Nonopiate (nonnarcotic) pain medications are given for mild to moderate pain. These drugs can generally be purchased over the counter (OTC) and may include acetaminophen, aspirin, and nonsteroidal antiinflammatory drugs (NSAIDs), such as ibuprofen (Motrin). It is best to check with a healthcare professional before taking any OTC medication. NSAIDs can slow blood clotting, especially if the individual is on chemotherapy due to drug interactions.

For moderate to severe pain, opiate (narcotic) medications may be given. These drugs include morphine (MS Contin), fentanyl (Duragesic), hydromorphone (Dilaudid), and oxycodone (Percocet, OxyContin). Individuals must have a prescription for these medications, and the medications are generally time released, meaning their effects last more than a few hours. Nonopioids may be used along with opioids for moderate to severe pain. Opiate medications may cause side effects such as drowsiness and constipation. Their use may also cause addiction, both physical and psychological, in a short length of time. For breakthrough pain, immediate-release opiates may be given, such as oral morphine (Oramorph) or oxycodone (Roxicodone). A prescription is required for these medicines. A short-acting opioid, which relieves breakthrough pain quickly, needs to be used with a long-acting opioid for persistent pain. It is important to tell a doctor or pharmacist if taking any OTC medication, as some OTC medicines may contain acetaminophen

(Tylenol). Some prescription pain medications, such as oxycodone/acetaminophen combination (Percocet) or hydrocodone/acetaminophen (Lortab, Vicodin) may also contain acetaminophen, thereby increasing the potential for acetaminophen-induced liver toxicity.

Individuals who take opiates for pain sometimes find that over time they need to take larger doses. This may be due to an increase in the pain or the development of drug tolerance. Drug tolerance occurs when the body gets used to the medicine and does not relieve the pain as well as it once did. Many individuals do not develop a tolerance to opiates. If tolerance does develop, usually small increases in the dose or a change in the kind of medicine will help relieve the pain. Increasing the doses of opiates to relieve increasing pain or to overcome drug tolerance does not always lead to addiction. Alcohol should be avoided when taking medications for pain due to a potential for interactions. Using alcohol in combination with pain medications can lead to overdose symptoms such as weakness, difficulty in breathing, confusion, anxiety, or more severe drowsiness or dizziness. It is recommended to use caution when driving automobiles or operating heavy machinery when taking opiate pain medications. Medications for pain may also cause nausea and vomiting in sensitive individuals.

For tingling and burning pain associated with some cancers, antidepressant medications (such as amitriptyline [Elavil]) or anticonvulsant medications (such as gabapentin [Neurontin]) may be used. Both these medications may cause drowsiness and sedation.

For pain caused by swelling, steroid medications, including prednisone (Deltasone), may be used. Side effects of steroid medications include edema (swelling) and a decline in immune system function.

Pain medications may be given by several different routes, including orally (by mouth), topically (on the skin), and rectally (into the anus as a suppository). Pain medications may also be given by injection, including subcutaneous (injected just under the skin using a small needle), intravenous (injection directly into the vein through a needle), intrathecal (placed directly into the fluid around the spinal cord), or epidural injection (into the space around the spinal cord). Patient-controlled analgesia (PCA) pumps may also be used. PCA pumps help control the amount of pain medicine an individual takes. When pain relief is needed, the individual can receive a preset dose of pain medicine by pressing a button on a computerized pump that is connected to a small tube placed in the body in a minor surgical technique.

Nondrug Treatments for Pain: Nondrug treatments are now widely used to help manage cancer pain. There are many techniques that are used alone or along with medicine. Some individuals find they can take a lower dose of medicine with such techniques. These methods include acupuncture, art therapy, focusing, healing touch, prayer, psychotherapy, transcutaneous electrical nerve stimulation, and yoga. See the Integrative Therapies section of this monograph for more information on these techniques.

Support Groups

Resources exist that provide cancer patients and their loved ones with an opportunity to learn ways of coping with the uncertainty that cancer brings and links to support groups that give them a chance to meet others who face similar issues. Support groups offer patients and loved ones emotional support, an opportunity to learn ways of coping with the uncertainty and changes in their lives, a chance to meet others who face similar issues, and a time to explore issues faced by all cancer survivors. Support groups for cancer patients can be located by asking a healthcare provider, such as a doctor or social worker, for more information.

INTEGRATIVE THERAPIES
Strong Scientific Evidence

Vitamin A: Vitamin A is a fat-soluble vitamin that is derived from two sources: preformed retinoids and provitamin carotenoids. Retinoids, such as retinal and retinoic acid, are found in animal sources such as livers, kidneys, eggs, and dairy produce. Carotenoids, like beta-carotene (which has the highest vitamin A activity), are found in plants such as dark-green or yellow vegetables and carrots.

The prescription drug all-trans-retinoic acid (ATRA [Vesanoid]) is a vitamin A derivative that is an established treatment for acute promyelocytic leukemia and improves median survival in this disease. Treatment should be under strict medical supervision. Vitamin A supplements should not be used simultaneously with ATRA due to a risk of increased toxicity.

Good Scientific Evidence

Psychotherapy: Psychotherapy is an interactive process between a person and a qualified mental health professional (psychiatrist, psychologist, clinical social worker, licensed counselor, or other trained practitioner). There is good evidence that psychotherapy can enhance cancer patients' quality of life by reducing emotional distress and aiding in coping with the stresses and challenges of cancer. Therapy may be supportive-expressive therapy, cognitive therapy, or group therapy. Studies conflict on whether therapy improves self-esteem, death anxiety, self-satisfaction, etc. While some patients seek psychotherapy in hopes of extending survival, there is no conclusive evidence of effects on medical prognosis.

Unclear or Conflicting Scientific Evidence

Acupuncture: Acupuncture, or the use of needles to manipulate the "chi," or body energy, originated in China over 5,000 years ago. There has been limited research on acupuncture for cancer pain, and the research that was done was shown to have mixed results. More studies are needed to determine potential benefits. Evidence from several small studies supports the use of acupuncture at a specific point on the wrist (P6), which helps reduce the nausea and vomiting associated with chemotherapy.

Aloe: Transparent gel from the pulp of the meaty leaves of *Aloe vera* has been used topically for thousands of years to treat wounds, skin infections, burns, and numerous other dermatologic conditions. Preliminary research suggests that aloe may help prevent or aid in the regression of cancerous tumors. Additional research is needed in this area. Caution is advised when taking aloe supplements, as numerous adverse effects, including a laxative effect, cramping, dehydration, and drug interactions, are possible. Aloe should not be used if the patient is pregnant or breastfeeding unless otherwise directed by a doctor.

American Pawpaw: Evidence supporting the use of the American pawpaw (*Asimina triloba*) tree for the treatment of cancer in humans is largely anecdotal and subjective. Use in humans has reported minimal side effects, and evidence from animal and in vitro studies suggests that American pawpaw extract does have some anticancer activity. Pawpaw standardized extract has been used for 18 months in patients with various forms of cancer. No well-designed studies on the long-term effects of pawpaw extracts have been conducted. Pawpaw should not be used if the patient is pregnant or breastfeeding unless otherwise directed by a doctor.

Antineoplastons: Antineoplastons are a group of naturally occurring peptide fractions isolated from human blood and urine. Antineoplastons were observed by Stanislaw Burzynski in the late 1970s and found to be absent in the urine of cancer patients. There is inconclusive scientific evidence regarding the effectiveness of antineoplastons in the treatment of cancer. Several preliminary human studies (case series, phase I/II trials) have examined antineoplaston types A2, A5, A10, AS2-1, and AS2-5 for a variety of cancer types. It remains unclear if antineoplastons are effective or what doses may be safe. Until better research is available, no clear conclusion can be drawn.

Arabinoxylan: Arabinoxylan is made by altering the outer shell of rice bran using enzymes from *Hyphomycetes mycelia* mushroom extract. Arabinoxylan has been found to improve immune reactions in diabetes and cancer patients. Arabinoxylan products may contain high calcium and phosphorus levels, which may be harmful for patients with compromised renal (kidney) function.

Aromatherapy: Healing with fragrant oils has been used for thousands of years. Aromatherapy is often used in people with chronic illnesses (frequently in combination with massage), with the intention to improve quality of life or well-being. There is not enough scientific evidence in this area to form a firm conclusion about the effectiveness of aromatherapy. Essential oils are not for internal use.

Art Therapy: Art therapy involves the application of a variety of art modalities, including drawing, painting, clay, and sculpture. Art therapy enables the expression of inner thoughts or feelings when verbalization is difficult or not possible. Limited evidence suggests that family caregivers of cancer patients may benefit from art therapy to help them cope with the stress of caregiving. Possible benefits include reduced stress, lowered anxiety, increased positive emotions, and increased positive communication with cancer patients and healthcare professionals. Art therapy may also reduce pain and other symptoms in cancer patients. More studies are needed to determine how best to use this form of intervention with this population.

Astragalus: Astragalus (*Astragalus membranaceus*) has been used in Chinese medicine for centuries for its immunity-enhancing properties. Although early laboratory and animal studies report increased immune cell function and reduced cancer cell growth associated with the use of astragalus, there is no reliable human evidence in these areas. A recent study reports that astragalus-based Chinese herbal medicine may increase effectiveness of platinum-based chemotherapy (such as cisplatin [Platinol]) when combined with chemotherapy. Astragalus is also sometimes used with the intention to reduce side effects of cancer treatments, such as fatigue and weight loss. Due to a lack of well-designed research, a firm conclusion cannot be drawn.

Bee Pollen: Bee pollen is considered a highly nutritious food because it contains a balance of vitamins, minerals, proteins, carbohydrates, fats, enzymes, and essential amino acids. Research has found that bee pollen may reduce some adverse effects of cancer treatment, but additional studies are needed before a firm recommendation can be made. Caution is advised when taking bee pollen supplements as allergic reactions may occur in sensitive individuals. Bee pollen should not be used if the patient is pregnant or breastfeeding unless otherwise directed by a doctor.

Bitter Melon: Bitter melon (*Momordica charantia*) is used in the traditional Ayurvedic form of medicine from India for lowering blood sugar levels. Research has also found that bitter melon extracts may be beneficial in cancer therapies. MAP30, a protein isolated from bitter melon extract, is reported to possess anticancer effects in laboratory studies. Potential anticancer effects have not been studied appropriately in humans. Caution is advised when taking bitter melon supplements, as numerous adverse effects, including blood sugar lowering and drug interactions, are possible. Bitter melon should not be used if the patient is pregnant or breastfeeding unless otherwise directed by a doctor.

Black Tea: Black tea (*Camellia sinensis*) is from the same plant as green tea, but processed differently and contains more caffeine than green tea. Several studies have explored a possible association between regular consumption of black tea and rates of cancer in populations. This research has yielded conflicting results, with some studies suggesting benefits and others reporting no effects. Laboratory and animal studies report that components of tea, such as polyphenols, have antioxidant properties and effects against tumors. Effects in humans remain unclear, and these components may be more common in green tea rather than in black tea. Some animal and laboratory research suggests that components of black tea may actually be carcinogenic, or cancer causing, although effects in humans are not clear. Overall, the relationship of black tea consumption and human cancer remains undetermined.

Bromelain: Bromelain is a sulfur-containing proteolytic digestive enzyme that is extracted from the stem and the fruit of the pineapple plant (*Ananas comosus*). There is not enough information to recommend for or against the use of bromelain in the treatment of cancer, either alone or in addition to other therapies. Caution is advised when taking bromelain supplements, as numerous adverse effects, including blood thinning and drug interactions, are possible.

Cat's Claw: Originally used in Peru, the use of cat's claw (*Uncaria tomentosa*) has been said to date back to the Inca civilization, possibly as far back as 2,000 years. Cat's claw has antiinflammatory properties, and several low-quality studies suggest it may slow tumor growth; however, this research is early and has not identified specific types of cancer that may benefit. A few studies suggest that cat's claw may also boost the immune system. Caution is advised when taking cat's claw supplements, as numerous adverse effects, including blood thinning and drug interactions, are possible. Cat's claw should not be used if the patient is pregnant or breastfeeding unless otherwise directed by a doctor.

Copper: Copper is a mineral that occurs naturally in many foods, including vegetables, legumes, nuts, grains, and fruits as well as shellfish, avocado, and beef (organs such as liver). Preliminary research reports that lowering copper levels theoretically may arrest the progression of cancer by inhibiting blood vessel growth (angiogenesis). Copper intake has not been identified as a risk factor for the development or progression of cancer. Copper is potentially unsafe when used orally in higher doses than the recommended dietary allowance. Copper supplements should not be used if the patient is pregnant or breastfeeding unless otherwise directed by a doctor.

Cranberry: Several laboratory studies have reported positive effects of proanthocyanidins, flavonoid components of cranberry (*Vaccinium macrocarpon*) and other fruits such as blueberries, grape seed, and pomegranate, on health. Based on a small amount of laboratory research, cranberry has been proposed for cancer prevention, but studies are needed in humans before a recommendation can be made.

Echinacea: The evidence from a small number of randomized trials evaluating efficacy of echinacea in the treatment of radiation-induced leukopenia (decrease in white blood cells) is equivocal. Studies have used the combination product Esberitox, which includes extracts of *Echinacea* (*Echinacea purpurea* and *pallida*) root, white cedar (*Thuja occidentalis*) leaf, and wild indigo (*Baptisia tinctoria*) root.

Essiac: Essiac contains a combination of herbs, including burdock root (*Arctium lappa*), sheep sorrel (*Rumex acetosella*), slippery elm inner bark (*Ulmus fulva*), and Turkish rhubarb (*Rheum palmatum*). The original formula was developed by the Canadian nurse Rene Caisse (1888-1978) and is thought to be effective in cancer therapies, although there is currently no evidence for any type of cancer. Different brands may contain variable ingredients, and the comparative effectiveness of these formulas is not known. None of the individual herbs used in Essiac has been tested in rigorous human cancer trials, although some components have antitumor activity in laboratory studies. Caution is advised when taking Essiac supplements, as numerous adverse effects, including drug interactions, are possible. Essiac should not be used if the patient is pregnant or breastfeeding unless otherwise directed by a doctor.

Focusing: Focusing (experiential therapy) is a method of psychotherapy that involves being aware of one's feelings surrounding a particular issue and understanding the meaning behind words or images conveyed by those feelings. Early evidence suggests that focusing may improve the mood and body attitude of cancer patients. Firm recommendations cannot be made until well-designed clinical trials are available.

Garlic: Preliminary human studies suggest that regular consumption of garlic (*Allium sativum,* particularly aged garlic) may reduce the risk of developing several types of cancer. Some studies use multi-ingredient products, so it is difficult to determine if garlic alone may play a beneficial role. Further well-designed human clinical trials are needed to conclude whether eating garlic or taking garlic supplements may prevent or treat cancer. Caution is advised when taking garlic supplements, as numerous adverse effects, including an increased risk of bleeding and drug interactions, are possible.

Ginseng: Several human studies suggest that Asian ginseng (*Panax ginseng*) may reduce the risk and progression of various organ cancers, especially if ginseng powder or extract is used. Results may have been affected by other lifestyle choices in people who use ginseng, such as exercise or dietary habits. Asian ginseng is also reported to help protect against radiation damage, increase immunity and well-being, and decrease fatigue. Additional trials are necessary before a clear conclusion can be reached. Caution is advised when taking ginseng supplements, as numerous adverse effects, including an increased risk of drug interactions, are possible. Ginseng should not be used if the patient is pregnant or breastfeeding unless otherwise directed by a doctor.

Green Tea: Green tea is made from the dried leaves of *Camellia sinensis,* a perennial evergreen shrub. Green tea has a long history of use in health and longevity, dating back to China approximately 5,000 years ago. Although used for centuries to help prevent diseases, the relationship of green tea consumption and human cancer remains inconclusive. Evidence from well-designed clinical trials is needed before a firm recommendation can be made in this area.

Healing Touch: Preliminary data suggest healing touch may be of benefit in cancer patients for inducing relaxation and improving quality of life. However, due to weaknesses in design and the small number of studies, data are insufficient to make definitive recommendations. Studies with stronger designs are needed.

Hoxsey Formula: "Hoxsey formula" is a misleading name because it is not a single formula, but rather a therapeutic regimen consisting of an oral tonic and topical (on the skin) preparations. The tonic is individualized for cancer patients based on general condition, location of cancer, and previous history of treatment. An ingredient that usually remains constant for every patient is potassium iodide. Other ingredients are then added and may include licorice, red clover, burdock, stillingia root, berberis root, pokeroot, cascara, Aromatic USP 14, prickly ash bark, and buckthorn bark. A red paste may be used, which tends to be caustic (irritating), and contains antimony trisulfide, zinc chloride, and bloodroot. A topical yellow powder may be used and contains arsenic sulfide, talc, sulfur, and a "yellow precipitate." A clear solution may also be administered and contains trichloroacetic acid. There are no well-designed human studies available evaluating the safety or effectiveness of Hoxsey formula. Caution is advised when taking the Hoxsey formula supplements, as numerous adverse effects, including an increased risk of drug interactions, are possible. Hoxsey formula should not be used if the patient is pregnant or breastfeeding unless otherwise directed by a doctor.

Hydrazine Sulfate: Hydrazine is an industrial chemical marketed as having the potential to repress weight loss and cachexia (muscle wasting) associated with cancer and to improve general appetite status. In large randomized, controlled trials, hydrazine has not been found effective for improving appetite, reducing weight loss, or improving survival in adults. The National Cancer Institute sponsored studies of hydrazine sulfate that claimed efficacy in improving survival for some patients with advanced cancer. Trial results found that hydrazine sulfate did not prolong survival for cancer patients. The FDA has received requests from individual physicians for approval to use hydrazine sulfate on a case-by-case "compassionate use" basis on the chance that patients with no other available effective therapy might benefit. The overall controversy in the use of hydrazine sulfate is ongoing, and relevance to clinical practice is unknown. The use of hydrazine sulfate needs to be evaluated further before any recommendations can be made. Side effects have been reported, including nausea, vomiting, stomach cramping, and diarrhea.

Lycopene: High levels of lycopene are found in tomatoes and in tomato-based products. Tomatoes are also sources of other nutrients such as vitamin C, folate, and potassium. Several laboratory and human studies examining tomato-based products and blood lycopene levels suggest that lycopene may be associated with a lower risk of developing cancer and may help stimulate the immune system. However, due to a lack of well-designed human research using lycopene supplements, this issue remains unclear.

Maitake Mushroom: Maitake is the Japanese name for the edible fungus *Grifola frondosa*. Maitake has been used traditionally both as a food and for medicinal purposes. Early studies in the laboratory as well as in humans suggest that beta-glucan extracts from maitake may increase the body's ability to fight cancer. These studies have not been well designed, and better research is needed before the use of maitake for cancer can be recommended.

Melatonin: There are several early-phase and controlled human trials of melatonin in patients with various advanced stage malignancies, including brain, breast, colorectal, gastric, liver, lung, pancreatic, and testicular cancer, as well as lymphoma, melanoma, renal cell carcinoma, and soft-tissue sarcoma. Currently, no clear conclusion can be drawn in this area. There is not enough definitive scientific evidence to discern if melatonin is beneficial against any type of cancer, whether it increases (or decreases) the effectiveness of other cancer therapies, or if it safely reduces chemotherapy side effects. Melatonin is not to be used for extended periods of time. Caution is advised when taking melatonin supplements, as numerous adverse effects, including drug interactions, are possible.

Mistletoe: Mistletoe is one of the most widely used unconventional cancer treatments in Europe. Extracts have been studied for a variety of human cancers, including bladder, breast, cervical, central nervous system, colorectal, head and neck, liver, lung, lymphatic, ovarian, and renal (kidney) cancers as well as melanoma and leukemia. Efficacy has not been conclusively proven for any one condition, and in fact some studies have shown a lack of efficacy in certain preparations for a variety of cancers. Larger, well-designed clinical trials are needed. Caution is advised when taking mistletoe supplements, as numerous adverse effects, including nausea, vomiting, and drug interactions, are possible. Mistletoe should not be used if the patient is

pregnant or breastfeeding unless otherwise directed by a doctor.

Moxibustion: Moxibustion is a healing technique employed across the diverse traditions of acupuncture and oriental medicine for over 2,000 years. Moxibustion uses the principle of heat to stimulate circulation and break up congestion or stagnation of blood and chi. Moxibustion is more closely related to acupuncture as it is applied to specific acupuncture points. More studies are needed.

Oleander: Laboratory studies of oleander (*Nerium oleander*) suggest possible anticancer effects, although reliable research in humans is not currently available. There are reports that long-term use of oleander may have positive effects in patients with leiomyosarcoma, Ewing's sarcoma, and prostate or breast cancer. More research is needed.

Omega-3 Fatty Acids: Omega-3 fatty acids are essential fatty acids found in some plants and fish. There should be a balance of omega-6 and omega-3 fatty acids for health. Randomized, controlled trials are necessary before a clear conclusion can be drawn. Caution is advised when taking omega-3 supplements, as numerous adverse effects, including an increase in bleeding and drug interactions, are possible. Omega-3 supplements should not be used if the patient is pregnant or breastfeeding unless otherwise directed by a doctor.

Prayer, Initial studies in patients with cancer (such as leukemia) report variable effects on disease progression or death rates when intercessory prayer is used. Better quality research is necessary before a firm conclusion can be drawn. Prayer helps give individuals suffering from cancer a sense of hope.

Reishi Mushroom: Reishi (*Ganoderma lucidum*) has been shown to have antineoplastic and immunomodulatory effects in animal studies. One clinical trial and two case reports exist on advanced cancer patients using Ganopoly, a *Ganoderma lucidum* polysaccharide extract. Results show improved quality of life and enhanced immune responses, which are typically reduced or damaged in cancer patients receiving chemotherapy and/or radiation therapy. The authors are closely related to the manufacturer of Ganopoly. Well-designed long-term studies are needed to confirm these results and potential side effects.

Seaweed: Bladderwrack (*Fucus vesiculosus*) is a brown seaweed that grows on the northern coasts of the Atlantic and Pacific oceans and the North and Baltic seas. Bladderwrack appears to suppress the growth of various cancer cells in animal and laboratory studies. Currently, there are no reliable human studies available to support a recommendation for use in cancer. Bladderwrack should not be used if the patient is pregnant or breastfeeding, or has hyperthyroidism (increased thyroid hormone), unless otherwise directed by a doctor.

Selenium: Selenium is a trace mineral found in soil, water, and some foods, and it is an essential element in several metabolic pathways. Several studies suggest that low levels of selenium (measured in the blood or in tissues such as toenail clippings), may be a risk factor for developing cancer, particularly prostate cancer. Population studies suggest that people with cancer are more likely to have low selenium levels than healthy matched individuals, but in most cases it is not clear if the low selenium levels are a cause or merely a consequence of disease. It remains unclear if selenium is beneficial in the treatment of any type of cancer.

Shark Cartilage: For several decades, shark cartilage has been proposed as a cancer treatment. Studies have shown shark cartilage or the shark cartilage product AE-941 (Neovastat) to block the growth of new blood vessels, a process called antiangiogenesis, which is believed to play a role in controlling growth of some tumors. There have also been several reports of successful treatments of end-stage cancer patients with shark cartilage, but these have not been well designed or included reliable comparisons to accepted treatments.

Many studies have been supported by shark cartilage product manufacturers, which may influence the results. In the United States, shark cartilage products cannot claim to cure cancer, and the FDA has sent warning letters to companies that promote products in this way. Without further evidence from well-designed human trials, it remains unclear if shark cartilage is of any benefit in cancer, and patients are advised to check with their doctor and pharmacist before taking shark cartilage.

Shiitake Mushroom: Shiitake (*Lentinus edodes*) has been taken by mouth for boosting the immune system, decreasing cholesterol levels, and for antiaging. Lentinan, derived from shiitake, has been injected as an adjunct treatment for cancer and HIV infection. Laboratory, animal, and human studies of lentinan have shown positive results in cancer patients when used in addition to chemotherapy drugs. Further well-designed clinical trials on all types of cancer are required to confirm these results.

Soy: Soy (*Glycine max*) contains compounds that have been effective against tumors. Genistein, an isoflavone found in soy, has been found in laboratory and animal studies to possess anticancer effects, such as blocking new blood vessel growth (antiangiogenesis), acting as a tyrosine kinase

inhibitor (a mechanism of many new cancer treatments), or causing cancer cell death (apoptosis). Until reliable human research is available, it remains unclear if dietary soy or soy isoflavone supplements are beneficial, harmful, or neutral in people with various types of cancer. Caution is advised when taking soy supplements, as numerous adverse effects, including an increased risk of drug interactions, are possible.

Transcutaneous Electrical Nerve Stimulation (TENS): TENS is a noninvasive technique in which a low-voltage electrical current is delivered through wires from a small power unit to electrodes located on the skin. Although TENS has been used with some success in pain associated with cancer, there is not enough reliable evidence to draw a firm conclusion in this area.

Thiamin (Vitamin B₁): Thiamin deficiency has been observed in some cancer patients, possibly due to increased metabolic needs. It is not clear if lowered levels of thiamin in such patients may actually be beneficial. Currently, it remains unclear if thiamin supplementation plays a role in the management of any particular type(s) of cancer.

Traditional Chinese Medicine (TCM): The ancient Chinese philosophy of Taoism provided the basis for the development of Chinese medical theory. TCM uses over 120 different herbs in cancer treatment depending upon the type and cause of the cancer. Studies have reported significant benefits, including reducing tumors, reducing treatment side effects, and improved response to treatment. More studies of stronger design are needed before TCM can be recommended with confidence as an adjunct to cancer treatment, although centuries of traditional use in cancer cannot be discounted.

Turmeric: Turmeric (*Curcuma longa*) is commonly used for its antiinflammatory properties. Several early animal and laboratory studies report anticancer (colon, skin, breast) properties of curcumin. Many mechanisms have been considered, including antioxidant activity, antiangiogenesis (prevention of new blood vessel growth), and direct effects on cancer cells. Currently, it remains unclear if turmeric or curcumin has a role in preventing or treating human cancers. There are several ongoing studies in this area. Caution is advised when taking turmeric supplements, as numerous adverse effects, including an increased risk of bleeding and drug interactions, are possible.

Vitamin C (Ascorbic Acid): Dietary intake of fruits and vegetables high in vitamin C has been associated with a reduced risk of various types of cancer in population studies (particularly cancers of the mouth, esophagus, stomach, colon, or lung). However, it is not clear that it is specifically the vitamin C in these foods that is beneficial, and vitamin C supplements have not been found to be associated with this protective effect. Experts have recommended increasing dietary consumption of fruits and vegetables high in vitamin C, such as apples, asparagus, berries, broccoli, cabbage, melon (cantaloupe, honeydew, watermelon), cauliflower, citrus fruits (lemons, oranges), fortified breads/grains/cereal, kale, kiwi, potatoes, spinach, and tomatoes. Vitamin C has a long history of adjunctive use in cancer therapy, and although there have not been any definitive studies using intravenous (or oral) vitamin C, there is evidence that it has benefit in some cases. Better-designed studies are needed. Large doses (greater than 2 grams) may cause diarrhea and gastrointestinal upset.

Vitamin E: There is no reliable scientific evidence that vitamin E is effective as a treatment for any specific type of cancer. Caution is merited in people undergoing treatment with chemotherapy or radiation because it has been proposed that the use of high-dose antioxidants may actually reduce the anticancer effects of these therapies. This remains an area of controversy, and studies have produced variable results. Patients interested in using high-dose antioxidants such as vitamin E during chemotherapy or radiation should discuss this decision with their medical oncologist or radiation oncologist. Caution is advised when taking vitamin E supplements, as numerous adverse effects, including an increased risk of bleeding and drug interactions, are possible.

Yoga: Yoga is an ancient system of relaxation, exercise, and healing with origins in Indian philosophy. Several studies in cancer patients report enhanced quality of life, less sleep disturbance, decreased stress symptoms, and changes in cancer-related immune cells after patients received relaxation, meditation, and gentle yoga therapy. Yoga is not recommended as a sole treatment for cancer but may be helpful as an adjunct therapy.

Fair Negative Scientific Evidence

Integrative therapies used in cancer therapies that have fair negative scientific evidence include apricot (*Prunus armeniaca*), beta-carotene, flaxseed and flaxseed oil (*Linum usitatissimum*), hypnotherapy, and iridology.

Traditional or Theoretical Uses that Lack Scientific Evidence

Integrative therapies with historical or theoretical uses in cancer but lack sufficient clinical evidence include acerola (*Malpighia glabra, Malpighia punicifolia*),

aconite (*Aconitum napellus*), African wild potato (*Hypoxis hemerocallidea*), alfalfa (*Medicago sativa*), andrographis (*Andrographis paniculata Nees,* Kan Jang, SHA-10), L-arginine, ashwagandha (*Withania somnifera*), asparagus (*Asparagus officinalis*), barley (*Hordeum vulgare*), bilberry (*Vaccinium myrtillus*), boron, bupleurum (*Bupleurum falcatum*), chicory (*Cichorium intybus*), dehydroepiandrosterone, feverfew (*Tanacetum parthenium*), garcinia (*Garcinia cambogia*), holy basil (*Ocimum sanctum*), hydroxycitric acid, kava kava (*Piper methysticum*), licorice (*Glycyrrhiza glabra*), neem (*Azadirachta indica*), ozone therapy, PC-SPES, podophyllum (*Podophyllum peltatum*), pycnogenol (*Pinus pinaster*), rehmannia (*Rehmannia glutinosa*), spiritual healing, sweet almond (*Prunus amygdalus dulcis*), thymus extract, watercress (*Nasturtium officinale*), and yew (*Taxus* spp.).

PREVENTION

Chemical Exposure Reduction: If individuals work with chemicals, such as is the case with hairdressers, printers, and painters, they should follow all safety instructions to avoid exposure. If individuals have their own well for water, they may wish to have it tested for contaminants such as lead and arsenic. Local health departments can be a source of water testing.

Exercise and Weight Control: Controlling weight and exercising regularly can reduce the risk of developing cancer. The American Cancer Society recommends at least 30 minutes of physical activity five or more days a week if the individual can tolerate it.

Fruits, Vegetables, and Whole Grains: Fruits, vegetables, and whole grains contain vitamins, minerals, fiber, and antioxidants, which may help protect from developing various types of cancer. Eating five or more servings of fresh fruits and vegetables every day is important for health. A variety of produce should be included in the individual's diet such as kale, chard, spinach, dark green lettuce, peppers, and squashes.

Limit Alcohol Consumption: Consuming moderate to heavy amounts of alcohol, such as more than one drink a day for women and two for men, may increase the risk of developing certain cancers, such as colon and breast cancer. This is particularly true if the individual has a close relative, such as a parent, child, or sibling with cancer.

Limit Fat, Especially Saturated Fat: People who eat high-fat diets may have a higher rate of cancer, such as colon cancer. It is important to limit saturated fats from animal sources such as red meat. Other foods that contain saturated fat include milk, cheese, ice cream, coconut and palm oils. It is best to restrict the total fat intake to about 30% of the daily calories, with no more than 10% coming from saturated fats.

Screening Tests: It is best to follow the early detection screening guidelines to help find colon, breast, prostate, and other cancers.

Smoking Cessation: Smoking can increase the risk of cancers such as lung and bladder.

Vitamins and Minerals: Calcium, magnesium, pyridoxine (vitamin B_6), and folic acid may help reduce the risk of colorectal cancer. Good food sources of calcium include skim or low-fat milk and other dairy products, shrimp, and soy products such as tofu and soy milk. Magnesium is found in leafy greens, nuts, peas, and beans. Food sources of vitamin B_6 include grains, legumes, peas, spinach, carrots, potatoes, dairy foods, and meat. Folic acid is found in dark leafy greens such as spinach and lettuce, and in legumes, melons, bananas, broccoli, and orange juice.

CONDITIONS: Common Cold/Respiratory Tract Infection, Bronchitis, Sinusitis

BACKGROUND

The common cold, or acute viral nasopharyngitis, is a viral infection of the upper respiratory system, which may involve the nose, throat, sinuses, eustachian tubes (connects the ears to the throat), trachea (windpipe), larynx (voice box), and bronchial tubes (airways).

Colds are one of the leading causes of doctor visits and missed days from school and work. According to the Centers for Disease Control and Prevention, 22 million school days are lost annually in the United States as a result of the common cold. Over the course of a year, people in the United States suffer one billion colds, according to some estimates.

Americans spend about $2.9 billion on over-the-counter (OTC) drugs in addition to $400 million on prescription medicines annually for the symptomatic relief from colds.

It is estimated that the average person contracts more than 50 colds during a lifetime. Anyone can get a cold, although preschool and grade school children catch them more frequently than do adolescents and adults. One of the main reasons that colds are so common among children is because they are often in close contact with each other in daycare centers and schools. In families with children in school, the number of colds per child can be as high as 12 a year. Also, the thymus gland, which produces immune system cells, is immature in children. Subsequently they have decreased resistance to bacterial and viral infections such as colds.

Adults average about two to four colds annually, although the range varies widely. Women, especially those aged 20-30 years, experience more colds than men, possibly due to closer contact with children. Based on studies, on average, people older than 60 have less than one cold a year.

In the United States, most colds occur during the fall and winter. Beginning in late August or early September, the rate of colds increases slowly over a few weeks and remains high until March or April, when it declines. The seasonal variation may relate to the opening of schools and to cold weather, which prompt people to spend more time indoors and increase the chances that viruses will spread from person to person.

Seasonal changes in relative humidity also may affect the prevalence of colds. The most common cold-causing viruses survive better when humidity is low during the colder months of the year. Cold weather also may make the inside lining of the nose drier and more vulnerable to viral infection.

RISK FACTORS AND CAUSES

The cause of developing a cold is due to a viral infection, including rhinoviruses, coronaviruses, adenoviruses, echoviruses, respiratory syncytial viruses, and coxsackieviruses, which can infect the upper respiratory system. Although over 100 different viruses can cause colds, 30-50% are caused by rhinoviruses.

The nose contains shelflike structures called turbinates, which help trap particles (dust, dander, dirt, and viruses) entering the nasal passages. Material deposited in the nose is transported by cilia, which are hairlike structures that sweep particles to the back of the throat within 10-15 minutes of exposure. Viruses attach to receptors on epithelial (outer layer of skin) cells. In response to infection, the immune system triggers a series of events, including release of inflammatory cytokines (a group of proteins that help regulate inflammation, blood cell production, and immunity), such as interleukin (IL)-6, IL-8, and granulocyte-macrophage colony-stimulating factor, fluid leakage (runny nose), mucous membrane swelling (stuffy nose), increased mucous production, and stimulation of sneeze and cough reflexes. Nasal symptoms can begin as early as two hours after exposure, while cough and sore throat symptoms usually begin 10-12 hours following exposure to the virus. In the early stages of a cold, when the number of infecting viruses is still low, it may be possible for the body to build an effective immune response that prevents the cold from worsening. Keeping the number of viruses, called viral load, low decreases the ability of the cold virus to replicate (multiply) and cause infection.

The most common means of infection is from direct contact with the cold virus, such as an individual touching environmental surfaces (including telephones, computer keyboards, and stair rails) that have cold germs on them and then touching the eyes or nose. If an individual is physically exhausted or overtired, the chances of becoming a victim to the cold virus increase due to a impairment in immunity, or the decreased ability of the immune system to fight off infection.

Colds are also easily transmitted (by coughing or sneezing) by inhaling droplets of mucus contaminated with cold viruses. Mucus is a thick, slippery secretion of the inner lining or organs (called mucous membranes) in the body, including the nostril, ears, anus, and lips. The cold virus is spread when the infected mucus drops come in contact with other individual's noses and eyes, occurring this way more frequently than through the mouth.

Social Activity: Individuals exposed to large amounts of people during the day are also exposed to many viruses. Children attending school or playing with other kids, traveling in airplanes or buses, and having large families increases the risk of exposure to a cold virus. Being around people that are sneezing and coughing increases the chances for getting a cold virus. Touching things that others frequently touch, such as railings and doors in public facilities, also increases the chances of developing a cold. An individual's workplace may also increase the chances of exposure to a cold virus. Healthcare workers (such as nurses, pharmacists, and doctors), day care workers, people that work in retail stores, and individuals in public office are exposed to many people daily, where the chances of viral exposure and developing a cold is increased.

Age: Children and infants (less than 14 years of age) are especially susceptible to colds. Their immune systems have not yet become adjusted to being exposed to various cold viruses and have not yet developed resistance to the viruses commonly encountered. Children also may not be as careful about cleanliness such as handwashing. Children tend to spend lots of time with other children (at play and school), making it easy for colds to spread. As they age, immunity develops to many of the common viruses that cause colds. Colds will generally occur less frequently with age.

Seasonal Changes: Both children and adults seem to be most susceptible to colds in fall and winter. In cold months when the air is very dry, people turn on their heating systems, drying the air even more. Dry air dehydrates the mucous membranes in the nose and throat, which are the first line of defense against the viruses. This allows the viruses to attack the tissue in the nose and throat. Individuals working in air conditioned offices tend to have more summer colds than people who do not work in air conditioned environments. Air conditioning dries out the air and the mucous membranes and can circulate viruses in the air.

Environmental Toxins: The risk of respiratory infections is increased by exposure to environmental toxins, including cigarette smoke, which can injure airways and damage the cilia (tiny hairlike structures that help keep the airways clear). Physically engaging in smoking or breathing in passive (secondhand) smoke can damage the cilia. Toxic fumes, industrial smoke, and other air pollutants are also environmental risk factors.

Lowered Immunity: Individuals with lowered immunity, such as those with the human immunodeficiency virus (HIV) or cancer, and individuals taking certain medications such as chemotherapy, are at greater risk of developing colds. Colds can be severe in these individuals due to poor immune status.

Medications: Drug therapies, including corticosteroid (steroid) treatments, chemotherapy, or other medications that suppress the immune system also increase the risk of developing an infection from a cold virus.

Stress: Stress can lower the resistance to infection by depressing the immune system. Stress causes the adrenal glands to increase the production of the stress hormone called cortisol. During normal stressful circumstances, cortisol production is a healthy response of the body. Chronic (long-term) stress, however, causes the levels of cortisol to stay increased, leading to decreased immunity, hyperinsulinemia (the inability of the body to process insulin), and an increase in blood pressure. Stress during menopause may also increase the chances of catching a cold due to impaired immunity.

Too Much Exercise: High-intensity or endurance exercises appear to suppress the immune system while they are being performed. Some highly trained athletes, for instance, report being susceptible to colds after strenuous exercise.

Malnutrition: Low vitamin and mineral levels, such as vitamins A, E, C and the B vitamins as well as selenium and zinc, may decrease immunity and increase the chances of getting a cold. Very-low-fat diets also appear to lower the immune system.

Lack of Sleep: Sleep helps the body recharge. Proper sleep (eight hours of uninterrupted sleep for an adult) can help keep the body's immune system healthy and fight off colds.

SIGNS AND SYMPTOMS

Symptoms of a common cold usually appear about one to three days after exposure to a cold virus. Signs and symptoms of a common cold may include runny or stuffy nose, itchy or sore throat, dry cough, facial pressure due to sinuses (hollow bones in the front of the face), slight body aches or a mild headache, sneezing, itchy and watery eyes, low-grade fever (less than 102° F), and mild fatigue (tiredness).

Nasal discharge may become thicker as a common cold runs its course. What makes a cold different from other viral infections (such as influenza) is that the individual generally will not have a high fever or colored sputum. They are also unlikely to experience significant fatigue from a common cold.

Colds last on average for one week. Mild colds may last only two or three days while severe colds may last for up to two weeks. Cough due to a cold can last for hours or days.

DIAGNOSIS

Colds are usually diagnosed clinically by the presence of typical symptoms, including runny or stuffy nose, itchy or sore throat, dry cough, nasal congestion, facial pressure (sinuses), slight body aches or a mild headache, sneezing, itchy and watery eyes, low-grade fever (less than less than 102° F), and mild fatigue (tiredness).

If the symptoms worsen after one to two weeks, a doctor will examine the individual's head, neck, and lungs for signs and symptoms of more serious respiratory illnesses, such as pneumonia or bronchitis. Upon presentation, a doctor may perform a throat culture or blood test to rule out infections secondary to bacteria such as *Streptococcus* (strep throat).

Often confused with influenza, the common cold is caused by different types of viruses and usually does not result in a significantly higher body temperature. A high fever (above 102° F) is a very reliable indicator of the flu. Hay fever may also cause many of the same symptoms as a cold, including runny or stuffy nose, cough, and scratchy throat.

Allergies to dander, dust, molds, or pollens (allergic rhinitis or hay fever) also can cause a runny nose, although this usually induces symptoms more persistent than the common cold.

COMPLICATIONS

Bacterial Infections: Colds can occasionally lead to bacterial infections of the middle ear, throat, or sinuses, requiring treatment with antibiotics. High fever (greater than 102° F), significantly swollen glands, severe sinus pain, and a cough that produces colored mucus may indicate a complication or more serious illness requiring a visit to a doctor. Colds also can produce colored mucus, and a doctor will have to determine if the mucus is infected from a cold virus or another infection, such as influenza or bacteria. Samples of the mucus are taken and studied under a microscope to determine the exact cause of the infection.

Sinusitis: From 0.5-5% of people with colds develop sinusitis, an infection in the sinus cavities (air-filled spaces in the front of the skull), including pressure, nasal stuffiness, and headache. Sinusitis is usually mild, but if it becomes severe, antibiotics generally eliminate further problems. In rare cases, however, sinusitis can be serious.

Bronchitis and Pneumonia: The common cold poses a risk for bronchitis and pneumonia in nursing home patients and other people who may be susceptible to infection. Some experts believe that the rhinovirus may play a more significant role than the flu in causing lower respiratory infections in such individuals.

Wheezing: Rhinovirus infection often triggers asthma attacks in individuals with asthma.

Acute Ear Infection (Otitis Media): The most frequent complication of common colds in children is otitis media, an ear infection in which bacteria infect the space behind the eardrum. Typical signs and symptoms of otitis media include earaches and, in some cases, green or yellow discharge from the nose, or the return of a fever following a common cold. Children who are too young to verbalize their distress may simply cry or pull on the affected ear.

TREATMENT

There is no cure for the common cold. OTC cold preparations may be used for symptoms.

Healthcare professionals recommend seeking medical attention if a patient has a fever of 102° F or higher; the fever is accompanied by aches, extreme fatigue, sweating, chills, and a cough with colored phlegm; or symptoms get worse instead of better or last more than 10 days. These are symptoms of a more serious viral illness such as influenza.

With a child that has a cold, medical attention is recommended if symptoms include a fever of 102° F or higher with chills or sweating, a fever that lasts more than 72 hours, vomiting or abdominal pain, unusual sleepiness, severe headache, difficulty breathing, persistent crying, ear pain, or a persistent cough.

Pharmacological Therapy

Pain Relievers and Fever Reducers: For fever, sore throat, body aches, and headache, acetaminophen (Tylenol) or ibuprofen (Advil, Motrin) may be used OTC. Acetaminophen can cause liver damage, especially if taken chronically or in doses that exceed four grams daily. Healthcare professionals recommend carefully following dosing guidelines when giving acetaminophen to children, as dosing can be confusing. Also, it is recommended to never give aspirin to children ages three to 12. Aspirin may play a role in causing Reye's syndrome, a rare but potentially fatal illness in children.

Nasal Decongestants: Nasal decongestants are useful medications for the common cold. Nasal decongestants help dilate (open) swollen mucous membranes of the nasal passages so the individual can breathe easier. Nasal decongestants include tablets, sprays, inhalers, and nose drops. Nasal decongestants include the oral decongestant pseudoephedrine (Sudafed), nasal sprays oxymetazoline (Afrin) and phenylephrine (Neo-Synephrine), and the nasal inhalers propyl-hexedrine (Benzedrex) or levmetamfetamine (Vicks Vapor Inhaler). They are safe for most patients, but they do have many side effects and conditions in which they should not be used, including in people with heart disease, high blood pressure, thyroid disease, glaucoma (increased pressure in the eyes), diabetes, seizure disorders, enlarged prostate, or by individuals using a monoamine oxidase inhibitor (type of antidepressant). Stinging, burning, sneezing, increased nasal discharge, drying of the nostrils, and altered taste may occur. If these effects continue or become bothersome, inform a doctor. Other side effects include rapid or pounding heartbeat, dizziness, trouble sleeping, shaking of the hands, and tremors. Healthcare professionals recommend not using decongestants while pregnant or breastfeeding. If symptoms get worse, a doctor may need to evaluate the situation.

Over time, decongestant nose drops, inhalers, and sprays can actually cause rebound congestion, which means the nasal passages are not able to function normally without using these medications. Prolonged use can also cause chronic inflammation of the mucous membranes. Decongestant nasal drops and sprays are not used for more than three days, which helps to stop the potential of nasal rebound.

There is widespread national abuse of pseudo-ephedrine tablets as a drug to make methamphetamine (crystal meth or meth), an illegal drug. Metham-phetamine is a highly addictive, synthetically produced central nervous system stimulant with effects similar to cocaine. Meth is the most prevalent synthetic drug manufactured in the United States and is easily produced in home laboratories using common store-bought chemicals. The ease of manufacturing meth and its highly addictive potential have caused the use of the drug to increase throughout the nation. Its use has reached epidemic levels in many parts of the country. National and state laws have attempted to stem this criminal activity by establishing limits on sales of pseudoephedrine. The pharmacist or pharmacy representative may ask for a name and address in many states to prove that the pseudoephedrine is purchased legitimately as a decongestant. There may also be limits on the how much pseudoephedrine can be purchased in one transaction as well as over a certain time period.

Pseudoephedrine products may not be available in all states OTC and may need to be purchased from behind the pharmacy counter. Also, a new oral nasal decongestant formulation (Sudafed PE) is available that decreases the potential for abuse. Sudafed PE contains the nasal decongestant phenylephrine and not pseudoephedrine.

Antihistamines: Antihistamines dry up excess nasal secretions (mucus), and in this way help to tempora-rily stop a runny nose. But they can also cause side effects such as dry mouth, constipation, and drowsi-ness as well as confusion and increased risk of falls if administered to elderly patients. Nonsedating antihistamines include fexofenadine (Allegra) and cetirizine (Zyrtec). Antihistamines that cause sedation include diphenhydramine (Benadryl), clemastine (Tavist), chlorpheniramine (Chlor-Trimeton), and brompheniramine (Dimetane).

Cough Syrups: Nonprescription cough syrups, containing various combinations of antihistamines, decongestants, and cough suppressants, are available OTC for symptomatic relief of cough associated with a cold. Many doctors strongly discourage the use of these combination medications for any child younger than age two, in whom accidental overdoses could be fatal. Coughs associated with a cold usually last less than two to three weeks. If a cough lasts longer than three weeks, see a doctor. Cough due to colds in adults may be safely treated for as long as seven days. If the cough is productive (brings up mucus), the ingredient guaifenesin can help break up the chest congestion (water intake is also important). If the cough is dry and hacking, a cough suppressant (dextromethorphan) can stop the cough.

Lozenges: Sore throat caused by a cold may be self-treated if the pain is minor. Experts recommend not self-treating a sore throat for more than two days. If a sore throat lasts more than seven days, healthcare professionals recommend seeing a doctor. Lozenges for sore throat contain active ingredients such as the anesthetics benzocaine, menthol, dyclonine, phenol/sodium phenolate, and hexylresorcinol. Phenol/sodium phenolate and hexylresorcinol also have antibacterial properties.

Antivirals: A few studies have investigated the use of antiviral medications to treat rhinovirus, including interferon alfa-2a and interferon gamma. These drugs are expensive and have to be refrigerated and injected. The most common side effect of interferon alfa-2a or alfa-2b therapy is a flulike reaction with fever, fatigue, irritability, chills, headaches, and muscle aches. These effects should become less severe and less frequent as therapy progresses.

Pleconaril (Picovir) is an antiviral drug in clinical testing that targets picornaviruses, the viruses that cause the majority of common colds such as rhinoviruses. Pleconaril has been reported to be effective in an oral form, but it causes severe adverse effects, including liver and kidney failure. An intranasal form with less side effects is currently under development.

Antibiotics: Healthcare professionals do not recommend using antibiotics to treat a cold. Antibiotic resistance has been called one of the world's most pressing public health problems. It is caused by the overprescribing of antibiotics for conditions that will not respond to antibiotics, such as outer ear infections and viral infections, including colds and influenza.

Others: Ipratropium bromide (Atrovent), a prescription nasal spray, significantly reduced nasal drainage and sneezing in studies of naturally occurring colds. The main side effects included nasal dryness, occasional epistaxis (nosebleeds), and headache. The duration of relief from nasal stuffiness is thought to be over three hours. Nedocromil (Tilade) and sodium cromoglycate (Cromolyn), prescription drugs used in the nose, have been reported to reduce the severity of the rhinovirus upper respiratory tract infections (a common cold).

Nonpharmacological Therapy

Nondrug therapy can help reduce cold symptoms and is recommended by healthcare professionals for all infants younger than nine months. Patients of all ages benefit from rest and increased intake of fluids. The American Academy of Pediatrics highly recommends the use of calibrated measuring devices for the administration of all liquid medications to children and infants.

Saline Nasal Drops: Isotonic saline nasal drops are recommended for infants. Healthcare professionals recommend one to two drops in each nostril 15-20 minutes before feeding and bedtime and repeated 10 minutes later. Adults and children may also use saline nasal drops (Ocean nasal spray) to relieve dry and inflamed nasal passages.

Nasal Bulb Aspirator: A nasal bulb aspirator may be used to gently suction mucus and aid in clearing the nasal passages in infants and young children. Nasal bulb aspirators use gentle suction to remove excess mucus from the nasal passages. They can be purchased without a prescription at pharmacies and most retail outlets.

Elevating the Head: Elevating the head of an infant's or child's bed may facilitate the drainage of secretions. Parents and caregivers should be cautioned, however, never to place pillows around or under an infant's head due to increased risk of suffocation.

Humidification: A cool mist vaporizer will add moisture to the air, relieving symptoms such as sore throat and congestion. Hot steam humidifiers are not recommended because of the risk of scalding. Humidifiers and vaporizers must be cleaned frequently to deter growth of bacteria and other pathogens. Infants and young children also benefit from exposure to warm, steamy air, which helps to clear nasal and bronchial passages of mucus and to ease breathing, especially at night. Parents can hold the infant or child on their lap outside the shower while running a warm or hot shower to generate steam. The child should not be placed in the water.

Petroleum Jelly: Petroleum jelly may be applied on skin underneath the nose if it becomes raw from repeated wiping.

INTEGRATIVE THERAPIES
Strong Scientific Evidence

Andrographis: Andrographis (*Andrographis paniculata*) has been widely used in Indian (Hindu) folk medicine and Ayurvedic forms of medicine. A combination of andrographis with Siberian ginseng or eleuthero (*Eleutherococcus senticosus*), called Kan Jang, may be effective in the treatment of acute upper respiratory tract infections including sinusitis (inflammation of the sinuses), a common symptom of colds. In a clinical study, this treatment was given for five days, and was shown to improve fever, muscle soreness, cough, sore throat, and headache.

Good Scientific Evidence

Sage: Sage mouthwashes and gargles have been approved for use against sore throat in Germany by the German Commission E. Additional study is needed comparing sage to standard therapies.

Vitamin C: Vitamin C, or ascorbic acid, is a water-soluble vitamin that is necessary in the body to form collagen in bones, cartilage, muscle, and blood vessels and aids in the absorption of iron. Dietary sources of vitamin C include fruits and vegetables, particularly citrus fruits, such as oranges. Scientific studies generally suggest that vitamin C does not prevent the onset of cold symptoms. However, in a subset of studies in people living in extreme circumstances, including soldiers in subarctic exercises, skiers, and marathon runners, significant reductions in the risk of developing colds by approximately 50% have been reported. This area merits additional study. Large doses of vitamin C may cause gastrointestinal upset, including diarrhea.

Unclear or Conflicting Scientific Evidence

Andrographis: Based on clinical evidence, andrographis may prevent upper respiratory tract infection during the winter months if taken on a daily basis. Additional high-quality clinical study is needed to reach a conclusion on whether andrographis may be effective in prevention of upper respiratory tract infections.

Boneset: Boneset (*Eupatorium perfoliatum*) is native to eastern North America and was used by Native Americans to treat fevers. Boneset is used homeopathically in very dilute amounts. Homeopathic boneset was found in one study to decrease the symptoms associated with a cold. Homeopathic medicines do not have side effects due to the very small amount of substance, such as boneset, used in their preparation.

Chamomile: Chamomile (*Matricaria recutita*) has been used medicinally for thousands of years and is widely used in Europe. It is a popular treatment for numerous ailments, including sleep disorders, anxiety, and digestion/intestinal conditions. In an early study, inhalation of steam with chamomile extract was reported to help common cold symptoms. Further research is needed to confirm these results. Caution is advised when taking chamomile supplements, as adverse effects including drowsiness are possible.

Echinacea: Echinacea (*Echinacea angustifolia, E. purpurea, E. pallida*) is one of the most widely used herbal supplements in the world. Echinacea seems to improve the body's natural immune system during colds and flu. However, preliminary studies have mixed results in using echinacea for preventing the common cold in adults. Although multiple low-quality studies have previously suggested that adults taking echinacea by mouth when cold symptoms begin may reduce the length and severity of symptoms, a clinical trial in July 2005 did not demonstrate any clinical benefit. Recent meta-analyses are conflicting; one suggested that standardized extracts of echinacea were effective in the prevention of symptoms of the common cold after clinical inoculation compared with placebo, whereas the other reported no such benefit. Further research is needed. Also, initial research suggests that echinacea may not be helpful in children for treatment of upper respiratory infections. Additionally, development of rash has been associated with echinacea use, and therefore the risks may outweigh the potential benefits in this population. Caution is advised when taking echinacea supplements, as adverse effects including drug interactions are possible. Echinacea

supplements should not be used if pregnant or breastfeeding unless otherwise directed by a doctor.

Elder: Elder (*Sambucus nigra*) has been reported to have antiviral and antibacterial activity in laboratory studies. There is a small amount of research on the combination herbal product, Sinupret, which is a German product that contains elder and several other herbs in patients with bronchitis. This formula contains elder flowers (*Sambucus nigra*) as well as gentian root, verbena, cowslip flower, and sorrel. Although benefits have been suggested, due to design problems with this research, no clear conclusion can be drawn either for Sinupret or elder in the management of bronchitis. Sinupret has also been reported to have beneficial effects when used with antibiotics to treat sinus infections, although the majority of this evidence is not high quality and requires confirmation with better research.

Euphorbia: One short clinical trial involving senior patients with chronic bronchitis with *Euphorbia helioscopia* showed a significant effect on patients. However, this is only one short trial done in a specific population of senior patients; longer and larger trials are needed to evaluate the effect of *Euphorbia helioscopia* in a wider range of patients.

Garlic: Garlic (*Allium sativum*) supplements may reduce the severity of upper respiratory tract infections, including colds. However, this has not been demonstrated in well-designed human studies. Garlic may improve the immune system's ability to fight off infection, such as a cold virus. Caution is advised when taking garlic supplements, as adverse effects including an increase in bleeding and drug interactions are possible. Garlic supplements should not be used if pregnant or breastfeeding unless otherwise directed by a doctor.

Goldenseal: Goldenseal (*Hydrastis canadensis*) has become a popular treatment for the common cold and upper respiratory tract infections and is often added to echinacea in commercial herbal cold remedies. Animal and laboratory research suggests that the goldenseal component berberine has effects against bacteria and inflammation. However, due to the very small amount of berberine in most goldenseal preparations, it is unclear whether goldenseal contains enough berberine to have the same effects. Caution is advised when taking goldenseal supplements, as adverse effects including drug interactions are possible. Goldenseal supplements should not be used if pregnant or breastfeeding, unless otherwise directed by a doctor.

Guided Imagery: Therapeutic guided imagery may be used to help patients relax and focus on images associated with personal issues they are confronting. Experienced guided imagery practitioners may use an interactive, objective guiding style to encourage patients to find solutions to problems by exploring their existing inner resources. Biofeedback is sometimes used with imagery to enhance meditative relaxation. Interactive guided imagery groups, classes, workshops, and seminars are available, as well as books and audiotapes. Preliminary research in children suggests that stress management and relaxation with guided imagery may reduce the duration of symptoms due to upper respiratory tract infections, including colds. Additional research is needed to confirm these results.

Hydrotherapy: Hydrotherapy is broadly defined as the external application of water in any form or temperature (hot, cold, steam, liquid, ice) for healing purposes. It may include immersion in a bath or body of water (such as the ocean or a pool), use of water jets, douches, application of wet towels to the skin, or water birth. These approaches have been used for the relief of various diseases and injuries or for general well-being. There is preliminary evidence that daily showers with warm water followed by cold water, or cold water alone, may reduce the duration and frequency of common cold symptoms. Additional research is needed in this area before a clear conclusion can be drawn.

Kiwi: Kiwi (*Actinidia deliciosa, A. chinensis*) may be beneficial in lung conditions such as upper respiratory infections (including colds). However, scientific data are lacking. One survey study suggests that kiwi, and other fruits high in vitamin C, may have a protective effect on lung conditions in children, especially wheezing. However, properly controlled studies are lacking at this time.

Mistletoe: Mistletoe (*Viscum album*) and Iscador (preparation of *Viscum album* whole extract) have been reported to improve clinical symptoms and markers of immune function in children with recurrent respiratory disease exposed to the Chernobyl nuclear accident. There is insufficient evidence to recommend for or against mistletoe therapy for recurrent respiratory disease in general. Caution is advised when taking mistletoe supplements, as adverse effects including drug interactions are possible. Mistletoe supplements should not be used if pregnant or breastfeeding unless otherwise directed by a doctor. Mistletoe should not be used with seizure disorders, glaucoma (increased pressure in the eyes), diabetes, or hyperthyroidism (high thyroid hormone).

Moxibustion: Moxibustion is the application of heat to various points on the body. It is widely used traditionally in China for respiratory tract infections, including colds, in children. However, at this time evidence is insufficient.

Nasal Irrigation: The three forms of nasal irrigation therapies used in clinical trials have been saline lavage, which uses a warm liquid solution of salt water; humidified warm air lavage (in hyperthermia or low body temperature); and large-particle nebulized aerosol therapy, which uses an aerosolized (droplets spread in the air) saline solution. Occasionally, antibiotics are added to the solution. Nasal saline irrigation is still the main treatment for acute rhinitis (runny nose) in infants since excessive usage of decongestant nose drops is contraindicated in early childhood. Studies support the usage of hypertonic saline for nasal irrigation. There is good evidence in support of nasal irrigation for allergic rhinitis and sinusitis. There is promising early evidence for using nasal irrigation in treating common colds, respiratory symptoms from occupational exposure, and in postoperative care following sinus or nasal surgeries.

Peppermint: Peppermint (*Mentha piperita*) is a flowering plant that grows throughout Europe and North America. Peppermint is widely cultivated for its fragrant oil. Peppermint oil has been used historically for numerous health conditions, including common cold symptoms, cramps, headache, indigestion, joint pain, and nausea. Menthol, a constituent of peppermint oil, is sometimes included in inhaled preparations for nasal congestion, including "rubs" that are applied to the skin and inhaled. High-quality research is lacking in this area. Use of essential oils is not for internal use.

Slippery Elm: Slippery elm (*Ulmus fulva*) is commonly used to treat sore throats, most typically taken as a lozenge. While anecdotally reported to be effective, supporting evidence is largely based on traditional evidence and the fact that components of slippery elm appear to possess soothing properties for the throat. Scientific evidence is necessary in this area before a clear conclusion can be drawn. Slipper elm throat lozenges are safe in recommended dosages.

Vitamin E: Daily supplementation with oral vitamin E does not appear to affect the incidence, duration, or severity of pneumonia (lower respiratory tract infections) in elderly nursing home residents or alter patterns of antibiotic use, although there may be a protective effect against colds (upper respiratory tract infections). Additional research is warranted. Caution is advised when taking vitamin E supplements, as adverse effects, including an increase in bleeding and drug interactions, are possible. Vitamin E supplements should not be used if pregnant or breastfeeding unless otherwise directed by a doctor.

Zinc: Zinc lozenges are advertised as decreasing the symptoms, length, and severity of a cold. However, there are contradictory results regarding the efficacy of zinc formulations in treating duration and severity of common cold symptoms. Although zinc might be beneficial in the treatment of cold symptoms, more studies are needed to clarify which zinc formulations may be most effective, which rhinoviruses are affected by zinc, and if nasal sprays provide a useful alternative application route for zinc treatment. A recent study found no significant differences between zinc nasal spray and placebo. Negative results may be the cause of using doses of zinc that are too low or the presence of compounds like citric or tartaric acid, which may reduce efficacy of zinc. All nasal sprays may cause changes in taste and smell in sensitive individuals, even resulting in the temporary or permanent loss of these senses.

Fair Negative Scientific Evidence

Echinacea: Initial research suggests that echinacea may not be helpful in children for alleviation of cold symptoms, possibly because parents are not able to recognize the onset of common cold symptoms soon enough to begin treatment, or because the dose of echinacea for use in children is not clear. There are fundamental differences in causes of upper respiratory tract infection symptoms in children versus adults (bacterial versus viral causes, different viruses, different sites of infection, etc.). Until additional research is available, echinacea cannot be considered effective in children for the treatment of upper respiratory infections. Furthermore, development of rash has been associated with echinacea use, and therefore the risks may outweigh the potential benefits for children.

Vitamin C: More than 30 clinical trials including more than 10,000 participants have examined the effects of taking daily vitamin C on cold prevention. Overall, no significant reduction in the risk of developing colds has been observed. In people who developed colds while taking vitamin C, no difference in severity of symptoms has been seen overall, although a very small significant reduction in the duration of colds has been reported (approximately 10% in adults and 15% in children). Laboratory experiments in which volunteers are infected with respiratory viruses while taking vitamin C have yielded differing results, but overall report small or no significant differences in symptom severity following infection.

Additionally, numerous studies have examined the effects of starting vitamin C for treatment of the common cold after the onset of cold symptoms. Overall, no significant benefits have been observed. Initial evidence from one study reports possible benefits with high doses of vitamin C taken at the onset of symptoms, but without additional evidence this remains indeterminate. At this time, the scientific evidence does not support this use of vitamin C.

PREVENTION

Cleanliness: Children and adults need to understand the importance of handwashing. Healthcare professionals recommend carrying a bottle of alcohol-based hand rub containing at least 60% alcohol for times when soap and water are not available. These gels kill most germs and are safe for older children to use themselves. Use cautiously, as the overuse of antibacterial cleansers can cause damage to normal bacteria that reside on the skin.

Keeping the kitchen and bathroom countertops clean, especially when someone in the family has a common cold, is important. Children's toys should be washed before and after play when a cold is present in the house.

Avoiding Spreading the Virus: Sneezing and coughing into tissues keeps the viruses from spreading. Tissues are discarded right away, and then the hands are washed. Children should sneeze or cough into the bend of their elbow when they do not have a tissue. Avoiding close, prolonged contact with anyone who has a cold is recommended by healthcare professionals. Wearing a facemask, purchased at a local pharmacy, can help in the prevention of spreading or catching a cold virus.

Fluids: Water, unsweetened juices (100% juice), hot teas, and warm soups (especially chicken soup) are all good choices to drink during a cold. Alcohol, caffeine, and cigarette smoke should be avoided as they may cause dehydration and aggravate the symptoms of a cold, including a runny and stuffy nose.

Sleep Quality: Plenty of sleep and rest helps the body recover from a cold. Healthcare professionals recommend at least eight hours of uninterrupted sleep (not waking up).

Temperature and Humidity: Keeping the room warm but not overheated where the individual with a cold lives is important. If the air is dry, a cool-mist humidifier or vaporizer can moisten the air and help ease congestion and coughing. A clean humidifier may help to prevent the growth of bacteria and molds.

CONGESTIVE HEART FAILURE (CHF)

BACKGROUND

Congestive heart failure (CHF), or heart failure, is a condition in which the heart is unable to adequately pump blood throughout the body and/or unable to prevent blood from accumulating, or "backing up," into the lungs.

In most cases, CHF is a process that occurs over time, when an underlying condition damages the heart or makes it work too hard, weakening the organ. Health conditions that may lead to CHF include coronary artery disease, hypertension (high blood pressure), or arrhythmias.

Symptoms of heart failure include shortness of breath and abnormal fluid retention, which usually results in swelling in the feet and legs.

According to the American Heart Association nearly five million individuals experience heart failure and about 550,000 new cases are diagnosed each year in the United States. Heart failure becomes more prevalent with age, and the number of cases is expected to grow as the overall age of the population increases.

CAUSES AND RISK FACTORS

The heart consists of four chambers: the right atrium, the left atrium, the right ventricle, and the left ventricle. The heart also has four major valves: the mitral valve, the tricuspid valve, the aortic valve, and the pulmonary valve. Atria are relatively thin-walled chambers that receive blood from the circulatory system and from the lungs. Ventricles are muscular chambers that pump blood into the circulatory system and into the lungs.

Blood passes from the atria into the ventricles through two processes. During the resting phase, when the ventricles are not contracting, the tricuspid and mitral valves open and allow some of the blood that has accumulated in the atria to flow passively through the valves into the ventricles. Then, the atria contract and actively pump blood out through the valves and into the ventricles. Once the ventricles fill with blood, they contract, pumping blood to the lungs and the rest of the body.

When the left ventricle cannot adequately pump blood out of the left atrium, or when one or more of the heart valves becomes leaky or narrowed, blood can back up into the lungs, causing left-sided heart failure. When this occurs, the lungs become congested with fluid (called pulmonary edema), causing difficulty breathing and interfering with the movement of oxygen from the lungs into the bloodstream, causing fatigue.

When an abnormality or condition affects the flow of blood through the right ventricle, pressure in the blood vessels increases and fluid is forced from the blood vessels into body tissues. This right-sided heart failure causes swelling (edema), usually in the feet and legs, and sometimes in the abdomen.

Coronary Artery Disease and Heart Attack: Coronary artery disease is the most common form of heart disease and the most common cause of heart failure. Over time, arteries that supply blood to the heart muscle narrow from a buildup of fatty deposits, a process called atherosclerosis. The buildup containing fats and clotting factors is called a plaque. Blood moves slowly through narrowed arteries, leaving some areas of the heart muscle chronically deprived of oxygen-rich blood. These areas of the heart may become weak from the lack of oxygen and pump less vigorously. In many cases, the blood flow to the muscle is just enough to keep the muscle alive but not functioning well. A heart attack occurs if an unstable plaque ruptures, causing a blood clot to completely block blood flow to an area of the heart muscle. A heart attack results in the death of heart muscle, which can quickly weaken the heart's pumping ability. Sometimes coronary artery disease is limited to the small coronary arteries. If these arteries become blocked, this won't cause a heart attack, but over time, it can gradually weaken the heart.

Hypertension (High Blood Pressure): Blood pressure is the force of blood pumped by the heart through the arteries. If blood pressure is high, the heart has to work harder than it should to circulate blood throughout the body. Over time, the heart muscle may become thicker to compensate for the extra work it must perform. In some cases, the heart will enlarge. Eventually, the heart muscle may become either too stiff or too weak to effectively pump blood.

Defective Heart Valves: The four valves of the heart keep blood flowing in the proper direction through the heart. A damaged valve forces the heart to work harder to keep blood flowing as it should. Over time, this extra work can weaken the heart.

Cardiomyopathy: Cardiomyopathy is a serious disease in which the heart muscle becomes inflamed and does not work as well as it should. There may be multiple causes, including viral infections, alcohol abuse, and the toxic effect of drugs such as cocaine or doxorubicin (Adriamycin) used for chemotherapy.

In addition, whole-body diseases that may lead to inflammation, such as lupus or thyroid problems, can also damage heart muscle.

Myocarditis: Myocarditis is an inflammation of the heart muscle. Myocarditis is most commonly caused by a virus and can lead to left-sided heart failure. The virus most often associated with myocarditis is coxsackievirus B, but other viruses may include adenovirus, parvovirus B19, echovirus, influenza virus, Epstein-Barr virus, and rubella virus. Human immunodeficiency virus can directly infiltrate the heart muscle and cause myocarditis. Other causes of myocarditis include bacteria (such as *Staphylococcus aureus*), parasites (such as *Trypanosoma cruzi* and *Toxoplasma* spp.), fungi (such as *Candida albicans*), exposure to certain chemicals (such as arsenic and hydrocarbons), medications that may cause allergic or toxic reactions (such as cocaine or penicillin), and systemic diseases causing inflammation (including lupus).

Congenital Heart Defects: Congenital heart defects are structural problems with the heart present at birth. Genetic defects contribute to the risk of certain types of heart diseases (such as arrhythmias or valve problems), which in turn may lead to heart failure. Estimates suggest that about one million Americans have a congenital heart defect. Approximately 35,000 babies in the United States are born with a heart defect each year.

Arrhythmias: Arrhythmias, or abnormal heart rhythms, may cause the heart to beat too fast. This creates extra work for the heart. Over time the heart may weaken, leading to heart failure.

Other Conditions: Health conditions, such as diabetes, severe anemia (lack of red blood cells to carry oxygen to tissues), hyperthyroidism (high thyroid hormone levels), hypothyroidism (low thyroid hormone levels), emphysema (lung disease that involves damage to the air sacs in the lungs), pulmonary edema (fluid in the lungs), hemochromatosis (an inherited disease in which too much iron builds up in the body), and amyloidosis (a group of diseases in which one or more organ systems in the body accumulate deposits of abnormal proteins such as C-reactive protein), may also contribute to heart failure. Kidney disease can contribute to heart failure due to an increase in high blood pressure and fluid retention.

Heart failure may develop during the last the months of pregnancy or several months after pregnancy. The cause of this is not well understood, but it may be due to an abnormal immune system response.

Viral infections may cause idiopathic heart failure or heart failure in which there is never an identified cause. Bacterial infections, such as pneumonia, may lead to CHF.

Exposure to toxins, such as alcohol or cocaine, may also lead to CHF. An example of drug-induced CHF is with encainide hydrochloride (Enkaid). Encainide is a drug used for arrhythmias (irregular heartbeats), but in susceptible individuals, its use may lead to CHF.

Obesity may also lead to CHF. Obesity promotes diabetes, hypertension (high blood pressure), and dyslipidemia (high cholesterol levels). These conditions are risk factors for developing coronary artery disease and, ultimately, CHF.

Sleep apnea, or the inability to breathe properly at night, results in low blood oxygen levels and increased risk of abnormal heart rhythms. Both of these problems can weaken the heart and lead to CHF.

The condition affects 1% of people aged 50 years and older and about 5% of those aged 75 years and older. African Americans experience heart failure twice as often as Caucasians. About 10% of patients diagnosed with heart failure die within one year, and about 50% die within five years of diagnosis.

CHF is equally frequent in men and women, and annual incidence approaches 10 per 1,000 population after 65 years of age. Survival following diagnosis of CHF is worse in men than women, but even in women, only about 20% survive much longer than eight to 12 years.

SIGNS AND SYMPTOMS

CHF is chronic (long term) and generally occurs slowly. Congestion, or the backing up of blood, occurs in the liver, abdomen, lower extremities, and lungs. The backing up of blood causes symptoms such as shortness of breath, fatigue, and swelling (particularly in the legs and feet). Other symptoms develop as the body tries to compensate for the heart's reduced pumping ability. The heart beats faster, its muscle thickens, and the ventricles may stretch to accommodate more blood. Damage to the ventricles may cause them to pump out of sync, further reducing the efficient delivery of blood to the body. Symptoms of CHF include a dry, hacking cough, especially when lying down; confusion, sleepiness, and disorientation may occur in older individuals; dizziness, fainting, fatigue, or weakness; fluid buildup, especially in the legs, ankles, and feet; increased urination at night; nausea; abdominal swelling, tenderness, or pain; weight gain due to fluid buildup; weight loss as nausea causes a loss of appetite and as the body fails to absorb food well; rapid breathing, bluish skin, and feelings of restlessness, anxiety, and suffocation; shortness of breath and lung congestion as the blood backs up in the lungs; and wheezing and spasms of the airways similar to asthma.

DIAGNOSIS

Physical Examination and Medical History: During a physical examination, a doctor will look for underlying causes of the problem and assess heart function. A stethoscope is used to detect murmurs (abnormal heart sounds) that may indicate a leaky or narrowed valve, and to detect fluid accumulation in the lungs. The doctor also looks for enlarged veins in the neck and for edema (swelling) in the legs, particularly the ankles, feet, and/or the abdomen.

A patient history may include information about risk factors, such as family medical history, past surgeries and medications, history of chest pain, high blood pressure (including treatments), heart attack, recent viral illness, or recent pregnancy.

Blood Tests: Blood tests may include blood cell counts to test for conditions such as anemia (low red blood cells); electrolyte levels, including sodium, potassium, and calcium; nutrient levels, such as vitamins and trace minerals; tests for kidney function, including blood urea nitrogen and creatinine levels; and testing for homocysteine and/or C-reactive protein, both markers of inflammation and heart disease. The diagnostic test marker for CHF is N-terminal prohormone brain natriuretic peptide. Brain natriuretic peptide is a hormone produced at higher levels by the failing heart muscle.

Electrocardiogram: An electrocardiogram (ECG) is a noninvasive test used to measure electrical activity in the heart. Electrical sensors called leads are attached to predetermined positions on the arms, legs, and chest to record electrical activity and help assess heart function. The heart's rhythm of contraction is controlled by the sinoatrial (SA) node, often called the pacemaker. Electrical impulses generated from the SA node spread through the heart via a nodal tissue pathway that coordinates the events leading to a heartbeat. The conduction system initiates and coordinates the muscular activity of the heart.

Echocardiogram: An echocardiogram, or echo, is an ultrasound examination of the heart that produces detailed images of the organ. It can be used to detect abnormalities in the structure of the heart and to measure the amount of blood ejected from the heart. During an echocardiogram, a microphone-like device (transducer) is used to transmit and receive ultrasonic waves that travel through the chest wall to the heart and are reflected back to the transducer. The reflected sound waves are translated into images of the heart, including the valves, chambers, and walls.

An echocardiogram also is used to measure the pressure change (gradient) between the left ventricle and the aorta to assess thickening of the walls of the heart, to evaluate pumping function, and to measure the amount of dilation (increased diameter) of the left ventricle.

Chest X-Ray: A chest x-ray is used in identifying the buildup of fluid in the lungs. Also, the heart usually enlarges in CHF, which may be visible on the x-ray film.

Cardiac Catheterization: Cardiac catheterization may be performed in individuals with angina and in those with a history of heart attack to determine if coronary heart disease is causing heart failure. Cardiac catheterization produces angiograms (such as x-ray images) of the coronary arteries and the left ventricle, and can be used to monitor heart function.

Cardiac catheterization involves injecting a small amount of radioactive dye, called a contrast agent, into the left ventricle through a catheter (a thin flexible tube). A special camera is then used to determine how much of the dye is ejected from the heart with each beat. The infusion of dye typically produces a characteristic "hot flash" sensation throughout the body that lasts 10-15 seconds.

Stress Test: In some individuals, a less invasive procedure called a stress test is used to assess the possibility of coronary heart disease. If the results of this procedure suggest the presence of coronary artery disease, a subsequent referral for cardiac catheterization is likely.

Several types of stress tests may be used by doctors to access heart function. In some cases, the individual simply walks on a treadmill while connected to an ECG. Another type uses intravenous (or in the veins) medication, usually dipyridamole (Persantine), which reproduces the stress of exercise on the heart.

Nuclear Stress Test: Nuclear stress tests involve injecting a radioactive substance, most commonly technetium or Tc-99m sestamibi (Cardiolite), into a vein. A special camera is then used to obtain images of the heart during rest and immediately following exercise on a treadmill as the radioactivity flows through the heart. The radioactivity levels used are not harmful.

A nuclear test, called a radionuclide ventriculography or multiple gated acquisition (MUGA) scan, allows doctors to see how much blood the heart pumps with each beat, called the ejection fraction. The MUGA scan gives an accurate and reproducible means of measuring and monitoring the actual amount of blood ejected from the heart. The tests use a small amount of radioactive material injected into the veins. A special camera detects the radioactive material as it flows through the heart. Individuals with an allergy to iodine or shellfish have special considerations and may not be able to have this test because the dye contains iodine. The use of medications, including the antihistamine diphenhydramine (Benadryl) and/or prednisone (Delatasone), prior to the administration of the dyes (contrast media), may help to prevent or decrease the chance of an allergic reaction.

Classifying Heart Failure: Results of these tests help doctors determine the cause of CHF and develop a program to treat the heart. To determine the best course of treatment, doctors may classify heart failure using one of two scales. The New York Heart Association scale classifies heart failure in categories from one to four. In class I heart failure, the mildest form, individuals can perform everyday activities and not feel winded or fatigued. Individuals with class II have slight limitation of physical activity and ordinary physical activity may result in fatigue, palpitation, shortness of breath, or chest pain. Those with class III have marked limitation of physical activity, and less than ordinary activity causes fatigue, palpitation, shortness of breath, or chest pain. Class IV is the most severe, and individuals are short of breath even at rest. The American College of Cardiology scale uses letters A-D. The system includes a category for individuals who are at risk of developing heart failure. Early stage heart failure includes stage A (individuals are at risk for developing heart failure without evidence of heart dysfunction) and stage B (there is evidence of heart dysfunction without symptoms). Advanced stage heart failure includes stage C (there is evidence of heart dysfunction with symptoms) and stage D (there are symptoms of heart failure despite maximal therapy). Doctors can use these classifications to identify the risk factors and begin early, more aggressive treatment to help prevent or delay heart failure.

COMPLICATIONS

CHF can affect many organs of the body. For example, the weakened heart muscles may not be able to supply enough blood to the kidneys, which then begin to lose their normal ability to excrete salt (sodium) and water. This diminished kidney function can cause the body to retain more fluid. The lungs may become congested with fluid (pulmonary edema) and the person's ability to exercise is decreased. Fluid may likewise accumulate in the liver, thereby impairing its ability to rid the body of toxins and produce essential proteins. The intestines may become less

efficient in absorbing nutrients and medicines. Over time, untreated CHF will affect virtually every organ in the body. The lack of blood flow to the heart can lead to irreversible damage to the heart muscle.

Chest pain (angina) is an indicator of a heart attack (myocardial infarction). A heart attack can cause sudden death.

TREATMENT

Treatment for CHF varies and involves reducing symptoms, treating the underlying cause of the condition when possible, and using medications to prevent further deterioration of heart function.

Lifestyle Changes

Lifestyle changes can help reduce symptoms such as fatigue, shortness of breath, and edema (swelling). These modifications may include dietary changes (such as a restricted salt intake of less than 2,000 mg daily), abstinence from alcohol, smoking cessation, and regular exercise (under the supervision of a doctor).

Medications

A combination of medications is used to treat CHF. Depending on the symptoms, individuals with CHF may take one, two, or more of these drugs. Several types of medications have proved useful in the treatment of heart failure, including angiotensin-converting enzyme (ACE) inhibitors, angiotensin receptor blockers (ARBS), beta-blockers, digoxin, diuretics, and aldosterone antagonists.

ACE Inhibitors: ACE inhibitors are medications that dilate or widen blood vessels to lower blood pressure, improve blood flow, and decrease the workload on the heart. ACE inhibitors include enalapril (Vasotec), lisinopril (Prinivil, Zestril), and captopril (Capoten).

Side effects of ACE inhibitors include chronic, nonproductive cough (occurs in about 10% of patients), dizziness or weakness (caused by low blood pressure), increased potassium levels, skin rashes, and sudden swelling of the lips, face, and cheeks (if this occurs, the patient must seek medical attention immediately).

Angiotensin II Receptor Blockers (ARBs): ARBS have many of the beneficial effects of ACE inhibitors, but they do not cause a persistent cough. They may be an alternative for individuals who cannot tolerate ACE inhibitors. ARBs include losartan (Cozaar) and valsartan (Diovan).

Digoxin (Lanoxin): Digoxin (Lanoxin) increases the strength of the heart muscle contractions. Digoxin

C

also tends to slow the heartbeat. Digoxin reduces heart failure symptoms and improves the individual's ability to live with the CHF. Side effects are rare but may include blurred vision, cardiac problems (such as arrhythmias or heart block), diarrhea, headaches, loss of appetite, hypotension (low blood pressure), and nausea and vomiting.

Beta-Blockers: Beta-blockers are a class of drugs that slows the heart rate and reduces blood pressure. Beta-blockers include carvedilol (Coreg), metoprolol (Lopressor), and propranolol (Inderal). These medicines also reduce the risk of some abnormal heart rhythms. Beta-blockers may reduce signs and symptoms of heart failure and improve heart function. Beta-blockers are started at low doses that are gradually increased over a period of several months. During the first several weeks of treatment, some patients experience worsening symptoms due to a decrease in oxygen circulation in the body. Other side effects include low blood pressure, difficulty breathing, sexual dysfunction, nausea, and weakness with exertion.

Diuretics: Diuretics, or water pills, make individuals urinate more frequently and keep fluid from collecting in the body. Commonly prescribed diuretics for heart failure include hydrochlorothiazide (Diuril) and furosemide (Lasix). Diuretics also decrease fluid in the lungs, helping individuals breathe more easily. Side effects include frequent urination and low potassium blood levels. Because of this, blood tests are performed periodically and a potassium supplement is prescribed if blood levels are low. Individuals may be asked to eat more fruits high in potassium, such as bananas and oranges, while on diuretic therapy.

Aldosterone Antagonists: Aldosterone antagonists are primarily potassium-sparing diuretics, but they have additional properties that help the heart work better, may reverse scarring of the heart, and may help individuals with severe heart failure live longer. Aldosterone antagonists include spironolactone (Aldactone) and eplerenone (Inspra). Unlike other diuretics, spironolactone can raise the level of potassium in the blood to dangerous levels. Healthcare professionals recommend eliminating high-potassium foods, such as bananas, lentils, nuts, peaches, potatoes, salmon, tomatoes, and watermelon while taking aldosterone antagonists.

Others: A medication called BiDil is a single pill that combines hydralazine and isosorbide dinitrate, both of which dilate and relax the blood vessels. BiDil increases survival when added to standard therapy in African American individuals with advanced heart failure. This is the first drug studied and approved for a specific racial group. Further studies will be necessary to determine if this combination medicine will be helpful for others with heart failure. Side effects may include blurred vision, dry mouth, irregular heartbeat, blood in the urine or stools, numbness or tingling in the arms or legs, and fainting.

Doctors often prescribe other heart medications, such as 3-hydroxy-3-methylglutaryl coenzyme A reductase inhibitors (statin) drugs, for cholesterol reduction. Statin drugs include atorvastatin (Lipitor) and lovastatin (Mevacor). They may cause liver problems or muscle pain. Antiarrhythmic drugs may also be prescribed to control irregular heartbeats, including diltiazem (Cardizem, Cardizem CR) and verapamil (Calan, Calan SR).

Individuals may be hospitalized for a few days if complications arise as a result of CHF symptoms. While in the hospital, individuals may receive additional medications such as intravenous (or into the veins) dobutamine (Dobutrex), milrinone, (Primacor), and nitroglycerin. These drugs work quickly to help the heart pump better and relieve symptoms. Individuals may also receive supplemental oxygen through a mask or small tubes placed in the nose. If severe heart failure is present, the individual may need to use supplemental oxygen long term.

Individuals hospitalized with severe CHF may be given an intravenous drug called nesiritide (Natrecor). Nesiritide is a synthetic version of a naturally occurring hormone in the body called brain natriuretic peptide (BNP). BNP is secreted in high levels by the heart in response to a failing heart. However, it is not clear if nesiritide is better than other intravenous medications for severe heart failure. Studies are ongoing to evaluate the safety and effectiveness of nesiritide in heart failure.

Other Treatments

Aquapheresis: In some cases, heart failure persists or worsens in spite of treatment. An ultrafiltration process called aquapheresis, which uses a mechanical system called the Aquadex FlexFlow (CHF Solutions, Brooklyn Park, Minn.), may be used to remove excess fluids and salt in CHF individuals who do not respond to lifestyle modifications and medication. In this treatment, blood is withdrawn using catheters (small tubes) inserted into veins in the arm, leg, or neck. The blood is then passed through a filter that removes excess fluid and is returned to the body. Studies have reported that ultrafiltration can remove more fluid at a faster rate than medication. The length of each treatment depends on the rate at which fluid can be removed from the body and the amount that must be removed.

Angioplasty: CHF caused by reduced blood flow in the heart as a result of blockages (plaques) in one or more coronary arteries may be treated using coronary angioplasty. In this procedure, a hollow tube (catheter) is inserted through an artery (usually the femoral artery in the groin), into the coronary artery, and to the blockage. A small balloon is then inserted through the catheter and is inflated to open the blocked artery. There is a slight risk for damage to the artery during angioplasty, but heart failure symptoms usually improve following the procedure. Stenting is used along with balloon angioplasty. Stenting involves placing a meshlike metal device into an artery at a site narrowed by plaque. The stent is mounted on a balloon-tipped catheter, threaded through an artery, and positioned at the blockage. The balloon is then inflated, opening the stent. Then, the catheter and deflated balloon are removed, leaving the stent in place. The opened stent keeps the vessel open and stops the artery from collapsing. Re-closure may occur with both balloon angioplasty and stenting. Doctors will prescribe blood thinning medications to help keep the arteries open, including aspirin, warfarin (Coumadin), and clopidogrel (Plavix).

Coronary Artery Bypass Graft (CABG) Surgery: CABG surgery may be recommended if the individual has severe coronary artery disease in addition to CHF. This may improve the blood supply to the heart. CABG surgery uses blood vessel grafts, which usually come from the patient's own arteries and veins located in the chest, leg, or arm. The graft goes around the clogged artery to create new pathways for oxygen-rich blood to flow to the heart. Some problems associated with CABG include a heart attack (occurs in 5% of patients), stroke (occurs in 5%, with the risk greatest in those over 70 years old), blood clots, death (occurs in 1-2% of individuals), and wound infection (occurs in 1-4%). Infection is most often associated with obesity, diabetes, or having had a previous CABG. In about 30% of patients, post-pericardiotomy syndrome can occur anywhere from a few days to six months after surgery. The symptoms of this syndrome are fever and chest pain. Symptoms can be treated with medications, including antibiotics (for infection), nitroglycerin, and antiinflammatory drugs. The incision in the chest or the graft site (if the graft was from the leg or arm) can be itchy, sore, numb, or bruised. Some individuals report memory loss, loss of mental clarity, or "fuzzy thinking" following a CABG.

Implantable Cardiac Defibrillator (ICD): An ICD may be used to treat severe heart failure. An ICD is a small electronic device that is surgically implanted under the skin in the chest to monitor heart rhythm. When an abnormal rhythm is detected, the defibrillator delivers an electrical "shock" to the heart to restore normal heart rhythm.

Intra-Aortic Balloon Pump (IABP): An IABP is a device that is inserted through an artery in the groin (femoral artery) and then placed within the main artery (aorta). An IABP is an inflatable balloon that expands and deflates in coordination with each heartbeat. It can be left in place for days to weeks and decreases the strain on the heart and increases blood flow throughout the body.

Valve Replacement Surgery: Individuals with heart failure caused by an abnormal heart valve may require valve repair or valve replacement surgery. These are open-heart procedures in which an abnormal valve is repaired or replaced with a porcine valve (from pig tissue), a mechanical valve (made of synthetic material), or a homograft valve (from a human donor). Complications include bleeding, blood clots, infection, kidney failure, stroke, heart attack, and death. A homograft valve is preferred, as these valves are not associated with a significant risk for blood clot formation and, thus, do not require blood thinner therapy. Most individuals remain in the hospital for a week after surgery and recovery takes approximately three to four weeks, after which most patients can resume leisure activities and many return to work. Approximately 60% of individuals who have valve replacement have a ten-year postsurgery survival rate.

Left Ventricular Assist Device: A left ventricular assist device is a mechanical pump that is surgically implanted in the upper abdomen to bypass the left ventricle and pump blood throughout the body. This device may be used in patients with end-stage heart failure who are awaiting heart transplantation. Long-term use of the device in patients with severe heart failure is being explored and defined.

Pacemaker: If individuals with CHF experience arrhythmias that will not respond to medication therapy, the arrhythmias may be corrected with a pacemaker. A pacemaker is a small, battery-powered device that is usually implanted near the collarbone. Pacemakers can be surgically placed into the chest (a permanent pacemaker) through a small incision, or they can be worn outside the body (a temporary pacemaker) and attached to the heart through a wire that is threaded through a neck vein. Temporary pacemakers are used only while an individual is in the hospital.

The surgery needed to implant a permanent pacemaker is considered a minor surgical procedure. The procedure may take one to two hours to complete.

The area where the pacemaker will be inserted will be numbed with an injection of an anesthetic such as lidocaine (Xylocaine). The individual should not feel any pain during the procedure, and should inform the doctor or staff if he or she is having pain so that more anesthetic medication may be given. One or more electrode-tipped wires run from the pacemaker through the blood vessels to the inner heart. If the heart rate is too slow or if it stops, the pacemaker sends out electrical impulses that stimulate the heart to beat at a steady, proper rate. The more advanced pacemakers can monitor and pace either the atria or ventricles (or both) in proper sequence to maximize the amount of blood being pumped from the heart. The pacemaker's batteries may need to be changed every five to ten years. It is recommended by the American Heart Association to limit exposure to devices that may interfere with pulse generators such as cellular phones, CB radios, electric blankets, and microwaves.

It is normal for the surgical wound to be somewhat painful and swollen for a few days after the procedure. This can usually be controlled with medications, such as tramadol (Ultram) or ibuprofen (Motrin). The wound may also appear mildly red for a few days; however, if the area of redness enlarges, a doctor should be notified due to the potential for a serious infection. If there are no other problems, most individuals who have a permanent pacemaker surgically implanted can go home the next day. They can usually return to normal activities within six weeks. For several weeks after having a pacemaker implanted, the individual may be asked not to lift more than five pounds or raise the affected arm over the shoulder.

Heart Transplant: In some cases, despite the use of optimal therapies as described above, the individual's condition continues to deteriorate due to progressive CHF. In selected individuals, heart transplantation is a viable treatment option. Candidates for a heart transplant are generally under age 70, do not smoke, and do not have severe or irreversible diseases affecting the other organs. Additionally, a transplant is done only when it is clear that the individual's prognosis on continued medical treatment is poor. Transplant patients require close medical follow-up while taking necessary drugs that suppress the immune system because of the risk of rejection of the transplanted heart. They must even be monitored for possible development of coronary artery disease in the transplanted heart.

Although there are thousands of patients on waiting lists for a heart transplant at any given time, the number of operations performed each year is limited by the number of available donor organs. For these reasons, heart transplantation is a realistic option in only a small subset of the large numbers of patients with CHF.

INTEGRATIVE THERAPIES
Strong Scientific Evidence

Hawthorn: Hawthorn (*Crataegus* spp.), a flowering shrub of the rose family, has an extensive history of use in cardiovascular disease dating back to the first century. Increased blood flow to the heart and heart performance has been observed in animals when given hawthorn supplements. One randomized, human clinical trial indicates that hawthorn may be effective in decreasing frequency or severity of anginal symptoms. Hawthorn has not been tested in the setting of concomitant drugs such as beta-blockers or ACE inhibitors, which are often the standard of care. At this time, there is insufficient evidence to recommend for or against hawthorn's use in coronary artery disease or angina. Hawthorn supplements should not be used if pregnant or breastfeeding unless otherwise directed by a doctor.

Good Scientific Evidence

Berberine: Berberine is a bitter-tasting, yellow, plant alkaloid with a long history of medicinal use in Chinese and Ayurvedic medicine. Berberine is present in the roots, rhizomes, and stem bark of various plants, including *Hydrastis canadensis* (goldenseal), *Coptis chinensis* (coptis or goldenthread), *Berberis aquifolium* (Oregon grape), *Berberis vulgaris* (barberry), and *Berberis aristata* (tree turmeric). Preliminary clinical research suggests that berberine, in addition to a standard prescription drug regimen for chronic CHF, may improve quality of life, heart function, and mortality. Further research is necessary. Berberine has been reported to cause nausea, vomiting, hypertension (high blood pressure), respiratory failure, and paresthesias (abnormal sensations such as numbness or tingling). Berberine is used with caution in individuals with diabetes.

Coleus: Coleus species have been used in Asian traditional medicine for several indications. Since the 1970s, research was predominantly concentrated on forskolin, a root extract of *Coleus forskohlii*. A small number of studies suggest that forskolin may improve cardiovascular function in patients with cardiomyopathy. However, these trials are small and of poor quality. Larger studies are needed.

Creatine: Creatine is naturally synthesized in the human body from amino acids primarily in the kidney and liver and transported in the blood for use by muscles. Cardiac creatine levels are reported as depressed in chronic heart failure. Several studies report that creatine supplementation is associated with improved heart muscle strength, body weight, and endurance in patients with heart failure. However, it is not clear what dose may be safe or effective. Supplementation is also reported to increase creatine in skeletal muscle in these patients, helping to increase strength and endurance. Well-designed studies comparing creatine with drugs used to treat heart failure are needed.

Selenium: Selenium is a trace metal that has been reported to have antioxidant properties. Keshan disease is cardiomyopathy (heart disease) restricted to areas of China in people having an extremely low selenium status. Prophylactic administration of sodium selenite has been shown to significantly decrease the incidence of this disorder.

Unclear or Conflicting Scientific Evidence

Arginine: Arginine, or L-arginine, is considered a semi-essential amino acid, because although it is normally synthesized in sufficient amounts by the body, supplementation is sometimes required. There is initial evidence from several studies that arginine when taken orally or by injection improves exercise tolerance and blood flow in arteries of the heart. Benefits have been reported in some patients with coronary artery disease and angina. Studies of arginine in patients with CHF have shown mixed results. Some studies report improved exercise tolerance. Additional studies are needed to confirm these findings before a firm conclusion can be drawn. L-arginine is generally considered safe in recommended dosages.

Astragalus: Astragalus (*Astragalus membranaceus*) is used in combination with other herbs in Chinese medicine to treat various heart diseases. There are several human case reports of reduced symptoms and improved heart function and diuretic ("water pill") effects, although these are not well described. High-quality human research is needed. Astragalus is used with caution in individuals with blood sugar regulation problems and those taking drugs to suppress immunity.

Ayurveda: Ayurveda, which originated in ancient India over 5,000 years ago, is probably the world's oldest system of natural medicine. Preliminary evidence suggests that sodium nimbidinate, made from the traditional Ayurvedic herb Nimba/Neem/Arishta (*Azadirachta indica*), may be an effective diuretic in patients with CHF. More studies are needed to confirm this effect.

Coenzyme Q10 (CoQ10): CoQ10 is produced by the human body and is necessary for the basic functioning of cells. The evidence for CoQ10 in the treatment of heart failure is controversial and remains unclear. Different levels of disease severity have been studied (New York Heart Association classes I-IV). Better research is needed in this area, studying effects on quality of life, hospitalization, and death rates. There is also conflicting evidence from research on the use of CoQ10 in patients with dilated or hypertrophic cardiomyopathy. CoQ10 is generally safe in recommended dosages, but further studies are needed.

Ginseng: A clinical study on the effect of *Panax ginseng* on CHF did not show a clear benefit of combining digoxin with ginseng. The relatively small study size and the use of a drug instead of a standardized extract limit the value of the evidence. Ginseng may also lower blood pressure. Caution is used when taking ginseng supplements, as adverse effects including drug interactions are possible. Ginseng supplements are not used if pregnant or breastfeeding unless otherwise directed by a doctor.

L-Carnitine: L-carnitine, carnitine, or acetyl-L-carnitine is an amino acid found in the body. Although preliminary results are promising, there is insufficient available clinical evidence for the use of L-carnitine in CHF.

Oleander: Extracts of *Thevetia peruviana* (also known as *Thevetia neriifolia*) and *Nerium oleander* have been observed to possess cardiac glycoside properties since the mid-1900s. Human clinical studies began in the 1930s, but have largely been abandoned due to the significant gastrointestinal toxicity of thevetin and peruvoside preparations. These glycosides have been staples of CHF therapy in China and Russia for decades, but data supporting use are scant, and no high-quality comparative studies to other better-tolerated cardiac glycoside preparations appear to exist. Notably, cardiac glycosides have not been shown to improve mortality in patients with CHF, although well-tolerated and widely used drugs such as digoxin have been demonstrated to alleviate symptoms and reduce frequency of hospitalization. Oral oleander ingestion cannot be recommended, particularly in its unprocessed "natural form" as an herbal remedy. The therapeutic to toxic window appears to be extremely narrow.

Passionflower: An extract containing passionflower and hawthorn has been studied in people with CHF for the treatment of shortness of breath and difficulty exercising. Individuals using this combination of herbs have experienced improvements in these symptoms.

However, any positive effects may have resulted from hawthorn, which is more commonly used for CHF. High-quality human research of passionflower alone and compared to prescription drugs used for this condition is needed. Passionflower extracts may cause drowsiness in sensitive individuals. Care is recommended when driving an automobile or operating heavy machinery while taking passionflower.

Taurine: Taurine is a nonessential amino acid–like compound, taurine is found in high abundance in the tissues of many animals, especially sea animals, and in much lower concentrations in plants, fungi, and some bacteria. Preliminary study suggests that taurine may be beneficial as an adjunct to traditional medications for symptoms of CHF. Taurine appears to be safe in recommended dosages.

Thiamin: Thiamin (also spelled thiamine) is a water-soluble B-complex vitamin, previously known as vitamin B_1 or aneurine. Thiamin was isolated and characterized in the 1920s, and thus was one of the first organic compounds to be recognized as a vitamin. Chronic severe thiamin deficiency can cause heart failure (wet beriberi), a condition that merits thiamin supplementation. It is not clear that thiamin supplementation is beneficial in patients with heart failure due to other causes.

Thymus Extract: The thymus is a lobular gland located under the breastbone near the thyroid gland. It reaches its maximum size during early childhood and plays a large role in immune function. Preliminary evidence suggests that thymus extract may increase left ventricular function, exercise tolerance, and survival. Additional study is needed in this area. It is important to use high-quality thymus gland supplements.

Fair Negative Scientific Evidence

Guided Imagery: Therapeutic guided imagery may be used to help individuals relax and focus on images associated with personal issues they are confronting. Preliminary human research reports no benefits of guided imagery in CHF.

Traditional or Theoretical Uses that Lack Sufficient Evidence

Integrative therapies traditionally used in CHF but that lack sufficient scientific evidence include acupuncture, aloe (*Aloe vera*), buchu (*Agathosma betulina*), dandelion (*Taraxacum officinale*), danshen (*Salvia miltiorrhiza*), dong quai (*Angelica sinensis*), ginkgo (*Ginkgo biloba*), horse chestnut (*Aesculus hippocastanum*), horsetail (*Equisetum arvense*), omega-3 fatty acids, fish oil, alpha-linolenic acid, scotch broom (*Cytisus scoparius*), tai chi, valerian (*Valeriana officinalis*), and vitamin E.

PREVENTION

Smoking Cessation: Smoking damages blood vessels, reduces the amount of oxygen in the blood, and makes the heartbeat faster. If an individual smokes, a doctor can help recommend a program to help him or her quit. Individuals are not considered for a heart transplant if smoking is continued.

Weight Control: It is recommended that individuals weigh themselves each morning after urination but before breakfast. Notify a doctor if there is a weight gain of three or more pounds in a day. Weight gain may indicate fluid build-up.

Being overweight contributes to other risk factors for stroke, such as high blood pressure, cardiovascular disease, and diabetes. Weight loss of as little as 10 pounds may lower blood pressure and improve cholesterol levels.

Exercise can lower blood pressure, increase the level of high-density lipoprotein ("good cholesterol"), and improve the overall health of blood vessels and heart. It also helps control weight, control diabetes, and reduce stress. Cardiac rehabilitation programs exist for individuals recovering from heart surgery. Cardiac rehabilitation is a medically supervised program to help heart patients recover quickly and improve their overall physical, mental, and social functioning. The goal is to stabilize, slow, or even reverse the progression of cardiovascular disease, thereby reducing the risk of heart disease, another cardiac event, or death. Cardiac rehabilitation programs include counseling so the individual can understand and manage the disease process; an exercise program; counseling on nutrition; helping the patient modify risk factors such as high blood pressure, smoking, high blood cholesterol, physical inactivity, obesity, and diabetes; providing vocational guidance to enable the patient to return to work; information on physical limitations; lending emotional support; and counseling on appropriate use of prescribed medications. A doctor can help initiate an exercise program and cardiac rehabilitation tailored to the individual with CHF.

Salt Restriction: Too much sodium (from salt) contributes to water retention, which makes the heart work harder. Excess sodium may causes shortness of breath and swollen legs, ankles, and feet. For individuals with heart failure the recommended sodium intake is no more than 2,000 mg daily. Some substitutes or "lite" salts contain a mixture of salt and other compounds. To get that familiar salty taste, individuals may use too much of the substitute and actually not reduce sodium intake. In addition, many salt substitutes contain potassium chloride. Too much potassium can be harmful. A dietitian can help outline a healthy, low-salt diet.

Stress Management: Stress can cause an increase in blood pressure along with increasing the blood's tendency to clot. Managing stress can be vital to keeping a heart healthy.

Diet Modification: Eating healthy foods is important. A heart-healthy diet should include five or more daily servings of fruits and vegetables, foods rich in soluble fiber (such as oatmeal and beans), foods rich in calcium (dairy products, spinach), soy products (such as tempeh, miso, tofu, and soy milk), and foods rich in omega-3 fatty acids, including cold water fish, such as salmon, mackerel, and tuna. Pregnant women and women who plan to become pregnant in the next several years should limit their weekly intake of cold water fish because of the potential for mercury contamination. Limiting red meats and high-fat foods (such as doughnuts, cookies, and chips) is recommended by healthcare professionals.

Alcohol: Excessive use of alcohol may weaken the heart muscle or increase the risk of abnormal heart rhythms, further worsening existing heart failure. Alcohol may also interact with some medications used to treat heart conditions. One glass of red wine daily may be beneficial for heart health.

Swelling: Leg, ankle, and foot edema can be improved by elevating the legs above heart level for 30 minutes three or four times per day. Leg elevation alone may be sufficient therapy for patients with mild venous insufficiency but is usually not adequate for more severe cases. In addition, it may not be practical for those who work to elevate their legs several times per day.

Leg edema (swelling) can also be prevented and treated with the use of compression stockings. Many types are available, including knee-high, thigh-high, and pantyhose. Knee-high stockings are sufficient for most individuals; thigh-high stockings are less desirable because they tend to provide too much pressure behind the knees, reducing blood flow in the veins and causing discomfort. The stockings should be put on as early as possible in the morning when edema is minimal. Healthcare professionals can help with choosing the right compression stocking for each individual.

Sleep: It is recommended that individuals with CHF who have shortness of breath sleep with their head propped up at a 45-degree angle using a pillow or a wedge.

CORONARY ARTERY DISEASE (CAD)

CONDITIONS: Coronary Artery Disease (CAD), Atherosclerosis

BACKGROUND

Coronary artery disease (CAD), also known as coronary heart disease (CHD), occurs when the coronary arteries (the blood vessels that supply oxygen-rich blood to the heart muscle) gradually become narrowed or blocked by plaque (a combination of fatty material, calcium, scar tissue, and proteins) deposits. The plaque deposits decrease the space through which blood can flow, leading to poor blood flow. As platelets (disk-shaped particles in the blood that aid clotting) come to the area, blood clots form around the plaque, causing the artery to narrow even further. Sometimes, the blood clot breaks apart, and blood supply is restored. In other cases, the blood clot (coronary thrombus) may totally block the blood supply to the heart muscle (coronary occlusion). This lack of blood flow (called ischemia) can "starve" some of the heart muscle and lead to chest pain (angina). A heart attack (myocardial infarction) results when blood flow is completely blocked, usually by a blood clot forming over a plaque that has ruptured. Unhealthy habits, such as a diet high in cholesterol and other fats, smoking, and lack of exercise accelerate the deposit of fat and calcium within the inner lining of coronary arteries.

CAD is the most common form of heart disease and the leading cause of death in men and women in the United States. CAD affects about 14 million men and women in the United States and claims more lives than the other seven leading causes of death combined.

Atherosclerosis: CAD is a type of atherosclerosis in which plaque builds up inside the arteries that carry blood to the heart. As the artery walls thicken, the passageway for blood narrows. Sometimes platelets gather at the narrow area and form a clot that decreases or prevents blood flow to the region of the heart supplied by the artery. Atherosclerosis can also lead to stroke (lack of oxygen) in the brain.

RISK FACTORS AND CAUSES

Causes of and risk factors associated with developing CAD include high cholesterol and low-density lipoprotein (LDL) levels in the blood, low levels of high-density lipoprotein (HDL), high blood pressure, smoking, diabetes mellitus, obesity, age, family history of heart disease, sedentary or inactive lifestyle, stress, and male gender.

SIGNS AND SYMPTOMS

Chest Pain: The most common symptom of CAD is chest pain, or angina (angina pectoris). Angina is described as a discomfort, heaviness, pressure, aching, burning, numbness, fullness, squeezing, or painful feeling. Angina that begins suddenly or lasts only a few seconds is less likely to be angina. Angina usually begins in the chest, but it can also start or spread to different areas of the body, such as down the left arm (most common site), to the left shoulder, to the neck or lower jaw, to the mid-back, or down the right arm. It can be mistaken for indigestion or heartburn, and the pain can be difficult to pinpoint. The chest pain associated with angina usually begins at a low level and then gradually increases over several minutes to a peak. Angina that occurs during activities will usually decrease when the activity is stopped. Angina may also be caused by the use of drugs such as cocaine or amphetamines, exposure to cold temperatures, anger, smoking, or eating a heavy meal.

Other symptoms that can occur with CAD include shortness of breath, palpitations (irregular heartbeats or arrhythmias), a fast heartbeat (tachycardia), weakness or dizziness, nausea, and increased sweating.

Heart Attack: A heart attack (myocardial infarction) may also occur, and the symptoms in men and women may differ. A study found that many women reported warning symptoms one month prior to having a heart attack. These symptoms included unusual fatigue, sleep disturbances, and shortness of breath. Only 30% reported chest pain, which the majority of men report.

Unfortunately, sometimes a heart attack is the first sign of CAD. According to the Framingham Heart Study, over 50% of men and 63% of women who died suddenly of CAD (mostly from heart attack) had no previous symptoms of this disease.

Some individuals who have CAD and insufficient blood flow to the heart muscle (ischemia) do not have any symptoms. This is called silent ischemia. In rare instances a patient may even have a silent heart attack, which is a heart attack without symptoms.

DIAGNOSIS

Physical Examination and Tests: Risk factors of stroke are evaluated, including high blood pressure, high cholesterol levels, calcium levels, diabetes, medications, elevated levels of homocysteine and/or C-reactive protein (CRP, a marker of inflammation), and obesity.

Cardiac Stress Test: A stress test determines how well the blood is flowing to the heart during exercise compared to resting. The patient either walks on a treadmill or is given an intravenous (in the veins) medication that simulates exercise (usually dipyridamole [Persantine]) while connected to an electrocardiograph machine. A nuclear stress test involves the injection of radioactive isotopes (most commonly technetium or Tc-99m sestamibi), and then blood flow to and from the heart is visualized using a type of camera.

Carotid Ultrasonography: This procedure evaluates blood flow using a wandlike device (transducer) that sends high-frequency sound waves into the neck to determine if there is any narrowing or clotting in the carotid arteries.

Arteriogram: Arteriogram (or angiogram) views arteries in the heart, brain, kidney, and many other parts of the body not normally seen in x-rays. A thin, flexible tube (catheter) is inserted through a small incision, usually in the groin area. The catheter is manipulated through the major arteries and into the carotid or vertebral artery. A dye is then injected through the catheter to provide x-ray images of the arteries.

Computerized Tomographic Angiography (CTA): In CTA, a dye is injected into the blood and x-ray beams create a three-dimensional image of the blood vessels in the neck and brain. CTA is used to look for aneurysms or blood vessel malformations and to evaluate arteries for narrowing. CT scanning, which is done without dye, can provide images of the brain and show hemorrhages, but without as much detailed information regarding the blood vessels.

Magnetic Resonance Imaging (MRI): MRI uses a strong magnetic field to generate a three-dimensional view of the brain. This test is sensitive for detecting an area of brain tissue damaged by an ischemic stroke (lack of blood flow and oxygen to the brain). Magnetic resonance angiography (MRA) uses this magnetic field and a dye injected into the veins to evaluate arteries in the neck and brain.

COMPLICATIONS

The lack of blood flow to the heart can lead to irreversible damage to the heart muscle.

Invasive surgery may be required, such as coronary artery bypass graft surgery.

Chest pain (angina) may lead to a heart attack (myocardial infarction), which may cause sudden death.

TREATMENT

Treatment aims to balance blood supply to the heart with maintaining oxygen demand and preventing worsening CHD.

Medications: Various medications can be used to prevent CAD and to treat the symptoms. These include platelet inhibitors (to "thin" the blood) such as aspirin (81-325 mg daily, may cause bleeding) or clopidogrel (Plavix), beta-blockers (decrease the heart rate and blood pressure; reducing the heart's demand for oxygen, which may cause fatigue) such as metoprolol (Lopressor, Toprol), nitroglycerin (increases the oxygen available to the heart by dilating coronary arteries; may cause headache), calcium channel blockers (slow heart rate and dilate coronary blood vessels; may slow heart rate) such as amlodipine (Norvasc) or diltiazem (Cardizem), angiotensin-inhibiting drugs or angiotensin-converting enzyme inhibitors (dilate blood vessels and increase oxygen to the heart; may cause cough) such as lisinopril (Prinivil, Zestril) or ramipril (Altace), and statins or 3-hydroxy-3-methylglutaryl coenzyme A (HMG-CoA) reductase inhibitors (help lower cholesterol levels; may cause liver problems or muscle pain) such as atorvastatin (Lipitor) or lovastatin (Mevacor).

Interventional Procedures: Common interventional procedures to treat CAD include balloon angioplasty (percutaneous transluminal coronary angioplasty) and stent placement (using a wire mesh that expands in the blood vessel, allowing more blood to flow normally). These procedures are considered nonsurgical because they are done by a cardiologist through a tube or catheter that is inserted into a blood vessel. Several types of balloons, stents (some contain anticlotting medications), and/or catheters are available to treat the plaque within the vessel wall. The physician chooses the type of procedure based on individual patient needs.

Coronary Artery Bypass Graft (CABG) Surgery: CABG surgery is when one or more blocked blood vessels is bypassed by a graft and normal blood flow is restored to the heart. These grafts usually come from the patient's own arteries and veins located in the chest, leg, or arm. The graft goes around the clogged artery to create new pathways for oxygen-rich blood to flow to the heart. Some problems associated with CABG include a heart attack (occurs in 5% of patients), stroke (occurs in 5%, with the risk greatest in those over 70 years old), blood clots, death (occurs in 1-2% of individuals), and sternal wound infection (occurs in 1-4%). Infection is most often associated with obesity, diabetes, or having had a previous CABG. In about 30% of patients, post-pericardiotomy syndrome can occur anywhere from a few days to six months after surgery. The symptoms of this syndrome are fever and chest pain, and it can be treated with medications (antibiotics, nitroglyccrin, and antiinflammatory drugs). The incision in the chest or the graft site (if the graft was from the leg or arm) can be itchy, sore, numb, or bruised. Some individuals report memory loss, loss of mental clarity or "fuzzy thinking" following a CABG.

Alternate CABG Methods: Alternate methods of CABG have been developed in recent times. Off-pump coronary artery bypass surgery (OPCAB) is a technique of performing bypass surgery without the use of cardiopulmonary bypass (the heart-lung machine). Further refinements to OPCAB have resulted in minimally invasive direct CAB, which is a technique of performing bypass surgery through a very small incision (cut). This procedure also eliminates many of the problems associated with conventional CABG, including major wound healing and infection.

Transmyocardial Laser Revascularization: Transmyocardial laser revascularization is a treatment that helps improve blood flow to areas of the heart not treated by angioplasty or surgery. A special carbon dioxide laser is used to create small channels in the heart muscle, improving blood flow in the heart. Frequently, it is performed along with CABG but on occasion has been done alone.

Enhanced External Counterpulsation (EECP): Individuals with persistent angina (chest pain) symptoms who have exhausted the standard treatments without successful results may be candidates for enhanced EECP. EECP may stimulate the openings or formation of small branches of blood vessels in the heart, which creates a natural bypass around narrowed or blocked arteries.

Angiogenesis: Angiogenesis means growing new blood vessels. Investigators are studying several substances that, if administered through the vein or directly into the heart, will trigger the production of new blood vessels, increasing blood flow to the heart muscle.

INTEGRATIVE THERAPIES
Strong Scientific Evidence

Beta-Sitosterol: Beta-sitosterol is one of the most common dietary phytosterols (plant sterols) found and synthesized exclusively by plants such as fruits, vegetables, soybeans, breads, and peanuts and peanut products. Many studies in humans and animals have demonstrated that supplementation of beta-sitosterol into the diet decreases total serum cholesterol as well as LDL cholesterol. Caution is advised when taking beta-sitosterol supplements, as numerous adverse

effects including drug interactions are possible. Beta-sitosterol supplements are not generally used during pregnancy or breastfeeding unless otherwise advised by a doctor.

Psyllium: Psyllium, also referred to as ispaghula, is derived from the husks of the seeds of *Plantago ovata*. Psyllium contains a high level of soluble dietary fiber and is the chief ingredient in many commonly used bulk laxatives, such as Metamucil and Serutan. Psyllium is well studied as a cholesterol-lowering agent with generally modest reductions seen in blood levels of total cholesterol and LDL ("bad cholesterol"). Effects have been observed following eight weeks of regular use. Psyllium does not appear to have significant effects on HDL ("good cholesterol") or triglyceride levels. Because only small reductions have been observed (total cholesterol and LDL), people with high cholesterol should discuss the use of more potent agents with their healthcare providers. Effects have been observed in adults and children, although long-term safety in children is not established. Psyllium may decrease the absorption of many prescription medications, nonprescription medications, and dietary supplements.

Good Scientific Evidence

Barley: The Food and Drug Administration has announced that whole grain barley and barley-containing products are allowed to claim that they reduce the risk of CHD. To qualify for the health claim, the barley-containing foods must provide at least 0.75 grams of soluble fiber per serving of the food.

Policosanol: Policosanol is a cholesterol-lowering natural mixture of higher aliphatic primary alcohols isolated and purified from sugar cane wax. Policosanol has been used to treat hypercholesterolemia (high cholesterol levels), and numerous studies have analyzed the effects of policosanol on cholesterol levels. There is a plausible, well-described mechanism supporting its use. Notably, most human studies have been conducted in Cuba, and many have been conducted by the same author(s). At this time, the evidence supporting the efficacy of this agent is compelling, although greater acceptance in the U.S. market may await completion of a large, well-conducted, randomized trial in the United States. Caution is advised when taking policosanol, as adverse effects including drug interactions are possible. Policosanol supplements should not be used if pregnant or breastfeeding unless otherwise directed by a doctor.

C

Unclear or Conflicting Scientific Evidence

Acupuncture: The practice of acupuncture, or the insertion of needles into various points on the body, originated in China 5,000 years ago. Some research has suggested that acupuncture might help reduce distress and symptoms of angina, but this has not been consistently shown in other studies.

Arginine: Arginine, or L-arginine, is considered a semiessential amino acid, because although it is normally synthesized in sufficient amounts by the body, supplementation is sometimes required. There is initial evidence from several studies that arginine when taken orally or by injection improves exercise tolerance and blood flow in arteries of the heart. Benefits have been reported in some patients with CAD and angina. Studies also suggest that arginine supplementation after myocardial infarction (heart attack) may decrease heart damage, but further research is needed to confirm these findings. L-arginine is generally safe in recommended dosages.

Astragalus: Astragalus products are derived from the roots of *Astragalus membranaceus* or related species, which are native to China. In Chinese medicine, herbal mixtures containing astragalus have been used to treat heart diseases. There are several human case reports of reduced symptoms and improved heart function, although these are not well described. High-quality human research is necessary before a conclusion can be drawn. Caution is advised when taking astragalus supplements, as adverse effects including drug interactions are possible. Astragalus supplements should not be used if pregnant or breastfeeding unless otherwise directed by a doctor.

Ayurveda: Evidence indicates that Ayurveda's comprehensive purification and detoxification regime known as panchakarma in heart disease patients may lead to increased vasoactive intestinal polypeptide (a vasodilator), acute reduction in total cholesterol, reduction in lipid peroxide (a measure of free radical damage), and a significant reduction in anxiety.

Arjuna: Arjuna (*Terminalia arjuna*) is a type of bark powder that is traditionally used as an anti-ischemic and cardioprotective agent in hypertension and ischemic heart diseases. Evidence has been found that it may reduce cholesterol and lipid peroxide levels as well as have significant antioxidant action that is comparable to vitamin E in CHD patients. Further research is needed before a firm conclusion can be drawn.

Beta-Glucan: Beta-glucan is a soluble fiber derived from the cell walls of algae, bacteria, fungi, yeast, and plants. It is commonly used for its cholesterol-lowering effects. Numerous trials have examined the effects of oral beta-glucan on cholesterol. Small reductions in total and LDL cholesterol ("bad" cholesterol) have been reported. Little to no significant changes have been noted to occur on triglyceride levels or HDL ("good" cholesterol) levels. The sum of existing positive evidence is suggestive and not definitive. Caution is advised when taking beta-glucan supplements, as numerous adverse effects including drug interactions are possible. Beta-glucan supplements are not generally used during pregnancy or breastfeeding unless otherwise advised by a doctor.

Betaine: Betaine is found in most microorganisms, plants, and marine animals. Its main physiological functions are to protect cells under stress and act as a source of methyl groups, which are needed for many biochemical pathways. Betaine is also found naturally in many foods and is most highly concentrated in beets, spinach, grain, and shellfish. Overall, betaine supplementation may produce significant reductions in homocysteine, a known risk factor of CAD, but additional studies are needed. Betaine supplements should not be used if pregnant or breastfeeding unless otherwise directed by a doctor.

Bilberry: Bilberry (*Vaccinium myrtillus*), also known as the European blueberry, is widely used as an antioxidant for general health. Bilberry has been used traditionally to treat heart disease and atherosclerosis (hardening of the arteries). There is some laboratory research in this area, but there is no clear information in humans. Caution is advised when taking bilberry supplements, as adverse effects, including an increase in bleeding and drug interactions, are possible. Bilberry supplements should not be used if pregnant or breastfeeding unless otherwise directed by a doctor.

Coenzyme Q10 (CoQ10): CoQ10 is produced by the human body and is necessary for the basic functioning of cells. Preliminary small human studies suggest that CoQ10 may reduce angina and improve exercise tolerance in people with clogged heart arteries. Several studies also suggest that the function of the heart may be improved after major heart surgeries such as CABG or valve replacement when CoQ10 is given to patients prior to or during the surgery. CoQ10 is generally safe in recommended dosages, but further studies are needed.

Cordyceps: *Cordyceps sinensis* is a fungus found mainly in China, Nepal, and Tibet. Cordyceps supplements may lower total cholesterol and triglyceride levels, although these changes may not be permanent or long lasting. Longer studies with follow-up are needed to determine the long-term effects of cordyceps on hyperlipidemia. Caution is advised when taking cordyceps supplements, as adverse effects including drug interactions are possible. Cordyceps supplements should not be used if pregnant or breastfeeding unless otherwise directed by a doctor.

Garlic: Garlic (*Allium sativum*) is traditionally used for heart health. Multiple studies in humans have reported small reductions in total blood cholesterol and LDL ("bad cholesterol") over short periods of time (four to 12 weeks). It is not clear if there are benefits after this amount of time. Effects on HDL ("good cholesterol") are also unclear. This remains an area of controversy, and well-designed, longer studies are needed in this area. Caution is advised when taking garlic supplements, as adverse effects, including an increase in bleeding and drug interactions, are possible. Garlic supplements should not be used if pregnant or breastfeeding unless otherwise directed by a doctor.

Ginseng: Asian ginseng, or *Panax ginseng,* has been used for more than 2,000 years in Chinese medicine for various health conditions. Several studies from China report that ginseng in combination with various other herbs may reduce symptoms of CAD. Ginseng may also lower blood pressure. Caution is advised when taking ginseng supplements, as adverse effects including drug interactions are possible. Ginseng supplements should not be used if pregnant or breastfeeding unless otherwise directed by a doctor.

Green Tea: Green tea is made from the dried leaves of *Camellia sinensis,* a perennial evergreen shrub. Green tea has a long history of use, dating back to China approximately 5,000 years ago. Green tea, black tea, and oolong tea are all derived from the same plant, just processed differently. There is evidence that regular intake of green tea may lower cholesterol levels and reduce the risk of heart attack or atherosclerosis (clogged arteries). Caution is advised when taking green tea supplements, as adverse effects including drug interactions are possible. Green tea supplements should not be used if pregnant or breastfeeding unless otherwise directed by a doctor.

Hawthorn: Hawthorn (*Crataegus* spp.), a flowering shrub of the rose family, has an extensive history of use in cardiovascular disease dating back to the first century. Increased blood flow to the heart and heart performance have been observed in animals when given hawthorn supplements. One randomized clinical trial indicates that hawthorn may be effective in decreasing frequency or severity of anginal symptoms. Hawthorn has not been tested in the setting of concomitant drugs such as beta-blockers or angiotensin-converting enzyme inhibitors, which are often the standard of care. At this time, there is insufficient evidence to recommend for or against hawthorn's use in CAD or angina. Caution is advised when taking hawthorn supplements, as adverse effects including drug interactions are possible. Hawthorn supplements should not be used if pregnant or breastfeeding unless otherwise directed by a doctor.

Kudzu: Kudzu (*Pueria lobota*) is well known to people in the Southeastern United States as an invasive weed, but it has been used in Chinese medicine for centuries. Kudzu has a long history of use in the treatment of cardiovascular disorders, including angina, acute myocardial infarction, and heart failure. A small number of poorly designed trials found kudzu to reduce the frequency of angina events in human subjects. Overall, the studies have been methodologically weak. Caution is advised when taking kudzu supplements, as adverse effects including drug interactions are possible. Kudzu supplements should not be used if pregnant or breastfeeding unless otherwise directed by a doctor.

Kundalini Yoga: Kundalini yoga is one of many traditions of yoga that share common roots in ancient Indian philosophy. It is comprehensive in that it combines physical poses with breath control exercises, chanting (mantras), meditations, prayer, visualizations, and guided relaxation. One case series report suggests that breathing techniques used in Kundalini yoga may help people with angina pectoris reduce symptoms and the need for medication. A specific breathing technique of Kundalini yoga reputed to help prevent heart attacks was examined in one study to determine its effects on heart function. The technique is as follows: one breath per minute of respiratory exercise with slow inspiration for 20 seconds, breath retention for 20 seconds, and slow expiration for 20 seconds. This occurs for 31 consecutive minutes. The technique was found to stabilize the heart's electrical wave patterns, which may have preventive value in heart health.

L-Carnitine: L-carnitine, or acetyl-L-carnitine, is an amino acid found in the body. Evidence from clinical trials suggests that L-carnitine is effective in reducing symptoms of angina; however, carnitine may not offer further benefit when patients continue conventional therapies. Additional studies are needed to confirm these findings. L-carnitine is generally safe when used in recommended dosages.

Niacin: Niacin, also known as vitamin B_3 or nicotinic acid, is a well-accepted treatment for high cholesterol. Multiple studies show that niacin (not niacinamide) has significant benefits on levels of HDL ("good cholesterol"), with better results than prescription drugs such as statins. There are also benefits on levels of LDL ("bad cholesterol"), although these effects are less dramatic. A combination therapy with niacin and a statin may increase the effects on LDL. The use of niacin for the treatment of dyslipidemia secondary to type 2 diabetes has been controversial because of the possible worsening glycemic control. Individuals should check with a physician and pharmacist before starting niacin.

Omega-3 Fatty Acids: Omega-3 fatty acids are essential fatty acids found in some plants and fish. There should be a balance of omega-6 and omega-3 fatty acids for health. There is strong scientific evidence from human trials that omega-3 fatty acids from fish or fish oil supplements significantly reduce blood triglyceride levels. Fish oil supplements have reported small improvements in HDL ("good cholesterol"), but increases (worsening) in LDL ("bad cholesterol") are observed. Several well-conducted randomized, controlled trials report that in people with a history of heart attack, regular consumption of oily fish or fish oil/omega-3 supplements reduces the risk of nonfatal heart attack, fatal heart attack, sudden death, and all-cause mortality (death due to any cause). Most patients in these studies were also using conventional heart drugs, suggesting that the benefits of fish oils may add to the effects of other therapies. Preliminary studies also report reductions in angina (chest pain) associated with fish oil intake. Better research is necessary before a firm conclusion can be drawn. Caution is advised when taking omega-3 supplements, as numerous adverse effects, including an increase in bleeding and drug interactions, are possible. Omega-3 supplements should not be used if pregnant or breastfeeding unless otherwise directed by a doctor.

Prayer: Prayer has far-reaching healing effects that are hard to study. Initial studies in patients with heart disease report variable effects on severity of illness, complications during hospitalization, procedure outcome, or death rates when intercessory prayer is used.

Psychotherapy: Psychotherapy is an interactive process between a person and a qualified mental health professional, such as a psychiatrist, psychologist, clinical social worker, licensed counselor, or other trained practitioner. Its purpose is the exploration of thoughts, feelings, and behavior for the purpose of problem solving or achieving higher levels of functioning. Alexithymia, or the inability to express

one's feelings may influence the course of CHD. Educational sessions and group psychotherapy may decrease alexithymia and reduce cardiac events.

Quercetin: Quercetin is one of the almost 4,000 bioflavonoids (antioxidants) that occur in foods of plant origin, such as red wine, onions, green tea, apples, berries, and Brassica vegetables (cabbage, broccoli, cauliflower, turnips). Several of the effects of flavonoids that have been observed in laboratory and animal studies suggest that they might be effective in reducing cardiovascular disease risk. Studies in humans using polyphenol compounds from red grapes showed improvement in endothelial function in patients with CHD. Antioxidant and cholesterol-lowering effects are proposed.

Red Yeast Rice: Red yeast rice is the product of yeast (*Monascus purpureus*) grown on rice and is served as a dietary staple in some Asian countries. It contains several compounds collectively known as monacolins, substances known to inhibit cholesterol synthesis. One of these, monacolin K, is a potent inhibitor of HMG-CoA reductase and is also known as lovastatin (Mevacor). Preliminary evidence reports that taking red yeast rice by mouth may result in cardiovascular benefits and improve blood flow. Since the 1970s, human studies have reported that red yeast lowers blood levels of total cholesterol, LDL ("bad cholesterol"), and triglyceride levels. Caution is advised when taking red yeast rice supplements, as adverse effects including drug interactions are possible. Red yeast rice supplements should not be used if pregnant or breastfeeding unless otherwise directed by a doctor. Red yeast rice should not be used in people with liver problems or in heavy alcohol users.

Reishi: Reishi (*Ganoderma lucidum*) is a fungus (mushroom) that grows wild on decaying logs and tree stumps. Reishi has been used in traditional Chinese medicine for more than 4,000 years to treat liver disorders, high blood pressure, arthritis, and other ailments. A reishi supplement was reported to improve the major symptoms of CHD such as angina (chest pain), palpitations (irregular heartbeats), shortness of breath, high blood pressure, and high cholesterol in patients. Long-term studies are needed to evaluate the efficacy and safety of reishi in CHD. Caution is advised when taking reishi supplements, as adverse effects, including an increase in bleeding and drug interactions, are possible. Reishi supplements should not be used if pregnant or breastfeeding unless otherwise directed by a doctor.

Relaxation Therapy: Relaxation techniques include behavioral therapeutic approaches that differ widely in philosophy, methodology, and practice. The primary goal is usually nondirected relaxation. Most techniques share the components of repetitive focus (on a word, sound, prayer phrase, body sensation, or muscular activity), adoption of a passive attitude towards intruding thoughts, and return to focus.

Resveratrol: Resveratrol is found in over 70 plant species, including nuts, grapes, pine trees, certain vines, and red wine. Resveratrol is used as an antioxidant in various health conditions, including heart disease prevention. Laboratory animal studies suggest resveratrol helps restore blood flow to the heart. Well-designed clinical trials in humans using resveratrol are needed. Caution is advised when taking resveratrol supplements, as adverse effects, including an increase in bleeding and drug interactions, are possible. Resveratrol supplements should not be used if pregnant or breastfeeding unless otherwise directed by a doctor.

Safflower: Safflower yellow injection may improve both western and traditional Chinese medicine symptoms for angina pectoris and CAD. More high-quality studies with safflower are needed to establish the effect of safflower yellow injection.

Soy: Soy (*Glycine max*) is a member of the pea family and has been a dietary staple in Asian countries for at least 5,000 years. Numerous human studies report that adding soy protein to the diet can moderately decrease blood levels of total cholesterol and LDL ("bad" cholesterol). Small reductions in triglycerides may also occur, while HDL ("good" cholesterol) does not seem to be significantly altered. Dietary soy protein has not been proven to affect long-term cardiovascular outcomes such as heart attack or stroke. Soy products such as tofu are high in protein and are an acceptable source of dietary protein. Caution is advised when taking soy supplements, as adverse effects including drug interactions are possible. Soy supplements should not be used if pregnant or breastfeeding unless otherwise directed by a doctor.

Tai Chi: Tai chi is a system of movements and positions believed to have developed in twelfth century China. Tai chi techniques aim to address the body and mind as an interconnected system and are traditionally believed to have mental and physical health benefits that improve posture, balance, flexibility, and strength. There is evidence that suggests tai chi decreases blood pressure and cholesterol as well as enhances quality of life in patients with chronic heart failure. Most studies have used elderly Chinese patients as their population; therefore, additional research is needed before a firm conclusion can be drawn.

Traditional Chinese Medicine: Traditional Chinese medicine herb combinations have been found to improve some markers of CHD. More studies of better design are needed before recommendations can be made.

Tribulus: Preliminary research suggests that tribulus (*Tribulus terrestris*) may be beneficial to patients with CHD. Additional study is needed to further evaluate its clinical effectiveness.

Vitamin B$_{12}$: Vitamin B$_{12}$ (or cyanocobalamin) is an essential water-soluble vitamin that is commonly found in a variety of foods such as fish, shellfish, meats, and dairy products. Vitamin B$_{12}$ is frequently used in combination with other B vitamins in a vitamin B–complex formulation. Folic acid, pyridoxine (vitamin B$_6$), and vitamin B$_{12}$ supplementation can reduce total homocysteine levels (a known risk factor of CAD). This reduction does not seem to help with secondary prevention of death or cardiovascular events, such as stroke or myocardial infarction in people with a prior stroke history. More evidence is needed to fully explain the association of total homocysteine levels with vascular risks and the potential use of vitamin supplementation.

Vitamin B$_6$: Vitamin B$_6$, or pyridoxine, is found in cereal grains, legumes, vegetables (carrots, spinach, peas), potatoes, milk, cheese, eggs, fish, liver, meat, and flour. Mild deficiencies of this B vitamin are common. Vitamin B$_6$ may help lower homocysteine levels. Also, decreased vitamin B$_6$ concentrations arc also associated with increased plasma levels of CRP. CRP is an indicator of inflammation that is associated with increased cardiovascular morbidity in epidemiologic studies.

Vitamin E: Vitamin E is a fat-soluble vitamin with antioxidant properties. Vitamin E has been suggested and evaluated in patients with angina, although possible benefits remain unclear. Vitamin E has been proposed to have a role in preventing or reversing atherosclerosis by inhibiting oxidation of LDL ("bad cholesterol"). Several population studies have suggested that a high dietary intake of vitamin E and high blood concentrations of alpha-tocopherol are associated with lower rates of heart disease. While the Cambridge Heart Antioxidant Study supported this hypothesis, the more recent prospective Heart Outcomes Prevention Evaluation (HOPE) study did not. This area remains controversial.

Yoga: Yoga is an ancient system of relaxation, exercise, and healing with origins in Indian philosophy. Several human studies suggest that yoga is helpful in people with heart disease, but it is unclear if yoga reduces the risk of heart attack or death, or if yoga is better than other forms of exercise such as lifestyle or dietary changes. Yoga may be a useful addition to standard therapies (such as medications for blood pressure or cholesterol) in people at risk for heart attacks, but further research is necessary.

Traditional or Theoretical Uses Lacking Sufficient Evidence

Other supplements that may have benefit in reducing the risk of developing or in treating CAD include alfalfa (*Medicago sativa*), aortic acid, ashwagandha (*Withania somnifera*), astaxanthin, avocado (*Persea americana*), berberine, chamomile (*Matricaria recutita, Chamaemelum nobile*), coleus (*Coleus forskohlii*), copper, creatine, danshen (*Salvia miltiorrhiza*), dehydroepiandrosterone, elder (*Sambucus nigra*), fenugreek (*Trigonella foenum-graecum*), flaxseed and flaxseed oil (*Linum usitatissimum*), folate (folic acid), gamma oryzanol, globe artichoke (*Cynara scolymus*), goldenseal (*Hydrastis canadensis*), grapefruit (*Citrus paradisi*), guggul (*Commiphora mukul*), gymnema (*Gymnema sylvestre R.Br.*), honey, horny goat weed (*Epimedium grandiflorum*), *Lactobacillus acidophilus*, lemongrass (*Cymbopogon* spp.), lycopene, macrobiotic diet, meditation, milk thistle (*Silybum marianum*), nopal (*Opuntia* spp.), ozone therapy, pantethine (pantothenic acid derivative), physical therapy, pomegranate (*Punica granatum*), probiotics, pycnogenol (*Pinus pinaster* spp. *atlantica*), red clover (*Trifolium pratense*), rhubarb (*Rheum officinale, Rheum palmatum*), scotch broom (*Cytisus scoparius* Link.), selenium, spirulina, sweet almond (*Prunus amygdalus dulcis*), taurine, transcutaneous electrical nerve stimulation, turmeric (*Curcuma longa Linn.*), vitamin D, white horehound (*Marrubium vulgare*), wild yam (*Dioscoreaceae villosa*), and zinc.

PREVENTION

High Blood Pressure (Hypertension) Control: One of the most important things that can be done for prevention of CAD is to reduce high blood pressure. Blood pressure should be a systolic reading of 120 and a diastolic reading of 80 (120/80 mm Hg). Exercising, managing stress, maintaining a healthy weight, and limiting sodium and alcohol intake are all ways to keep blood pressure in check. Medications to treat hypertension, such as diuretics, angiotensin-converting enzyme inhibitors, and angiotensin receptor blockers may be used.

Cholesterol and Saturated Fat Intake Reduction: Eating less cholesterol and fat, especially saturated fat, may reduce the amount of plaque in arteries.

Most people should aim for an LDL level below 130 mg/dL. If there are other risk factors for heart disease, the target LDL may be below 100 mg/dL. If the individual is at a very high risk for heart disease, such as having a previous heart attack, an LDL level below 70 mg/dL may be optimal. Statin drugs (HMG-CoA reductase inhibitors) can be prescribed to help maintain healthy cholesterol levels.

Platelet Inhibitors: In otherwise healthy men older than 50 years, an aspirin 325 mg every other day prevents myocardial infarction (at a rate of two men per 1,000) but not stroke. In otherwise healthy women older than 45 years, an aspirin 100 mg every other day prevents ischemic stroke (at a rate of three women per 1,000) but not myocardial infarction. Platelet inhibitors, or antiaggregants (prevent platelet clumping), such as aspirin may increase in the risk of gastrointestinal bleeding. Other platelet inhibitors include dipyridamole (Persantine), ticlopidine (Ticlid), and clopidogrel (Plavix). A 15% relative risk reduction in vascular events (stroke, death, and myocardial infarction) has been documented for aspirin compared with placebo.

Smoking Cessation: Smoking is a major risk factor for CAD. Nicotine constricts blood vessels and forces the heart to pump harder. A buildup of carbon monoxide reduces oxygen in the blood and damages the lining of the blood vessels.

Diabetes Control: Managing diabetes with diet, exercise, weight control, and medication is essential. Strict control of blood sugar may reduce damage to the heart.

Flu Shots: Flu shots for patients with chronic cardiovascular disease are now used routinely.

Weight Control: Being overweight contributes to other risk factors for stroke, such as high blood pressure, cardiovascular disease, and diabetes. Weight loss of as little as 10 pounds may lower blood pressure and improve cholesterol levels.

Exercise: Exercise can lower blood pressure, increase the level of HDL cholesterol ("good cholesterol"), and improve the overall health of blood vessels and heart. It also helps control weight, control diabetes, and reduce stress. Thirty minutes daily of exercise is normally recommended.

Stress Management: Stress can cause an increase in blood pressure along with increasing the blood's tendency to clot. Managing stress can be vital to keeping a heart healthy.

Diet: Eat healthy foods. A brain-healthy diet should include five or more daily servings of fruits and vegetables, foods rich in soluble fiber (such as oatmeal and beans), foods rich in calcium (dairy products, spinach), soy products (such as tempeh, miso, tofu, and soy milk), and foods rich in omega-3 fatty acids, including cold water fish, such as salmon, mackerel, and tuna. Pregnant women and women who plan to become pregnant in the next several years should limit their weekly intake of cold water fish because of the potential for mercury contamination. The U.S. Food and Drug Administration has announced that whole grain barley and barley-containing products are allowed to claim that they reduce the risk of CAD.

DEPRESSION

BACKGROUND

Depression, or depressive disorder, is an illness that involves the body, mood, and thoughts. Depression is considered a mood disorder. Imbalances in three neurotransmitters (brain chemicals), serotonin, norepinephrine, and dopamine, are linked to depression. Depression affects the way a person eats and sleeps, the way one feels about oneself, and the way one thinks about life situations. Unlike normal emotional experiences of sadness, loss, or passing mood states, depressive disorders are persistent and can significantly interfere with an individual's thoughts, behavior, mood, activity, and physical health.

Depressive disorders affect approximately 18.8 million American adults or about 9.5% of the U.S. population age 18 and older in a given year. This includes major depressive disorder (severe depression), dysthymic disorder (mild to moderate depression), and bipolar disorder (manic-depressive). Among all medical illnesses, major depression is the leading cause of disability in the U.S. and many other developed countries.

Without treatment, symptoms can last for weeks, months, or years. Appropriate treatment, however, can help most people who suffer from depression.

Children and teenagers can also suffer from depression. Depression in the young is defined as an illness when the feelings of depression persist and interfere with a child or adolescent's ability to function. About 5% of children and adolescents in the general population suffer from depression at any given point in time. Children under stress, who experience loss, or who have trouble with attention, learning, conduct, or anxiety disorders are at a higher risk for depression.

RISK FACTORS AND CAUSES

Neurotransmitter Imbalances: Studies suggest that a low or high level of neurotransmitters such as serotonin, norepinephrine, or dopamine cause depression. Studies have found evidence that a change in the sensitivity of the receptors on nerve cells to these neurotransmitters may be one issue, along with an imbalance in the amounts of neurotransmitters. Balancing neurotransmitters with drug therapy is the current focus for treatment of major depression.

Heredity: Researchers have identified several genes that may be involved in bipolar disorder and are looking for genes linked to other types of depression. But not everyone with a family history of depression develops the disorder and, conversely, people with no family history of the disorder can become depressed.

Gender: Depression occurs twice as frequently in women as in men for reasons that are not fully understood. Hormonal changes such as menstrual cycle changes, postpartum period, premenopause, pregnancy, childbirth, miscarriage, and menopause are the most likely causes of depression.

Although men are less likely to suffer from depression than women, six million men in the United States are affected by the illness. Men are less likely to admit to depression. The rate of suicide in men is four times that of women, though more women attempt it.

Stress: Stressful life events, particularly a loss or threatened loss of a loved one or a job, can trigger depression.

Medications: Long-term use of certain medications, such as some drugs used to control high blood pressure, sleeping pills, or birth control pills, may cause symptoms of depression in some people.

Illnesses: Having a chronic illness, such as heart disease, stroke, diabetes, cancer, or Alzheimer's disease, puts an individual at a higher risk of developing depression. Having an underactive thyroid (hypothyroidism), even mildly, also can cause depression. Physical trauma (damage) to the brain can also trigger depression.

Personality: Certain personality traits, such as having low self-esteem and being overly dependent, self-critical, pessimistic, and easily overwhelmed by stress, can make an individual more vulnerable to depression.

Postpartum Depression: It is common for mothers to feel a mild form of distress that usually occurs a few days to weeks after giving birth. During this time the woman may have feelings of sadness, anger, anxiety, irritability, and incompetence. A more severe form of the baby blues, called postpartum depression, also can affect new mothers.

Hormones: Women experience depression about twice as much as men, which leads researchers to believe hormonal factors may play a role in the development of depression.

Alcohol, Smoking, and Drug Abuse: Abuse of alcohol, cigarettes, and recreational drugs such as cocaine, methamphetamine (crystal meth), ecstasy, and marijuana can lead to depression.

Previous Depression: More than half of those who experience a single episode of depression will continue to have episodes that occur as frequently as once or even twice a year. Without treatment, the frequency of depressive illness as well as the severity of symptoms tend to increase over time. Left untreated, depression can lead to suicide.

SIGNS AND SYMPTOMS

The onset of the first episode of depression may not be obvious if it is gradual or mild. The symptoms of depression represent a significant change from how a person functioned before the illness. Symptoms of depression can either be mild, moderate, or severe.

Loss of Interest in Normal Daily Activities: An individual may lose interest in or pleasure from activities that they used to enjoy.

Depressed Mood: The individual may feel sad, helpless, or hopeless and may have crying spells.

Sleep Disturbances: Sleeping too much or having problems sleeping can be a sign of depression. Waking in the middle of the night or early in the morning and not being able to get back to sleep are typical.

Impaired Thinking or Concentration: The individual may have trouble concentrating or making decisions or have problems with memory.

Weight Changes: An increased or reduced appetite and unexplained weight gain or loss may indicate depression.

Agitation: The individual may seem restless, agitated, irritable, and easily annoyed.

Fatigue (Tiredness): Weariness and a lack of energy nearly every day are common signs of depression. The individual may feel as tired in the morning as when going to bed the night before.

Low Self-Esteem: Feelings of worthlessness and excessive guilt are common symptoms of depression.

Loss of Sexual Interests: If the individual was sexually active before developing depression, he or she may notice a dramatic decrease in the level of interest in having sexual relations.

Preoccupation with Death: The individual may have a persistent negative view of his or her situation in life and the future. They may have thoughts of death, dying, or suicide.

Other Physical Symptoms: Depression can also cause a wide variety of physical complaints, such as gastrointestinal problems (indigestion, constipation, or diarrhea), headache, and backache. Many people with depression also have symptoms of anxiety, including restlessness, inability to concentrate, and loss of sleep.

Depression in Children and the Elderly: Children, teens, and older adults may react differently to depression. In these groups, symptoms may take different forms or may be masked by other conditions. Kids may pretend to be sick, worry that a parent is going to die, perform poorly in school, refuse to go to school, or exhibit behavioral problems. The elderly may be more willing to discuss the physical symptoms of depression instead of their emotional difficulties, including constant complaining about aches and pains.

Suicidal Thoughts: Suicidal thoughts may accompany depression. Anyone who has suicidal feelings, talks about suicide, or attempts suicide should be taken seriously and should receive immediate help from a mental health specialist. Certain warning signs may indicate serious depression and the possibility of suicide. Danger signs include pacing, agitated behavior, frequent mood changes and sleeplessness for several nights; actions or threats of assault, physical harm, or violence; threats or talk of death or suicide, such as "I don't care anymore," or "You won't need to worry about me much longer"; withdrawal from activities and relationships; putting affairs in order, such as saying goodbye to friends, giving away prized possessions, or writing a will; a sudden brightening of mood after a period of being depressed, or unusually risky behavior, such as buying or handling a gun or driving recklessly can be indicators of suicidal thinking.

TYPES OF DEPRESSION

Major Depression: This type of depression lasts more than two weeks. Symptoms may include overwhelming feelings of sadness and grief, loss of interest or pleasure in activities usually enjoyed, and feelings of worthlessness or guilt. This type of depression may result in poor sleep, a change in appetite, severe fatigue, and difficulty concentrating. Severe depression may increase the risk of suicide.

Atypical Depression: Individuals with atypical depression, as opposed to major depression, experience improved mood when something good happens. In addition, two of the following symptoms occur to have atypical depression: an increase in appetite or weight gain (as opposed to the reduced appetite or weight loss of "typical" depression), excessive sleeping (as opposed to insomnia), leaden paralysis (a severe form of fatigue or tiredness), and sensitivity to rejection.

Dysthymia: Dysthymia is a less severe depression (mild to moderate) than major but a more chronic form of depression. Signs and symptoms usually are not disabling, and periods of mild depression can alternate with short periods of feeling normal. Having dysthymia places an individual at an increased risk of major depression. To be considered having dysthymia, the first two years of depressed mood cannot include any episodes of major depression. In addition, no underlying cause of depressed mood, such as a general medical condition (premenstrual syndrome, menopause, or coronary heart disease) or substance abuse, may be present. The symptoms of dysthymia and the associated signs of depression cause significant distress or impairment in social, occupational, and other important areas of functioning. When a major depressive episode occurs on top of dysthymia, healthcare professionals may refer to the resultant condition as double depression.

Adjustment Disorders: Having a loved one die, losing a job, or receiving a diagnosis of cancer or another disease can cause an individual to feel tense, sad, overwhelmed, or angry. Eventually, most people come to terms with the lasting consequences of life stresses, but some do not; this is called an adjustment disorder. Adjustment disorders are forms of depression that occur when the response to a stressful event or situation causes signs and symptoms of depression. Some people develop an adjustment disorder in response to a single event such as a parent or spouse dying. In others, it stems from a combination of stressors. Adjustment disorders can be acute (lasting less than six months) or chronic (lasting longer). Doctors classify adjustment disorders based on the primary signs and symptoms of depression.

Bipolar Disorder: Having recurrent episodes of depression and elation (mania) is characteristic of bipolar disorder. Because this condition involves emotions at both extremes (poles), it's called bipolar disorder or manic-depressive disorder. Mania affects judgment, causing individuals to make unwise decisions. Some people have bursts of increased creativity and productivity during the manic phase. The number of episodes at either extreme may not be equal. Some people may have several episodes of depression before having another manic phase, or vice versa.

Seasonal Affective Disorder (SAD): SAD is a pattern of depression related to changes in seasons and a lack of exposure to sunlight. SAD usually occurs in winter. It may cause headaches, irritability, and a low energy level. SAD is not a chronic (long-term) depressive disorder.

Postpartum Depression: According to the American College of Obstetricians and Gynecologists, about 10% of new moms experience postpartum depression,

a more severe form of depression that can develop within the first six months after giving birth. For women with postpartum depression, feelings such as sadness, anxiety and restlessness can be so strong that they interfere with daily tasks. Rarely, a more extreme form of depression known as postpartum psychosis can develop. Symptoms of this psychosis include a fear of harming oneself or one's baby, confusion and disorientation, hallucinations and delusions, and paranoia.

Premenstrual Dysphoric Disorder (PMDD): PMDD occurs when depressive symptoms, such as crying, tiredness, and sadness, occur one week prior to menstruation and disappear after menstruation.

DIAGNOSIS

History and Physical Examination: To diagnosis depression the doctor must first rule out all other disease possibilities. Typically, the diagnosis begins with a medical history, including questions about the duration, severity, and characteristics of symptoms. The physician will ask about diet, stress, any medications currently being taken, and changes in sleep patterns. Questionnaires may be used to determine the level of depression.

Diagnosis also involves ruling out other mental health conditions that may produce symptoms similar to depression. These may include other mood disorders, such as bipolar, schizophrenia, attention deficit–hyperactivity disorder, and borderline personality disorder.

A diagnosis of depressive disorder is based on criteria found in the Diagnostic and Statistical Manual of Mental Disorders IV, developed by the American Psychiatric Association.

Laboratory Tests: Blood tests can determine if the levels of neurochemicals (brain chemicals), including serotonin, dopamine, and norepinephrine, are healthy. Tests may be ordered to rule out other causes, such as blood or urine tests to determine the balance of salts and sugar in the blood, hormone function, blood cell counts, and drug and alcohol levels. Computerized tomography scan, positron emission tomography, or magnetic resonance imaging of the head may be ordered to check for blood clots, bleeding, or tumors. A spinal tap (lumbar puncture) may be ordered to get a sample of spinal fluid to determine if a brain infection, such as meningitis or encephalitis (both forms of brain inflammation), exists. These tests may rule out other conditions that may be present (such as brain tumor or other disease) and may determine if imbalances in neurochemistry are present.

COMPLICATIONS

About half of the people who have a first episode of depression will have another episode within 10 years. The risk of further bouts of depression is higher than in someone who has never been depressed.

Alcohol and drug abuse are very common among people with depression.

Depressive disorder can have devastating effects on relationships as complete isolation and withdrawal during depression are common.

Suicide may be a complication of untreated, mistreated, or misdiagnosed depression. Women attempt suicide more often than men do, but men are much more likely to succeed in killing themselves. The rate of suicide is four times greater for men. Men over 70 are the most likely to commit suicide. Calling a local suicide hotline, such as the National Suicide Prevention Lifeline at 1-800-273-8255, can help someone thinking of suicide.

TREATMENT

Treatment for depression usually involves a combination of drug and psychological therapies.

Psychotherapy: Psychotherapy involves talking to a healthcare professional about one's problems and life situation. There are several types of psychotherapy that have been shown to be effective for depression, including cognitive-behavioral therapy and interpersonal therapy. Research has shown that mild to moderate depression can often be treated successfully with either of these therapies used alone. However, severe depression appears more likely to respond to a combination of psychotherapy and medication.

Cognitive-Behavioral Therapy (CBT): CBT helps to change the negative thinking and unsatisfying behavior associated with depression while teaching individuals how to unlearn the behavioral patterns that contribute to their depression.

Interpersonal Therapy (IPT): IPT focuses on improving troubled personal relationships and on adapting to new life roles that may have been associated with a person's depression.

Medications: Drugs used for depression often take two to four weeks to start having an effect and six to 12 weeks to have their full effect. The first antidepressant medications were introduced in the 1950s. Research has reported that imbalances in neurotransmitters like serotonin, dopamine, and norepinephrine can be improved with antidepressant use.

Selective Serotonin Reuptake Inhibitors (SSRIs): SSRIs act specifically on the neurotransmitter (brain chemical) serotonin. Serotonin is mainly involved with mood balance. SSRIs are the most common agents prescribed for depression worldwide. These agents increase the amount of serotonin that is available for use by the brain. SSRIs include fluoxetine (Prozac), sertraline (Zoloft), paroxetine (Paxil), citalopram (Celexa), escitalopram (Lexapro), and fluvoxamine (Luvox).

Serotonin and Norepinephrine Reuptake Inhibitors (SNRIs): SNRIs are the second most popular antidepressants worldwide. These agents increase the amount of both serotonin and norepinephrine. SNRIs include venlafaxine (Effexor) and duloxetine (Cymbalta). SSRIs and SNRIs tend to have fewer side effects than other types of antidepressants. Side effects include nausea, nervousness, insomnia, diarrhea, rash, agitation, or sexual side effects (problems with arousal or orgasm).

Norepinephrine-Dopamine Reuptake Inhibitors (NDRIs): NDRIs act by increasing the amounts of dopamine and norepinephrine available to the brain. Bupropion (Wellbutrin) is commonly used as an antidepressant in this class.

Tricyclic Antidepressants (TCAs): TCAs are older antidepressants that are not used as frequently now. They work similarly to the SNRIs but have other properties that result in very high side effect rates compared to almost all other antidepressants. They are sometimes used in cases where other antidepressants have not worked. TCAs include amitriptyline (Elavil), desipramine (Norpramin), doxepin (Sinequan), imipramine (Norpramin, Tofranil), nortriptyline (Pamelor, Aventyl), and protriptyline (Vivactil). TCAs cause side effects that include dry mouth, constipation, bladder problems, sexual problems, blurred vision, dizziness, drowsiness, skin rash, and weight gain or loss.

Monoamine Oxidase Inhibitors (MAOIs): MAOIs are seldom used now for depression. They also increase amounts of serotonin, norepinephrine, and dopamine for the brain to use in mood stabilization. They can sometimes be effective for people who do not respond to other medications or who have atypical depression with marked anxiety, excessive sleeping, irritability, hypochondria (health anxiety), or phobic (obsessive) characteristics. However, they are the least safe antidepressants to use, as they have important medication interactions, including causing dangerously high blood pressure, and require adherence to a diet free of tyramine, a chemical found in certain foods such as fish (especially dried and salted), chocolate, alcoholic beverages (Chianti wine), and fermented foods such as cheese and soy sauce, sauerkraut, and processed meat. MAOIs include phenelzine (Nardil), isocarboxazid (Marplan), and tranylcypromine sulfate (Parnate). A range of other, less serious side effects occur, including weight gain, constipation, dry mouth, dizziness, headache, drowsiness, insomnia, and sexual side effects (problems with arousal or satisfaction).

Other: Mirtazapine (Remeron) is an antidepressant used commonly in the elderly that helps cause weight gain. A common side effect is drowsiness. Often psychiatrists will combine antidepressants with each other or with agents that are not antidepressants themselves. A class of drugs called atypical antipsychotic agents, including aripiprazole (Abilify), olanzapine (Zyprexa), quetiapine (Seroquel), ziprasidone (Geodon), and risperidone (Risperdal), may be used. Side effects for these drugs are high, including excessive sedation and tardive dyskinesia (a nervous system disorder causing facial grimaces, lip smacking, and uncontrollable shaking). According to the American Diabetes Association, certain antipsychotic drugs may increase the risk of diabetes, obesity, and high blood pressure.

Stimulants, such as methylphenidate (Ritalin) or dextroamphetamine (Dexedrine) can be added. Stimulants may cause dry mouth, disturbances in sleep patterns, nervousness, anxiousness, and weight loss.

Mood-stabilizing medications may be prescribed, including lithium (Eskalith, Lithobid), valproic acid (Depakene), divalproex (Depakote), and carbamazepine (Tegretol), to treat bipolar depression. Medications called atypical antipsychotics such as olanzapine (Zyprexa), risperidone (Risperdal), and quetiapine (Seroquel) were initially developed for treatment of psychotic disorders.

Hormone Therapy: For women with postpartum depression or PMDD, hormonal replacement with estrogen and/or progesterone may help with depression. However, there is an increased risk of heart disease and cancer (breast and ovarian) with the use of these medications.

Electroconvulsive Therapy (ECT): ECT involves the use of electrical current to stimulate various parts of the brain and is used mainly in people who have episodes of major depression associated with suicidal tendencies or in people whose medication has proved to be ineffective. ECT profoundly affects brain metabolism and blood flow to various areas of the brain. How that correlates to easing depression remains unknown, but this therapy is often highly effective. Safety of ECT is controversial, and adverse effects such as confusion, memory loss, headache, hypotension (low blood pressure), and tachycardia (increased heart rate) may occur.

Light Therapy: This therapy may help if the individual has SAD. This disorder involves periods of depression that recur at the same time each year, usually when days are shorter in the fall and winter. Scientists believe fewer hours of sunlight may increase levels of melatonin, a brain hormone thought to induce sleep and depress mood. Treatment in the morning with a specialized type of bright light, which suppresses production of melatonin, may help with this disorder. Melatonin is a hormone for the sleep-wake cycle and may be decreased during depression.

Mild Depression: If mild depression is diagnosed, antidepressant drugs are not usually recommended as a first treatment. Exercise seems to help some people with depression. Talking through feelings using counseling may also be helpful for mild depression. Talking to a friend or relative, self-help reading material, or a local self-help group are good choices. If the depression is mild but there is a past history of depression, antidepressants may be used.

Chronic (long-term) mild depression or dysthymia (present for two or more years) is more likely in people over 55 years and can be difficult to treat. Individuals diagnosed with dysthymia are usually started on a course of antidepressants.

Moderate Depression: If mild depression does not improve, antidepressants or talking treatments are generally used. Research has shown that antidepressants and psychological therapies are equally effective in treating mild or moderate depression, but having the two types of treatment together does not seem to offer any extra benefits.

Severe Depression: If severe depression is diagnosed, antidepressant therapy together with psychotherapy are usually used in combination.

Although major depression can be a devastating illness, it is highly treatable. Between 80-90% of individuals diagnosed with major depression can be effectively treated and return to their usual daily activities and feelings.

Hospitalization: Depression is a serious medical illness. Urgent care and hospitalization may be necessary when individuals seem to be a danger to themselves or others, or if they are psychotic. A person experiencing extreme major depression should be brought to the hospital immediately to prevent suicide or possible violence to another person. An acute episode is treated with medications and a low-stimulation environment. Depending on the individual's symptoms and history, longer term hospitalization may be required.

INTEGRATIVE THERAPIES

Strong Scientific Evidence

Music Therapy: Music has been referred to as an ancient tool of healing. Many different forms of music intervention have been used to reduce depression and anxiety in a variety of medical conditions and medical procedures. There is evidence that music therapy may increase responsiveness to antidepressant medication. In elderly adults with depression, a home-based program of music therapy may have long-lasting effects. In depressed adult women, music therapy may lead to reductions in heart rate, respiratory rate, blood pressure, and depressed mood.

St. John's Wort: Extracts of St. John's wort (*Hypericum perforatum*) have been recommended traditionally for a wide range of medical conditions, with the most common modern-day use being the treatment of depression. St. John's wort has been extensively studied in Europe over the last two decades, with more recent research in the United States. Short-term studies (one to three months) suggest that St. John's wort is more effective than placebo (sugar pill), and equally effective as TCAs in the treatment of mild-to-moderate major depression. Comparisons to the more commonly prescribed SSRIs, such as fluoxetine (Prozac) or sertraline (Zoloft), are more limited. However, other data suggest that St. John's wort may be just as effective as SSRIs with fewer side effects. Safety concerns exist as with most conventional and complementary therapies. Studies of St. John's wort for severe depression have not provided clear evidence of effectiveness.

In published studies, St. John's wort has generally been well tolerated at recommended doses for up to one to three months. The most common adverse effects include gastrointestinal upset, skin reactions, fatigue/sedation, restlessness or anxiety, sexual dysfunction (including impotence), dizziness, headache, and dry mouth. Caution is advised when taking St. John's wort, as numerous adverse effects including many drug interactions are possible. Drug interactions with St. John's wort can have severe consequences. One small study reported elevated thyroid stimulating hormone levels to be associated with taking St. John's wort. St. John's wort should not be used if pregnant or breastfeeding unless otherwise directed by a doctor.

Good Scientific Evidence

5-Hydroxytryptophan (5-HTP): Supplement use of 5-HTP may help balance serotonin in the body. Serotonin is the brain chemical associated with sleep, mood, movement, eating, and nervousness. While cells outside the brain, such as platelets in the blood and some cells in the intestine, produce and utilize serotonin, all serotonin used by brain cells must be made within the neurons themselves. When serotonin is not properly constructed within the brain, the result can be irritability, aggression, impatience, anxiety, and depression. It has been suggested that 5-HTP may reduce psychotic symptoms and mania or aid in panic disorder when used short term (up to one year), but studies in people with schizophrenia have shown different results. Caution is advised when taking 5-HTP supplements, as numerous adverse effects including drug interactions are possible. 5-HTP is not recommended during pregnancy or breastfeeding unless otherwise advised by a doctor.

Art Therapy: Art therapy enables the expression of inner thoughts or feelings when verbalization is difficult or not possible. It involves the application of a variety of art modalities, including drawing, painting, clay, and sculpture. Art therapy may be an effective intervention for hospitalized, suicidal adolescents. There is evidence that it can be used to aid in developing a sense of identity and optimism about the future. It may also aid in relaxation and willingness to communicate and may result in shorter hospitalization.

Dehydroepiandrosterone (DHEA): DHEA is a hormone made in the human body that serves as precursor to male and female sex hormones (androgens and estrogens). The majority of clinical trials investigating the effect of DHEA on depression support its use for this purpose under the guidance of a healthcare provider. Further research is needed to confirm these results. Few side effects are reported when DHEA supplements are taken by mouth in recommended doses. Side effects may include fatigue, nasal congestion, headache, acne, or rapid/irregular heartbeats. In women, the most common side effects are abnormal menses, emotional changes, headache, and insomnia. Individuals with a history of abnormal heart rhythms, blood clots or hypercoagulability, and those with a history of liver disease should avoid DHEA supplements. Caution is advised when taking DHEA supplements, as numerous drug interactions are possible. DHEA is not recommended during pregnancy or breastfeeding.

Psychotherapy: Psychotherapy is an interactive process between a person and a qualified mental health professional (psychiatrist, psychologist, clinical social worker, licensed counselor, or other trained practitioner). A broad range of psychotherapies are effective for the treatment of depression, including behavior therapy, CBT, and IPT. Brief dynamic therapy, marital therapy, and family therapy may work best, depending on the patient's problems and circumstances. Although prescription medication is the most effective treatment for bipolar disorder, psychotherapy may help patients take their medication, prevent relapses, and reduce suicidal behavior.

Yoga: Yoga is an ancient system of relaxation, exercise, and healing with origins in Indian philosophy. Several human studies support the use of yoga for depression in both children and adults. Although this preliminary research is promising, better studies are needed.

Unclear or Conflicting Scientific Evidence

Acupressure: Acupressure, or shiatsu, has been used in China for thousands of years for health and healing. Several studies suggest that fatigue and depressive mood may improve with acupressure therapy. Further research is necessary to confirm these findings.

Acupuncture: Acupuncture, or the use of needles to manipulate the "chi" or body energy, originated in China over 5,000 years ago. A small number of studies have sought to compare acupuncture with antidepressant medications used in depression. More studies are needed on this use.

Aromatherapy: Fragrant oils have been used for thousands of years. Aromatherapy is a technique in which essential oils from plants are used with the intention of preventing or treating illness, reducing stress, or enhancing well-being. Preliminary research suggests that lavender (*Lavandula officinalis*) aromatherapy may be helpful as an adjunct to prescription antidepressant medications. Additional research is necessary before a firm conclusion can be drawn.

Ayurveda: Ayurveda, which originated in ancient India over 5,000 years ago, is probably the world's oldest system of natural medicine. Early evidence suggests that a traditional Ayurvedic formula containing extracts of four Indian herbs, Ashvatha, Kapikachu, Dhanvayasa, and Bhuriphali, may have benefits similar to conventional antidepressant medication. Further studies are needed to confirm these results.

Folic Acid: Folic acid, or folate, deficiency has been found among many individuals suffering from depression and has been linked to poor response to antidepressant therapies. Folate supplements have been used for enhancing treatment response to antidepressants. Limited clinical research suggests that folic acid is not effective as a replacement for conventional antidepressant therapy. Folate appears to be well tolerated in recommended doses. Blood tests can determine if an individual is low in vitamins such as folic acid.

Ginkgo: Preliminary study of SAD suggests that ginkgo (*Ginkgo biloba*) is not effective in preventing the development of depression during the winter months. Other research in elderly patients with depression shows possible minor benefits. Ginkgo may also help in decreasing sexual side effects such as loss of libido in individuals taking antidepressants. Overall, there is not enough evidence to form a clear conclusion. Caution is advised when taking ginkgo supplements as numerous adverse effects including an increase in bleeding and drug interactions are possible. Ginkgo is not recommended during pregnancy or breastfeeding, unless otherwise advised by a doctor.

Healing Touch (HT): Preliminary data from one small study suggest a series of HT sessions over time may contribute to reducing depression. However, data are insufficient to form definitive conclusions, and studies of better design are needed.

Kundalini Yoga: Kundalini yoga is one of many traditions of yoga that share common roots in ancient Indian philosophy. It is comprehensive in that it combines physical poses with breath control exercises, chanting (mantras), meditations, prayer, visualizations, and guided relaxation. It is an elaborate system focused on healing and "purifying" the mind, body, and emotions. There is evidence from one small clinical trial where Kundalini yoga was practiced of benefit in depression. More trials are needed to establish whether this is a viable therapy for depression before a recommendation can be made.

L-Carnitine: L-carnitine (also known as acetyl-L-carnitine) is an antioxidant and may help blood flow as well as neurological function. Although the results are promising there is insufficient evidence to support the use of acetyl-L-carnitine in the treatment of depression. Well-designed clinical trials with adequate subject number are required. Caution is advised when taking acetyl-L-carnitine supplements as numerous adverse effects including drug interactions are possible.

Massage: Various forms of therapeutic superficial tissue manipulation have been practiced for thousands of years across cultures. Massage is relaxing and may decrease stress. There is insufficient evidence to determine if massage is beneficial in patients with depression. Additional research is necessary in order to form a scientifically based recommendation.

Melatonin: There is limited study of melatonin given to patients with sleep disturbances associated with bipolar disorder (such as insomnia or irregular sleep patterns). No clear benefits have been reported. Depression may be associated with neuroendocrine and sleep abnormalities, such as reduced time before dream sleep (random eye movement latency). Melatonin has been suggested for the improvement of sleep patterns in patients with depression, although research is limited in this area. Further studies are needed before a clear conclusion can be reached. Melatonin is not to be used for extended periods of time. Caution is advised when taking melatonin supplements as numerous adverse effects including drug interactions are possible. Melatonin is not recommended during pregnancy or breastfeeding unless otherwise advised by a doctor.

Omega-3 Fatty Acids: Essential fatty acids (including omega-3 fatty acids) have many roles in the body, including proper nerve and brain function. There have been several studies on the use of omega-3 fatty acids in depression; however, not enough reliable evidence is available to form a clear conclusion or replace standard treatments. Omega-3 fatty acids found in fish oils are normally used. It is important to choose quality fish oil supplements, as heavy metals have been reported in some fish oil supplements. The label should say if the product has been tested for heavy metal contamination (such as lead and mercury).

Qi Gong: Qi gong is a type of traditional Chinese medicine that is thought to be at least 4,000 years old. Preliminary study shows that qi gong may be beneficial for relieving stress. Available data remain inconclusive, yet thousands of years of effectiveness in China for stress and anxiety must be appreciated.

Reiki: Reiki is a Buddhist practice that is approximately 2,500 years old. It is used for stress reduction and relaxation and is administered by "laying on hands" and moving around the "energy" of the body. There is evidence that Reiki can reduce symptoms of distress when compared to placebo. More information is needed before a conclusion can be drawn.

Relaxation Therapy: Relaxation therapy includes self-control relaxation, paced respiration, and deep breathing. There is promising early evidence from human trials supporting the use of relaxation to reduce symptoms of depression, although effects appear to be short lived. Better quality research is necessary before a firm conclusion can be drawn.

Riboflavin (Vitamin B$_2$): Riboflavin is a water-soluble vitamin that is involved in many processes in the body and is necessary for normal cell function, growth, and energy production. Adequate nutrient supplementation with riboflavin may be required for the maintenance of adequate cognitive function. Treatment with B vitamins, including riboflavin, has been reported to improve depression scores in patients taking TCAs.

S-**Adenosylmethionine (SAMe):** SAMe is normally formed in the body from the essential amino acid methionine. SAMe supplements are used in depression and mood disorders. SAMe has been studied for use in depression for many decades. However, the majority of trials that have been performed have significant methodological flaws limiting their clinical usefulness. A small number of randomized, placebo-controlled trials suggest an antidepressant effect that is greater than that observed with placebo. Although some studies have suggested that SAMe has a more rapid onset of action in depression than TCAs, it is uncertain whether these effects result in improved patient outcomes. Large randomized, placebo-controlled trials that compare SAMe to other antidepressants such as the SSRIs are needed. Until these trials are available, it is difficult to justify the use of SAMe in patients with depression since there are many effective antidepressants available to this patient population. Caution should be used when taking SAMe supplements as drug interactions are possible. SAMe is not recommended during pregnancy or breastfeeding unless otherwise advised by a doctor.

Tai Chi: Tai chi is a system of movements and positions believed to have developed in twelfth century China. Tai chi techniques aim to address the body and mind as an interconnected system and are traditionally believed to have mental and physical health benefits to improve posture, balance, flexibility, and strength. Preliminary research suggests that tai chi may alleviate depression, anger, and fatigue. Better studies are needed before conclusions can be drawn.

Vitamin B$_6$ (Pyridoxine): Some research suggests that pyridoxine supplementation alone or in combination with high doses of other B vitamins might help with depression. Pyridoxine helps increase the "calming" neurochemicals serotonin and gamma-aminobutyric acid levels in the blood, possibly benefiting people in dysphoric mental states. Well-designed clinical trials are needed to confirm potential benefit. Vitamin B$_6$ may be found in a multivitamin or a B-complex vitamin supplement.

PREVENTION

Healthcare providers recommend that an individual suffering from depression reduce stress and try to develop regular sleep patterns. Sleep disturbances may signal the early phase of a depressive episode.

Learn to recognize the early warning signs and triggers of depression. Warning signs of relapse vary from patient to patient and may include thoughts of death or slight changes in sleep patterns (a common indicator), mood, energy, self-esteem, sexual interest, concentration, willingness to take on new projects, and dress or grooming.

DIABETES

CONDITIONS: Diabetes, Maturity-Onset Diabetes of the Young (MODY), Metabolic Syndrome, Type 1 Diabetes, Type 2 Diabetes

BACKGROUND

Diabetes, also known as diabetes mellitus, is a chronic health condition where the body is unable to produce enough insulin and properly break down sugar (glucose) in the blood. Glucose comes from food and is used by the cells for energy. Glucose is also made in the liver. Insulin is a hormone produced by the pancreas, a large gland behind the stomach. Insulin is needed to move sugar into the cells where it can be used for energy needed for body processes.

After digestion of food, glucose passes into the bloodstream. For glucose to get into cells, insulin must be present. Throughout the pancreas are clusters of cells called the islets of Langerhans. Islets are made up of several types of cells, including beta cells that make insulin. When normal individuals eat, beta cells in the pancreas automatically produce the right amount of insulin to move glucose from blood into the cells of the body. In individuals with diabetes, however, the pancreas either produces little or no insulin, or the cells do not respond appropriately to the insulin that is produced. Glucose builds up in the blood, overflows into the urine, and passes out of the body in the urine. Thus, the body loses its main source of fuel even though the blood contains large amounts of glucose. Glucose may also interact with cells, especially those in very narrow blood vessels. This process may lead to neuropathies and decreased immune function.

With type 1 diabetes, the body does not make any insulin. With type 2 diabetes, the more common type, the body does not make or use insulin properly. Without enough insulin, glucose stays in the blood and causes a condition called hyperglycemia, or high blood sugar levels.

Diabetes is associated with long-term complications that affect almost every part of the body. The disease often leads to blindness, heart and blood vessel disease, stroke, kidney failure, amputations, and nerve damage. Uncontrolled diabetes can complicate pregnancy, and birth defects are more common in babies born to women with diabetes. Pregnant women can temporarily develop gestational diabetes, a type of diabetes that begins late in pregnancy.

In 2007, an estimated 20.8 million children and adults in the United States, or 7% of the population, had diabetes mellitus. An estimated 14.6 million have been diagnosed with diabetes (both type 1 and type 2), while 6.2 million people (or nearly one-third) are unaware that they have type 2 diabetes.

Diabetes is widely recognized as one of the leading causes of death and disability in the United States. The U.S. Centers for Disease Control and Prevention recognize diabetes as the sixth leading cause of death in the United States, with over 72,000 deaths in 2004.

TYPES AND CAUSES

Prediabetes: Individuals with prediabetes have blood glucose levels that are higher than normal but not high enough for a diagnosis of diabetes. This condition raises the risk of developing type 2 diabetes, heart disease, and stroke.

Prediabetes is also called impaired fasting glucose (IFG) or impaired glucose tolerance (IGT), depending on the test used to diagnose it. Some individuals have both IFG and IGT. In IFG, glucose levels are a little high when it has been several hours after eating. In IGT, glucose levels are a little higher than normal right after eating.

Prediabetes is becoming more common in the United States, according to estimates provided by the U.S. Department of Health and Human Services. Many individuals with prediabetes go on to develop type 2 diabetes within 10 years.

Type 1 Diabetes: Type 1 diabetes is an autoimmune disease. An autoimmune disease results when the body's immune system that fights infection begins to attack a part of the body. In diabetes, the immune system attacks and destroys the insulin-producing beta cells in the pancreas. The pancreas then produces no insulin. An individual with type 1 diabetes must take insulin daily for proper blood sugar control.

It is not known exactly what causes the body's immune system to attack the beta cells, but researchers believe that autoimmune, genetic, viral, and environmental factors may be involved. Type 1 diabetes accounts for about 5-10% of cases of diagnosed diabetes in the United States. Type 1 diabetes develops most often in children and young adults but can appear at any age.

Symptoms of type 1 diabetes usually develop over a short period, although beta cell destruction can begin years earlier. Symptoms may include increased thirst and urination, constant hunger, weight loss, blurred vision, and extreme fatigue. If not diagnosed and treated with insulin, a person with type 1 diabetes can develop a condition called diabetic ketoacidosis or a low blood pH due to the accumulation of ketones in the blood. Diabetic ketoacidosis may lead to a coma if not treated appropriately.

Type 2 Diabetes: The most common form of diabetes is type 2 diabetes. About 90-95% of individuals with diabetes have type 2. This form of diabetes is most often associated with older age, obesity, family history of diabetes, previous history of gestational diabetes (diabetes developed during pregnancy), physical inactivity, and certain ethnicities. About 80% of individuals with type 2 diabetes are overweight.

Type 2 diabetes is increasingly being diagnosed in children and adolescents. When type 2 diabetes is diagnosed, the pancreas is usually producing enough insulin, but for unknown reasons the body cannot use the insulin effectively. This is a condition called insulin resistance. After several years of making extra insulin because the body cannot use it efficiently, insulin production decreases. The result is the same as for type 1 diabetes—glucose builds up in the blood and the body cannot make efficient use of its main source of fuel.

Insulin also normally shuts down the ability of the liver to produce glucose. In individuals with type 2 diabetes, however, insulin is unable to inhibit sugar production in the liver, either because the pancreas is not producing enough insulin or because insulin's signal cannot be detected.

The symptoms of type 2 diabetes develop gradually. Their onset is not as sudden as in type 1 diabetes. Symptoms may include fatigue, frequent urination, increased thirst and hunger, weight loss, blurred vision, and slow healing of wounds or sores. Some individuals have no symptoms.

Type 2 diabetes can be treated with diet, exercise, and oral prescription medications but may require insulin shots.

Hyperinsulinemia: Hyperinsulinemia is when an individual has too much insulin in the blood. Hyperinsulinemia is not diabetes but may lead to type 2 diabetes if not managed appropriately. Hyperinsulinemia is a sign of an underlying problem that is causing the pancreas to secrete excessive amounts of insulin. The most common cause of hyperinsulinemia is insulin resistance, a condition in which the body is resistant to the effects of insulin and the pancreas tries to compensate by making more insulin. Rarely, hyperinsulinemia is caused by a tumor of the insulin-producing cells of the pancreas (insulinoma) or excessive numbers of insulin-producing cells in the pancreas (nesidioblastosis). Hyperinsulinemia may not have signs or symptoms unless it causes low blood sugar (hypoglycemia).

Metabolic Syndrome: Metabolic syndrome, also known as syndrome X or insulin resistance syndrome, is a set of abnormalities in which type 2 diabetes (insulin resistant) or hyperinsulinemia is almost always present. Insulin resistance causes the tissues to stop responding to insulin. If an individual has insulin resistance, the body will make more and more insulin, but because the tissues do not respond to it, the body will not be able to use glucose (sugar) properly. Insulin resistance often occurs with other health problems, such as diabetes, high cholesterol, high blood pressure, and heart attack. When a person has many of these problems together, doctors call it insulin resistance syndrome. Metabolic syndrome includes hypertension (high blood pressure), hyperlipidemia (high cholesterol), large waist size, an increase in cortisol (stress hormone), abnormalities in blood clotting, and an increase in inflammatory responses. A high rate of cardiovascular disease is associated with the metabolic syndrome.

Diabetes Insipidus (DI): DI is a rare disease, not widely diagnosed, in which the kidneys produce abnormally large volumes of dilute urine. DI is caused by a deficiency of the antidiuretic hormone (ADH), also known as vasopressin. DI can also be caused by insensitivity of the kidneys to ADH. DI is different from diabetes mellitus, which involves insulin problems and high blood sugar. The symptoms can be similar, such as extreme thirst and frequent urination. However, DI is related to how the kidneys handle fluids. Urine and blood tests can determine which is present.

Gestational Diabetes: Some women develop gestational diabetes late in pregnancy. Although this form of diabetes usually disappears after the birth of the baby, women who have had gestational diabetes have a 20-50% chance of developing type 2 diabetes within five to 10 years. Maintaining a reasonable body weight and being physically active may help prevent development of gestational diabetes turning into type 2 diabetes.

As with type 2 diabetes, gestational diabetes occurs more often in some ethnic groups and among women with a family history of diabetes. Gestational diabetes is caused by the hormones of pregnancy or a shortage of insulin. Women with gestational diabetes may not experience any symptoms. When a woman has diabetes and her blood sugar is poorly controlled and too high, excess amounts of sugar are transported to the baby. Since the baby does not have diabetes, the fetus is able to increase the production of insulin substantially in order to use this extra sugar. This abnormal cycle of events can result in several complications including macrosomia (large baby, over 8.8 pounds), neonatal hypoglycemia (low blood sugar), stillbirth, and birth defects (such as brain, spinal cord, or heart conditions).

The only treatment for gestational diabetes is insulin, as oral antidiabetic medications cannot be used in pregnancy due to the possible risks.

Maturity-Onset Diabetes of the Young (MODY): MODY is a type of diabetes that is caused by genetic mutations. MODY may occur during childhood or adolescence but may be misdiagnosed as type 1 or type 2 diabetes or may be unidentified until the patient is an adult. Research indicates that the genetic mutations responsible for MODY interfere with normal pancreatic secretion of insulin. Currently, six gene mutations have been identified as causative factors for MODY, each of which produces several different forms of MODY, named MODY 1 to MODY 6. Each type of MODY has different signs and symptoms, clinical manifestations, complications, and treatments.

It has been estimated that 1-5% of diabetes cases in the United States are MODY. MODY typically presents during a patients 20s, usually before the age of 25. Patients at risk for MODY have a strong family history of diabetes and/or have developed diabetes before middle age. In contrast to clinical manifestations in other forms of diabetes, MODY patients are typically not overweight and are sometimes able to be treated with meal planning, oral diabetes medications, or low doses of insulin. It is recommended for these patients to work closely with their healthcare providers to determine the best treatment based on the specific type of MODY diagnosed.

RISK FACTORS

Type 1 Diabetes

Family History: Having a family history of the disease increases the chance that an individual will develop antibodies to the insulin-making cells (beta cells) in the pancreas. But being genetically predisposed to type 1 diabetes does not mean that the individual will develop diabetes. Only about 10-15% of individuals with type 1 diabetes have a family history of the disease. If the father has the disease, a child has a 6% risk of developing it. If a sibling has the disease, a child has a 5% risk of developing it. If the mother has the disease, a child has a 2% risk of developing it. If an identical twin has the disease, the other twin has a 30-50% risk of developing it. If both a parent and one sibling have the disease, a child has a 30% risk of developing it.

Ethnicity: Caucasian individuals have an increased risk for developing type 1 diabetes compared to African-Americans, Asians, or Latinos.

Presence of Islet Cell Antibodies in the Blood: People who have both a family history of type 1 diabetes and islet cell antibodies in their blood are likely to develop the disease.

Viral Infections During Childhood: A child who has certain viral infections, particularly Coxsackie B infections, has a risk almost six times greater of developing type 1 diabetes than children who have not had this type of viral infection. However, this does not mean that the child will definitely develop type 1 diabetes. It is unclear how these infections lead to type 1 diabetes.

Lack of Breastfeeding: Children who have a genetic tendency for type 1 diabetes and stop breastfeeding before three months of age or who are given cow's milk formula before four months of age have a slightly increased risk for developing type 1 diabetes. Children who have a sibling with diabetes and drink more than two eight-ounce glasses of cow's milk per day during childhood may have a four times greater risk of developing antibodies for type 1 diabetes, increasing the risk of developing the disease. Doctors are uncertain how cow's milk actually plays a role in the development of type 1 diabetes. Insulin in the cow's milk may be a factor.

Type 2 Diabetes

Age: The risk of developing type 2 diabetes begins to rise significantly at about age 45 and rises considerably after age 65 years. This may be due to a decrease in exercise, loss of muscle mass, and increased weight. However, type 2 diabetes is increasing dramatically among children, adolescents, and younger adults.

Family History: The risk of type 2 diabetes increases if a parent or sibling has type 2 diabetes.

Pregnancy: Developing gestational diabetes increases the risk of developing type 2 diabetes later in life. Also, giving birth to a baby weighing more than nine pounds increases the risk of developing type 2 diabetes. About 3-8% of pregnant women in the United States develop gestational diabetes.

Inactivity: The less active an individual is, the greater the risk of developing type 2 diabetes. Physical activity helps control weight, uses glucose as energy, and makes cells more sensitive to insulin.

Prediabetes: Prediabetes is a condition in which the blood sugar level is higher than normal, but not high enough to be classified as type 2 diabetes. Left untreated, prediabetes often progresses to type 2 diabetes. Recent research has shown that some long-term damage to the body, especially the heart and circulatory system, may already be occurring during prediabetes. There are 54 million people in the United States who have prediabetes.

Ethnicity: Certain ethnic groups, such as African-Americans, Native Americans, Latinos, and Japanese Americans, have a greater risk of developing type 2 diabetes than Caucasians.

Weight: Being overweight is a primary risk factor for type 2 diabetes. The more fatty tissue, the more resistant cells become to insulin. Fat cells actually produce hormones, such as leptin and adiponectin, which decrease insulin tissue sensitivity, potentially leading to diabetes mellitus type 2.

Metabolic Syndrome: Metabolic syndrome, including high blood pressure, high cholesterol levels, and abdominal obesity, increases the chances of developing type 2 diabetes.

Maturity-Onset Diabetes of the Young (MODY)

Patients at risk for MODY have a strong family history of diabetes and/or have developed diabetes before middle age. There is a 50% chance for a child to inherit MODY if either parent has MODY. In the field of genetics, this is called autosomal dominant inheritance. MODY is also referred to as a monogenic form of diabetes, which describes its ability to be inherited by a single pair of genes.

SIGNS AND SYMPTOMS

Type 1 Diabetes

Symptoms of type 1 diabetes are often dramatic and come on very suddenly. Type 1 diabetes is usually recognized in childhood or early adolescence, often in association with an illness (such as a virus) or injury. The initial symptoms of type 1 diabetes are an increased production of urine, excessive thirst, fatigue, tiredness, loss of weight, increased appetite, feeling sick, blurred vision, and infections such as thrush or irritation of the genitals.

Type 1 diabetics can develop diabetic ketoacidosis. Ketoacidosis is a serious condition where the body has dangerously high levels of ketones. Ketones are substances that are made when the body breaks down fat for energy. Normally, the body gets the energy it needs from carbohydrates. However, stored fat is broken down and ketones are made if the diet does not contain enough carbohydrates to supply the body with sugar (glucose) for energy, or if the body cannot use blood sugar (glucose) properly, as in diabetes. Symptoms of ketoacidosis include nausea and vomiting. Dehydration and often serious disturbances in blood levels of potassium follow. Without treatment, ketoacidosis can lead to coma and death.

Type 2 Diabetes

Symptoms of type 2 diabetes are often subtle and may be attributed to aging or obesity. An individual may have type 2 diabetes for many years without knowing it. Individuals with type 2 diabetes can develop hyperglycemic hyperosmolar nonketotic syndrome, which is characterized by no or few ketones and high glucose in the blood

Some individuals who have type 2 diabetes have patches of dark, velvety skin in the folds and creases of their bodies, usually in the armpits and neck. This condition, called acanthosis nigricans, is a sign of insulin resistance.

If not properly treated, type 2 diabetes can lead to complications such as blindness, kidney failure, heart disease, and nerve damage.

MODY

MODY may occur during childhood or adolescence but may be misdiagnosed as type 1 or type 2 diabetes, or may be unidentified until the patient is an adult. Individuals with MODY may have little to no symptoms of diabetes, or have only mild symptoms, or may have mild to significant hyperglycemia. MODY patients are typically not overweight and generally do not have similar risk factors as seen with type 2 diabetes, such as hypertension (high blood pressure) or hyperlipidemia (elevated serum lipids).

Many patients with MODY do not have any symptoms of diabetes and may be diagnosed with high serum glucose while in the process of discovering other disorders. Other symptoms may include increased thirst and urination. It is recommended that individuals who have mild to moderate hyperglycemia identified before the age of 30, a family history of diabetes, and low insulin requirements be tested for MODY.

Common Symptoms of Type 1 and Type 2 Diabetes

Fatigue: In diabetes, the body is inefficient and sometimes unable to use glucose for fuel. The body switches over to metabolizing fat, partially or completely, as a fuel source. This process requires the body to use more energy. The end result is feeling fatigued or constantly tired.

Unexplained Weight Loss: Individuals with diabetes are unable to process many of the calories in the foods they eat. Therefore, they may lose weight even though they eat an apparently appropriate or even excessive amount of food. Losing sugar and water in the urine and the accompanying dehydration also contributes to weight loss.

Excessive Thirst (Polydipsia): An individual with diabetes develops high blood sugar levels. The body tries to counteract this by sending a signal to the brain to dilute the blood, which translates into thirst. The body encourages more water consumption to dilute the high blood sugar back to normal levels and to compensate for the water lost by excessive urination.

Excessive Urination (Polyuria): Polyuria is frequent urination. Another way the body tries to get rid of the extra sugar in the blood is to excrete it in the urine. This can also lead to dehydration because excreting the sugar carries a large amount of water out of the body along with it.

Excessive Eating (Polyphagia): Polyphagia is excessive hunger. If the body is able, it will secrete more insulin in order to try to deal with the excessive blood sugar levels. One of the functions of insulin is to stimulate hunger. Therefore, higher insulin levels lead to increased hunger and eating. Despite increased caloric intake, the person may gain very little weight or may even lose weight.

Poor Wound Healing: White blood cells are important in defending the body against bacteria and also in cleaning up dead tissue and cells. High blood sugar levels prevent white blood cells from functioning normally. When these cells do not function properly, wounds take much longer to heal and become infected more frequently.

Vascular Problems: Long-term high blood sugar levels are associated with thickening of blood vessels, which prevents good circulation and body tissues from getting enough oxygen and other nutrients.

Infections: Certain infection syndromes, such as frequent yeast infections, skin infections, and frequent urinary tract infections, may result from suppression of the immune system by diabetes and by the presence of glucose in the tissues, which allows bacteria to grow well. They can also be an indicator of poor blood sugar control in a person known to have diabetes.

Altered Mental Status: Agitation, unexplained irritability, inattention, extreme lethargy, or confusion can all be signs of very high blood sugar, ketoacidosis, hyperosmolar hyperglycemia nonketotic syndrome, or hypoglycemia (low sugar). These merit the immediate attention of a medical professional. Call a healthcare provider or 911.

Blurry Vision: The primary cause of legal blindness in the working population of the United States today is diabetes mellitus. Blurry vision is not specific for diabetes but is frequently present with high blood sugar levels.

COMPLICATIONS

Diabetes mellitus (diabetes) can affect many major organs in the body, including the heart, blood vessels, nerves, eyes, and kidneys. Keeping blood sugar levels close to normal most of the time can dramatically reduce the risk of these complications.

Short-Term Complications

Short-term complications of diabetes, such as a high blood sugar level, require immediate care. Left untreated, these conditions can cause seizures and loss of consciousness (coma).

Hyperglycemia: Hyperglycemia is a condition of high blood sugar levels. Blood sugar levels can rise for many reasons, including eating too much, experiencing stress, or not taking enough insulin or medications. It is important to check blood sugar levels often and watch for signs and symptoms of high blood sugar, including frequent urination, increased thirst, dry mouth, blurred vision, fatigue, and nausea. If hyperglycemia is present, adjustment to meal plans, medications, or both may be necessary. If blood sugar levels are persistently above 250 mg/dL, consulting a doctor immediately is recommended by healthcare providers. Diabetic hyperosmolar syndrome, a life-threatening condition in which sky-high blood sugar causes blood to become thick and syrupy, may be present.

Diabetic Ketoacidosis: Diabetic ketoacidosis is characterized by high levels of ketones in the blood. If the cells are starved for energy, the body may begin to break down fat. This produces toxic substances known as ketones. It is important to watch for loss of appetite, nausea, vomiting, fever, stomach pain, and a sweet, fruity smell on the breath, especially if the blood sugar level has been consistently higher than 250 mg/dL. Diabetic ketoacidosis is more common in type 1 diabetes than type 2.

Hypoglycemia: Hypoglycemia is a condition of low blood sugar. If blood sugar levels drop below the target range, it is known as low blood sugar. Blood sugar levels can drop for reasons including skipping a meal, getting more physical activity than normal, or taking too much diabetic medication. It is important to check blood sugar levels regularly and to watch for early signs and symptoms of low blood sugar, including sweating, shakiness, weakness, hunger, dizziness, and nausea. Later signs and symptoms include slurred speech, drowsiness, and confusion. If signs or symptoms of low blood sugar are present, it is recommended by healthcare providers to eat or drink something that will quickly raise blood sugar levels, such as fruit juice, glucose tablets, hard candy, or regular (not diet) soda. If consciousness is lost, a family member or close contact may need to give an emergency injection of glucagon, a hormone that stimulates the release of sugar into the blood.

Glucagon is a medication that is prescribed to some individuals with blood sugar regulation problems.

Long-Term Complications

Long-term complications of diabetes develop gradually. The earlier the individual develops diabetes and the less controlled the blood sugar levels are, the higher the risk of complications. Eventually, diabetes complications may be disabling or even life threatening.

Heart and Blood Vessel Disease: Diabetes dramatically increases the risk of various cardiovascular problems, including coronary artery disease with chest pain (angina), heart attack, stroke, narrowing of the arteries (atherosclerosis), and high blood pressure. According to the American Heart Association, approximately 75% of individuals who have diabetes die of some type of heart or blood vessel disease. Diabetic microangiopathy is the damage to very small blood vessels due to high blood sugar levels. Microangiopathy causes the walls of very small blood vessels (capillaries) to become so thick and weak that they bleed, leak protein, and slow the flow of blood. Diabetics may develop microangiopathy with thickening of capillaries in many areas, including the eyes, feet, legs, and kidneys.

Diabetic Neuropathy: Diabetic neuropathy, or nerve damage, occurs due to excess blood sugar levels that can injure the walls of the tiny blood vessels (capillaries) that nourish the nerves, especially in the legs. Diabetic neuropathy can cause tingling, numbness, burning, or pain that usually begins at the tips of the toes or fingers and over a period of months or years gradually spreads upward. Left untreated, the individual can lose all sense of feeling in the affected limbs. Diabetic neuropathy is a common cause of limb amputations. The injuries to the skin occur and are not felt, due to neuropathy, until infection progresses too far to save the tissue, especially the toes and feet. Damage to the nerves that control digestion can cause problems with nausea, vomiting, diarrhea, or constipation. For men, erectile dysfunction may also occur as a result of poor blood flow to the penis and nerve damage, both caused by diabetes.

Diabetic Nephropathy: Diabetic nephropathy causes kidney damage and is a complication of diabetes that is caused by uncontrolled high blood sugar. High blood sugar damages the filtering system of the kidneys. Over time, the damage can lead to kidney failure. Diabetic nephropathy is the most common cause of kidney failure in the United States. Severe damage can lead to kidney failure or irreversible end-stage kidney disease, requiring dialysis or a kidney transplant.

Eye Damage: Chronic high blood sugar levels damage sensitive blood vessels in the eye, resulting in blurry vision and vision damage. Diabetes can damage the blood vessels of the retina (diabetic retinopathy), potentially leading to blindness. The primary cause of legal blindness in the working population of the United States today is diabetes mellitus. Diabetes also increases the risk of other serious vision conditions, such as cataracts and glaucoma.

Foot Ulcers: Nerve damage in the feet or poor blood flow to the feet increases the risk of various foot complications, including diabetic foot ulcers. Left untreated, cuts and blisters can become serious infections. Severe damage might require toe, foot, or even leg amputation.

Skin and Mouth Conditions: Diabetes may leave the individual more susceptible to skin problems, including bacterial infections, fungal infections, and itching. Gum infections also may be a concern, especially if there is a history of poor dental hygiene.

Osteoporosis: Diabetes may lead to lower than normal bone mineral density, increasing the risk of osteoporosis. Osteoporosis is a disease in which bones become fragile and more likely to break. If not prevented or if left untreated, osteoporosis can progress painlessly until a bone breaks.

Alzheimer's Disease (AD): Type 2 diabetes may increase the risk of AD. AD is a progressive degenerative disease of the nervous system that leads to dementia and eventually death. The more uncontrolled blood sugar levels are, the greater the risk of developing AD. Researchers have found that cardiovascular problems caused by diabetes may contribute to dementia by blocking blood flow to the brain or causing strokes (neurological damage caused by lack of oxygen to the brain). Other possibilities are that too much insulin in the blood leads to brain-damaging inflammation, or lack of insulin in the brain deprives brain cells of glucose.

Gastroparesis: Gastroparesis is a disorder that affects people with both type 1 and type 2 diabetes. In gastroparesis, movement of food through the stomach slows or stops completely. The muscles in the wall of the stomach work poorly or not at all, preventing the stomach from emptying properly. This can interfere with digestion and cause nausea and vomiting, problems with blood sugar control, and malnutrition.

Depression: Studies report that individuals with diabetes have a greater risk of depression than individuals without diabetes. Causes underlying the association between depression and diabetes are unclear. Depression may develop because of stress but also may result from the metabolic effects of diabetes on the brain. Studies suggest that people with diabetes who have a history of depression are more likely to develop diabetic complications than those without depression.

DIAGNOSIS

The main diagnostic test for diabetes is taking a blood test to measure glucose, either when the individual has been fasting (not consuming food) or at other times of the day. Diagnostic tests are also used routinely during pregnancy to identify gestational diabetes. Some diabetes tests require obtaining a blood sample in a doctor's office.

Depending on the test used, the level of blood glucose can be affected by many factors, including eating or drinking (water is acceptable); taking medications that are known to raise blood sugar levels, such as oral contraceptives, some diuretics (water pills), and corticosteroids; or a recent injury, physical illness, or surgery that may temporarily alter blood sugar levels.

Fasting Blood Glucose Test: Fasting blood glucose testing checks blood glucose levels after fasting for between 12-14 hours. The individual can drink water during this time but should strictly avoid any other beverage. Individuals with diabetes may be asked to delay their diabetes medication or insulin dose until the test is completed. This test can be used to diagnose diabetes or prediabetes. The fasting plasma glucose is the preferred test for diagnosing diabetes due to convenience and is most reliable when done on an empty stomach in the morning, so the presence of food and natural biorhythms do not cause fluctuations in blood sugar levels.

If the fasting glucose level is 100-125 mg/dL, the individual has a form of prediabetes called IFG, meaning that the individual is more likely to develop type 2 diabetes but does not have the condition yet. A level of 126 mg/dL or above, confirmed by repeating the test on another day, means that the individual has diabetes.

Oral Glucose Tolerance Test (OGTT): During an OGTT, a high-glucose drink is given to the individual. Blood samples are checked at regular intervals for two hours. OGTTs are used when the results of the fasting blood glucose are borderline. They are also used to diagnose diabetes in pregnancy (gestational diabetes). This test can be used to diagnose diabetes or prediabetes.

Random Blood Glucose Test: Random blood glucose testing checks blood glucose levels at various times during the day. It does not matter when the

individual last ate. Blood glucose levels tend to stay constant in an individual who does not have diabetes. This test, along with an assessment of symptoms, is used to diagnose diabetes.

Fructosamine Testing: Doctors may measure the level of fructosamines, also known as glycated proteins, in serum or plasma to estimate average glucose levels in diabetic patients during the preceding two to three weeks. In diabetic patients, elevated blood glucose levels correlate with increased fructosamine formation. Fructosamine is formed due to a reaction between fructose and amino acid residues of proteins.

Fructosamine testing is often prescribed when changes are being made in a diabetes treatment plan and information is needed about how well the new plan is working. High levels of vitamin C (ascorbic acid), lipemia (high amount of fat in the blood), hemolysis (breakdown of red blood cells), and hyperthyroidism (high levels of thyroid hormones) can interfere with test results.

Hemoglobin A1c: Hemoglobin A1c, also known as glycated hemoglobin or glycosylated hemoglobin, indicates an individual's average blood sugar control over the last two to three months. Sugar (glucose) in the bloodstream can become attached to the hemoglobin (the part of the cell that carries oxygen) in red blood cells. This process is called glycosylation. Once the sugar is attached, it stays there for the life of the red blood cell, which is about 120 days. The higher the level of blood sugar, the more sugar attaches to red blood cells. The hemoglobin A1c test measures the amount of sugar sticking to the hemoglobin in the red blood cells. A1c is formed when glucose in the blood binds irreversibly to hemoglobin to form a stable glycated hemoglobin complex. A1c values are not subject to the fluctuations that are seen with daily blood glucose monitoring. Results are given in percentages.

The American Diabetes Association (ADA) recommends A1c as the best test to find out if an individual's blood sugar is under control over time. The test should be performed every three months for insulin-treated patients, during treatment changes, or when blood glucose is elevated. For stable patients on oral agents, healthcare professionals recommended testing A1c at least twice per year. The ADA currently recommends an A1c goal of less than 7.0%. Studies have reported that there is a 10% decrease in relative risk of microvascular complications, such as diabetic nephropathy or diabetic neuropathy, for every 1% reduction in hemoglobin A1c.

Gestational Diabetes Diagnosis: Gestational diabetes is diagnosed based on blood glucose levels measured during the OGTT. Glucose levels are normally lower during pregnancy, so the cutoff levels for diagnosis of diabetes in pregnancy are lower. Blood glucose levels are measured before a woman drinks a beverage containing glucose. Then levels are checked one, two, and three hours afterward. If a woman has two blood glucose levels meeting or exceeding any of the following numbers, she has gestational diabetes: a fasting blood glucose level of 95 mg/dL, a one-hour level of 180 mg/dL, a two-hour level of 155 mg/dL, or a three-hour level of 140 mg/dL.

MODY Diagnosis: Genetic testing can help diagnose MODY; however, commercially available genetic tests for MODY are not widely available. In a MODY test a blood sample is collected, and the DNA is isolated and analyzed for mutations characteristic of MODY. Genetic testing may be helpful in selecting specific treatments for MODY, depending on the specific genetic mutation involved. Prenatal testing may also be available for diagnosis of MODY. As each type of MODY has different clinical manifestations, it is recommended for patients to work with their healthcare providers to discuss testing options, to determine whether genetic testing is appropriate, and to decide which genetic tests are necessary.

TREATMENT

Treatment for diabetes is a lifelong commitment of monitoring blood sugar, taking insulin if prescribed, maintaining a healthy weight, eating healthy foods, and exercising regularly. The goal is to keep your blood sugar level as close to normal as possible to delay or prevent complications. In fact, tight control of blood sugar levels can reduce the risk of diabetes-related heart attacks and strokes by more than 50%.

Lifestyle Choices

If an individual has been diagnosed with diabetes, healthy lifestyle choices, including diet and exercise, are necessary. These healthy choices will help to improve glycemic (blood sugar) control and prevent or minimize complications of diabetes.

Diet: A healthy diet is important in controlling blood sugar levels and preventing diabetes complications. Eat a consistent, well-balanced diet that is high in fiber, low in saturated fat, and low in concentrated sweets. A consistent diet that includes roughly the same number of calories at about the same times of day helps a healthcare provider prescribe the correct dose of medication or insulin.

What and how much an individual eats will affect his or her blood sugar level. Blood sugar is typically highest one to two hours after a meal. One way individuals with diabetes can manage their food intake to keep their blood glucose as close to normal as possible is by calculating how many grams of carbohydrate they eat. Carbohydrates tend to have the greatest effect on blood glucose. The balance between the amount of carbohydrate eaten and the available insulin determines how much the blood glucose level goes up after meals or snacks. To help control their blood glucose, individuals should know which foods contain carbohydrates, the size of a "serving" of different foods, and how many carbohydrate servings to eat each day. A dietician can help individuals work out a dietary plan that is right for them.

Foods that contain carbohydrates include grains, pasta, and rice; breads, crackers, and cereals; starchy vegetables, including potatoes, corn, peas, and winter squash; legumes such as beans, peas, and lentils; fruits and fruit juices; milk and yogurt; and sweets and desserts. Nonstarchy vegetables such as spinach, kale, broccoli, salad greens, and green beans are very low in carbohydrates. Carbohydrate counting can ensure that the right amount of carbohydrate is eaten at each meal and snack.

The amount of food an individual eats is also closely related to blood glucose control. If an individual eats more food than is recommended on a meal plan, blood glucose goes up. Although foods containing carbohydrates have the most impact on blood glucose, most foods will have some effect.

Exercise and Weight Control: Regular exercise, in any form, can help reduce the risk of developing diabetes. Physical activity moves sugar from the blood into the cells. The more active an individual is, the lower the blood sugar level. Activity can also reduce the risk of developing complications of diabetes such as heart disease, stroke, kidney failure, blindness, and leg ulcers. Exercise will also help to keep blood sugar at a relatively even level and avoid excessively low or high blood sugar levels, which can be dangerous and even life threatening. As little as 20 minutes of walking, three times a week, has a proven beneficial effect. No matter how light or how long, some exercise is better than no exercise. If the individual has complications of diabetes, such as eye, kidney, or nerve problems, they may be limited both in type of exercise and amount of exercise that can safely be performed without worsening the condition. Individuals taking insulin may need to lower the insulin dose before unusual physical activity and exercise. A doctor will help in determining these changes.

If the individual is overweight, losing even ten pounds can reduce the risk of diabetes. To keep weight in a healthy range, it is recommended by healthcare professionals to focus on permanent changes to eating and exercise habits. A dietitian or a weight modification program can help individuals reach their goals.

Self-Monitoring Blood Glucose: Checking blood sugar levels frequently, at least before meals and at bedtime, is important in controlling diabetes. Even if the individual takes insulin and eats on a rigid schedule, the amount of sugar in the blood can change unpredictably. Depending on what type of insulin therapy the individual is prescribed, such as single-dose injections, multiple-dose injections, or an insulin pump, the individual may need to check and record blood sugar levels up to four or more times a day. Careful monitoring is the only way to make sure that the blood sugar level remains within target range. A range of 90-130 mg/dL before meals is suggested for most individuals with diabetes. A doctor will tell the individual what his or her target range should be.

Also, results should be recorded in a logbook that should include insulin or oral medication doses and times, when and what was eaten, when and for how long exercise occurred, and any significant events of the day, such as high or low blood sugar levels and how the problem was treated. A daily blood sugar logbook or diary is invaluable to the healthcare team in seeing how the individual is responding to medications, diet, and exercise in the treatment of diabetes.

Better equipment now available makes testing blood sugar levels less painful and less complicated. Medicare now pays for diabetic testing supplies, as do many private insurers and Medicaid.

A doctor or healthcare team will help the individual decide what type of meter to buy. There are more than 20 types of meters available on the market. Examples include Accu-Chek (Hoffman-La Roche AG, Basel, Switzerland) and OneTouch (LifeScan, Inc., Milpitas, Calif.). Meters vary in size, weight, test time, blood sample requirements, memory capabilities, and other special features. Most meters can measure blood glucose with only a one- or two-step process. Most also incorporate no-wipe technology, which means users do not have to wipe off excess blood after applying a blood drop to the reagent strip. In addition, many meters now require only a very small amount of blood, thus decreasing the problems with bleeding often seen in advanced diabetics and the elderly and the fear and pain of wounds from the lancet.

A few of the newer meters offer the option of obtaining blood samples from alternate sites, such as a forearm instead of a fingertip. This can benefit patients who find constant lancet wounds on their fingers difficult to tolerate. The fingers have many nerve endings and are a very painful site for testing, although they are the most reliable. More complex meters have features to aid in identifying trends and to graph reports for more comprehensive data tracking, particularly for patients who test several times a day.

In order to get an accurate blood glucose result, the individual needs to make sure that the meter is clean, that its code matches the test strips, that the finger is clean, and that an adequate-size drop of blood is being tested. Before pricking the finger, it is recommended by healthcare professionals to wash the hands with warm water, shake the hands below the waist, and squeeze the finger a few times.

GlucoWatch: In 2001, the U.S. Food and Drug Administration (FDA) approved the GlucoWatch (Cygnus, Inc., Redwood City, Calif.), a watch-like device that helps individuals with diabetes measure their blood glucose via tiny electric currents. It draws small amounts of fluid from the skin and measures blood glucose levels three times per hour for up to 12 hours. The GlucoWatch is considered a first step toward noninvasive, continuous glucose monitoring, but it does have some shortfalls. GlucoWatch is not considered as accurate as a blood test, so any measurements that fall outside of normal ranges will need to be re-tested with a fingerstick test.

Medications

Insulin and Oral Medications: Many individuals with diabetes can manage their blood sugar with diet and exercise alone, but some need diabetes medications or insulin therapy. In addition to diabetes medications, a doctor might prescribe low-dose aspirin therapy to help prevent heart and blood vessel disease. Aspirin prevents blood from clotting by blocking the production of thromboxane A_2, a chemical that platelets produce that causes them to clump. Aspirin accomplishes this by inhibiting the enzyme cyclooxygenase-1 that produces thromboxane A_2.

Many oral or injected medications can be used to treat type 2 diabetes. Some diabetes medications stimulate the pancreas to produce and release more insulin. Others inhibit the production and release of glucose from the liver, which means the individual needs less insulin to transport sugar into the cells.

Still others block the action of stomach enzymes that break down carbohydrates or make tissues more sensitive to insulin.

Medications: The decision about which medications are best depends on many factors, including blood sugar levels and the presence of any other health problems. Medications taken by mouth for diabetes and blood sugar regulation include:

Sulfonylureas: Sulfonylureas help the pancreas make more insulin, which then lowers blood glucose. They also help the body use the insulin it makes to better lower blood glucose. For these medications to work, the pancreas has to make some insulin. Possible side effects include hypoglycemia (low blood sugar levels), an upset stomach, a skin rash or itching, and weight gain. Examples of sulfonylurea medications include glimepiride (Amaryl), glyburide (DiaBeta), chlorpropamide (Diabinese), acetohexamide (Dymelor), glipizide (Glucotrol, Glucotrol XL), glyburide (Glynase, Micronase), tolbutamide (Orinase), and tolazamide (Tolinase).

Biguanides: Biguanides help lower blood glucose by making sure the liver does not make too much glucose. Biguanides also lower the amount of insulin in the body. Metformin (Glucophage) is currently the only biguanide available. Individuals may lose a few pounds when starting metformin. This weight loss can help control blood glucose. Metformin can also improve blood fat and cholesterol levels, which are often not normal if the individual has type 2 diabetes. Metformin does not generally cause blood glucose to get too low (hypoglycemia), unless it is combined with other medications that increase insulin. Metformin may cause nausea and vomiting if more than about two to four alcoholic drinks a week are consumed while on the medication. Other side effects include nausea, diarrhea, headache, and weakness. A metallic taste in the mouth may be noticed.

Alpha-Glucosidase Inhibitors: Alpha-glucosidase inhibitors are a class of oral medications for type 2 diabetes that decrease the absorption of carbohydrates from the intestine, resulting in a slower and lower rise in blood glucose throughout the day, especially right after meals. Before carbohydrates are absorbed from food, they must be broken down into smaller sugar particles like glucose by enzymes in the small intestine. One of the enzymes involved in breaking down carbohydrates is called alpha-glucosidase. By inhibiting this enzyme, carbohydrates are not broken down as efficiently and glucose absorption is delayed. The alpha-glucosidase inhibitors include acarbose (Precose) and miglitol (Glyset).

Thiazolidinediones: Thiazolidinediones help make the cells more sensitive to insulin. The insulin can then move glucose more efficiently from the blood into the cells for energy. Side effects of these medications may include weight gain, anemia (less red blood cells, which causes the blood to carry less oxygen than normal), and edema (fluid accumulation). More serious side effects include liver damage and chronic heart failure. A doctor will monitor the individual's liver function while taking thiazolidinediones. Examples of thiazolidinediones includes pioglitazone (Actos) and rosiglitazone (Avandia).

Meglitinides: Meglitinides help the pancreas make more insulin right after meals, which lowers blood glucose. A doctor might prescribe a meglitinide medication by itself or with metformin (Glucophage) if one medicine alone does not control blood glucose levels. Possible side effects of meglitinides include hypoglycemia (low blood sugar) and weight gain. Examples include repaglinide (Prandin).

D-Phenylalanine Derivative: D-phenylalanine derivatives help the pancreas make more insulin quickly and for a short time. Then the insulin helps lower blood glucose after eating a meal. These medications may cause blood glucose levels to drop too low. Doctors will check liver function while taking d-phenylalanine derivatives. An example of a d-phenylalanine derivative is nateglinide (Starlix).

Dipeptidyl-Peptidase 4 (DPP-4) Inhibitor: DPP-4 inhibitors enhance the body's own ability to control blood sugar levels, increase insulin when blood sugar is high, especially after eating, and reduce the amount of sugar made by the liver after eating. Sitagliptin (Januvia) is currently the only DPP-4 inhibitor available. Side effects of DPP-4 inhibitors include a runny or stuffy nose, sore throat, headache, nausea, stomach pain, or diarrhea.

Exenatide (Byetta): Exenatide (Byetta) is an injectable drug that reduces the level of sugar (glucose) in the blood. It is used for treating type 2 diabetes. Exenatide belongs in a class of drugs called incretin mimetics because these drugs mimic the effects of incretins. Incretins, such as human-glucagon-like peptide-1 (GLP-1), are hormones that are produced and released into the blood by the intestine in response to food. GLP-1 increases the secretion of insulin from the pancreas, slows absorption of glucose from the gut, and reduces the action of glucagon. Glucagon is a hormone that increases glucose production by the liver. All three of these actions reduce levels of glucose in the blood. In addition, GLP-1 reduces appetite. Exenatide is a synthetic (manmade) hormone that resembles and acts like GLP-1. In studies, exenatide-treated patients achieved lower blood glucose levels and experienced weight loss. Exenatide was approved by the FDA in May 2005.

Combination Medications: Some antidiabetic medications may be combined to provide glucose and insulin control. An example of a combination drug is glyburide combined with metformin (Glucovance). Side effects of combination drugs are similar to those associated with the individual drugs in the product.

Insulin: Insulin is a naturally occurring hormone secreted by the pancreas. Insulin is required by the cells of the body in order for them to remove and use glucose from the blood. Insulin may need to be taken by type 1 and type 2 diabetics. Because stomach enzymes interfere with insulin taken by mouth, insulin must be injected or inhaled. Often, insulin is injected using a fine needle and syringe or an insulin pen injector (a device that looks like an ink pen, except the cartridge is filled with insulin).

Individuals with diabetes mellitus have an inability to take up and use glucose from the blood and, as a result, the glucose level in the blood rises. In type 1 diabetes, the pancreas cannot produce insulin. Therefore, insulin therapy is needed. In type 2 diabetes, individuals produce insulin, but cells throughout the body do not respond normally to the insulin. Nevertheless, insulin also may be used in type 2 diabetes to overcome the resistance of the cells to insulin. By increasing the uptake of glucose by cells and reducing the concentration of glucose in the blood, insulin prevents or reduces the long-term complications of diabetes, including damage to the blood vessels, eyes, kidneys, and nerves. Insulin is administered by injection under the skin (subcutaneously). The subcutaneous tissue of the abdomen is preferred because absorption of the insulin is more consistent from this location than subcutaneous tissues in other locations.

There are several types of insulin, classified by how soon and how long they act. It is helpful to know when the insulin starts to work, its peak (when the insulin is working its hardest), and the duration (how long the insulin works). Premixed combinations of slower and fast-acting insulin are also available. Depending on the individual's needs, a doctor may prescribe a mixture of insulin types to use throughout the day and night. Insulin medications can be made from bovine, porcine, and recombinant human insulin sources. However, in the United States, bovine tissue–derived insulin is no longer available as of 1999 due to FDA concerns over the possible transmission of bovine spongiform encephalopathy (also known as mad cow disease), and most porcine-derived formulations have

been discontinued as well. Nearly all insulin on the market today is now produced from bacteria and is identical to human insulin.

Regular (rapid onset of action, short duration of action) and NPH (slower onset of action, longer duration of action) human insulin are the most commonly used preparations. Regular insulin has an onset of action (begins to reduce blood sugar) within 30 minutes of injection, reaches a peak effect at one to three hours, and has effects that last six to eight hours. NPH insulin is insulin with an intermediate duration of action. It has an onset of action starting about two hours following injection. It has a peak effect four to 12 hours after injection and a duration of action of 18-26 hours.

Lente insulin is also insulin with an intermediate duration of action. It has an onset of action two to four hours after injection, a peak activity six to 12 hours after injection, and a duration of action of 18-26 hours. Ultralente insulin is long-acting insulin with an onset of action four to eight hours after injection, a peak effect 10-30 hours after injection, and a duration of action of more than 36 hours.

An ultra-rapid-acting insulin, insulin lispro (Humalog), is a chemically modified, natural insulin. When compared to regular insulin, insulin lispro has a more rapid onset of action, an earlier peak effect, and a shorter duration of action. It reaches peak activity 0.5-2.5 hours after injection. Therefore, insulin lispro should be injected 15 minutes before a meal as compared to regular insulin, which is injected 30-60 minutes before a meal.

Insulin aspart (NovoLog) and insulin glargine (Lantus) are both human insulins that have had their chemical composition slightly altered. The chemical changes provide insulin aspart with a faster onset of action (20 minutes) and a shorter duration of action (three to five hours) than regular human insulin. It reaches peak activity one to three hours after injection. Insulin glargine has a slower onset of action (70 minutes) and a longer duration of action (24 hours) than regular human insulin. Its activity does not peak.

Premixed insulins are a combination of specific proportions of intermediate-acting and short-acting insulin in one bottle or insulin pen (the numbers following the brand name indicate the percentage of each type of insulin). Examples of premixed insulins include Humalog mix 75/25, NovoLog 70/30, Novolin 70/30, and Humulin 70/30.

Healthcare professionals recommend storing unopened bottles of insulin in the refrigerator; also, insulin should not be used after the expiration date. Insulin should not be frozen. Store bottles that are being used at room temperature (59-86° F) for 28-30 days. Discard after 30 days. Avoid exposing the bottles to temperature extremes (less than 36° F or more than 86° F). Regular insulin should not be used if it becomes cloudy in appearance. NPH insulin should not be used if it becomes clumped or crystallized or if the bottle becomes frosted. Make sure that dosages are rechecked whenever changing insulin. Get guidance from a healthcare professional before mixing insulins.

Insulin Pump: An insulin pump also may be an option. The pump is a device about the size of a cell phone worn on the outside of the body. A tube connects the reservoir of insulin to a catheter that is inserted under the skin of the abdomen. The pump is programmed to dispense specific amounts of insulin automatically. It can be adjusted to deliver more or less insulin depending on meals, activity level, and blood sugar level.

Inhaled Insulin: Inhaled insulin (Exubera) is also available. Inhaled insulin is a powdered form of insulin that is rapid acting, usually taken before a meal. It replaces only short-acting forms of injectable insulin, not the longer acting (basal) insulin that may be required as part of a diabetes treatment plan. Inhaled insulin is not approved for anyone younger than 18 and should not be used by individuals who smoke or who have given up cigarettes within the past six months. However, it is considered safe for individuals who live with smokers. Exubera is not recommended for individuals with asthma, bronchitis, emphysema, or any form of active lung disease. Baseline tests for lung function are recommended by healthcare providers before starting treatment, after the first six months of treatment, and every year thereafter, even if no pulmonary symptoms such as lung or breathing problems exist.

Surgery

Pancreas Transplant: Many individuals with type 1 diabetes can manage their disease by following a diet and exercise plan, monitoring blood glucose levels, and using insulin injections. But for some individuals, this is a difficult task, resulting in a number of serious short- and long-term complications. A pancreas transplant is the closest thing to restoring normal pancreas function. A pancreas transplant is not the best option for all people with type 1 diabetes, however, and is primarily recommended for individuals with kidney failure.

Pancreas transplants pose serious health risks and are not always successful. The individual will need to take immune-suppressing drugs, such as cyclosporine (Sandimmune), to prevent organ rejection. These drugs can have serious side effects, including a high risk of infection and organ injury. Because the side effects can be more dangerous than the diabetes, pancreas transplants are usually reserved for individuals whose diabetes cannot be controlled or those who have serious complications.

Other Surgeries: Islet transplantation is an experimental procedure where islets (special cells in the pancreas that make insulin) are taken from the pancreas of a deceased healthy organ donor. The islets are purified, processed, and transferred into the individual with type 1 diabetes. Once implanted, the beta cells in these islets begin to make and release insulin. Researchers hope that islet transplantation will help people with type 1 diabetes live without daily injections of insulin. Stem cell transplants may also offer help to those suffering from type 1 diabetes, but the benefits are controversial in the United States.

INTEGRATIVE THERAPIES
Good Scientific Evidence

Beta-Glucan: Beta-glucan is a soluble fiber derived from the cell walls of algae, bacteria, fungi, yeast, and plants. It is commonly used for its cholesterol-lowering effects. There are several human trials supporting the use of beta-glucan for glycemic (blood sugar) control. Although early evidence is promising, additional study is needed before a firm recommendation can be made. Beta-glucan has a generally regarded as safe status in the United States.

Ginseng: Several studies report a blood sugar-lowering effect of American ginseng (*Panax quinquefolium*) in individuals with type 2 diabetes, both on fasting blood glucose and on postprandial glucose levels. These results are promising, especially as ginseng does not seem to cause dangerous low blood sugar levels. Future research needs to evaluate long-term efficacy of American ginseng in treating type 2 diabetes compared to standard oral hypoglycemic drugs. American ginseng may increase the effects of blood sugar–lowering medications, including insulin.

Gymnema: Preliminary human research reports that gymnema (*Gymnema sylvestre*) may be beneficial in patients with type 1 or type 2 diabetes when it is added to diabetes drugs being taken by mouth or to insulin. Further studies of dosing, safety, and effectiveness are needed before a strong recommendation can be made. Gymnema may increase the effects of blood sugar–lowering medications, including insulin. Gymnema may alter the ability to detect sweet tastes.

D

Stevia: Stevia (*Stevia rebaudiana*) has been widely used for diabetes in South America and animal studies have had promising results. Studies report decreases in plasma glucose when stevia was taken in normal volunteers, but there is currently no conclusive evidence of effectiveness when used for diabetes. Additional study is needed in this area to confirm these findings. Stevia may increase the effects of blood sugar–lowering medications, including insulin.

Unclear or Conflicting Scientific Evidence

Acupuncture: The practice of acupuncture originated in China 5,000 years ago. Today it is widely used throughout the world and is one of the main pillars of Chinese medicine. Although preliminary results are promising, there is a lack of well-designed studies to determine the contribution of acupuncture in diabetes.

Alfalfa: A small number of animal studies report reductions in blood sugar levels following ingestion of alfalfa (*Medicago sativa*). Human data are limited, and it remains unclear if alfalfa can aid in the control of sugars in patients with diabetes or hyperglycemia.

Aloe: Transparent gel from the pulp of the meaty leaves of *Aloe vera* has been used topically for thousands of years to treat wounds, skin infections, burns, and numerous other dermatological conditions. Dried latex from the inner lining of the leaf has traditionally been used as an oral laxative. Although some preliminary research for using aloe in diabetes is positive, study results are mixed. More research is needed to explore the effectiveness and safety of aloe in diabetics.

Arabinoxylan: Altering the outer shell of rice bran using enzymes from *Hyphomycetes mycelia* mushroom extract produces arabinoxylan compound. The product called MGN-3 (or BioBran in Japan) is a complex containing arabinoxylan as a major component. Although preliminary research is positive, there is currently a lack of scientific evidence investigating the role of arabinoxylan in diabetics. More study is needed.

Ashwagandha: Based on early study, ashwagandha (*Withania somnifera*) may decrease blood sugar levels. Additional evidence is required in this area.

Astragalus: Although there is experimental evidence that astragalus (*Astragalus membranaceus*) alone, and in combination with hypoglycemic medication, has significant hypoglycemic properties, the clinical studies are poorly designed and results inadequately presented. The clinical data suggest that astragalus-containing herbal remedies plus conventional therapy (oral hypoglycemics) in the treatment of type 2 diabetes are more effective than conventional oral hypoglycemics alone. More research is required in this area.

Atkins Diet: The Atkins diet proposes that, in order to lose weight, one should adopt an eating style that radically departs from the FDA MyPyramid. It proposes the elimination of most carbohydrates as a source of energy; in the place of carbohydrates, the diet advocates the significantly increased consumption of fats, including trans fats and hydrogenated oils.

Carbohydrate-restricted diets have been shown to have positive effects on serum insulin in both diabetics and nondiabetics and insulin requirements in diabetics. Preliminary evidence suggests that following the Atkins diet may result in improvements in metabolic parameters in insulin-resistant women. Furthermore, a decrease in hemoglobin A1c and medication requirements were noted in type 2 diabetics. Long-term safety studies are still required in this field, as well as additional well-designed clinical trials.

Banaba: Banaba (*Lagerstroemia speciosa*) is a medicinal plant that grows in India, Southeast Asia, and the Philippines. Preliminary research investigating the effects of banaba on diabetes report promising results. However, additional research is necessary before a firm conclusion can be made.

Barley: Barley (*Hordeum vulgare*) is a cereal used as a staple food in many countries. It is commonly used as an ingredient in baked products and soup in Europe and the United States. Barley malt is used to make beer and as a natural sweetener called malt sugar or barley jelly sugar. Preliminary evidence suggests that barley meal may improve glucose tolerance. Better research is necessary before a firm conclusion can be drawn.

Berberine: Berberine is a bitter-tasting, yellow, plant alkaloid with a long history of medicinal use in Chinese and Ayurvedic medicine. Berberine is present in the roots, rhizomes, and stem bark of various plants including goldenseal (*Hydrastis canadensis*). Historically, berberine has been suggested to aid in glycemic regulation. The safety and effectiveness of berberine for this indication remains unclear. More research is needed in this area.

Bilberry: Bilberry (*Vaccinium myrtillus*), a close relative of blueberry, has a long history of medicinal use. Bilberry has been used traditionally in the treatment of diabetes, and animal research suggests that bilberry leaf extract can lower blood sugar levels. Human research is needed in this area.

Biotin: Biotin is an essential water-soluble B vitamin. In preliminary research, biotin has been reported to decrease insulin resistance and improve glucose tolerance—both properties that may be beneficial in patients with types 2 (adult-onset) diabetes. However, there is not sufficient human evidence to form a clear conclusion in this area.

Bitter Melon: Bitter melon (*Momordica charantia*) has traditionally been used as a remedy for lowering blood glucose in patients with diabetes mellitus. Preliminary study has indicated that bitter melon may decrease serum glucose levels. However, because safety and efficacy have not been established, bitter melon should be avoided by diabetics except under the strict supervision of a qualified healthcare professional, including a pharmacist, with careful monitoring of serum blood sugars. Bitter melon may increase the effects of blood sugar–lowering medications, including insulin.

Burdock: Animal research and initial human studies suggest possible blood sugar–lowering effects of burdock (*Arctium lappa*) root or fruit. However, the available human research has not been well designed, and further study is needed.

Cinnamon: Several human studies support the use of cinnamon (*Cinnamomum* spp.) in diabetes. More research on the proposed health benefits of cinnamon supplementation is warranted.

Dandelion: There is limited animal research on the effects of dandelion (*Taraxacum officinale*) on blood sugar levels in animals. Effects in humans are not known.

Devil's Club: The hypoglycemic (blood sugar–lowering) effect is one of many reported uses for devil's club (*Oplopanax horridus*), which had a traditional use in diabetes and continues to be used for this condition. Although early evidence looks promising, additional high-quality trials are needed to make a firm recommendation.

Evening Primrose Oil: A small number of laboratory studies and theories suggest that evening primrose (*Oenothera biennis*) oil may be helpful in diabetes, but more information is needed.

Fenugreek: Fenugreek (*Trigonellafoenum-graecum*) has been found to lower serum glucose levels both acutely and chronically. Although promising, these data cannot be considered definitive, and at this time there is insufficient evidence to recommend either for or against fenugreek for type 2 diabetes. Additional study is warranted in this area.

Review of the literature also suggests a possible efficacy of fenugreek in type 1 diabetics. Although promising, these data cannot be considered definitive. At this time, there is insufficient evidence to recommend either for or against the use of fenugreek for type 1 diabetes.

Fig: Preliminary evidence suggests that fig (*Ficus carica*) has antioxidant properties and may be beneficial in type 1 diabetes. Additional study is warranted in this area.

Flaxseed: Human studies on the effect of flaxseed (*Linum usitatissimum*) on blood sugar levels report mixed results. More research is needed to determine the effect of flaxseed on blood sugar regulation.

Gotu Kola: Gotu kola is from the perennial creeping plant, *Centella asiatica* (formerly known as *Hydrocotyle asiatica*), which is a member of the parsley family. It is native to India, Madagascar, Sri Lanka, Africa, Australia, China, and Indonesia. Preliminary studies have suggested beneficial effects of the total triterpenoid fraction of *Centella asiatica* on subjective and objective parameters of venous insufficiency of the lower extremities. However, additional study is needed in this area.

Green Tea: Green tea is made from the dried leaves of *Camellia sinensis,* a perennial evergreen shrub. Green tea has a long history of use, dating back to China approximately 5,000 years ago. Green tea, black tea, and oolong tea are all derived from the same plant. More studies are required to determine if green tea and polyphenols have any therapeutic benefit for diabetes prevention or treatment.

Holy Basil: Holy basil (*Ocimum sanctum*) may have blood sugar–lowering effects and may be useful as an adjunct to dietary therapy and drug treatment in mild to moderate diabetes mellitus. It is unknown whether common culinary basil (*Ocimum basilicum*) would have similar effects. More research is warranted.

Honey: Early evidence suggests that honey may help lower blood sugar levels in diabetic patients. Additional study is warranted in this area.

Hydrotherapy: Hydrotherapy is broadly defined as the external application of water in any form or temperature (hot, cold, steam, liquid, ice) for healing purposes. It may include immersion in a bath or body of water (such as the ocean or a pool), use of water jets, douches, application of wet towels to the skin, or water birth. Although hydrotherapy is used by healthcare practitioners for diabetes support, there is insufficient research in this area.

Jackfruit: Jackfruit (*Artocarpus heterophyllus*), which refers to both a species of tree and its fruit, is native to southwestern India and Sri Lanka. Jackfruit was reportedly cultivated for food as early as the sixth century BC in India. Jackfruit leaves may improve glucose tolerance. However, there is little available research in this area. Additional study is needed.

D

Kudzu: Preliminary evidence suggests puerarin, a constituent of kudzu (*Pueraria lobata*), may improve insulin resistance. Insulin resistance is a condition in which the cells of the body become resistant to the effects of insulin and the normal response to a given amount of insulin is reduced. As a result, higher levels of insulin are needed in order for insulin to have its effects. Insulin resistance precedes the development of type 2 diabetes. Therefore, reversing insulin resistance can lessen chances of developing type 2 diabetes and heart disease. Additional study is needed before a firm conclusion can be made.

Lutein: Lutein is found in high levels in foods such as green vegetables, egg yolk, kiwifruit, grapes, orange juice, zucchini, squash, and corn. For some commercially available supplements, lutein is extracted from marigold petals. Currently, there is insufficient available evidence to recommend for or against the use of lutein for diabetes. Preliminary evidence is conflicting.

Maitake: Maitake is the Japanese name for the edible fungus *Grifola frondosa,* which is characterized by a large fruiting body and overlapping caps. Maitake has been used traditionally both as a food and for medicinal purposes. In animal studies, maitake extracts are reported to lower blood sugar levels. However, little is known about the effect of maitake on blood sugar in humans.

Milk Thistle: A small number of studies suggest possible improvements of blood sugar control using milk thistle (*Silybum marianum*) supplementation in cirrhotic patients with diabetes. However, more scientific evidence needs to be found.

Myrcia: Myrcia is a medium-sized shrub that grows in drier regions of the Amazon and other parts of Brazil. In Brazil, the common name pedra hume caá refers to three species of *Myrcia* plants that are used interchangeably: *Myrcia salicifolia, Myrcia uniflora,* and *Myrcia sphaerocarpa DC.* Myrcia has been used traditionally by indigenous tribes in the rainforest to treat diabetes. Human study has not confirmed a blood sugar–lowering benefit in type 2 diabetic patients. More research is warranted to make a strong recommendation.

Nopal: Traditionally, nopal, or prickly pear, has both food and medicinal uses. Animal studies have shown that nopal may reduce blood glucose levels in diabetes. Based on available clinical trial, there is some preliminary clinical evidence that prickly pear cactus can decrease blood glucose levels in patients with type 2 diabetes. However, the quality of available studies is low and more research needs to be performed.

Onion: One clinical trial found that fresh onion (*Allium cepa*) significantly decreased serum glucose levels in diabetics. More research is needed in this area to confirm these results.

Psychotherapy: Psychotherapy may improve blood sugar control in teens and adults with poorly controlled type 1 diabetes, especially if blood sugar problems are related to depression.

Cognitive behavior therapy may reduce depression and improve blood sugar level control in patients with type 2 diabetes. Therapy may be less effective in people with diabetes complications or poorly controlled blood sugar levels. More studies are needed.

Psyllium: Psyllium, also referred to as ispaghula, is derived from the husks of the seeds of *Plantago ovata*. Psyllium contains a high level of soluble dietary fiber and is the chief ingredient in many commonly used bulk laxatives, including products such as Metamucil. Several studies have examined the administration of psyllium with meals or just prior to meals in order to measure effects on blood sugar levels. Better evidence is necessary before a firm conclusion can be drawn. Psyllium-containing products may delay gastric emptying time and reduce absorption of some drugs. It is advised that drugs be taken at separate administration times from psyllium to minimize potential interactions (for example, one hour before or a few hours after taking psyllium).

Pycnogenol: Pycnogenol (Horphag Research, Berlin) is the patented trade name for a water extract of the bark of the French maritime pine (*Pinus pinaster* spp. *atlantica*), which is grown in coastal southwest France. Supplementation of Pycnogenol with conventional diabetes treatment may lower glucose levels and improve endothelial function. Also, supplementation with Pycnogenol may improve symptoms associated with diabetic microangiopathy. Further research is needed to confirm these results.

Red Clover: Red clover (*Trifolium pratense*) has been studied in patients with type 2 diabetes to determine potential benefits in diabetic complications such as high blood pressure and narrowing of the arteries and veins. Further research is needed. Red clover is not recommended during pregnancy and breastfeeding due to its estrogen-like activity.

Red Yeast Rice: Red yeast rice is the product of yeast (*Monascus purpureus*) grown on rice and is served as a dietary staple in some Asian countries. Early human evidence suggests the potential for benefits in diabetics. Additional study is needed. There is limited evidence about the side effects of red yeast. Mild headache and abdominal discomfort can occur. Side effects may be similar to those for the prescription drug lovastatin (Mevacor). Heartburn, gas, bloating, muscle pain or damage, dizziness, asthma, and kidney problems are possible. People with liver disease should not use red yeast products.

Reishi Mushroom: Reishi mushroom (*Ganoderma lucidum*), also known as ling zhi in China, grows wild on decaying logs and tree stumps. Based on animal studies that demonstrated the blood sugar and lipid-lowering activities of *Ganoderma lucidum* (ling zhi, reishi mushroom), a clinical study was conducted to evaluate the effect of Ganopoly versus placebo in diabetic patients. The treatment of Ganopoly slightly decreased the levels of plasma glucose and glycosylated hemoglobin and improved other markers for diabetes. The authors are closely related to the manufacturer of Ganopoly. Long-term studies with larger sample size are needed to evaluate the efficacy and safety of Ganopoly in treating diabetic patients. Reishi may increase bleeding in sensitive individuals, including those taking blood thinning medications such as aspirin or warfarin (Coumadin).

Safflower: Lipid (fat) abnormalities are commonly associated with diabetes, and complications of atherosclerotic disease are frequently associated with diabetes. Safflower (*Carthamus tinctorius*) oil may negatively affect glucose metabolism due to the extra intake of energy or fat, but these effects may be less pronounced than in fish oil.

Seaweed: *Fucus vesiculosus* is a brown seaweed that grows on the northern coasts of the Atlantic and Pacific oceans and the North and Baltic seas. Its name is sometimes used for *Ascophyllum nodosum,* which is another brown seaweed that grows alongside *Fucus vesiculosus*. These species are often included in kelp preparations along with other types of seaweed. Based on animal research, extracts of bladderwrack may lower blood sugar levels. However, there are no reliable human studies available to support a recommendation for use in diabetes. Seaweeds may alter thyroid hormone levels.

Soy: Several small studies have examined the effects of soy (*Glycine max*) supplements on blood sugars in people with type 2 ("adult onset") diabetes. Results are mixed, with some research reporting decreased blood glucose levels and other trials noting no effects. Overall, research in this area is not well designed and better information is needed before the effects of soy on blood sugars can be clearly described.

Spirulina: The term spirulina refers to a large number of cyanobacteria, or blue-green algae. Spirulina is a rich source of nutrients, containing up to 70% protein, B-complex vitamins, phycocyanin, chlorophyll, beta-carotene, vitamin E, and numerous minerals. In fact, spirulina contains more beta-carotene than carrots. Preliminary study of people with type 2 diabetes mellitus reports that spirulina may reduce fasting blood sugar levels after two months of treatment. More research is needed before a firm conclusion can be drawn.

Taurine: Taurine is a nonessential amino acid–like compound. Taurine is found in high abundance in the tissues of many animals, especially sea animals, and in much lower concentrations in plants, fungi, and some bacteria. It has been proposed that diabetes patients have decreased taurine levels. Currently, there is limited available evidence to use taurine in the treatment of diabetes.

Vitamin D: Vitamin D is found in numerous dietary sources such as fish, eggs, fortified milk, and cod liver oil. The sun is also a significant contributor to our daily production of vitamin D and as little as 10 minutes of exposure is thought to be enough to prevent deficiencies. It has been reported that infants given calcitriol during the first year of life are less likely to develop type 1 diabetes than infants fed lesser amounts of vitamin D. Other related studies have suggested using cod liver oil as a source of vitamin D to reduce the incidence of type 1 diabetes. There is currently insufficient evidence to form a clear conclusion in this area.

In recent studies, adults given vitamin D supplementation were shown to improve insulin sensitivity. Further research is needed to confirm these results.

Vitamin E: Vitamin E is a fat-soluble vitamin with antioxidant properties. Vitamin E has been proposed for the prevention of types 1 or 2 diabetes; for the improvement of abnormal sugar control in diabetes; for prevention of platelet dysfunction and atherosclerosis in diabetes; for the correction of vitamin E deficiency in diabetic patients; and for the prevention of diabetic complications of the eye, kidneys, and nervous system (neuropathy, retinopathy, nephropathy). It is not clear that vitamin E is beneficial in any of these areas, and further evidence is necessary. Vitamin E may increase bleeding in sensitive individuals, including those taking blood-thinning medications such as aspirin or warfarin (Coumadin).

White Horehound: Animal studies and early human studies suggest that white horehound (*Marrubium vulgare*) may lower blood sugar levels. White horehound has been used for diabetes in some countries, including Mexico. Further well-designed human trials are needed.

Yoga: Yoga is an ancient system of relaxation, exercise, and healing with origins in Indian philosophy. Several preliminary human studies suggest that daily yoga may improve control of blood sugar levels in people with type 2 diabetes when it is added to standard drug therapy. It is not clear if yoga is better than any other form of exercise therapy. Better research is needed.

Zinc: Zinc formulations have been used since ancient Egyptian times to enhance wound healing, although the usefulness of this approach is only partially confirmed by clinical data of today. Diabetic patients typically have significantly lower serum zinc levels compared with healthy controls. Based on one randomized, controlled trial, zinc supplementation for type 2 diabetics may have beneficial effects in elevating their serum zinc level and in improving their glycemic control that is shown by decreasing their hemoglobin A1c concentration. Also, oral zinc supplementation may improve glycemic control and severity of peripheral neuropathy. Further research is needed.

Fair Negative Scientific Evidence

Coenzyme Q10: Preliminary evidence suggests that coenzyme Q10 does not affect blood sugar levels in patients with type 1 or type 2 diabetes and does not alter the need for diabetes medications.

Garlic: Animal studies suggest that garlic (*Allium sativum*) may lower blood sugar and increase the release of insulin, but studies in humans do not confirm this effect. Garlic may increase bleeding in sensitive individuals, including those taking blood-thinning medications such as aspirin or warfarin (Coumadin).

Omega-3 Fatty Acids (Fish Oil): The available scientific evidence suggests that there are no significant long-term effects of fish oil in patients with diabetes. Most studies in this area are not well designed.

Prayer: Prayer has not been shown to help prevent or treat diabetes or related health issues. Diabetes should be treated by a qualified healthcare professional using proven therapies.

Therapeutic Touch: There is initial research that therapeutic touch does not affect blood sugar levels in patients with type 1 diabetes mellitus.

Traditional or Theoretical Uses Lacking Sufficient Evidence

Integrative therapies used in diabetes or related conditions that have historical or theoretical uses but lack sufficient clinical evidence include 5-hydroxytryptophan, acerola (*Malpighia glabra, Malpighia punicifolia*), homeopathic aconite (*Aconitum napellus*), agave (*Agave americana*), annatto (*Bixa orellana*), applied kinesiology, asparagus (*Asparagus officinalis*), astaxanthin, beta-carotene, bovine colostrum, calamus (*Acorus calamus*), chelation therapy, chlorophyll, cordyceps (*Cordyceps sinensis*), detoxification therapy, fo-ti (*Polygonum multiflorum*), folic acid, garcinia (*Garcinia cambogia*), hydroxycitric acid, goldenseal (*Hydrastis canadensis*), grapefruit (*Citrus paradisi*), guided imagery, horsetail (*Equisetum arvense*), hydrazine sulfate, hypnotherapy, iridology, lemongrass (*Cymbopogon* spp.), lycopene, mangosteen (*Garcinia mangostana*), massage, methysulfonylmethane, music therapy, neem (*Azadirachta indica*), noni (*Morinda citrifolia*), pet therapy, qi gong, reflexology, reiki, relaxation therapy, rosemary (*Rosmarinus officinalis*), selenium, spiritual healing, turmeric (*Curcuma longa*), and vitamin C.

MANAGEMENT AND PREVENTION

Healthy lifestyle choices can help prevent type 2 diabetes and manage type 1 diabetes. Even if diabetes runs in the individual's family, diet and exercise can help prevent the disease. Healthy lifestyle choices can help individuals prevent potentially serious complications of diabetes, such as stroke, nerve damage, and heart disease.

Dental Health: Diabetes may leave individuals prone to gum infections. Healthcare professionals recommend brushing the teeth at least twice daily, flossing the teeth once a day, and schedule dental exams at least twice a year. Contacting a dentist right away if the gums bleed or look red or swollen is recommended.

Diet: It is important to choose foods low in fat and calories. Fresh fruits, vegetables, and whole grains. It is best to eliminate all refined carbohydrates (sugars and white flour) and hydrogenated oils. Limiting the amount of high-sugar beverages, such as soft drinks and fruit punches, is recommended by healthcare professionals. Avoid high-fat foods like ice cream, butter, and high-fat meats. Decreasing the consumption of milk and dairy products may also help with blood sugar control. Lean poultry and fish should be eaten more often than red meat. It is best not to cook with butter, margarine, lard, and hydrogenated oils. Olive oil or vegetable oils such as safflower are recommended by healthcare professionals.

Eating healthy foods and exercising regularly can also help control high blood pressure and high cholesterol levels.

Alcohol consumption should be limited to no more than one drink per day for women, two per day for men, and none if there is difficulty controlling alcohol intake (addiction) or uncontrolled blood sugar levels.

Foot Health: Healthcare professionals recommend to wash the feet daily in lukewarm water and top dry them gently, especially between the toes. It is important to moisturize the feet with lotion. Checking the feet every day for blisters, cuts, sores, redness, or swelling is important. It is recommended to consult a doctor if a sore or other foot problem that does not heal within a few days exists.

Glucagon Kit: Keeping a glucagon kit nearby in case of a low blood sugar emergency is important. Glucagon is an important hormone involved in carbohydrate metabolism. Produced by the pancreas, it is released when the glucose level in the blood is low (hypoglycemia), causing the liver to convert stored glycogen into glucose and release it into the bloodstream. The action of glucagon is thus opposite to that of insulin, which instructs the body's cells to take in glucose from the blood in times of satiation. An injection of glucagon will raise blood sugar levels.

Identification Tags: Healthcare professionals recommend that individuals with diabetes wear a tag or bracelet identifying the condition.

Ketones: Individuals can test to see if the body is making ketones by doing a simple urine test. There are several products available for ketone testing that can be purchased without a prescription. Common product names include Ketostix, Chemstrip K, and Acetest. The test result can be negative or show small, moderate, or large quantities of ketones. Healthcare professionals recommend testing for ketones during the following situations: anytime the blood glucose is over 250 mg/dL for two checks in a row; when the individual is ill (often illness, infections, or injuries will cause sudden high blood glucose and this is an especially important time to check for ketones); when the individual is planning to exercise and the blood glucose is over 250 mg/dL; and when pregnant, individuals should test for ketones each morning before breakfast and anytime the blood glucose is over 250 mg/dL. As long as blood glucose levels are not too high, the presence of ketones is not a problem. Untreated high blood glucose with ketones can lead to a life-threatening condition called diabetic ketoacidosis. If the ketone test is positive, healthcare providers recommend calling a doctor immediately.

Physical Activity and Weight Control: Healthcare professionals recommend 30 minutes of moderate physical activity a day when tolerated. Taking a brisk daily walk, riding a bike, or swimming laps are good exercises for individuals with diabetes. Losing weight is very important in maintaining healthy blood sugar levels.

Studies have reported that individuals can lower the risk of developing diabetes by losing 5-7% of body weight through diet and increased physical activity. Diet and exercise resulting in a 5-7% weight loss (approximately 10-14 pounds in an individual weighing 200 pounds) can lower the incidence of type 2 diabetes by nearly 60%.

Proper Glucose Control: The single best thing an individual can do is to keep blood sugar levels within the suggested range every day. The only way to do this is through a combination of regular blood sugar checks (self blood glucose monitoring), a balanced diet low in simple sugars and fat and high in complex carbohydrates and fiber, and appropriate medical treatment. A nutritionist, a doctor, and others on the healthcare team will help set up appropriate diabetes treatment strategies for the individual.

Regular Doctor Visits: Scheduling regular health checkups is important. However, regular diabetes checkups are not meant to replace yearly physicals or routine eye exams. Doctors will look for any diabetes-related complications, such as neuropathy, as well as screen for other medical problems. An eye care specialist will check for signs of retinal damage, cataracts, and glaucoma.

Smoking Cessation: Smoking cigarettes or use of any other form of tobacco raises the risks for developing complications from diabetes, such as heart attack, stroke, nerve damage, and kidney disease. Smoking damages blood vessels and contributes to heart disease, stroke, and poor circulation in the limbs. Smokers who have diabetes are three times more likely to die of cardiovascular disease than are nonsmokers who have diabetes, according to the ADA. A doctor can help plan a strategy to stop smoking or to stop using other types of tobacco.

Stress Reduction: Chronic stress can lead to the adrenal glands releasing the stress hormone cortisol. Chronic release of cortisol can lead to health problems such as blood sugar regulation problems such as hyperinsulinemia, high cholesterol levels, inflammation, poor immunity, and obesity. Stress can be controlled through integrative therapies, such as meditation, breathing, yoga, and certain herbs and vitamins. Getting plenty of rest may also help with decreasing stress and improving immunity. High blood sugar levels can weaken the immune system.

CONDITIONS: Gallbladder/Pancreas Disorders, Cholecystitis, Cholestasis, Gallbladder Attack/Biliary Colic, Gallstones, Gilbert's Syndrome, Pancreatitis

BACKGROUND

The biliary tract is a system of organs and tubes (ducts) that help transport a digestive fluid, called bile, from the liver to the small intestine. Bile, which is produced in the liver and stored in the gallbladder, is needed to break down and absorb fats in foods. Gallbladder disorders, also called biliary tract disorders, occur when there is a disruption in this process. For instance, the most common gallbladder disorder is gallstones. This occurs when the bile becomes too concentrated and tiny particles in the fluid form a stonelike mass in the ducts that blocks proper bile flow.

The pancreas, which is located behind the stomach, is another organ that helps break down foods that are consumed. The pancreas produces enzymes that are released into the small intestine to break down proteins, carbohydrates, and lipids (fats) in food. A section of the pancreas also produces insulin and glucagon; both help regulate the amount of sugar in the blood. Pancreatitis is a common pancreatic disorder that occurs when the organ becomes inflamed.

Most gallbladder and pancreatic disorders can be successfully treated with medications and/or surgery.

CHOLECYSTITIS

Overview: Cholecystitis is the inflammation of the gallbladder wall and nearby abdominal lining.

Causes: Most cases of cholecystitis occur when a gallstone becomes lodged in the cystic duct, which is the tube that connects the gallbladder to the common bile duct. Other less common causes include bacterial infections in the bile duct system, tumors of the liver or pancreas, or decreased blood supply to the gallbladder. Diabetics have an increased risk of developing a decreased blood supply to the gallbladder.

Symptoms: Symptoms may develop suddenly or gradually over the course of several years. Most cholecystitis attacks last one to two days. Common symptoms include severe pain in the upper right part of the abdomen after meals that usually lasts for several hours, nausea, vomiting, mild fever, rigid abdominal muscles, yellowing of the skin and eyes (jaundice), and loose, light-colored bowel movements. In rare cases, cholecystitis may cause itching, especially in the hands and feet.

Diagnosis: There are several tests available to detect abnormalities of the gallbladder. After a detailed medical history and physical examination are performed, the healthcare provider determines the appropriate tests needed to diagnose the underlying cause.

An ultrasound, which involves rubbing a wand-like instrument (called a transducer) over the lower abdomen, may be performed to take pictures of the gallbladder. Patients may also undergo a computerized tomography (CT) scan that takes pictures of the internal organs. A dye is often injected into the patient before the CT scan is performed to help the healthcare provider view the tubes and organs of the biliary system in more detail.

An endoscopic retrograde cholangiopancreatography (ERCP) may be performed at a hospital to check for problems in the liver, gallbladder, bile ducts, and pancreas. During the procedure, a thin, flexible tube with a camera at the tip (called an endoscope) is inserted through the mouth and into the small intestine until it reaches the biliary ducts and pancreas. A small plastic tube is then inserted through the endoscope and a colored dye is injected. This allows the healthcare provider to see detailed images of the biliary tract.

If the patient has a fever in addition to cholecystitis symptoms, a blood culture may be performed to diagnose an infection. A sample of the patient's blood is analyzed for the presence of disease-causing microorganisms.

Treatment: Treatment depends on the underlying cause. Infections are treated with medications called antibiotics. The specific dose and type of antibiotic used depends on the specific type and severity of the infection.

If a gallstone is causing the condition, the gallbladder is usually surgically removed. If the gallbladder is removed, patients can expect a full recovery. Complications are rare but may include damage to the common bile duct, bleeding, and infection. Nonsurgical procedures, such as bile salt tablets and sound wave therapy, are only considered if the patient is unable to undergo surgery or the stone is primarily made up of cholesterol. This is because gallstones usually recur when nonsurgical procedures are used.

CHOLESTASIS

Overview: Cholestasis occurs when the flow of digestive fluid produced by the liver (called bile) is either limited or stopped at some point between the liver and the small intestine. As a result, a waste product, called bilirubin, leaks into the bloodstream where it accumulates.

Bilirubin is yellow to green in color. When it leaks into the bloodstream, it may cause the skin and eyes to become yellow in color.

Causes: Cholestasis may be caused by problems in or outside of the liver. For instance, acute liver inflammation (hepatitis), alcoholic liver disease, primary biliary cirrhosis, cirrhosis of the liver, certain medications (e.g., birth control pills or an antipsychotic and antinausea drug called chlorpromazine), hormonal changes during pregnancy, and cancer that has spread to the liver may cause cholestasis.

Problems outside of the liver, such as gallstones, narrowing of a bile duct, cancer of a bile duct, cancer of the pancreas, and inflammation of the pancreas (pancreatitis), may cause cholestasis.

Symptoms: Many times the only symptom noticed is itchy skin (especially on the hands and feet). This is because waste products from the bile leak into the bloodstream and irritate the skin. Other symptoms may include yellowing of the eyes and skin (jaundice), light-colored stools, oily and foul-smelling stools (steatorrhea), dark urine, abdominal pain, vomiting, loss of appetite, and fever.

Bile is needed to emulsify fats as well as calcium, vitamin D, and vitamin K from foods. This process allows the intestines to absorb important nutrients. When not enough bile is released into the intestine, these vitamins are unable to be absorbed into the blood. If left untreated, these nutrient deficiencies may lead to the development of weak or brittle bones or increased bleeding.

Diagnosis: Blood tests can confirm a diagnosis of cholestasis. Patients with the disorder typically have high levels of two liver enzymes: alkaline phosphatase and gamma-glutamyl transpeptidase. Patients with cholestasis generally have three times the normal amount of alkaline phosphatase in their blood. Healthy individuals have 44-147 international units of alkaline phosphatase per liter of blood and 0-51 international units of gamma-glutamyl transpeptidase.

A healthcare provider may be able to tell if the condition is caused by an obstruction inside or outside of the liver after a detailed medical history and physical examination. If the patient has a history of hepatitis or alcoholism or is taking new drugs, an obstruction in the liver is usually suspected. If the physical examination shows that the gallbladder is rigid or painful, an obstruction outside of the liver is suspected.

Additional tests, such as a CT scan, magnetic resonance imaging (MRI) scan, or ultrasound, may be performed to help determine the underlying cause of the condition. If it is suspected that the ducts in the liver are blocked, a liver biopsy may be performed to confirm a diagnosis. If it is suspected that the bile ducts are blocked, either an ERCP or magnetic resonance cholangiopancreatography is performed. Both of these tests provide detailed images of the gallbladder ducts.

Treatment: Treatment of cholestasis depends on the underlying cause.

If a gallstone is blocking the flow of bile, the gallbladder is usually surgically removed. If the gallbladder is removed, patients can expect a full recovery. Complications are rare but may include damage to the common bile duct, bleeding, and infection. During the procedure, a flexible tube called an endoscope is inserted through the anus. Additional surgical tools are inserted through the tube to remove the gallbladder. Nonsurgical procedures, such as bile salt tablets and sound wave therapy, are only considered if the patient is unable to undergo surgery or the stone is primarily made up of cholesterol. This is because gallstones usually recur when nonsurgical procedures are used.

If a medication (e.g., birth control pills or chlorpromazine) is the suspected cause, a healthcare provider may recommend switching to an alternative drug. Patients should not stop taking their medications or change their doses without first consulting their healthcare providers.

If hepatitis is causing the condition, symptoms will resolve once the swelling and/or infection resolves. In general, there are few treatment options for hepatitis. Patients may receive medications, including antivirals and immunomodulators (e.g., interferons), but they are not always effective.

Calcium, vitamin D, and/or vitamin K supplements may be necessary if the patient has nutritional deficiencies. Patients should only take supplements under the strict supervision of their healthcare providers.

In addition, a medication called cholestyramine (Questran) may be taken by mouth to reduce itchiness associated with cholestasis. This medication binds with certain substances in the bile, preventing them from being reabsorbed to irritate the skin. It remains unknown if cholestyramine is safe for pregnant or breastfeeding women.

Patients with cholestasis should avoid substances that may be toxic to the liver, including certain medications (e.g., chlorpromazine) and alcohol, because they may worsen symptoms.

G

GALLBLADDER ATTACKS

Overview: A gallbladder attack, also called gallbladder colic, is characterized by pain and nausea and may accompany many types of gallbladder disorders.

Causes: A gallbladder attack may occur when a gallstone moves through the biliary tract towards the small intestine or if the gallbladder becomes inflamed (a condition called cholecystitis). An attack may also be the result of cholestasis, which occurs when the flow of bile is blocked or if the gallbladder becomes inflamed (cholecystitis).

Symptoms: Gallbladder attacks generally last one to four hours. Common symptoms include dull, sharp, or excruciating pain on the right side of the abdomen, as well as nausea, vomiting, and bloating. The gallbladder, which is located in the lower right side of the abdomen, is usually tender to the touch. It is common for pain to radiate to the right shoulder blade.

Diagnosis: A healthcare provider will be able to tell if a patient is having gallbladder attacks after a detailed medical history and physical examination are performed. The next step is to determine the underlying cause of the symptoms.

Blood tests are usually performed to determine if the patient has cholestasis. Patients with cholestasis typically have high levels of two liver enzymes: alkaline phosphatase and gamma-glutamyl transpeptidase. Healthy individuals have 44-147 international units of alkaline phosphatase per liter of blood and 0-51 international units of gamma-glutamyl transpeptidase per liter of blood.

A CT scan, MRI scan, or ultrasound may also be performed. These tests produce images of the internal organs and may help the healthcare provider detect abnormalities, such as gallstones, that may be causing the gallbladder attack.

ERCP may be performed at a hospital to check for problems in the liver, gallbladder, bile ducts, and pancreas. During the procedure, a thin, flexible tube with a camera (called an endoscope) is inserted through the mouth into the small intestine until it reaches the bile ducts and pancreas. A small plastic tube is inserted through the endoscope and a colored dye is injected. This allows the healthcare provider to see detailed images of the biliary tract.

Treatment: Treatment of gallbladder attacks depends on the underlying cause. For instance, if a gallstone is causing a gallbladder attack, the gallbladder is usually surgically removed. Antibiotics may be prescribed if an infection is the cause. The type of antibiotic used depends on the specific type of infection and severity of the condition. If a medication is the suspected cause, a healthcare provider may recommend an alternative dose or different medication.

GALLSTONES (CHOLELITHIASIS)

Overview: Gallstones, also called cholelithiasis, develop when small particles of the bile in the gallbladder solidify into a stonelike mass. Sometimes gallstones are too large to pass through the biliary ducts and the stone becomes stuck inside the tubes in the gallbladder. In such cases, surgery is necessary to remove the gallbladder.

Causes: Bile consists of bile salts and a fatty compound called lecithin. Lecithin is needed to dissolve the cholesterol in the bile excreted by the liver. Individuals may develop gallstones if there is more cholesterol in the bile than can be dissolved. It is important to note that cholesterol in the blood is not related to cholesterol in the liver. If patients have high levels of cholesterol in the liver it does not mean that they have high levels of cholesterol in the blood. In healthy individuals, the liver is able to control the amount of cholesterol produced in order to keep levels constant. Therefore, cholesterol-lowering drugs cannot prevent gallstones from developing.

Gallstones may also develop if the gallbladder does not empty completely or often enough. When this happens, the bile may become too concentrated. This is especially common among pregnant women because high levels of estrogen during pregnancy increases bile cholesterol levels and decreases the number of the times the gallbladder empties. Also, eating too little fat or not eating for extended periods of time may also increase the risk of gallstones because it causes the gallbladder to empty less frequently.

Symptoms: If the biliary ducts become blocked with a gallstone, bile flow is disrupted. As a result, the bile duct muscles continually contract to try to force the bile through the tubes. This causes a sudden, steady, moderate, or intense pain in the abdomen (called biliary colic or a gallbladder attack). Most pain is felt in the upper or middle abdomen. In some cases, the pain may radiate to the right shoulder blade. Although pain may develop at any time, it is usually felt a couple hours after eating. Pain may last anywhere from 15 minutes to several hours. Some patients may develop nausea and vomiting during an attack. Once the pain goes away, patients may continue to feel a mild aching or soreness in the abdomen for about one day.

Diagnosis: There are several tests available to diagnose gallstones. An ultrasound is typically performed. During the procedure, a wandlike device, called a transducer, is rubbed over the abdomen. Sound waves produce images of the internal organs, including the gallbladder, and the healthcare provider is able to detect gallstones. Additional tests may also be performed, such as a CT scan. A CT scan produces detailed images of the internal organs.

A radionuclide scan (also called a cholescintigraphy, hydroxyl iminodiacetic acid scan, or HIDA scan) may be performed. During a radionuclide scan, the patient is injected with a radioactive dye, called HIDA, because it accumulates in the liver and biliary system. Pictures of the abdomen are then taken. This dye is visible in the ducts and organs in the abdomen. If a gallstone is present in the cystic duct, the dye will not make it all the way to the gallbladder. The amount of radiation emitted during the test is less than that of an x-ray. However, most healthcare providers do not perform this test in pregnant or breastfeeding mothers unless it is absolutely necessary.

Treatment: If the gallstone is blocking a biliary duct, the gallbladder is usually surgically removed. A procedure called endoscopic sphincterotomy is most often performed. During the procedure, which is performed at a hospital, the patient receives general anesthesia. Then, a thin, flexible tube called an endoscope is inserted through the patient's anus. Additional surgical tools are inserted through the tube to remove the gallbladder. The gallbladder may also be removed through an incision in the abdomen. However, this type of surgery is performed less often because it is more invasive and requires a longer recovery time than an endoscopic sphincterotomy.

Once the gallbladder is removed, patients can expect a full recovery. Some patients may experience more frequent bowel movements and/or looser-than-normal stools or diarrhea. In some cases, these symptoms may gradually improve over time. Complications are rare but may include damage to the common bile duct, bleeding, and infection.

Nonsurgical procedures, such as bile salt tablets or sound wave therapy, are only considered if the patient is unable to undergo surgery or if the stone is primarily made up of cholesterol. This is because gallstones usually recur when nonsurgical procedures are used. Bile salt tablets called ursodiol (Actigall) may be taken by mouth to dissolves cholesterol gallstones. In order to prevent gallstones from recurring, most patients need to take the medication daily for the rest of their lives.

Patients with cholesterol gallstones may undergo a procedure called extracorporeal shock wave lithotripsy. Sound waves (shock waves) are used to break the stone into smaller pieces. Patients receive sedatives and/or anesthesia before the procedure. The patient will either be partially submerged in a tub of water or will lie on a soft cushion. Patients wear headphones because the shock waves are loud. High-energy sound waves then pass through the patient's body and break the stone into smaller pieces. The healthcare provider usually uses x-rays or an ultrasound to ensure that the stone breaks down. Treatment usually lasts for about one hour. Patients then take ursodiol (Actigall) daily for the rest of their lives to help prevent the gallstones from recurring.

Side effects of shock wave therapy include blood in the urine, bruising on the abdomen or back, bleeding around the kidney or nearby organs, and pain when the stone fragments are passed in the urine. This therapy is not recommended for pregnant women or patients with cholecystitis or cholangitis.

GILBERT'S SYNDROME

Overview: Gilbert's syndrome is a common inherited disorder that occurs when the liver is unable to properly process the yellow-green pigments in bile (called bilirubin). The increased levels of bilirubin in the bloodstream may lead to yellowing of the skin (jaundice), but the liver itself remains normal. In fact, this condition is so mild that is not usually considered a disease.

Causes: Gilbert's syndrome is an inherited disorder, which is why it is more common among men than women. The condition is passed down as an autosomal dominant trait. This means patients only need to inherit one copy of the mutated gene in order to develop Gilbert's syndrome.

Several factors may worsen symptoms of Gilbert's syndrome by slightly increasing the amount of bilirubin in the blood. Examples include illnesses (e.g., the common cold or the flu), fasting or skipping meals, menstruation, dehydration, or overexertion.

Symptoms: Gilbert's syndrome rarely causes any symptoms. Some patients may periodically develop a condition called jaundice, which causes the skin and eyes to appear yellow.

Although some patients experience periods of fatigue and abdominal pain, it is unclear if they are related to Gilbert's syndrome.

Diagnosis: Gilbert's syndrome is diagnosed after a blood test. Patients with the condition will have more than 0.3-1.9 milligrams of total bilirubin per deciliter of blood and more than 0-0.3 milligrams of direct bilirubin per deciliter of blood. However, levels of bilirubin normally fluctuate throughout the day. Therefore, if Gilbert's syndrome is strongly suspected but initial results are normal, repeat testing may be recommended at a different time of day.

Treatment: Gilbert's syndrome generally does not require treatment. Even if a patient experiences periods of jaundice, each symptomatic episode is very mild and will go away in a few days.

PANCREATITIS

Overview: Pancreatitis is severe inflammation of the pancreas. When the pancreas becomes inflamed, the digestive enzymes in the organ become active too soon. Instead of becoming active in the intestines, they become active inside the pancreas, where they can cause organ damage.

Once the underlying cause is treated, most patients experience a full recovery. However, if the condition is left untreated, scarring may occur in the pancreas. Once the organ becomes scarred, the condition cannot be reversed and the patient will require long-term treatment to manage the symptoms.

Causes: Alcohol is the leading cause of pancreatitis. Individuals who drink heavily for many years have an increased risk of developing it. It is not clear exactly how alcohol affects the pancreas. However, researchers have found that alcohol causes digestive enzymes to be released sooner than normal. Alcohol also increases the permeability of the small ducts. As a result, the pancreatic digestive enzymes are able to damage healthy tissues inside the pancreas. In addition, alcohol abuse has been shown to cause protein plugs, which may develop into gallstones.

Gallstones are another common cause of pancreatitis. Gallstones develop when small particles of the bile in the gallbladder solidify into a stonelike mass. Sometimes the gallstones move from the gallbladder to a small tube called the common bile duct. This common bile duct connects to another tube called the pancreatic duct. If the stone blocks the pancreatic duct, it causes the pancreas to become inflamed. If left untreated, enzymes may leak from the pancreas and damage healthy tissues.

Some medications, including antibiotics such as pentamidine (Pentam) and the anti-HIV drug didanosine (Videx), have been shown to cause pancreatitis. Also, studies have shown that some drugs, including the antiretroviral tenofovir (Viread) and the anticancer drug hydroxyurea (Droxia, Hydrea), may increase the amount of didanosine in the blood, which further increases the risk of pancreatitis.

Symptoms: Acute symptoms of pancreatitis appear suddenly and may lasts for several hours or even days. Common symptoms include nausea, rapid pulse, fever, vomiting, and severe abdominal pain and swelling. The abdomen may be tender when touched. Drinking alcohol causes the symptoms to worsen.

If the underlying cause of pancreatitis is not treated, the condition may become chronic (long term). Common symptoms of chronic pancreatitis include nausea, vomiting, fever, and unintentional weight loss. Chronic pancreatitis may lead to temporary diabetes, malnutrition, and severe pain.

Diagnosis: A blood test may be performed to determine if there are elevated levels of the pancreatic enzymes amylase and lipase in the blood. Patients with pancreatitis will test positive for these enzymes.

Imaging studies, such as an abdominal x-ray or CT scan, may be performed to determine whether the pancreas is larger than normal. Both of these tests, which are performed at a hospital, produce images of the internal organs. Patients with pancreatitis will have an inflamed pancreas.

An ERCP may be performed at a hospital to evaluate the damage of the pancreas. During the procedure, a thin, flexible tube with a camera is inserted through the mouth into the small intestine until it reaches the bile ducts and pancreas. During the test, a small tissue sample may be removed and analyzed in a laboratory for infections or cancer. Because this procedure may damage the pancreas if not performed by a qualified physician, it is only conducted if all other tests are inconclusive. There is also a slight risk of infection.

Treatment: There is no cure for chronic pancreatitis. However, alcohol avoidance and pain medications can effectively relieve symptoms of the condition.

Acute pancreatitis usually improves after about one week of treatment.

If a medication, such as pentamidine (Pentam) or the anti-HIV drug didanosine (Videx), is suspected to be causing acute pancreatitis, a healthcare provider may recommend switching to an alternative dose or medication. Patients should not stop taking medications or take different dosages without first consulting their healthcare providers.

Antimicrobials are used to treat infections that cause pancreatitis. Antibiotics are used to treat bacterial infections, antifungals are used to treat fungal infections, and antivirals are used to treat viral infections. The exact type of medication and length of treatment depends on the type and severity of the infection as well as the patient's overall health.

If a gallstone is causing acute pancreatitis, the gallbladder is usually surgically removed. A surgical procedure, called endoscopic sphincterotomy, is most often performed. During the procedure, which is performed at a hospital, the patient receives general anesthesia and is asleep during the surgery. Then, a thin, flexible tube, called an endoscope, is inserted through the patient's anus. Additional surgical tools are inserted through the tube to remove the gallbladder. Nonsurgical procedures are only considered if the patient is unable to undergo surgery or if the stone is primarily made up of cholesterol. This is because gallstones usually recur when nonsurgical procedures are used.

INTEGRATIVE THERAPIES

Good Scientific Evidence

Globe Artichoke: Globe artichoke is a perennial, thistle-like plant originating in southern Europe around the Mediterranean Sea. Globe artichoke leaf extract has been found to increase bile secretion in animal, human, and laboratory studies. Additional human study is needed to make a firm recommendation for artichoke as a choleretic for patients who have cholestasis.

Use cautiously if allergic/hypersensitive to members of the Asteraceae or Compositae family (e.g., chrysanthemums, daisies, marigolds, ragweed, and arnica) due to possible cross-reactivity. Use cautiously with cholelithiasis or biliary/bile duct obstruction or kidney disease. Avoid if pregnant or breastfeeding.

Unclear or Conflicting Scientific Evidence

S-Adenosylmethionine (SAMe): SAMe is a natural substance found in every cell of the body. Currently, there is insufficient available evidence to determine if SAMe is an effective treatment for cholestasis in pregnant women. It is important to note that there is no information on the use of SAMe prior to the third trimester.

SAMe may be beneficial for pruritus (severe itching) and serum bilirubin levels associated with cholestasis associated with nonpregnancy. However, additional study is needed.

Avoid if allergic to SAMe. Use cautiously with diabetes or anxiety disorders. Avoid with bipolar disorder. Avoid in the first and second trimesters of pregnancy or if breastfeeding due to a lack of safety information.

Soy: Soy is a subtropical plant native to southeastern Asia. This member of the pea family (Fabaceae) grows from one to five feet tall. Due to limited human study, there is not enough evidence to determine if soy is an effective treatment for cholelithiasis. Further research is needed before a recommendation can be made.

Avoid if allergic to soy. The effects of high doses of soy or soy isoflavones in humans are not clear and therefore are not recommended. There has been one case report of vitamin D–deficiency rickets in an infant nursed with soybean milk that was not specifically designed for infants. People who experience intestinal irritation from cow's milk may experience intestinal damage or diarrhea from soy. It is unknown if soy or soy isoflavones share the same side effects as estrogens (e.g., increased risk of blood clots). The use of soy is often discouraged in patients with hormone-sensitive cancers (e.g., breast cancer or prostate cancer). Other hormone-sensitive conditions, such as endometriosis, may also be worsened. Patients taking blood-thinning drugs like warfarin or aspirin should check with their doctors and pharmacists before taking soy supplements. Soy, as a part of the regular diet, is traditionally considered to be safe during pregnancy and breastfeeding, but there are limited scientific data.

Turmeric: Turmeric is a perennial plant native to India and Indonesia that is often used as a spice in cooking. Anecdotally, it has been observed that there is a low incidence of cholelithiasis in Indian populations. Animal research reports that adding the turmeric constituent, curcumin, to the diet reduces the incidence of chemically induced gallstones in mice, and it has been suggested that turmeric may inhibit the formation of cholesterol gallstones. Preliminary human data suggest that curcumin possesses cholagogue (gallbladder contracting) properties. This mechanism may play a role in the prevention of gallstones. However, use of turmeric may be inadvisable in patients with active gallstones.

Avoid if allergic to turmeric (curcumin), yellow food colorings, or plants belonging to the Curcuma or Zingiberaceae (ginger) families. Use cautiously with a history of bleeding disorders, immune system deficiencies, liver disease, or gallstones. Use cautiously if taking blood thinners like warfarin (Coumadin) or aspirin. Use cautiously if pregnant or breastfeeding.

White Horehound: The expert German panel, the Commission E, has approved white horehound as a choleretic for the treatment of dyspepsia (upset stomach) and lack of appetite. The evidence supporting this use is largely anecdotal and based on historical use, and there is currently insufficient scientific research to recommend for or against this use of white horehound.

Avoid if allergic to white horehound or any member of the Lamiaceae (mint) family. White horehound is generally considered safe when used to flavor foods. Use cautiously with diabetes, high/

low/unstable blood pressure, high levels of sodium in the blood, irregular heartbeats, or gastrointestinal disease. Use cautiously if taking diuretics. Avoid if pregnant or breastfeeding.

Zinc: Zinc formulations have been used since ancient Egyptian times to enhance wound healing. Zinc sulfate supplementation seemed to decrease serum unconjugated bilirubin levels in a small study. Well-designed clinical trials are needed to confirm these results.

Zinc is generally considered safe when taken at the recommended dosages. Avoid zinc chloride since studies have not been done on its safety or effectiveness. While zinc appears safe during pregnancy in amounts lower than the established upper intake level, caution should be used since studies cannot rule out the possibility of harm to the fetus.

Fair Negative Scientific Evidence

Iridology: Iridology is the study of the iris for diagnostic purposes. Conventional medicine regards iridology as an unsubstantiated alternative diagnostic technique, although some studies have suggested it may have some potential validity. Preliminary study examined the ability of iridologists to diagnose gallbladder disease from slide photographs of patients with the disease and found no evidence of agreement or diagnostic accuracy. There is no evidence supporting iridology as a diagnostic tool in gallbladder disease.

Iridology should not be used alone to diagnose disease. Studies of iridology have reported incorrect diagnoses, and potentially severe medical problems may thus go undiagnosed. In addition, research suggests that iridology may lead to inappropriate treatment.

PREVENTION

Avoid or minimize alcohol consumption because it may lead to pancreatitis.

Patients can reduce their risks of developing gallstones by maintaining a healthy body weight, exercising regularly, and consuming a reduced-fat, high-fiber diet that includes a variety of fresh vegetables, fruits, and whole grains.

Patients are encouraged not to smoke because it increases the risk of developing pancreatitis.

Patients who have a history of gallstones should take bile salt tablets, called ursodiol (Actigall), daily to prevent gallstones from recurring.

GASTROINTESTINAL DISORDERS

BACKGROUND

Gastrointestinal disorders occur when the digestive tract (gastrointestinal) does not function properly. As a result, patients may have difficulty digesting food, absorbing nutrients, or having normal bowel movements.

Several body parts, including the mouth, esophagus, stomach, small intestine, large intestine, and anus, make up the digestive (gastrointestinal) tract. The digestive process begins when food enters the mouth. When a person begins chewing food, digestive enzymes in the saliva break down the food before it is swallowed. The esophagus is a muscular tube that carries food and liquids from the mouth to the stomach. The stomach contains harsh enzymes that break down food so it can be absorbed by the body. Food then enters the small intestine, which contains three parts: the duodenum, jejunum, and ileum. Most of digestion occurs in the small intestine because it is responsible for absorbing nutrients from food. The remaining food then enters the colon, which also has three parts: the cecum, colon, and rectum. The large intestine absorbs any remaining water from indigestible food matter and eliminates the unusable food matter, or waste, from the body. The anus is the external opening of the rectum. It allows waste (feces) to be excreted from the body.

There are many different types of gastrointestinal disorders. Some gastrointestinal disorders affect multiple parts of the digestive tract, while others only affect the esophagus, abdomen/stomach, intestines, or anus/rectum. The severity of gastrointestinal disorders varies significantly, depending on the specific type of the disease. Some disorders, such as indigestion, are mild while others, such as Crohn's disease, are lifelong.

DISORDERS THAT AFFECT MULTIPLE PARTS OF THE GASTROINTESTINAL TRACT

Diarrhea: Diarrhea occurs when an individual has loose stools or watery stools. Diarrhea is a symptom of an underlying health problem, such as an infection, that prevents the intestines from properly absorbing nutrients from food. Acute diarrhea lasts a few days and affects nearly everyone at some point in their lives. Chronic diarrhea generally lasts longer than four weeks and may be a sign of a serious condition such as inflammatory bowel disease or gastroenteritis.

Diarrhea is usually caused by a viral, bacterial, or parasitic infection. Diarrhea that is caused by an infection (often called infectious diarrhea) may be passed from person to person. Viruses, such as the Norwalk virus, cytomegalovirus, viral hepatitis herpes simplex virus, and rotavirus, are the most likely to cause diarrhea. Infants and young children are most likely to develop diarrhea as a result of a rotavirus infection. If an individual consumes food or water that is contaminated with certain bacteria or parasites, he/she may develop diarrhea. This type of diarrhea is often called traveler's diarrhea because it frequently occurs in people who are traveling to developing countries. Common bacterial causes of diarrhea include *Campylobacter, Salmonella, Escherichia coli* (*E. coli*), *Shigella dysenteriae,* and *Clostridium difficile.* Common parasites that are known to cause diarrhea include *Giardia lamblia* and *Cryptosporidium.*

Diarrhea may be caused by a number of other factors, including lactose intolerance, certain medications (especially antibiotics and anti-HIV medications called antiretrovirals), artificial sweeteners called sorbitol and mannitol (commonly found in sugar-free products and many types of chewing gum), surgery, or other gastrointestinal disorders (such as irritable bowel syndrome).

Symptoms of diarrhea often include frequent and loose stools, abdominal pain or cramping, bloating, fever, excessive thirst, and dehydration. Diarrhea causes dehydration because the body loses water and salts. Infants and young children are at risk of developing severe dehydration as a result of diarrhea. Patient with severe diarrhea may be unable to control the passage of stool, a condition known as fecal incontinence. When a patient experiences frequent, severe, and bloody diarrhea, the condition is often called dysentery.

Diarrhea usually requires little to no medical treatment. Individuals with diarrhea should drink plenty of water. Patients may also benefit from drinks that contain electrolytes, including Pediatric Electrolyte, Pedialyte, or Enfalyte. Individuals should avoid diuretics, such as caffeine, because they worsen symptoms of dehydration. Certain foods, including rice, dry toast, and bananas, may help reduce symptoms of diarrhea. In addition, antidiarrheal medications, such as bismuth subsalicylate

(Pepto-Bismol, Bismatrol, Kaopectate), diphenoxylate atropine (Lomotil, Lofene, Lonox), or loperamide hydrochloride (Imodium), may also be taken to reduce diarrhea in patients older than three years of age. If diarrhea continues for longer than four days or blood is present in the stool, patients should visit their healthcare providers to determine the underlying cause. If an infection is causing symptoms, an antimicrobial medication may be prescribed. The specific type, dose, and duration of treatment depend on the severity and type of infection.

Irritable Bowel Syndrome (IBS): IBS, also called spastic colon, mucous colitis, spastic colitis, nervous stomach, or irritable colon, is a long-term condition that is characterized by abdominal pain, cramping, diarrhea, and constipation. IBS is a functional bowel disorder because the bowel appears normal but does not function properly. Although the exact cause of IBS is unknown, researchers believe that poor diet, neurotransmitter imbalances, and infections may contribute to the development of the disorder.

The colon contracts (colon motility) to move the contents inside the colon toward the rectum. During this passage, water and nutrients are absorbed into the body and waste is excreted as stool. A few times each day, contractions push the stool down the colon resulting in a bowel movement. In IBS patients, the muscles of the colon, sphincters, and pelvis do not contract properly. As a result, patients experience constipation or diarrhea. This causes symptoms of abdominal pain, cramping, bloating, and a sense of incomplete stool movement. Symptoms may improve after the patient has a bowel movement.

Health complications arising from IBS include hemorrhoids (aggravated by diarrhea and/or constipation), depression, weight loss, vitamin and mineral deficiencies, and psychosocial problems. Most people can control symptoms of IBS with diet, stress management, lifestyle modification, and prescribed medications. A medication called loperamide (Imodium) is commonly used to treat IBS patients with diarrhea. Laxatives, such as polyethylene glycol (MiraLAX), sorbitol, and lactulose (Cephulac), may be used. Phosphate enemas (Fleet Phospho-soda) and emollient enemas (Colace Microenema) have also been used. Suppositories, such as bisacodyl (Dulcolax), may also be taken. The most widely studied drugs for the treatment of abdominal pain are a group of drugs called antispasmodics, which cause muscle relaxation. Commonly used antispasmodics include hyoscyamine (Levsin, Levsinex), dicyclomine (Bentyl), and methscopolamine (Pamine). For some patients, however, IBS may be disabling. They

may be unable to work, attend social events, or even travel short distances due to urgency to defecate (pass stool) and/or pain in the colon.

Inflammatory Bowel Disease (IBD): IBD refers to two chronic diseases that cause inflammation of the intestines: ulcerative colitis and Crohn's disease. The cause of IBD remains unknown. However, current research indicates that IBD most likely involves a complex interaction of factors, including heredity, the immune system, and antigens in the environment. The symptoms of these two illnesses are very similar, which often makes it difficult to distinguish between the two. In fact, about 10% of colitis (inflamed colon) cases cannot be diagnosed as either ulcerative colitis or Crohn's disease. When physicians cannot diagnose the specific IBD, the condition is called indeterminate colitis.

IBD causes chronic inflammation in the gastrointestinal tract and may lead to complications, such as colon cancer. The most common symptoms of both ulcerative colitis and Crohn's disease are diarrhea (ranging from mild to severe), abdominal pain, decreased appetite, and weight loss. If the diarrhea is extreme, it may lead to dehydration, increased heartbeat, and decreased blood pressure. As food moves through inflamed areas of the gastrointestinal tract, it may cause bleeding. Continued loss of blood in the stool may result in low levels of iron in the blood, a condition called anemia. In addition, Crohn's disease may also cause intestinal ulcers, fever, fatigue, arthritis, eye inflammation, skin disorders, and inflammation of the liver or bile ducts. Ulcers may extend through the intestinal wall creating a fistula (an abnormal opening). If an internal fistula develops, food may not reach the area of the intestine involved in absorption. External fistulas in the anus may result in continuous bowel drainage onto the skin. Fistulas may also become infected, a condition that can be life threatening if left untreated. Symptoms of a fistula may include pain, fever, tenderness, itching, and general feeling of discomfort.

Toxic megacolon is a rare but potentially life-threatening complication of severe IBD. Toxic megacolon is characterized by a dilated colon (megacolon), abdominal distension (bloating), and occasionally fever, abdominal pain, or shock. In severe cases, the condition may cause the colon to become paralyzed. Toxic megacolon prevents the individual from having bowel movements. If the condition is not treated, the colon may rupture, resulting in peritonitis, a life-threatening condition that requires emergency surgery. Other complications may include dehydration, malnutrition, obstruction, ulcers, and anal fissures.

Many medications are used to treat IBD. Anti-inflammatories, such as sulfasalazine (Azulfidine), mesalamine (e.g., Asacol, Rowasa), olsalazine (Dipentum), and balsalazide (Colazal), help reduce inflammation. Corticosteroids, such as prednisone (Deltasone), have been shown to effectively reduce inflammation of the gastrointestinal tract in IBD patients. Medications, called immunosuppressants, have been used to treat IBD. Examples include azathioprine (Imuran), mercaptopurine (Purinethol), cyclosporine (e.g., Neoral, Sandimmune), and infliximab (Remicade). A fiber supplement, such as psyllium powder (Metamucil) or methylcellulose (Citrucel), may help relieve symptoms of mild to moderate diarrhea. Inflammation may cause the intestines to narrow, resulting in constipation. Laxatives may be taken to relieve symptoms of constipation. Oral laxatives, such as Correctol, and sigmoidoscopy have been used. A qualified healthcare provider may recommend acetaminophen (Tylenol) to relieve mild pain. Avoid nonsteroidal antiinflammatory drugs (NSAIDs), such as ibuprofen (Advil, Motrin) or naproxen (Aleve), as researchers have found a strong relationship between NSAIDs and IBD flare-ups. Therefore, NSAIDs should not be taken.

If all other treatments fail to relieve symptoms, a qualified healthcare provider may recommend surgery. Surgery is more commonly performed in ulcerative colitis patients because inflammation is limited to the colon. During the procedure, the entire colon and rectum are removed (proctocolectomy). A new procedure, known as ileoanal anastomosis, eliminates the need for recovered patients to wear a bag to collect stool. This new procedure involves attaching a pouch directly to the anus, allowing the patient to expel waste normally. However, the patient may have as many as five to seven watery bowel movements a day because there is no longer a colon to absorb water. From 25-40% of patients with ulcerative colitis eventually need surgery.

Indigestion (Nonulcer Dyspepsia): Indigestion, also called nonulcer dyspepsia (upset stomach), is a general term that describes discomfort in the upper abdomen. Patients who have indigestion typically suffer from several symptoms, including heartburn, bloating, belching, and nausea. Indigestion affects nearly everyone from time to time, and it is not considered a serious health condition. Indigestion may occur if a patient eats too much of a particular food (especially fatty or spicy foods) or eats too quickly. Alcohol, stress, and anxiety may also contribute to indigestion. Because indigestion is such a common condition, it generally does not require a diagnosis. However, patients who frequently experience indigestion should visit their healthcare providers because it may be a symptom of an underlying medical condition, such as acid reflux disease.

Antacids, such as calcium carbonate (e.g., Tums, Alka-Mints, Rolaids Calcium Rich), may be taken by mouth to treat symptoms of heartburn and upset stomach. Antiflatulent medications, such as alpha-galactosidase enzyme (Beano) or simethicone (Gas-X, Genasyme, Mylanta Gas Relief), may be taken by mouth to prevent and/or treat symptoms of bloating and flatulence (gas).

Monosodium Glutamate (MSG) Symptom Complex (Chinese Restaurant Syndrome): Monosodium glutamate symptom complex, also called Chinese restaurant syndrome, is a group of symptoms that some patients develop after eating Chinese foods. Symptoms typically include flushing, headache, sweating, facial pain or swelling, numbness or burning around the mouth, and chest pain. Although it has been suggested that a food additive in Chinese food called MSG may cause the reaction, it has not been proven. Since there are limited scientific data about the condition, it remains unknown if the frequency and amount of MSG exposure increase or decrease an individual's risk of experiencing symptoms.

Patients generally do not require treatment for MSG symptom complex because symptoms are mild and resolve on their own. However, if patients experience chest pain or difficulty breathing, they should seek immediate medical treatment because this may be a sign of a serious allergic reaction called anaphylaxis.

Diverticulosis and Diverticulitis: Diverticulosis refers to small, bulging pouches (diverticula) in any part of the digestive tract. Diverticula are most often found in the large intestine (colon). However, they may also develop in the esophagus, stomach, or small intestine.

Diverticulosis is a common condition that affects more than half of Americans who are older than 60 years of age. Most patients do not know they have diverticulosis because they do not experience any signs or symptoms of the condition. However, if the diverticula become infected or inflamed, the condition is called diverticulitis. Patients with diverticulitis typically experience intense abdominal pain, nausea, bloating, bleeding from the rectum, tenderness in the abdomen, difficulty or pain during urination, fever, and changes in bowel movements.

Diverticulitis is usually diagnosed after a computerized tomography (CT) scan is performed. A machine produces images of the internal organs in the abdomen. Inflamed diverticula will be apparent if the patient has diverticulitis.

G

Mild cases of diverticulitis can be treated with rest, changes in the diet, and antibiotics. Patients should not eat any fiber, including whole grains, fruits, and vegetables, for several days. This restricted diet gives the colon time to heal. Antibiotics, such as metronidazole (Flagyl), moxifloxacin (Avelox), ciprofloxacin (Cipro), amoxicillin/clavulanate (Augmentin), and imipenem (Primaxin) are commonly prescribed to kill the bacteria that are infecting the diverticula. Serious cases of diverticulitis may eventually require surgery to remove the infected part of the colon.

Peptic Ulcers: An ulcer is an open sore or break in a body tissue. Peptic ulcers develop on the inside lining of the stomach (gastric peptic ulcer), upper small intestine (duodenal peptic ulcer), or esophagus (esophageal peptic ulcer). Researchers have found that a bacterial infection with *Helicobacter pylori* is the most common cause of gastric and duodenal ulcers. Some medications, including aspirin and NSAIDs such as ibuprofen (Motrin, Advil), may also cause gastric and duodenal ulcers. In addition, smoking tobacco increases a patient's risk of developing ulcers. It remains unclear whether or not excessive alcohol consumption leads to an increased risk of ulcers.

Esophageal peptic ulcers are usually associated with acid reflux disease. Contrary to popular beliefs, diet and stress do not cause peptic ulcers. However, high levels of stress and acid foods and beverages, such as coffee, may aggravate symptoms of peptic ulcers. Peptic ulcers generally cause pain that may be felt anywhere from the chest to the stomach. Pain may last a few minutes to several hours. Symptoms are often the worst when the stomach is empty or at night. They may also come and go for a few days to weeks. Less common symptoms include vomiting blood, dark blood in the stools, nausea, vomiting, and unexplained weight loss.

Most ulcers are diagnosed after an x-ray is taken of the upper gastrointestinal tract. An endoscopy may also be performed. During the procedure, a thin tube with a camera (endoscope) is inserted into the mouth and into the digestive tract. This allows the healthcare provider to see if ulcers are present.

Patients take antibiotics, such as amoxicillin (Amoxil), clarithromycin (Biaxin), or metronidazole (Flagyl), if an *H. pylori* infection is causing peptic ulcers. Patients also take medications called acid blockers, which reduce the amount of acid in the stomach. As a result, the patient experiences less pain, and the gastrointestinal tract is able to heal. Examples of acid blockers include ranitidine (Zantac), famotidine (Pepcid), cimetidine (Tagamet),

and nizatidine (Axid). Patients should take their medications exactly as prescribed. If medication is not taken regularly or stopped too early, the ulcer may not heal properly. Also, during treatment, patients should not smoke, consume alcohol, or take NSAIDs because they may worsen symptoms.

Pyloric Stenosis: Pyloric stenosis is a rare condition that occurs when babies are born with abnormally large muscles at the opening at the bottom of the stomach (pylorus). The pylorus connects the stomach to the small intestine. Babies with pyloric stenosis are unable to transport food into the small intestine. This may lead to extremely forceful vomiting (also called projectile vomiting) that may contain blood, weight loss, dehydration, and electrolyte imbalances. Babies are usually hungry after vomiting. They may cry without tears because they are dehydrated.

The exact cause of pyloric stenosis remains unknown. However, researchers believe that genetics plays a role. Most patients are diagnosed and treated when they are three to 12 weeks old. Babies with pyloric stenosis need to have surgery as soon as possible to correct the pylorus. The surgical procedure, called pyloromyotomy, involves reducing the size of the pylorus muscles. Patients typically experience an improvement in symptoms about 24 hours after surgery.

Colic (Infancy): Colic is usually defined as crying for more than three hours a day, three days per week, for longer than three weeks in an otherwise healthy baby. It remains unknown what causes colic. However, researchers have suggested that it may be caused by gastrointestinal problems, such as lactose intolerance or an immature digestive system. This is because sometimes a colic episode stops after a baby passes gas or has a bowel movement. Other possible causes include maternal anxiety, differences in the way a baby is fed or comforted, and/or allergies. There is currently no treatment that has been proven to be effective for the treatment of colic in babies. Colic typically goes away once the baby reaches three months of age.

Biliary Colic: Biliary colic, also called a gallbladder attack, describes pain and nausea that accompanies many disorders that affect the gallbladder. The gallbladder is an organ that stores digestive fluids that are needed to break down fats in foods.

Biliary colic may occur when a gallstone moves through the biliary tract towards the small intestine. An attack may also be the result of cholestasis, which occurs when the flow of bile is blocked. Gallbladder attacks may also occur if the gallbladder becomes inflamed. Gallbladder attacks generally last one to four hours. Common symptoms include pain on the right side of the abdomen, nausea, vomiting, and bloating. The gallbladder, which is located in the lower right side of the abdomen, is usually tender to the touch. The pain may be dull, sharp, or excruciating. It is common for the pain to radiate to the right shoulder blade.

A healthcare provider will be able to tell if a patient is having gallbladder attacks after a detailed medical history and physical examination are performed. The next step is to determine the underlying cause of the symptoms. Blood tests and liver function tests may be performed to determine if the patient has cholestasis. If the patient's alkaline phosphatase levels are three times higher than normal, cholestasis is indicated. A CT scan, magnetic resonance imaging scan, or ultrasound may also be performed. These tests produce images of the internal organs and may help the healthcare provider detect abnormalities, such as gallstones, that may be causing the condition. An endoscopic retrograde cholangiopancreatography may be performed at the hospital to check for problems in the liver, gallbladder, bile ducts, and pancreas. During the procedure, a thin, flexible tube with a camera is inserted through the mouth into the small intestine. The tube then hooks into the bile duct, allowing the healthcare provider to see the biliary tract.

Treatment of gallbladder attacks depends on the underlying cause. For instance, a gallstone may need to be surgically removed if it is causing symptoms. Antibiotics may be prescribed if an infection is the cause. If a medication is the suspected cause, a healthcare provider may recommend an alternative medication.

Gastroenteritis: Gastroenteritis describes inflammation of the stomach and intestine that causes diarrhea, vomiting, and cramps. Gastroenteritis is often mistaken for the stomach flu or food poisoning because it causes similar symptoms. Although some doctors may call gastroenteritis the flu, gastroenteritis is not caused by any of the influenza viruses. An infection in the digestive tract may cause gastroenteritis. This may happen if patients consume foods or beverages that contain disease-causing bacteria, viruses, or parasites. In some cases, the food itself may irritate the patient's digestive tract. For instance, if a lactose-intolerant patient consumes a dairy product, the stomach and intestines become irritated, which may lead to gastroenteritis. In addition, some mediations, including aspirin, NSAIDs, some antibiotics, caffeine, laxatives, and steroids, may cause gastroenteritis.

Most patients recover quickly from gastroenteritis. However, babies and the elderly have a greatest risk of developing life-threatening complications, such as dehydration and poor nutrition. If an infection is causing gastroenteritis, patients take medications called antimicrobials to kill the disease-causing organisms. Commonly prescribed antimicrobials include ciprofloxacin (Cipro), trimethoprim/sulfamethoxazole (Bactrim), and rifaximin (Xifaxan, Redactiv, Flonorm). Adults may also take medications, called antiemetics, which reduce vomiting. Commonly prescribed antiemetics include promethazine (Phenergan, Anergan), prochlorperazine (Compazine), or ondansetron (Zofran). Antidiarrheals, such as diphenoxylate atropine (Lomotil, Lofene, Lonox) or loperamide hydrochloride (Imodium), may also be taken to reduce diarrhea in patients older than three years old.

Gaucher's Disease: Gaucher's disease is a rare, inherited disorder that occurs when a fatty substance called glucocerebroside accumulates in the spleen, liver, lungs, and bone marrow. In some cases, it also affects the functioning of the brain. Patients with Gaucher's disease are born with low levels of a digestive enzyme called glucocerebrosidase, which breaks down glucocerebroside. This deficiency causes glucocerebroside to build up in the body.

There are three types of Gaucher's disease: type I, type II, and type III. Type I is the most common form. It causes enlargement of the liver (hepatomegaly) and spleen (splenomegaly) and it may also affect the lungs and kidneys. When fat develops in the liver, it is often called hepatic steatosis. Type I may develop at any age. Type II is a fatal condition that develops during infancy and causes severe brain damage. Most children with type II Gaucher's disease die by the age of two years old. Type III causes the liver and spleen to enlarge and brain damage gradually occurs over time. Type III usually occurs in children and adolescents.

Gaucher's disease is diagnosed after a blood test. Patients with the disorder will have low levels of glucocerebrosidase in their blood.

There is currently no cure for Gaucher's disease. Patients with type I and type III Gaucher's disease take enzyme replacement therapy, which has been proven to effectively manage symptoms. However, there is no effective treatment to manage the symptoms of type II.

ESOPHAGEAL DISORDERS

Gastroesophageal Reflux Disease (GERD): GERD, also called acid reflux disease, occurs when liquid from the stomach backs up (regurgitates) into the esophagus. This liquid may contain stomach acids and bile. In some cases, the regurgitated stomach liquid can cause inflammation (esophagitis), irritation, and damage to the esophagus. It remains unknown exactly what causes GERD. Several factors, including hiatal hernias (when the stomach pushes up through a hole in the diaphragm muscle), abnormally weak contractions of the lower esophageal sphincter, and abnormal emptying of the stomach after a meal, have been associated with GERD.

Common symptoms of GERD include a burning sensation in the chest that may spread to the throat (heartburn), chest pain (especially when lying down), difficulty swallowing (dysphagia), regurgitating food or sour liquid, coughing, hoarseness, sore throat, and wheezing. Several factors may worsen symptoms of the condition. For instance, spicy foods, fatty foods, chocolate, caffeine, tomato sauce, carbonated beverages, mint, alcoholic beverages, large meals, lying down after eating, some medications (e.g., sedatives, tranquilizers, or blood pressure drugs), and cigarette smoking may worsen symptoms of GERD. Most cases of GERD can be diagnosed based on the patient's symptoms.

GERD is usually a lifelong condition because there is no cure for the disorder. Patients must take medications for the rest of their lives to manage symptoms. In addition, patients should not smoke because it may increase the amount of stomach acid and worsen symptoms. Patients with mild cases of GERD may be able to manage their symptoms with over-the-counter medications and changes in the diet. Patients may experience improvements in symptoms if they eat smaller meals and eliminate foods that are known to cause heartburn.

Antacids, such as Gelusil, Rolaids, Mylanta, Maalox, or Tums, may neutralize stomach acid and provide quick relief of GERD symptoms. However, they will not help the esophagus heal. Patients who take antacids frequently may experience diarrhea or constipation. Some over-the-counter H2 receptor blockers, such as cimetidine (Tagamet HB), famotidine (Pepcid AC), nizatidine (Axid AR), and ranitidine (Zantac 75), may also help provide quick relief of symptoms. These medications reduce the amount of stomach acid that is produced. Side effects of H2 receptor blockers, which are uncommon, may include changes in bowel movements, dry mouth, dizziness, or drowsiness. Proton pump inhibitors, such as omeprazole (Prilosec), may also be taken short term to help the esophagus heal. Patients should not take these medications long term unless they talk with their healthcare providers first.

Patients with persistent GERD may require prescription-strength medications to manage symptoms and prevent esophageal damage. H2 blockers, such as Axid, Pepcid, Tagamet, and Zantac, are commonly prescribed. Examples of prescription-strength proton pump inhibitors include esomeprazole (Nexium), lansoprazole (Prevacid), omeprazole (Prilosec), pantoprazole (Protonix), and rabeprazole (Aciphex).

Achalasia: Achalasia is a rare disease that occurs when the muscles of the esophagus are unable to relax. The esophageal sphincter, which is the muscle between the lower esophagus and stomach, is unable to relax enough to allow food to pass into the stomach. Also, the lower half of the esophagus does not contract and relax properly. As a result, the food is not properly pushed down into the stomach, and patients have difficulty swallowing food (dysphagia). The exact cause of achalasia remains unknown. Researchers believe that several factors, including infections, genetics, and abnormalities in the immune system, may contribute to the development of the condition.

The most common symptom of achalasia is difficulty swallowing solid foods and liquids. Some patients experience heavy sensations in the chests after eating that feels like chest pain. If food collects in the esophagus, it may cause irritation and lead to esophagitis (inflamed esophagus). Some patients may regurgitate their food if it is trapped in the esophagus. If regurgitated food enters the windpipe (trachea), it may cause infections such as pneumonia. Since patients have difficulty swallowing and consuming foods and beverages, they typically experience weight loss. Other complications may include malnutrition and dehydration.

Achalasia is usually diagnosed after a video esophagram is performed. During the procedure, the patient drinks a barium solution and video x-rays are taken of the esophagus. The healthcare provider is able to see if the barium enters the stomach properly. If the patient has achalasia, the barium will stay in the esophagus longer than normal. In addition, the lower end of the esophagus will be very narrow.

Some patients may experience an improvement in symptoms if they eat slowly, take small bites, and chew their food thoroughly. In addition, patients with achalasia usually take nitrates, such as isosorbide dinitrate (Isordil), and calcium-channel blockers, such as nifedipine (Procardia) or verapamil (Calan), to relax the muscles of the esophagus. These medications provide short-term relief of symptoms.

A procedure called forceful dilation, or stretching of the lower esophageal sphincter, is often needed to open the esophagus and allow food to enter the stomach. During the procedure, a tube with a balloon at the end is inserted into the patient's esophagus. The balloon is placed across the sphincter and inflated. As a result, the sphincter stretches out. Forceful dilation successfully treats 65-90% of patients with achalasia. The most serious complication of forceful dilation is rupture of the esophagus, which occurs in about 5% of patients. If a rupture occurs, antibiotics and/or surgery may be required. Forceful dilation is generally quicker and less expensive than surgery.

If forceful dilation is unsuccessful, a surgical procedure, called esophagomyotomy, may be performed. During the procedure, the sphincter is cut, which expands the esophagus and makes it easier for the patient to swallow. The procedure is more effective than forceful dilation. An estimated 80-90% of patients are treated successfully with esophagomyotomy. However, in some cases, dysphagia may return. The most common side effect of esophagomyotomy is GERD. In order to prevent GERD, the esophagomyotomy may be modified so that it does not completely cut the sphincter or the esophagomyotomy may be combined with antireflux surgery. Regardless of which surgery is performed, some healthcare providers recommend lifelong treatment with GERD medications, such as Axid, Pepcid, Tagamet, or Zantac. Other doctors only recommend lifelong treatment if GERD is diagnosed 24 hours after surgery.

Botox injections in the lower sphincter are the newest treatment for achalasia. The botulinum toxin is injected to weaken the sphincter. The effects of treatment usually last for several months. Patients may require additional injections. Patients who are elderly or unable to undergo surgery typically receive this treatment. It may also be performed to help patients gain weight and improve their nutritional status before surgery.

Esophageal Spasms: Patients may experience spasms in the esophagus. Esophageal spasms may cause difficulty swallowing, painful swallowing, sensation that something is stuck in the throat, heartburn, and chest pain. The exact cause of spasms remains unknown. However, eating hot or cold foods may contribute to the condition. GERD or heartburn may also play a role in the development of esophageal spasms.

Patients typically take nitrates, such as isosorbide dinitrate (Isordil), or calcium-channel blockers, such as nifedipine (Procardia) or verapamil (Calan), to relax the muscles.

ACUTE ABDOMEN AND STOMACH DISORDERS

Appendicitis: Appendicitis occurs when an organ in the lower right side of the abdomen, called the appendix, becomes inflamed and filled with pus. The cause of appendicitis is not always clear. In some cases, appendicitis may occur if food waste or a solid piece of stool becomes trapped in an opening near the appendix. It may also occur after an infection. The most common symptom of appendicitis is severe pain in the lower right-hand side of the abdomen. Additional symptoms may include nausea, vomiting, loss of appetite, low-grade fever, constipation, bloating or inability to pass gas, diarrhea, and abdominal swelling. Patients with appendicitis will have high levels of white blood cells in their blood. Imaging studies are also performed to determine if the appendix is enlarged.

Patients with appendicitis must have their appendix surgically removed as quickly as possible. Since the appendix has no known purpose, the patient's life is unaffected after the appendix is removed. If the appendix is not removed quickly, it may break open or rupture. If the appendix ruptures, it may lead to an infection in the lining of the abdominal cavity. Infections may cause a condition called peritonitis, which occurs when the abdominal lining becomes inflamed. If the appendix ruptures, the patient may start to feel better. However, soon after, the abdomen may swell because it becomes full of gas and fluid. At this point, the abdomen usually feels hard, tight, and tender to the touch. Severe pain also develops throughout the entire abdomen. Patients may be unable to pass gas or have a bowel movement. Additional symptoms of peritonitis include fever, thirst, and decreased urination.

Patients who have symptoms of peritonitis should seek immediate medical treatment. Even if the condition is treated quickly, it may be fatal. Patients will receive aggressive treatment with intravenous antibiotics. Surgery is necessary to remove the burst appendix. Patients will also receive all fluids and nutrition through injections until their condition is improved.

Stomach Inflammation (Gastritis): Stomach inflammation, also called gastritis, may develop suddenly (acute) or gradually over a longer period of time (chronic). Most cases of gastritis are caused by an infection with the same bacterium (*Helicobacter pylori*) that causes stomach ulcers. Gastritis may also be caused by traumatic injury or surgery, excessive alcohol consumption, and regular use of NSAIDs such as ibuprofen (Motrin, Advil) or naproxen (Aleve). A condition called bile reflux disease may also cause gastritis. This occurs when bile, a fluid that helps digest fats, enters the stomach. In rare cases, gastritis may occur when the body's own immune cells attack the stomach. It remains unknown what triggers this autoimmune reaction. The acid in the stomach may worsen symptoms of gastritis.

Symptoms of gastritis generally include a burning pain or aching in the upper abdomen that may worsen when food is eaten, nausea, vomiting, loss of appetite, bloating, feeling of fullness in the upper abdomen after eating, and weight loss. In some cases, gastritis may cause stomach bleeding. Symptoms of stomach bleeding include blood in the vomit and black or dark-colored stools. In some cases, gastritis may lead to ulcers and an increased risk of stomach cancer.

In most cases, patients fully recover quickly once treatment is started. Patients typically take antacids, such as Tums, Mylanta, or Rolaids, to help neutralize the stomach acid. This helps reduce symptoms of gastritis quickly. Acid blockers, such as cimetidine (Tagamet), ranitidine (Zantac), nizatidine (Axid), or famotidine (Pepcid), may be taken to reduce the amount of stomach acid that is produced. Proton pump inhibitors, such as omeprazole (Prilosec), lansoprazole (Prevacid), rabeprazole (Aciphex), and esomeprazole (Nexium), may also be taken to reduce the amount of stomach acid produced. If an infection with *H. pylori* is causing gastritis, patients generally receive a combination of antibiotics and proton pump inhibitors. Commonly prescribed antibiotics include amoxicillin (Amoxil), clarithromycin (Biaxin), and metronidazole (Flagyl).

Hypochlorhydria (Low Stomach Acid): Hypochlorhydria occurs when patients have low levels of stomach acid, also called hydrochloric acid. The body needs stomach acid in order to break down foods so that they can be absorbed in the intestines. Natural aging, a poor diet, chronic use of certain medications, and past infection with the *Helicobacter pylori* bacteria may limit a patient's ability to produce hydrochloric acid. Hypochlorhydria may also be a symptom of an underlying medical condition such as Addison's disease, depression, asthma, eczema, gallstones, hepatitis, osteoporosis, psoriasis, thyroid disease, and autoimmune disorders.

If there is low acidity in the stomach, patients may only be able to partially digest food. This may lead to malnutrition. Symptoms of hypochlorhydria may include bloating, gas, belching, burning or dryness of the mouth, heartburn, multiple food allergies, rectal itching, redness or dilated blood vessels in the cheeks and nose, adult acne, hair loss (in women), iron deficiency, undigested foods in the stool, yeast infection, as well as diarrhea or constipation. Patients with hypochlorhydria also have an increased risk of developing infections in the gastrointestinal tract because it provides an ideal environment for disease-causing organisms, such as bacteria. Patients with hypochlorhydria take betaine hydrochloride or glutamic acid hydrochloride with meals and snacks. These medications increase the amount of stomach acid, which helps the body properly break down and digest foods.

Ileus: Ileus occurs when the small and/or large intestine is partially or completely blocked. Ileus is a nonmechanical blockage. Unlike mechanical blockages, which occur when the bowel is physically blocked, a nonmechanical blockage occurs when the rhythmic contractions that move material through the bowel, called peristalsis, stop. Ileus is usually associated with an infection of the peritoneum, which is the membrane that lines the abdomen. This is most common in infants and children. Intestinal surgery may lead to temporary ileus that lasts two to three days. Ileus may also be a complication of surgery on other body parts, such as the chest or joints. Other medical conditions, including kidney disease and heart disease, may cause ileus. Some chemotherapy drugs, such as vincristine (Oncovin, Vincasar PES, Vincrex) or vinblastine (Velban, Velsar), may cause ileus. Symptoms of ileus may include abdominal distention, abdominal cramping, nausea, vomiting, bloating or failure to pass gas, and difficulty having bowel movements.

Patients with ileus must receive nutrition and fluids intravenously to give the intestines time to heal. If an infection is causing the condition, antibiotics are prescribed. Other medications, including cisapride and vasopressin (Pitressin), may be prescribed to stimulate the intestines to contract and relax.

INTESTINAL DISORDERS

Celiac Disease (Nontropical Sprue): Celiac disease, also called nontropical sprue, is a digestive disorder that occurs when an individual's immune system overreacts to gluten, a protein found in wheat, rye, barley, and oats. When a patient with the disease eats food that contains gluten, the immune cells flood to the stomach and intestine to destroy the gluten. However, among these immune cells are autoantibodies that attack the lining of the intestine by mistake. As a result, the intestinal lining becomes damaged.

It has not been determined what triggers this reaction in celiac patients. However, celiac disease is associated with autoimmune disorders, such as lupus. Autoimmune disorders occur when the patient's immune system mistakenly identifies body cells as harmful invaders, such as bacteria. As a result, the immune cells in celiac patients attack the patient's intestinal cells when gluten is consumed. Celiac disease causes symptoms of abdominal pain and bloating after consuming gluten. Additionally, complications, including poor absorption, may occur if the patient continues to eat gluten-containing foods. When the intestinal lining is damaged, patients have difficulty absorbing nutrients. Symptoms of poor nutrition include weight loss, diarrhea, abdominal cramps, gas, bloating, fatigue, foul-smelling or grayish stools that may be oily (steatorrhea), stunted growth in children, and osteoporosis (hollow, brittle bones).

If celiac disease is suspected, blood tests will be performed to determine whether or not the patient has autoantibodies associated with the disease. If autoantibodies are present, a positive diagnosis is made.

Although there is currently no cure for celiac disease, the condition can be managed with a gluten-free diet. Patients should avoid all foods that contain gluten. This includes any type of wheat (including farina, graham flour, semolina, and durum), barley, rye, bulgur, Kamut, kasha, matzo meal, spelt, and triticale. Therefore, foods such as bread, cereal, crackers, pasta, cookies, cake, pie, gravy, and sauce should be avoided unless they are labeled as gluten free. In general, patients who strictly follow a gluten-free diet can expect to live normal, healthy lives. Symptoms will subside several weeks after the diet is started, and patients will be able to absorb food normally once they avoid eating gluten. A dietician or certified nutritionist may help a patient with celiac disease develop a healthy diet. Patients with celiac disease may also find gluten-free cookbooks to be a helpful resource. Many products, including rice flour and potato flour, can be used as substitutes for gluten-containing flour.

Menkes Kinky Hair Disease: Menkes kinky hair disease, also called Menkes disease, is an inherited disorder that decreases the body's ability to absorb copper. Cells in the body need copper to function properly. The disease is characterized by sparse and coarse hair, short stature, and progressive deterioration of the nervous system. Symptoms develop during infancy. Babies with Menkes kinky hair disease show slightly slowed development for two to three months after birth. The baby's condition will worsen after this time and he/she will lose previously developed skills. Other symptoms include silver or colorless hair, seizures, and osteoporosis (hollow and brittle bones).

There is currently no cure for Menkes kinky hair disease. Patients may receive injections of copper. However, patients typically die by the age of 10.

Acrodermatitis Enteropathica: Acrodermatitis enteropathica is an inherited condition that occurs when the body is unable to absorb zinc. This trace element is necessary for the functioning of over 300 different enzymes and plays a vital role in an enormous number of biological processes. The exact cause of acrodermatitis enteropathica remains unknown. However, researchers believe that genetics may play a role.

Symptoms of acrodermatitis enteropathica may include red and swollen patches of dry and scaly skin, crusted or pus-filled blisters on the skin, swollen skin around the nails, mouth ulcers, red and glossy tongue, impaired wound healing, as well as hair loss on the scalp, eyelashes, and eyebrows. Additional symptoms may include pinkeye, sensitivity to light, decreased appetite, diarrhea, irritability, failure to grow, and depressed mood. A zinc deficiency can be diagnosed after a blood test.

Although there is no cure for the disorder, zinc supplements taken by mouth daily have been shown to effectively manage symptoms. Without treatment, acrodermatitis enteropathica will lead to death. Skin lesions usually heal one to two weeks after treatment is started. Other symptoms begin to improve within 24 hours.

ANORECTAL DISORDERS

Hemorrhoids: Hemorrhoids are inflamed veins in the anus and rectum. Hemorrhoids may develop inside or outside of the rectum, depending on the specific veins that are affected. Hemorrhoids are common, affecting nearly half of individuals who are older than 50 years of age. Hemorrhoids develop when there is increased pressure in the veins of the anus and rectum. This is often due to straining during constipation, sitting or standing for extended periods of time, pregnancy, childbirth, and diarrhea. Obese patients have an increased risk of developing hemorrhoids.

Internal hemorrhoids are not painful because pain nerves are not present inside the membranes of the rectum. However, internal hemorrhoids may cause bleeding when stools are passed. External hemorrhoids are usually painful. The veins outside of the rectum are swollen and may itch. Bleeding may occur, especially when straining to move the bowels. External hemorrhoids can be diagnosed after observing the inflamed veins. If internal hemorrhoids are suspected, a healthcare provider may examine the rectum with an anoscope, proctoscope, or sigmoidoscope.

Mild cases of hemorrhoids are usually treated with over-the-counter creams or ointments, such as Preparation H. Warm baths may also help improve symptoms. If a blood clot forms in a hemorrhoid, a healthcare provider can make a surgical incision to remove the clot. Rubber band ligation may be used to treat severe or persistent cases of hemorrhoids. During the procedure, small rubber bands are inserted around the base of the hemorrhoids. This cuts off the blood supply in the vein until the hemorrhoid falls off. During a procedure called sclerotherapy, a chemical is injected near the hemorrhoid to shrink the inflamed vein. If these therapies are ineffective, the hemorrhoids may be surgically removed in a process called hemorrhoidectomy.

Rectal Prolapse: Rectal prolapse occurs when the inner lining of the rectum, called the rectal mucosa, protrudes from the anus. Rectal prolapse occurs when the tissues that normally support that rectal mucosa become loose and allow the tissue to slip down through the anus. Without treatment, the condition may worsen and a large part of the rectum may protrude from the body through the anus. When this happens, the condition is called a complete prolapse. Most patients do not realize that they have rectal prolapse until it reaches this stage. Initially, the rectum may protrude during certain activities, such as coughing or laughing. Eventually, the prolapsed rectum may protrude more frequently or permanently.

Patients may be able to feel the tissue protruding out of the anus. Common symptoms of rectal prolapse include pain during bowel movements, mucus or bleeding from the protruding tissue, and inability to control bowel movements.

Most patients with rectal prolapse require surgery. The surgeon reattaches the rectum to the back side of the inner pelvis. Surgery may be performed through the abdomen or the perineum. Stool softeners, such as calcium docusate (Surfak) or sodium docusate (Colace), may help reduce pain and straining during bowel movements.

Rectal Inflammation (Proctitis): Rectal inflammation, also called proctitis, occurs when the lining of the rectum (rectal mucosa) becomes swollen. Patients with proctitis often experience rectal bleeding, anal and rectal pain, frequent urges to have a bowel movement, passing mucus through the rectum, feeling of rectal fullness, and diarrhea.

There are many potential causes of proctitis. The most common cause is sexually transmitted diseases, which are acquired through anal or oral-anal intercourse. Other causes may include IBD and bacterial infections, such as streptococcus. Less common causes include chemicals (such as hydrogen peroxide enemas), injury to the rectum, radiation therapy that is applied near the rectum (for conditions such as prostate or cervical cancer), and medications or objects that are inserted into the rectum.

Several tests may be performed to diagnose the underlying cause of proctitis. Blood tests may be performed to detect possible infections. A colonoscopy may be performed to examine the inside of the colon for abnormalities. Healthcare providers may also use a swab to collect a sample of fluid from the rectum or urethra. The sample is then tested for sexually transmitted diseases.

Most cases of proctitis are effectively treated and patients experience a full recovery. Treatment depends on the underlying cause of proctitis. If a bacterial infection is present, antibiotics, such as ciprofloxacin (Cipro), levofloxacin (Levaquin), penicillin, amoxicillin (Amoxil, Trimox), azithromycin (Zithromax), clarithromycin (Biaxin), or clindamycin (Cleocin), may be taken. If a viral infection (e.g., herpes) causes proctitis, antivirals, such as such as acyclovir (Zovirax), may be taken. Corticosteroids may be taken if radiation therapy is causing proctitis. If IBD is causing symptoms, antiinflammatories, such as sulfasalazine (Azulfidine), or antidiarrheals, such as psyllium powder (Metamucil), may be taken.

Laxative-Induced Colon Damage: Laxatives are medications that are used to stimulate bowel movements. They are primarily used to treat constipation. Patients who overuse laxatives may develop colon damage. Long-term use of laxatives may cause the muscles in the colon to become weak from lack of use. The nerves in the lining of the colon may also become damaged. As a result, this may slow intestinal mobility and cause constipation. Symptoms of laxative abuse include weight loss, hair loss, vomiting, abdominal pain, low energy, dehydration, dry eyes, headaches, mood swings, and bone pain. Therefore, patients should not take laxatives more frequently than the packaging label suggests. If symptoms persist, patients should consult their healthcare providers to diagnose and properly treat the underlying cause.

INTEGRATIVE THERAPIES
Good Scientific Evidence

Fennel: Fennel grows in the Mediterranean region. For centuries, fennel fruits have been used as herbal medicines in Europe and China. Fennel tea is often used to treat infants with digestive disorders.

It has a mild flavor and seems to be well tolerated. An emulsion of fennel seed oil and an herbal tea containing fennel have reduced infantile colic. Additional studies are warranted in order to confirm these findings.

Avoid if allergic or hypersensitive to fennel or other members of the Apiaceae family. Fennel is generally well tolerated. However, serious allergic reactions may occur. Use cautiously with diabetes. Avoid with epilepsy. Avoid in infants and toddlers. Avoid if pregnant or breastfeeding.

Hypnosis, Hypnotherapy: Hypnosis is a trancelike state in which a person becomes more aware and focused and is more open to suggestion. Hypnotherapy has been used to treat health conditions or to change behaviors. Early research suggests that hypnotherapy may lower the sensory and motor component of the gastrocolonic response in patients with IBS. Better studies are necessary to make a strong recommendation.

Use cautiously with mental illnesses (e.g., psychosis, schizophrenia, manic depression, multiple personality disorder, or dissociative disorders) or seizure disorders.

Peppermint: Peppermint is a flowering plant that grows throughout Europe and North America. Peppermint is most often grown for its fragrant oil. Peppermint may improve IBS symptoms. Additional study is necessary before a strong recommendation can be made.

Avoid if allergic or hypersensitive to peppermint or menthol. Peppermint is generally considered safe in nonallergic adults when taken in small doses. Use cautiously with glucose-6-phosphate dehydrogenase deficiency or gallbladder disease. Menthol, which makes up part of peppermint oil, is generally considered safe in nonallergic adults. However, doses of menthol greater than 1 gram per kilogram of body weight may be deadly in humans. Avoid if pregnant or breastfeeding.

Probiotics: Probiotics are beneficial bacteria and are sometimes called friendly germs. They help maintain a healthy intestine by keeping harmful bacteria and yeasts in the gut under control. Most probiotics come from food sources, especially cultured milk products. Probiotics can be taken as capsules, tablets, beverages, powders, yogurts, and other foods. Many varieties and combinations of probiotics have been studied in clinical trials for IBS. Findings frequently report reductions of symptoms, including pain, flatulence, bloating, and stool frequency. There is some evidence of reduced inflammation. The magnitude of benefit seen in most studies is modest. Not all studies, however, show beneficial effects. More studies are needed to determine the best protocols and what level of benefit can be expected.

Probiotics are generally considered safe and well tolerated. Avoid if allergic or hypersensitive to probiotics. Use cautiously if lactose intolerant.

Psyllium: Psyllium, also known as ispaghula, comes from the husks of the seeds of *Plantago ovata*. Psyllium contains a high level of soluble dietary fiber and is the main ingredient in many commonly used laxatives, such as Metamucil and Serutan. Psyllium has long been used as a chief ingredient in "bulk laxatives." Generally, an increase in stool weight, an increase in bowel movements per day, and a decrease in total gut transit time has been observed in most studies. Psyllium has been studied for the treatment of diarrhea, particularly in patients undergoing tube feeding. It has also been studied in addition to Orlistat therapy in hopes of decreasing gastrointestinal effects (diarrhea and oily discharge) of this weight loss agent. An effective stool-bulking effect has generally been found in scientific studies.

Avoid if allergic or hypersensitive to psyllium, ispaghula, or English plantain (*Plantago lanceolata*). Prescription drugs should be taken one hour before or two hours after psyllium. Use cautiously if pregnant or breastfeeding because psyllium may lower blood sugar levels.

Unclear or Conflicting Scientific Evidence

Acupressure, Shiatsu: During acupressure, finger pressure is applied to specific acupoints on the body. Acupressure is used around world for relaxation, wellness promotion, and the treatment of many health problems. A small study suggests that acupressure may improve gastrointestinal motility. Additional research is necessary before a firm conclusion can be drawn. With proper training, acupressure appears to be safe if self-administered or administered by an experienced therapist. No serious long-term complications have been reported, according to scientific data. Hand nerve injury and herpes zoster ("shingles") cases have been reported after shiatsu massage. Forceful acupressure may cause bruising.

Acupuncture: Acupuncture is commonly used throughout the world. According to Chinese medicine theory, the human body contains a network of energy pathways through which vital energy, called "chi," circulates. These pathways contain specific "points" that function like gates, allowing chi to flow through the body. Needles are inserted into these points to regulate the flow of chi. Illness and symptoms are thought to be caused by problems in the circulation of chi through the meridians. Although limited evidence suggests benefit may be possible, more studies are needed in order to make recommendations for or against acupuncture in IBS.

Needles must be sterile in order to avoid disease transmission. Avoid with valvular heart disease, infections, bleeding disorders, medical conditions of unknown origin, and neurological disorders. Avoid on areas that have received radiation therapy and during pregnancy. Avoid if taking drugs that increase the risk of bleeding (anticoagulants). Use cautiously with pulmonary disease (e.g., asthma or emphysema). Use cautiously in elderly or medically compromised patients, diabetics, or those with a history of seizures. Avoid electroacupuncture with arrhythmia (irregular heartbeat) and in patients with pacemakers.

Acustimulation: Acustimulation is different from acupuncture. However, Chinese acupuncture theory is used in acustimulation to locate points on the body where electrical stimulation is applied to reduce certain symptoms. Nausea and vomiting are believed to be the result of a disturbance in the normal nerve impulses passing between the brain and stomach. Acustimulation uses a mild electrical current at the wrist to restore normal signals between the brain and stomach, thus reducing nausea and vomiting. Western science explains acustimulation in terms of the nervous system rather than the circulation of chi, which is the basis of Chinese acupuncture theory. However, the chi pathways ("meridians") have certain parallels with the nervous system. This makes it possible to use acupuncture points to identify locations where electrical stimulation may influence certain responses of the nervous system. One small study suggests that acustimulation to the P6 wrist point and the ST36 point below the knee may help reduce symptoms and pain in patients with IBS. However, the design was weak and more studies are needed to determine benefits in IBS.

The only known side effect of acustimulation devices is slight skin irritation under the electrodes when the wristband is used. Switch wrists to prevent this from happening. Acustimulation devices should only be used on the designated area. Use cautiously with pacemakers. Avoid if the cause of medical symptoms is unknown. Keep acustimulation devices out of the reach of children.

Agrimony: Agrimony was one of the most famous vulnerary herbs with antiinflammatory and diuretic properties. The tannin content is responsible for many of its medicinal uses. The dried leaves can be used to make tea for drinking or as a throat gargle.

Agrimony has been used for many gastrointestinal conditions such as appendicitis, mild diarrhea, stimulation of appetite, and ulcers. Additional human study is needed to make a firm recommendation.

Avoid if allergic or hypersensitive to agrimony. Avoid with diarrhea that is caused by an underlying disease. Agrimony should only be used for mild and acute diarrhea. Avoid in patients who are susceptible to constipation. Use cautiously if taking anticoagulants or blood pressure–lowering drugs. Avoid if pregnant or breastfeeding.

Ayurveda: Ayurveda is a form of natural medicine that originated in ancient India more than 5,000 years ago. Ayurveda is an integrated system of techniques that uses diet, herbs, exercise, meditation, yoga, and massage or bodywork to achieve optimal health on all levels. A compound Ayurvedic preparation with *Aegle marmelos Linn. Correa* and *Bacopa monniera Linn.* is a traditional herbal preparation used for digestive disturbances and diarrhea. There is evidence from one study suggesting that this combination may have short-term benefits for patients with IBS, especially those with diarrhea. However, benefits may not be maintained in the long term. More studies are needed to evaluate this treatment.

There is preliminary evidence that the herb amalaki (*Emblica officinalis/Phyllanthus emblica*), a fruit used in a variety of Ayurvedic remedies, including the popular general tonic Chyavanaprash, may reduce symptoms of gastritis and dyspepsia (upset stomach). There is also evidence that the Ayurvedic herb *Asparagus racemosus* (Shatavari) may reduce gastric emptying time at a rate comparable to that of the drug metoclopramide, which is commonly used for dyspepsia. Some of this research has been with healthy subjects, however, and further clinical trials are needed using the above remedies to evaluate their efficacy.

Ayurvedic herbs should be used cautiously because they are potent and some constituents can be potentially toxic if taken in large amounts or for a long time. Some herbs imported from India have been reported to contain high levels of toxic metals. Ayurvedic herbs can interact with other herbs, foods, or drugs. A qualified healthcare professional should be consulted before taking. Use guggul cautiously with peptic ulcer disease. Avoid sour food, alcohol, and heavy exercise with guggul. Mahayograj guggul should not be taken for long periods of time. Pippali (*Piper longum*) should be taken with milk and avoided with asthma. Avoid sweet flag and amalaki (*Emblica officinalis*) at bedtime. Avoid *Terminalia chebula* (harda) if pregnant. Avoid Ayurveda with traumatic injuries, acute pain, advanced disease stages, and medical conditions that require surgery.

Bacopa (*Bacopa Monnieri*): *Bacopa monnieri* leaf extract is called brahmi in Ayurvedic medicine. It is widely used in India, especially for enhancing memory, pain relief, and epilepsy. Preliminary evidence suggests that bacopa and bael fruit used in combination may treat IBS. However, additional studies using bacopa alone are needed before bacopa can be recommended for IBS.

Avoid if allergic/hypersensitive to *Bacopa monnieri,* its constituents, or any member of the Scrophulariaceae (figwort) family. Use cautiously with drugs or herbs that are broken down by the liver, thyroid drugs, calcium-blocking drugs, or sedatives. Avoid if pregnant or breastfeeding.

Belladonna: Belladonna has been used for centuries to treat many medical conditions. Belladonna has been used historically for the treatment of IBS, and in theory its mechanism of action should be effective for some of the symptoms. However, of the few studies that are available, none clearly shows that belladonna alone (not as part of a mixed product) provides this effect.

Avoid if allergic to belladonna or plants of the Solanaceae (nightshade) family (e.g., bell peppers, potatoes, or eggplants). Avoid with a history of heart disease, high blood pressure, heart attack, abnormal heartbeat (arrhythmia), congestive heart failure, stomach ulcer, constipation, stomach acid reflux (serious heartburn), hiatal hernia, gastrointestinal disease, ileostomy, colostomy, fever, bowel obstruction, benign prostatic hypertrophy (enlarged prostate), urinary retention, glaucoma (narrow angle), psychotic illness, Sjögren's syndrome, dry mouth (xerostomia or salivary gland disorders), neuromuscular disorders such as myasthenia gravis, or Down's syndrome. Avoid if pregnant or breastfeeding.

Chamomile: Chamomile is an herb that has an applelike smell and taste. Chamomile is a common tea. Chamomile is used traditionally for numerous gastrointestinal conditions, including digestion disorders, "spasm" or colic, upset stomach, flatulence (gas), ulcers, and gastrointestinal irritation. However, currently there is no reliable human research available in any of these areas. Additional study is needed. Chamomile is reputed to have antispasmodic activity, but there is little research to substantiate this claim. Additional research evaluating chamomile alone is needed.

Avoid if allergic to chamomile or any related plants such as aster, chrysanthemum, mugwort, ragweed, or ragwort. Stop use two weeks before and immediately after surgery/dental/diagnostic procedures with bleeding risks. Use cautiously if driving or operating machinery. Avoid if pregnant or breastfeeding.

Chiropractic: Chiropractic care focuses on how the relationship between musculoskeletal structure (mainly the spine) and bodily function (mainly nervous system) affects health. Chiropractors use many techniques, including spinal manipulative therapy, diet, exercise, x-rays, and others (e.g., interferential and electrogalvanic muscle stimulation). There is not enough reliable scientific evidence to make a conclusion about the effects of chiropractic techniques in the management of infantile colic.

Use extra caution during cervical adjustments. Use cautiously with acute arthritis, conditions that cause decreased bone mineralization, brittle bone disease, bone softening conditions, bleeding disorders, and migraines. Use cautiously with the risk of tumors or cancers. Avoid with symptoms of vertebrobasilar vascular insufficiency, aneurysms, unstable spondylolisthesis, or arthritis. Avoid if taking drugs that increase the risk of bleeding. Avoid in areas of paraspinal tissue after surgery. Avoid if pregnant or breastfeeding due to a lack of scientific data.

Clay: Clay has been used medicinally for centuries in Africa, India, and China. There is not enough scientific evidence to recommend the medicinal use of clay by mouth in patients with gastrointestinal disorders. Some clay preparations have been found to be similar to Kaolin and Kaopectate, which are used to treat gastrointestinal disturbances, including diarrhea. However, overall, there are significant potential risks that accompany the use of clay, including intestinal blockage and injury and lead poisoning. There is not enough scientific research to support a recommendation for play with modeling clay as an effective therapeutic intervention in children with constipation and encopresis (fecal incontinence).

There are no reports of allergy to clay in the available scientific literature. However, in theory, allergy/hypersensitivity to clay, clay products, or constituents of clay may occur. Avoid if pregnant or breastfeeding.

Copper: Copper is a mineral that occurs naturally in many foods, including vegetables, legumes, nuts, grains, fruits, shellfish, avocado, beef, and animal organs. Menkes kinky hair disease is a rare disorder of copper transport/absorption. Copper supplementation may be helpful in this disease, although further research is necessary before a clear management recommendation can be made.

Avoid if allergic/hypersensitive to copper. Avoid use of copper supplements during the early phase of recovery from diarrhea. Avoid with hypercupremia, genetic disorders affecting copper metabolism (e.g., Wilson's disease, Indian childhood cirrhosis, or idiopathic copper toxicosis), or HIV/AIDS. Use water cautiously if it contains more than six milligrams of copper per liter. Use cautiously with anemia, arthralgias, or myalgias. Use cautiously if taking birth control pills. Use cautiously if at risk for selenium deficiency. The U.S. recommended dietary allowance (RDA) is 1,000 micrograms for pregnant women. The RDA is 1,300 micrograms for nursing women.

Globe Artichoke: Globe artichoke is a popular phytomedicine in Europe. It is purported to possess diuretic, choleretic, antidyspeptic, lipid-lowering, and antioxidant properties. There is insufficient available evidence to recommend for or against the use of artichoke in relieving the symptoms of IBS.

Use cautiously if allergic/hypersensitive to members of the Asteraceae or Compositae families (e.g., chrysanthemums, daisies, marigolds, ragweed, or arnica) due to possible cross-reactivity. Use cautiously with cholelithiasis, biliary/bile duct obstruction, or kidney disease. Avoid if pregnant or breastfeeding.

Hypnosis, Hypnotherapy: Hypnosis is a trancelike state in which a person becomes more aware and focused and is more open to suggestion. Hypnotherapy has been used to treat health conditions or to change behaviors. Early research indicates that gut-oriented hypnosis may have a beneficial effect on shortening gastric emptying both in dyspeptic and in healthy subjects. Additional study is needed before a firm conclusion can be drawn.

Use cautiously with mental illnesses (e.g., psychosis, schizophrenia, manic depression, multiple personality disorders, or dissociative disorders) or seizure disorders.

Lactobacillus acidophilus: Lactobacilli are bacteria that normally live in the human small intestine and vagina. Human studies report mixed results in the improvement of IBS symptoms after taking *Lactobacillus acidophilus* by mouth.

One human study using *L. acidophilus* in combination with another bacterium (*Bifidobacterium infantis*) in infants reported fewer cases of necrotizing enterocolitis (severe inflammation of the gut) and no complications related to treatment. Additional research is necessary in this area before a conclusion can be drawn.

Lactobacillus acidophilus may be difficult to tolerate if allergic or hypersensitive to dairy products. Avoid with a history of an injury or illness of the intestinal wall, immune disease, or heart valve surgery. Avoid if taking prescription drugs, such as corticosteroids, because there is a risk of infection. Use cautiously with heart murmurs. Antibiotics or alcohol may destroy *Lactobacillus acidophilus*. Therefore, it is recommended that *Lactobacillus acidophilus* be taken three hours after taking antibiotics or drinking alcohol. Some individuals can use antacids, such as famotidine (Pepcid) or esomeprazole (Nexium), to decrease the amount of acid in the stomach one hour before taking *Lactobacillus acidophilus*.

Lycopene: Lycopene is a carotenoid found in tomatoes. It is also present in human serum, liver, adrenal glands, lungs, prostate, colon, and the skin. Multiple studies have examined whether intake of tomatoes or tomato-based products helps prevent digestive tract cancers, including oral, pharyngeal, esophageal, gastric, colon, and rectal. Results have been inconsistent, with some studies reporting significant benefits and others finding no effects. Research that specifically studies lycopene supplements is limited, and more research is needed in this area before a conclusion can be drawn.

Avoid if allergic to tomatoes or to lycopene. Due to a lack of conclusive data, avoid if pregnant or breastfeeding.

Peppermint Oil: Peppermint is a flowering plant that grows throughout Europe and North America. Peppermint is most often grown for its fragrant oil. There is currently a lack of sufficient evidence to recommend for or against the use of a peppermint oil compress for abdominal distention.

Avoid if allergic or hypersensitive to peppermint or menthol. Peppermint is generally considered safe in nonallergic adults when taken in small doses. Use cautiously with glucose-6-phosphate dehydrogenase deficiency or gallbladder disease. Menthol, which makes up part of peppermint oil, is generally considered safe in nonallergic adults. However, doses of menthol greater than one gram per kilogram of body weight may be deadly in humans. Avoid if pregnant or breastfeeding.

Psyllium: Psyllium, also known as ispaghula, comes from the husks of the seeds of *Plantago ovata*. Psyllium contains a high level of soluble dietary fiber and is the main ingredient in many commonly used laxatives (like Metamucil and Serutan). Psyllium preparations have been studied for more than 20 years in the treatment of IBS symptoms. Results of these trials have been conflicting. In some cases, insoluble fiber may worsen the clinical outcome.

Avoid if allergic or hypersensitive to psyllium, ispaghula, or English plantain (*Plantago lanceolata*). Prescription drugs should be taken one hour before or two hours after psyllium. Use cautiously if pregnant or breastfeeding because psyllium may lower blood sugar levels.

Reflexology: Reflexology involves the application of manual pressure to specific points or areas of the feet that are believed to correspond to other parts of the body. Reflexology is often used with the intention to relieve stress or prevent/treat physical disorders. Preliminary study of reflexology in humans with IBS has not yielded definitive results. Better research is needed in this area before a recommendation can be made.

Avoid with recent or healing foot fractures, unhealed wounds, or active gout flares affecting the foot. Use cautiously and seek prior medical consultation with osteoarthritis affecting the foot or ankle or severe vascular disease of the legs or feet. Use cautiously with diabetes, heart disease, pacemakers, unstable blood pressure, cancer, active infections, past episodes of fainting (syncope), mental illness, gallstones, or kidney stones. Use cautiously if pregnant or breastfeeding. Reflexology should not delay diagnosis or treatment with more proven techniques or therapies.

Relaxation Therapy: Relaxation techniques include behavioral therapeutic approaches that differ widely in philosophy, methodology, and practice. The primary goal is usually nondirected relaxation. Most techniques share the components of repetitive focus (on a word, sound, prayer phrase, body sensation, or muscular activity), adoption of a passive attitude towards intruding thoughts, and return to the focus. Early research in humans suggests that relaxation may aid in the prevention and relief of IBS symptoms. Large, well-designed trials are needed to confirm these results.

Avoid with psychiatric disorders such as schizophrenia/psychosis. Jacobson relaxation (flexing specific muscles, holding that position, then relaxing the muscles) should be used cautiously with illnesses such as heart disease, high blood pressure, or musculoskeletal injury. Relaxation therapy is not recommended as the sole treatment approach for potentially serious medical conditions and should not delay the time to diagnosis or treatment with more proven techniques.

Rhubarb: In traditional Chinese medicine, rhubarb is used as an ulcer remedy and it is considered a bitter, cold, dry herb used to "clear heat" from the liver, stomach, and blood. One double-blind controlled trial examined the effect of the herbal extract Amaro Medicinale (Giuliani Pharma, Milan, Italy) and its constituents, including rhubarb, on mild gastrointestinal disturbances. Although the herbal extract and a combination of rhubarb and gentian seem promising, higher quality studies with rhubarb as a monotherapy are need to discern rhubarb's effect on gastrointestinal disturbances.

Avoid if allergic/hypersensitive to rhubarb, its constituents, or related plants from the Polygonaceae family. Avoid using rhubarb for more than two weeks because it may induce tolerance in the colon, melanosis coli, laxative dependence, pathological alterations to the colonic smooth muscles, and substantial loss of electrolytes. Avoid with atony, colitis, Crohn's disease, dehydration with electrolyte depletion, diarrhea, hemorrhoids, insufficient liver function, intestinal obstruction or ileus, IBS, menstruation, preeclampsia, kidney disorders, ulcerative colitis, or urinary problems. Avoid handling rhubarb leaves, as they may cause contact dermatitis. Avoid rhubarb in children under age 12 due to water depletion. Use cautiously with bleeding disorders, heart conditions, coagulation therapy, constipation, or a history of kidney stones or thin or brittle bones. Use cautiously if taking antipsychotic drugs or oral drugs, herbs, or supplements (including calcium, iron, and zinc). Avoid if pregnant or breastfeeding.

Saccharomyces Boulardii: *Saccharomyces boulardii* is a type of yeast that does not cause disease in humans. One clinical trial exists to support treatment with *Saccharomyces boulardii* for IBS. Additional study is required before a firm recommendation can be made

Avoid if allergic or hypersensitive to yeast, *Saccharomyces boulardii, Saccharomyces cerevisiae,* or other species in the Saccharomycetaceae family. Use cautiously in immunocompromised or critically ill patients. Use cautiously with indwelling central venous catheters, colitis, cancer, or constipation. Use cautiously in the elderly, in individuals undergoing chemotherapy, and in infants. Use cautiously if taking antidiarrheal agents. Avoid with a yeast infection. Avoid if pregnant or breastfeeding.

Selenium: Selenium is a mineral found in soil, water, and some foods. Low selenium status has been demonstrated in several malabsorptive syndromes and in some digestive and gastrointestinal allergic conditions. There is some evidence that children with food allergies have a higher risk of selenium deficiency. There is no clear benefit of selenium supplementation as a therapy for malabsorptive syndromes, although vitamin supplementation in general may be warranted.

G

Avoid if allergic or sensitive to products containing selenium. Avoid with a history of nonmelanoma skin cancer. Selenium is generally regarded as safe for pregnant or breastfeeding women. However, animal research reports that large doses of selenium may lead to birth defects.

Slippery Elm: Slippery elm is native to eastern Canada and the eastern and central United States. Its name refers its slippery consistency when the inner bark is chewed or mixed with water. Slippery elm has been traditionally used to treat inflammatory conditions of the digestive tract such as gastritis, peptic ulcer disease, and enteritis. It may be taken alone or in combination with other herbs. Additional study is needed in this area before a clear conclusion can be drawn.

Avoid if allergic or hypersensitive to slippery elm. Avoid if pregnant or breastfeeding.

Transcutaneous Electrical Nerve Stimulation (TENS): TENS is a noninvasive technique in which a low-voltage electrical current is delivered through wires from a small power unit to electrodes located on the skin. There is conflicting evidence from clinical trials on the effectiveness of TENS in postoperative ileus. Well-designed, large studies are needed before a recommendation can be made.

Avoid with implantable devices such as defibrillators, pacemakers, intravenous infusion pumps, or hepatic artery infusion pumps. Use cautiously with decreased sensation (e.g., neuropathy) or seizure disorders. Avoid if pregnant or breastfeeding.

PREVENTION

Patients should not take laxatives more frequently than the packaging label suggests. If symptoms persist, patients should consult their healthcare providers to diagnose and properly treat the underlying cause.

Patients who have a history of indigestion should eat smaller, more frequent meals to help prevent symptoms. Limiting spicy, fried, or fatty foods may also reduce the risk of indigestion.

Patients should not consume excessive amounts of alcohol because it irritates the stomach. Abusing alcohol may cause inflammation or bleeding in the stomach.

Patients are encouraged not to smoke because smoking damages the protective lining of the stomach. Smoking increases an individual's risk of developing gastritis and ulcers. In addition, smoking increases the amount of stomach acid and delays healing, which increases a patient's risk of developing stomach cancer.

Patients should limit their use of nonsteroidal antiinflammatory drugs (NSAIDS) such as ibuprofen (Motrin, Advil) because they may cause stomach inflammation and bleeding as well as ulcers.

Patients should properly wash all produce thoroughly before eating to reduce the risk of developing gastrointestinal infections.

Individuals who are in areas of the world that have poor sanitation should only drink bottled water to avoid the risk of gastrointestinal infections. If this is not possible, individuals should boil their water before drinking it. This kills any disease-causing bacteria or parasites that may be living in the water.

Patients should only consume dairy products that have been pasteurized. This reduces the risk of developing a gastrointestinal infection that may cause diarrhea.

Individuals should avoid or limit their intake of the artificial sweeteners sorbitol and mannitol because they may cause diarrhea. These artificial sweeteners are commonly found in sugar-free products and chewing gum.

Patients with gastrointestinal disorders should take their medications exactly as prescribed in order to prevent complications from occurring.

GENITOURINARY DISORDERS

CONDITIONS: Genitourinary Disorders, Incontinence, Urinary Tract Infection (UTI), Interstitial Cystitis, Neurogenic Bladder

BACKGROUND

Genitourinary disorders are illnesses that occur when the urinary organs and genital organs are not functioning properly. These disorders may be the result of aging, illness, or injury. There are many organs involved in urination, including two kidneys, two ureters, the bladder, two sphincter muscles, and the urethra. The kidneys, a pair of organs located on the left and right side of the abdomen, are an essential component of the urinary tract. The kidneys are responsible for removing toxins, chemicals, and waste products from the blood. Urine then leaves the kidneys and travels down two tubes called ureters. The muscles in the ureter walls constantly tighten and relax to bring urine into the bladder. Small amounts of urine enter the bladder approximately every 10-15 seconds. The bladder is a hollow muscular organ. The bladder stretches until it is full with urine. Healthy adults can hold up to 16 ounces (two cups) of urine in their bladders for two to five hours. Muscles, called sphincters, prevent urine from leaking out of the bladder. When the bladder is full, nerves send a message to the brain, which then causes the patient to feel the urge to urinate. During urination, the brain signals the muscles in the bladder to contract and the sphincter muscles to relax. This causes urine to empty out of the bladder.

Examples of genitourinary disorders include interstitial cystitis, neurogenic bladder, kidney stones, pelvic inflammatory disease (PID), prolapsed uterus, urinary incontinence, and urinary tract infection (UTI). In addition to causing urinary problems, many of these conditions may also affect the reproductive organs, including the uterus, cervix, fallopian tubes, and vagina in women and the testicles, epididymis (tubular organ where sperm collect after leaving the testis), prostate gland, and penis in males. Treatment of genitourinary disorders depends on the specific type and severity of the disorder. If left untreated, some disorders, including PID, may lead to infertility. Therefore, patients who have symptoms of genitourinary disorders should visit their healthcare providers as soon as possible.

COMMON TYPES AND CAUSES

Interstitial Cystitis: Interstitial cystitis, also called painful bladder syndrome or frequency-urgency-dysuria syndrome, is a long-term inflammatory condition that causes frequent urination and bladder pain. In healthy individuals, the bladder will expand until it is full. Once this happens, the brain receives a message from the pelvic nerves, which causes patients to feel the urge to urinate. Patients with interstitial cystitis feel the urge to urinate more often than they should. Although interstitial cystitis can affect anyone, it is most common among women.

The exact cause of interstitial cystitis remains unknown. Most experts believe that patients are born with a leaky epithelium, which is the protective lining of the bladder. If toxic or harmful substances enter the bladder through the epithelium, it may cause irritation and lead to cystitis. It has also been suggested that the interstitial cystitis is the result of inheritance, infections, allergic reactions, or autoimmunity. Autoimmunity occurs when the immune system, which normally fights against disease and infection, mistakenly attacks body cells. However, further research is needed to verify these theories.

Neurogenic Bladder: A neurogenic bladder occurs when the pelvic nerves do not function properly. This may lead to either an overactive or underactive bladder. There are many potentially causes of a neurogenic bladder. Some of the most common causes include diabetes, infections, tumors, heavy metal poisoning, vaginal childbirth, stroke, multiple sclerosis, and brain or spinal cord injuries. Some patients are born with genetic nerve problems that cause the condition.

Kidney Stones (Renal Calculi): Kidney stones, also called renal calculi, urolithiasis, or nephrolithiasis, usually develop when the urine becomes too concentrated (urine acidification). As a result, minerals and other substances in the urine form hard crystals in the kidneys. Over time, these crystals may combine to form a small, hard mass or stone. There are four types of kidney stones that can develop: calcium stones (calcium oxalate stones), struvite stones, uric acid stones, and cystine stones.

Calcium stones are the most common type of kidney stones, accounting for 80% of cases. Calcium stones develop when there are high levels of calcium (hypercalcemia) and oxalate in the blood. Patients who consume excessive amounts of vitamin D or have overactive thyroids may have high levels of calcium in the blood. Patients who consume large amounts of oxalic acid or undergo intestinal bypass surgery may have high levels of oxalate in the blood.

Struvite stones are usually caused by chronic UTIs. The bacteria that cause these infections release enzymes that increase the amount of ammonia in the urine. This excess ammonia may form large, sharp stones that may damage the kidneys.

Uric acid stones form when there is excess uric acid in the urine. Uric acid is a byproduct of protein metabolism. These stones are usually caused by a cancer treatment called chemotherapy. They may also develop in patients who eat high-protein diets. Some patients are genetically predisposed to develop uric acid stones.

Cystine stones develop in patients who have an inherited disorder called cystinuria. This disorder causes the kidneys to release too many amino acids. The excess amino acids then form stones.

Pelvic Inflammatory Disease (PID): PID is an infection of the female reproductive organs that causes pain and swelling. If left untreated, PID may lead to long-term pelvic pain. It may also result in infertility or complications during pregnancy. PID usually develops when a sexually transmitted bacteria enter the uterus and reproduce in the upper genital tract. The most common bacteria that cause PID also cause the sexually transmitted diseases (STDs) gonorrhea and chlamydia.

Prolapsed Uterus: If the uterus collapses into the vaginal canal, the condition is called a prolapsed uterus. There are many causes of a prolapsed uterus. Weakened pelvic muscles caused by aging may lead to a prolapsed uterus. Vaginal childbirth and medical conditions, such as such as chronic cough, straining from constipation, pelvic tumors, or an accumulation of fluid in the abdomen, may also cause the condition.

Urinary Incontinence: Urinary incontinence describes the inability to control the bladder. The bladder spontaneously empties all or some of the urine. Incontinence is a symptom of an underlying illness. Incontinence may be temporary or permanent, depending on the cause.

Most children, especially those younger than seven years old, experience nighttime incontinence, also called bedwetting or nocturnal enuresis. This may happen because the child's bladder is still developing and it cannot hold all of the urine that is produced during sleep. Very young children may be unable to recognize when they have full bladders. This is because the nerves that control the bladder take a long time to develop. Adults may also wet the bed. Other causes of bedwetting in children and adults may include stress, UTIs, sleep apnea, diabetes, and chronic constipation. In addition, alcohol, caffeine, dehydration, overhydration, bladder irritation, medications (such as sleeping pills, antidepressants, or diuretics), UTIs, and constipation may lead to temporary incontinence.

Urinary incontinence may also be a long-term symptom of an underlying medical condition. For instance, pregnant women may experience incontinence because their bodies are going through hormonal and weight changes. Vaginal childbirth may damage the pelvic nerves and supportive tissues and muscles that are involved in bladder control. Aging is also associated with urinary incontinence because the bladder muscles become weaker over time. Also, elderly women produce less estrogen, a hormone that helps keep the lining of the bladder and urethra healthy. Other medical conditions, including inflamed prostate gland (prostatitis), enlarged prostate, prostate cancer, bladder stones, neurological disorders (such as Parkinson's disease or multiple sclerosis), and tumors that block the urinary tract may lead to urinary incontinence.

Urinary Tract Infections (UTIs): A UTI is an infection of the urinary system. UTIs may affect any part of the urinary tract, including the kidneys, ureters, bladder, and urethra. However, most infections involve the lower tract, which includes the urethra and the bladder. Infections may cause swelling, especially of the urethra (urethritis), bladder (cystitis), epididymis (epididymitis), or one or both testicles (orchitis). When a UTI causes cystitis, the condition is sometimes called honeymoon cystitis. If bleeding occurs with an inflamed bladder, the condition is called hemorrhagic cystitis.

Infections typically develop when bacteria or viruses enter the urinary system through the urethra. Once inside the bladder, the disease-causing microorganism begins multiplying. Females are more likely to develop UTIs than males. This is because the female's urethra is much closer to the anus than the male's. The anus harbors many disease-causing organisms that may cause UTIs.

Patients with UTIs typically experience a full recovery with treatment. However, if the patient does not receive treatment, the infection may spread to the kidneys where it can cause permanent damage.

Signs and Symptoms

Interstitial Cystitis: Symptoms of interstitial cystitis vary among patients. Individual patients may also experience changes in the severity of symptoms over time. For instance, stress, menstruation, allergies, and sexual activity may worsen symptoms. Common symptoms include a frequent urge to urinate and passing small amounts of urine many times a day. Patients with severe interstitial cystitis may urinate more than 50 times in one day. Patients may experience pain in the pelvis or perineum (area between the anus and genital organs). Some patients may experience pain during sexual intercourse. Males may also experience pain when they ejaculate. Some patients may experience either pain or frequent urination. However, most patients experience a combination of both symptoms.

Kidney Stones (Renal Calculi): If the kidney stone is small, patients do not experience any symptoms of the condition. However, if the stone is large enough to block the tubes inside the kidney, patients may experience an intense pain that often comes and goes. Pain may last anywhere from five to 15 minutes at a time. The pain usually begins in the lower back. As the stone moves from the kidney toward the bladder, the patients may feel pain near the abdomen, groin, or genitals. Additional symptoms may include blood in the urine, cloudy or foul-smelling urine, nausea, vomiting, and constant urge to urinate. In some patients, the kidney stone may cause an infection. Symptoms of an infection include fever and chills.

Neurogenic Bladder: Damaged or defective nerves may send signals to the bladder at the wrong time, causing the muscles to spontaneously contract. This causes the bladder to become overactive. Symptoms of an overactive bladder may include frequent urination, persistent urge to urinate, and spontaneous emptying of the bladder that cannot be controlled (incontinence). Urine may occasionally leak out in small amounts throughout the day. Other patients with neurogenic bladders may have underactive bladders. This happens when the nerves do not receive the message that the bladder is full or the message is too weak for the bladder to be completely emptied. When the nerves do not function properly, urine builds up in the bladder (urine retention). An overfull bladder may empty without warning. If the bladder is too full, it may back up and put pressure on the kidneys.

PID: Common symptoms of PID include pain in the lower abdomen and pelvis, irregular menstrual bleeding, foul-smelling vaginal discharge, lower back pain, fever, fatigue, diarrhea, vomiting, pain during intercourse, and difficulty or pain during urination.

Prolapsed Uterus: Symptoms of a prolapsed uterus vary depending on the severity of the condition.

Mild cases may not cause any symptoms. Common symptoms may include a feeling of fullness or pressure in the pelvis, lower back pain, sensation that something is falling out of the vagina, difficulty urinating or moving the bowels, and difficulty walking.

Urinary Incontinence: Patients with urinary incontinence are unable to control their bladders. Urine may leak out when the patient laughs, coughs, exercises, or lifts heavy weights. Small amounts of urine may leak out periodically throughout the day or night. Some patients may experience a sudden urge to urinate followed by an uncontrolled emptying of the bladder. Some patients may be unable to empty their bladders completely. As a result, urine may build up in the bladder until it cannot hold any more fluid. When this happens, the bladder spontaneously releases the urine. Some patients, especially children younger than seven years old, may be unable to control their bladders during sleep.

UTI: Common symptoms of a UTI include a constant urge to urinate, burning sensation during urination, blood in the urine (hematuria), cloudy or foul-smelling urine, and frequently passing small amounts of urine. If the bladder becomes inflamed the condition is called cystitis. Symptoms of cystitis may include pelvic pressure, pain in the lower abdomen, and painful and frequent urination. If the urethra becomes inflamed (urethritis), patients may experience a burning sensation during urination. Men with urethritis may experience penile discharge. If the epididymis becomes inflamed in males, symptoms may include scrotal pain, tenderness in one or both testicles, tenderness in the groin, painful urination, painful intercourse or ejaculation, blood in the semen, and swelling of one or both testicles (orchitis).

COMPLICATIONS

Infertility: Patients with PID may become infertile. Patients who wait to receive treatment have the greatest risk of becoming infertile. Therefore, patients who experience signs and symptoms of PID should visit their healthcare providers as soon as possible.

Pain: Up to 50% of females with PID develop chronic pelvic pain that may last for months or years. PID may cause scarring in the fallopian tubes and other organs that may lead to pain during exercise, ovulation, and sexual intercourse. Patients with interstitial cystitis may experience severe pain. This pain may worsen during sexual intercourse or ejaculation. This may affect sexual intimacy among couples. Medications are available to reduce these

G

symptoms. Patients should regularly visit their healthcare providers to ensure that their treatments are effective.

Skin Problems: Patients with urinary incontinency may develop skin rashes, infections, or sores.

Quality of Life: Patients who experience urinary incontinence may also suffer from a decreased quality of life. Patients may be less likely to travel or participate in activities because they are worried about having accidents. Patients with incontinence should visit their healthcare providers to diagnose and treat the underlying cause.

DIAGNOSIS

Interstitial Cystitis: A potassium sensitivity test is the standard diagnostic for interstitial cystitis. During the procedure, a flexible tube, called a catheter, is used to fill the bladder is with distilled water. Then, the bladder is filled with a potassium solution. After each solution is instilled into the bladder, the patient rates how much pain and urgency to urinate he or she feels. If the patient feels more pain or urgency to urinate with the potassium solution than with the water, the patient is diagnosed with interstitial cystitis. Although researchers are unsure whether the potassium solution indicates increased bladder permeability or hypersensitive sensory nerves, patients with interstitial cystitis have been shown to be sensitive to the solution. Healthy patients do not notice any difference between the two solutions.

Kidney Stones (Renal Calculi): Imaging studies, such as a computerized tomography (CT) scan or magnetic resonance imaging (MRI) scan, may be performed if kidney stones are suspected. These tests take pictures of the kidneys, allowing healthcare providers to detect kidney stones.

Neurogenic Bladder: If it is suspected that the patient has a neurogenic bladder, tests are performed to evaluate the bladder and nervous system. Tests may be performed to determine how much water the bladder can hold and whether it is able to empty completely and efficiently.

Imaging studies, including x-rays, CT scans, and MRI scans, may be performed to take pictures of the urinary tract and nervous system. The images may show abnormalities that indicate nerve damage. A healthcare provider may perform a test called an electroencephalograph to detect abnormalities in the brain that may be causing the condition. During the procedure, small electrodes are taped to the patient's forehead. The electrical signals from the brain are transmitted to a small monitor. If the signals are abnormal, a positive diagnosis is made. An electromyography (EMG) may also be performed to test the muscles and nerves of the bladder. During the procedure, a needle electrode is inserted through the skin and into the bladder muscle. The electrical activity detected by the electrode is displayed on a screen.

PID: PID is diagnosed after a pelvic examination, cervical cultures, and/or analysis of the vaginal discharge. During a pelvic exam, a small instrument called a speculum is inserted into the vagina and the healthcare provider is able to examine the vagina, cervix, and uterus. The reproductive organs, including the uterus, will appear inflamed during a pelvic exam. Cervical cultures and/or analyses of vaginal discharge are performed to detect the presence of bacteria that are known to cause PID. If bacteria are present, a positive diagnosis is made.

Prolapsed Uterus: A prolapsed uterus is diagnosed after a pelvic exam. Imaging studies, such as CT scans or MRI scans, are often needed to determine the severity of the condition.

Urinary Incontinence: Patients who experience urinary incontinence should visit their healthcare providers to determine the underlying cause. Since it is common for children younger than seven years old to wet the bed, they usually do not require a medical diagnosis. Several tests may be performed to diagnose the patient. A healthcare provider may ask the patient to record fluid intake, time of urination, and number of incontinence episodes over the course of several days.

A sample of urine may be collected from the patient to check for an infection. A sample of blood may be taken from the patient to check for medications or chemicals that may be causing incontinence. A postvoid residual measurement test may be performed to determine if the patient is able to empty the bladder. Patients urinate into a container that allows the healthcare provider to measure the amount of urine that is excreted. Then, the healthcare provider inserts a soft, thin tube into the urethra and bladder to drain any remaining urine. If there is a lot of urine left in the bladder, this may indicate that there is an obstruction (such as at tumor) or a problem with the muscles or nerves. A pelvic ultrasound may be performed to detect abnormalities in the urinary tract. During a pelvic ultrasound in females, a probe, called a transducer, is inserted into the vagina. The transducer sends pictures of the pelvic organs to a nearby camera. During a pelvic ultrasound in males, a transducer is inserted into the rectum, and pictures are taken of the pelvic organs, including the prostate and seminal vesicles. Urodynamic testing may also be performed to measure the pressure inside the bladder when it is empty and when it is filling. A catheter is inserted through the patient's urethra and into the bladder. The bladder is then filled with water. The pressure inside the bladder is monitored. This test allows the healthcare provider to measure the strength of the bladder muscle. A cystoscopy may be performed to detect possible abnormalities in the urinary tract. During the procedure, a thin tube with a camera, called a cystoscope, is inserted into the urethra and into the urinary tract. The cystoscope projects images of the urinary tract onto a screen.

UTI: A urine analysis is the standard diagnostic test for a UTI. A sample of the patient's urine is analyzed in a laboratory. If disease-causing microorganisms are present, a positive diagnosis is made. Pus and blood cells may also be detected in the urine, which suggest an infection.

Treatment

Antibiotics: Medications called antibiotics are used to treat UTIs and PID. Antibiotics, which are usually taken by mouth, kill the disease-causing microorganism. Severe infections that have spread to the kidneys may require hospitalization and intravenous antibiotics. Commonly prescribed antibiotics include amoxicillin (Amoxil, Trimox), nitrofurantoin (Furadantin, Macrodantin), trimethoprim (Proloprim), and trimethoprim/sulfamethoxazole (Bactrim, Septra). Symptoms usually start to improve after a few days of treatment. Patients should take medications exactly as prescribed. Even if symptoms appear to go away, patients should take all of their medication because there may still be bacteria in the body. Stopping medication early may allow the infection to return. Also, stopping medication early may lead to antibiotic resistance. The few remaining bacteria in the body that survive most of the antibiotic therapy are the most difficult to kill. If the bacteria become resistant to treatment, the medications will no longer be effective if taken in the future.

Pentosan (Elmiron): The only medication that is approved by the U.S. Food and Drug Administration for the treatment of interstitial cystitis is called pentosan (Elmiron). This drug may help fix the epithelium, which is the protective lining of the bladder. As a result, the drug may help prevent toxic substances from entering the bladder and causing irritation. Patients may experience reduction in pain after two to four months and decreases in urgency to urinate after about six months of treatment. Side effects may include upset stomach and hair loss. Avoid if pregnant, possibly pregnant, or if thinking

about becoming pregnant because pentosan may cause miscarriage.

Extracorporeal Shock Wave Lithotripsy (ESWL): If patients with kidney stones are unable to pass their stones by drinking extra fluids, a procedure called ESWL may be performed. This is the most commonly used procedure to remove kidney stones. Sound waves (shock waves) are used to break the stone into smaller pieces. Patients receive sedatives and/or anesthesia before the procedure. The patient will either be partially submerged in a tub of water or will lie on a soft cushion. Patients wear headphones because the shock waves are loud. High-energy sound waves then pass through the patient's body and break the stone into smaller pieces. The healthcare provider usually uses x-rays or an ultrasound to monitor the status of the stone. Treatment usually lasts for about one hour. Once the stone is broken into smaller pieces, it can be excreted in the urine. Side effects of treatment include blood in the urine, bruising on the abdomen or back, bleeding around the kidney or nearby organs, and pain when the stone fragments are passed in the urine.

Nonsteroidal Antiinflammatory Drugs (NSAIDs): Patients with interstitial cystitis may take NSAIDs such as ibuprofen (Motrin, Advil) to reduce pain and inflammation associated with the condition.

Tricyclic Antidepressants: Patients with interstitial cystitis may take tricyclic antidepressants, such as imipramine (Tofranil), by mouth to help relax the bladder. Although these medications are primarily prescribed to treat depression, they have also been shown to have muscle relaxant properties. As a result, tricyclic antidepressants may help reduce a patient's urge to urinate and minimize pain. Side effects may include dry mouth, constipation, bladder problems, sexual problems, blurred vision, dizziness, drowsiness, skin rash, and weight gain or loss.

Cystoscopy with Bladder Distention: Some patients with interstitial cystitis may undergo a procedure called cystoscopy with bladder distention. Patients receive anesthesia so they will not feel any pain during the procedure. A thin tube, called a cystoscope, is inserted through the urethra and into the bladder. Then water is infused into the bladder to stretch the bladder. If successful, the treatment will temporarily reduce frequent urges to urinate. If the patient has a positive response to treatment, the procedure may be repeated in the future. This procedure is generally well tolerated.

Anticholinergics: Medications called anticholinergics may be used to treat patients with overactive bladders. These drugs help relax the muscles of the bladder and prevent urine retention. The U.S. Food and Drug Administration has approved trospium chloride (Sanctura), darifenacin (Enablex), and solifenacin succinate (VESIcare) for the treatment of overactive bladders. Medications such as oxybutynin chloride (Ditropan, Oxytrol), tolterodine (Detrol), hyoscyamine (Levsin), and propantheline bromide (Pro-Banthine) have also been prescribed to treat overactive bladders. These drugs are usually taken by mouth daily to reduce symptoms. They are also available as patches that are applied to the skin. Side effects may include dry mouth, blurred vision, constipation, increased heartbeat, and flushing (reddening of the skin).

Bladder Training: Patients with underactive bladders may be able to control their bladders better with a type of therapy called bladder training. The patient records the amount of fluid intake, trips to the bathroom, and episodes of urine leakage every day over the course of several days to weeks. This record may have a pattern and patients may be able to avoid accidents by planning to use the bathroom at certain times of the day. Once patients gain control over their bladders, they may be able to increase the time between urination.

Kegel Exercises: Patients may be able to reduce symptoms of urinary incontinence by strengthening their urinary sphincter muscles. These muscles help control urination. To do Kegel exercises, squeeze the muscles that are used to stop urine flow for about three seconds. Then release and repeat several times. Patients can perform these exercises any time during the day.

Urethral Inserts: Urethral inserts are small, tampon-like disposable devices that females insert into the urethra. The urethra is the tube that releases urine out of the body. Therefore, urethral inserts help prevent urine from leaking out. These inserts, which are available by prescription, should not be used every day. Instead, they are usually used if a patient has predictable incontinent episodes. For instance, some patients may experience incontinence during exercise. When the females need to urinate, the device can be easily removed.

Pessary: Female patients with a prolapsed bladder or uterus that is causing urinary incontinence may be prescribed a pessary. This device is a stiff ring that is inserted into the vagina. The device holds up the bladder and helps prevent leakage. The pessary needs to be removed and cleaned daily in order to prevent infections.

Surgery: In severe cases of urinary incontinence, surgery may be considered. This treatment is usually reserved for patients who have not responded to other types of treatment. Surgery may be performed to enlarge the bladder. A part of the patient's bowel may be removed and added to the bladder to make it bigger. Although this surgery may improve symptoms of urinary incontinence, it may make it more difficult to empty the bladder. There is also a risk that the bladder may rupture, causing urine to leak into nearby tissues. Other potential risks include bladder infection and bladder/kidney stones. Patients with a prolapsed uterus require surgery to either remove or repair the uterus. When discussing treatment options, patients should tell their healthcare providers if they want to have children in the future. Patients can only become pregnant if they have a uterus. Therefore, if the patient wants to become pregnant one day, the healthcare provider will first try to repair the uterus before removing it.

Protective Pads and Garments: Patients with persistent urinary incontinence may benefit from protective pads and garments. Most products available today are similar in size to normal undergarments. They are not noticeable under clothing. These products are available at local drugstores, supermarkets, and medical supply stores. Panty liners or pads may be worn inside of undergarments to collect urine. Adult diapers are also available. Males who leak small amounts of urine throughout the day may use a drip collector. This is a small piece of padding that covers the penis. Children who wet the bed may wear diapers, such as Pull-Ups, during sleep. Children are able to take these diapers off like normal underwear, and they help keep bed linens clean and dry after an accident.

Catheter: If patients experience urinary incontinence because the bladder is unable to empty, a soft tube, called a catheter, may be recommended. The catheter is inserted into the urethra several times a day to drain the bladder. This helps prevent the bladder from spontaneously overflowing when it is full. It also helps prevent the urine from backing up and causing permanent kidney problems. Healthcare providers will show patients how to use catheters. Catheters will need to be removed and cleaned daily in order to prevent infections.

INTEGRATIVE THERAPIES

Good Scientific Evidence

Cranberry: Cranberries come from small evergreen shrubs with tart, red, edible berries. The berries are used in sauces, jellies, and drinks. There are multiple studies of cranberry (juice or capsules) for the prevention of UTIs in healthy women and nursing home residents. While no single study convincingly demonstrates the ability of cranberry to prevent UTIs, the sum total of favorable evidence combined with laboratory research tends to support this use. It is not clear what dosage is best. Patients should choose a juice that is made with 100% cranberry juice. Cranberry seems to work by preventing bacteria from sticking to cells that line the bladder. Contrary to prior belief, urine acidification (urine that is concentrated and has a lower-than-normal pH) does not appear to play a role. Notably, many studies have been sponsored by the cranberry product manufacturer Ocean Spray. Additional research is needed in this area before a strong recommendation can be made.

Avoid if allergic to cranberries, blueberries, or other plants of the genus *Vaccinium*. Sweetened cranberry juice may affect blood sugar levels. Use cautiously with a history of kidney stones. Avoid more than the amount usually found in foods if pregnant or breastfeeding.

Physical Therapy: The goal of physical therapy is to improve mobility, restore function, reduce pain, and prevent further injury. Many different techniques are used, including exercises, stretches, traction, electrical stimulation, and massage. A variety of techniques have been used to improve incontinence (loss of urinary control) such as pelvic floor neuromuscular electrostimulation combined with exercises, pelvic floor muscle exercises alone (Kegel exercises), vaginal cones, and vaginal balls. Vaginal balls should be thoroughly cleaned after each use. Outcome measures studied have included bladder volume, vaginal palpation, and perceptions of improvement. Overall, short-term improvements have been seen with pelvic floor exercises and vaginal balls. Physical therapy appeared more effective than biofeedback techniques based on one trial, but higher quality trials and comparisons with placebo are needed to confirm these results.

Not all physical therapy programs are suited for everyone, and patients should discuss their medical history with their qualified healthcare professionals before beginning any treatments. Based on the available literature, physical therapy appears generally safe when practiced by a qualified physical therapist. However, complications are possible. Physical therapy may aggravate preexisting conditions. Persistent pain and fractures of unknown origin have been reported. Physical therapy may increase the duration of pain or cause limitation of motion. Pain and anxiety may occur during the rehabilitation of patients with burns. Both morning stiffness and bone erosion have been reported in the physical therapy literature although causality is unclear. Erectile dysfunction has also been reported. All therapies during pregnancy and breastfeeding should be discussed with a licensed obstetrician/gynecologist before initiation.

Unclear or Conflicting Scientific Evidence

Acupressure, Shiatsu: During acupressure, finger pressure is applied to specific acupoints on the body. Acupressure is used around the world for relaxation, wellness promotion, and the treatment of many health problems. Early research suggests that acupressure may help treat children who wet the bed. However, further research is needed to confirm these initial findings.

With proper training, acupressure appears to be safe if self-administered or administered by an experienced therapist. No serious long-term complications have been reported, according to scientific data. Hand nerve injury and herpes zoster ("shingles") cases have been reported after shiatsu massage. Forceful acupressure may cause bruising.

Acupuncture: Acupuncture is commonly used throughout the world. According to Chinese medicine theory, the human body contains a network of energy pathways through which vital energy, called "chi," circulates. These pathways contain specific "points" that function like gates, allowing chi to flow through the body. Needles are inserted into these points to regulate the flow of chi. Acupuncture has been suggested as a possible treatment for patients who wet the bed. However, additional long-term studies are needed to determine whether or not this is an effective treatment. Early study in women suggests a reduced recurrence over six months and reduced residual urine (urine retained in the bladder after urination). Better-designed studies are needed to determine recommendations for this use.

Needles must be sterile in order to avoid disease transmission. Avoid with valvular heart disease, infections, bleeding disorders, medical conditions of unknown origin, or neurological disorders. Avoid on areas that have received radiation therapy and during pregnancy. Avoid if taking drugs that increase the risk of bleeding (anticoagulants). Use cautiously with pulmonary disease (such as asthma or emphysema). Use cautiously with a history of seizures, diabetes, or critical illnesses or if elderly. Avoid electroacupuncture with arrhythmia (irregular heartbeat) or in patients with pacemakers.

Bromelain: Bromelain is an herb that contains a digestive enzyme that comes from the stem and

G

the fruit of the pineapple plant. Additional research is needed to determine if bromelain can help treat UTIs.

Avoid if allergic to bromelain, pineapple, honeybee venom, latex, birch pollen, carrots, celery, fennel, cypress pollen, grass pollen, papain, rye flour, wheat flour, or other members of the Bromeliaceae family. Use cautiously with a history of bleeding disorders, stomach ulcers, heart disease, liver disease, or kidney disease. Use cautiously two weeks before and immediately after dental or surgical procedures. Use cautiously while driving or operating machinery. Avoid if pregnant or breastfeeding.

Chamomile: Chamomile is an herb that has an applelike smell and taste. The name chamomile is derived from the Greek kamai melon, which means ground apple. Chamomile is a common ingredient in tea. Preliminary research suggests that the combination of chamomile baths plus chamomile bladder washes and antibiotics is superior to antibiotics alone for hemorrhagic cystitis. Additional research is necessary before a conclusion can be reached.

Avoid if allergic to chamomile or any related plants, such as aster, chrysanthemum, mugwort, ragweed, or ragwort. Stop use two weeks before and immediately after surgery or dental or diagnostic procedures that have bleeding risks. Use cautiously if driving or operating machinery. Avoid if pregnant or breastfeeding.

Chiropractic: Chiropractic care focuses on how the relationship between musculoskeletal structure (mainly the spine) and bodily function (mainly nervous system) affects health. There is not enough reliable scientific evidence to ascertain the effects of chiropractic techniques in the management of nocturnal enuresis (bedwetting).

Use extra caution during cervical adjustments. Use cautiously with acute arthritis, conditions that cause decreased bone mineralization, brittle bone disease (osteoporosis), bone softening conditions, bleeding disorders, or migraines. Use cautiously with the risk of tumors or cancers. Avoid with symptoms of vertebrobasilar vascular insufficiency, aneurysms, unstable spondylolisthesis, or arthritis. Avoid if taking agents that increase the risk of bleeding. Avoid in areas of paraspinal tissue after surgery. Avoid if pregnant or breastfeeding due to a lack of scientific data.

Chlorophyll: Chlorophyll is responsible for the green color of plants. It can be obtained from green leafy vegetables (e.g., broccoli, Brussels sprouts, cabbage, lettuce, and spinach), algae, wheatgrass,

and numerous herbs (e.g., alfalfa, damiana, nettle, and parsley). Based on historical use, chlorophyll has been suggested to improve bodily odor in colostomy patients. Despite empirical use, clinical research with chlorophyll supplements did not support these findings. Further research is warranted.

Avoid if allergic or hypersensitive to chlorophyll or any of its metabolites. Use cautiously with photosensitivity, compromised liver function, diabetes, or gastrointestinal conditions or obstructions. Use cautiously if taking immunosuppressants or anti-diabetes agents. Avoid if pregnant or breastfeeding.

Cranberry: Cranberries come from small evergreen shrubs with tart, red, edible berries. The berries are used in sauces, jellies, and drinks. There is preliminary evidence that cranberry juice may reduce urine odor from incontinence or bladder catheterization. Further study is needed before a recommendation can be made. There are no well-designed human studies of cranberry for the treatment of UTIs. Laboratory research suggests that cranberry may not be an effective treatment when used alone, although it may be helpful as an adjunct to other therapies such as antibiotics.

Avoid if allergic to cranberries, blueberries, or other plants of the genus *Vaccinium*. Sweetened cranberry juice can affect blood sugar levels. Use cautiously with a history of kidney stones. Avoid more than the amount usually found in foods if pregnant or breastfeeding.

Dimethyl Sulfoxide (DMSO): DMSO is naturally found in vegetables, fruits, grains, and animal products. DMSO is available for both nonmedicinal and medicinal uses. The major clinical use of DMSO is to relieve symptoms of interstitial cystitis. DMSO may relieve the symptoms of inflammatory bladder disease. Further research is needed to confirm these results.

Avoid if allergic or hypersensitive to DMSO. Use cautiously with urinary tract cancer, liver disorders, or kidney dysfunction. Avoid if pregnant or breastfeeding.

Horseradish: Horseradish (*Armoracia rusticana*) is a hardy perennial plant of the Brassicaceae family, which includes mustard and cabbage. Several laboratory studies suggest that horseradish has antibiotic activity. One human study used a combination product made from horseradish root and nasturtium herb to treat common bacterial infections, including UTIs. Researchers found that the combination product was as effective as standard antibiotic therapy. However, further studies evaluating horseradish alone are needed.

Intravenous horseradish should be used cautiously. Use cautiously with bleeding disorders, high blood pressure, thyroid disorders, kidney disorders, gastro-intestinal conditions, or ulcers. Use cautiously if taking anticoagulants, antiplatelet drugs, blood pressure drugs, antiinflammatories, or thyroid hormones or if receiving cancer treatment. Avoid medicinal amounts of horseradish if pregnant or breastfeeding.

Hypnosis, Hypnotherapy: Hypnosis is a trancelike state in which a person becomes more aware and focused and is more open to suggestion. Hypnotherapy has been used to treat health conditions or to change behaviors. Studies have evaluated the effectiveness of hypnotherapy for the treatment of bedwetting. However, results are inconclusive. Further research is needed.

Use cautiously with mental illnesses such as psychosis, schizophrenia, manic depression, multiple personality disorders, or dissociative disorders. Use cautiously with seizure disorders.

Iodine: Iodine is an element that the human body needs to make thyroid hormones. Povidone-iodine bladder irrigation has been suggested as a way to prevent infections before catheters are removed. There is limited research in this area.

Reactions can be severe and deaths have occurred with exposure to iodine. Avoid iodine-based products if allergic or hypersensitive to iodine. Do no use for more than 14 days. Avoid Lugol solution and saturated solution of potassium iodide (SSKI, Pima) with hyperkalemia (high amounts of potassium in the blood), pulmonary edema (fluid in the lungs), bronchitis, or tuberculosis. Use cautiously when applying to the skin because it may irritate or burn tissues. Use sodium iodide cautiously with kidney failure. Avoid sodium iodide with gastrointestinal obstruction. Iodine is safe in recommended doses for pregnant or breastfeeding women. Avoid povidone-iodine for perianal preparation during delivery or postpartum antisepsis.

Magnet Therapy: Magnetic fields play an important role in Western medicine, including use for MRI, pulsed electromagnetic fields, and experimental magnetic stimulatory techniques. Several small preliminary studies have been conducted using electromagnetic stimulation therapy in patients with urinary incontinence (including both stress and urge incontinence). The premise of this approach is that by seating individuals in a chair unit with a magnetic coil, electromagnetic pulses can be created that induce contractions of pelvic floor muscles. A course of therapy may involve up to two 20-minute treatments per day over eight weeks. The available studies have not been randomized, placebo controlled, or adequately blinded, and the number of involved patients has been small. Therefore, although the initial results are promising, better quality studies are necessary before a clear conclusion can be drawn. Nonetheless, patients with persistent incontinence who have not had success with other approaches and who have been evaluated by a urologist may wish to pursue this approach with qualified healthcare professionals (who can explain the potential benefits and risks). Incontinence may occur for various reasons, some that are potentially serious, and women or men experiencing incontinence should be evaluated by their qualified healthcare practitioners.

Avoid with implantable medical devices like heart pacemakers, defibrillators, insulin pumps, or hepatic artery infusion pumps. Avoid with myasthenia gravis or bleeding disorders. Avoid if pregnant or breastfeeding. Magnet therapy is not advised as the sole treatment for potentially serious medical conditions and should not delay the time to diagnosis or treatment with more proven methods. Patients are advised to discuss magnet therapy with their qualified healthcare providers before starting treatment.

Moxibustion: Moxibustion is a therapeutic method in Chinese and Japanese acupuncture. The therapy involves burning an herb (usually mugwort) above the skin or on the acupuncture points to introduce heat into an acupuncture point and alleviate symptoms. It may be applied in the form of a cone, stick, or loose herb. It may also be placed on the head of an acupuncture needle to manipulate the temperature gradient of the needle. There is preliminary evidence from one study suggesting that moxibustion combined with acupuncture may help reduce urological symptoms in women with urethral syndrome (inflammation of the urethra resulting in painful urination). However, more studies are needed before definitive recommendations for or against this approach can be made.

Avoid with aneurysms, any kind of "heat syndrome," heart disease, convulsions, cramps, diabetic neuropathy, extreme fatigue, anemia, fever, or inflammatory conditions. Avoid over allergic skin conditions, ulcerated sores, skin adhesions, or inflamed areas or organs. Do not use over the face, genitals, head, or nipples. Avoid using immediately after exercise or taking a hot bath or shower. Use cautiously over large blood vessels and thin or weak skin. It is not advisable to bathe or shower for up to 24 hours after a moxibustion treatment. Avoid if pregnant or breastfeeding.

Peppermint: Peppermint is a flowering plant that grows throughout Europe and North America. Peppermint is most often grown for its fragrant oil.

G

Peppermint tea added to other therapies has been used in the treatment of UTIs. It is not clear if this is an effective treatment, and it is not recommended to rely on peppermint tea alone to treat this condition.

Avoid if allergic or hypersensitive to peppermint or menthol. Peppermint is generally considered safe in nonallergic adults when taken in small doses. Use cautiously with glucose-6-phosphate dehydrogenase deficiency or gallbladder disease. Menthol, which makes up part of peppermint oil, is generally considered safe in nonallergic adults. However, doses of menthol greater than 1 gram per kilogram of body weight may be deadly in humans. Avoid if pregnant or breastfeeding.

Probiotics: Probiotics are beneficial bacteria and are sometimes called friendly germs. They help maintain a healthy intestine and aid in digestion. They also help keep harmful bacteria and yeasts in the gut under control. Most probiotics come from food sources, especially cultured milk products. Probiotics can be taken as capsules, tablets, beverages, powders, yogurts, and other foods. Studies of *Lactobacillus* preparations have had mixed results. Evidence suggests that a combination of *Lactobacillus rhamnosus* GR-1 and *L. fermentum* RC-14 may reduce potentially harmful vaginal bacteria and yeast in healthy women. Other studies have found no benefit for women or preterm infants. More studies are needed to determine the effectiveness of probiotics in the prevention of urinary and urogenital tract infections.

Probiotics are generally considered safe and well tolerated. Avoid if allergic or hypersensitive to probiotics. Use cautiously if lactose intolerant.

Psychotherapy: Psychotherapy is an interactive process between a person and a qualified mental health professional. The patient explores thoughts, feelings, and behavior to help with problem solving. One small trial showed that psychotherapy may be more effective than either a bedwetting alarm or rewards in terms of children failing or relapsing. In another study, psychotherapy and a placebo were just as effective as psychotherapy combined with the medications piracetam and diphenylhydantoin, suggesting that psychotherapy may be used before drugs. Further research is needed to determine if psychotherapy is an effective treatment for bedwetting. People with unstable bladders (detrusor instability) or sensory urgency may benefit from psychotherapy. Early research suggests that psychotherapy may help reduce urgency, improve incontinence, and decrease nighttime urination, but probably not overall frequency. More research is needed in this area.

Psychotherapy cannot always fix mental or emotional conditions. Psychiatric drugs are some-times needed. In some cases, symptoms may get worse if the proper medication is not taken. Not all therapists are qualified to work with all problems. Use cautiously with serious mental illness or some medical conditions because some forms of psychotherapy may stir up strong emotional feelings and expression.

Saw Palmetto: Saw palmetto (*Serenoa repens* or *Sabal serrulata*) is used popularly in Europe for symptoms of enlarged prostate (benign prostatic hypertrophy). There is currently insufficient evidence to recommend for or against the use of saw palmetto for the management of hypotonic neurogenic bladder (also known as underactive or flaccid neurogenic bladder).

Avoid if allergic or hypersensitive to saw palmetto. Use cautiously with a history of health conditions involving the stomach, liver, heart, or lungs. Use cautiously with hormone-sensitive conditions or bleeding disorders. Use cautiously if taking anticoagulants (e.g., warfarin), hormonal drugs (e.g., finasteride), or birth control pills. Avoid if pregnant or breastfeeding.

Transcutaneous Electrical Nerve Stimulation (TENS): TENS is a noninvasive technique in which a low-voltage electrical current is delivered through wires from a small power unit to electrodes located on the skin. Further research is needed to determine if TENS is an effective treatment for patients with urinary incontinence/detrusor instability.

Avoid with implantable devices such as defibrillators, pacemakers, intravenous infusion pumps, or hepatic artery infusion pumps. Use cautiously with seizure disorders or decreased sensation, such as neuropathy. Avoid if pregnant or breastfeeding.

Thymus Extract: Thymus extracts for nutritional supplements are usually derived from young calves (bovine). Preliminary evidence from a controlled trial suggests that thymus extract reduces urinary tract reinfection, frequency, and infection persistence. Further evidence is required before recommendations can be made.

Avoid if allergic or hypersensitive to thymus extracts. Use bovine thymus extract supplements cautiously due to potential for exposure to the virus that causes "mad cow disease." Avoid use with an organ transplant or other forms of allografts or xenografts. Avoid with thymic tumors, myasthenia gravis (neuromuscular disorder), or untreated hypothyroidism. Avoid if taking immunosuppressants or hormonal therapy. Avoid if pregnant or breastfeeding. Thymic extract increases human sperm motility and progression.

Uva Ursi: Uva ursi (bearberry) is described as a small evergreen shrub with clusters of small white or pink bell-shaped flowers and dull orange berries. Uva ursi has long been used as a folk remedy to treat UTIs. The active ingredients in the herb are believed to be ursolic acid and isoquercitrin. Additional study is needed to make a firm conclusion in this area.

Avoid if allergic or hypersensitive to uva ursi (*Arctostaphylos uva-ursi*) or to other members of the Ericaceae family. Avoid with a history of anxiety, high blood pressure, glaucoma, impaired cerebral circulation, benign prostate tumor (with residual urine accumulation), pheochromocytoma, Grave's disease, or kidney disease. Use cautiously with liver disorders, gastrointestinal problems, or gallstones. Use cautiously if taking diuretics. Avoid if pregnant or breastfeeding.

Fair Negative Scientific Evidence

Cranberry: Cranberries come from small evergreen shrubs with tart, red, edible berries. The berries are used in sauces, jellies, and drinks. There is preliminary evidence that cranberry is not effective in preventing UTIs in children with neurogenic bladder.

Avoid if allergic to cranberries, blueberries, or other plants of the genus *Vaccinium*. Sweetened cranberry juice can affect blood sugar levels. Use cautiously with a history of kidney stones. Avoid more than the amount usually found in foods if pregnant or breastfeeding.

PREVENTION

Patients should drink plenty of water to reduce the risk of developing kidney stones.

Patients should empty their bladders when they feel the urge to urinate. Waiting a long time after the urge arises increases the risk of developing a UTI.

Patients should empty their bladders after intercourse. This helps reduce the risk of UTIs.

Children who wet the bed should avoid drinking fluids a few hours before bedtime.

Promptly treating STDs, such as gonorrhea, helps reduce the risk of developing PID.

Patients who have been diagnosed with PID should ask their sexual partner to be tested and treated for STDs. This can help prevent the patient from developing PID in the future.

Patients should practice safe sex and use condoms or other protective barriers during oral, anal, and vaginal sex.

GYNECOLOGICAL CANCERS

CONDITIONS: Gynecological Cancers, Cervical/Uterine Cancer, Endometrial Cancer, Ovarian Cancer, Vaginal Cancer, Vulvar Cancer

BACKGROUND

Gynecological cancer is cancer originating in the female reproductive organs. Gynecological cancers include cancer of the cervix, fallopian tubes, ovaries, uterus, vagina, and vulva. Gynecological cancer affects many women, with about 80,000 new cases diagnosed in the United States each year. About half of those cases are uterine cancer. The risk of getting cancer increases with age, and inherited gene mutations or a family history of cancer may increase the risk. Gynecological cancers can be benign (noncancerous) or malignant (cancerous). Ovarian cancer, with more than 22,000 new cases estimated per year, is the second most common gynecological cancer, and it accounts for more than 16,000 deaths annually. Gynecological cancer is a serious disease, but in the majority of cases it can be treated and cured. Gynecological cancer may be treated by specialized surgical procedures, radiation therapy, and/or chemotherapy.

TYPES

Cervical Cancer: Cervical cancer develops in the lining of the cervix, which is the lower part of the uterus (womb) entering the vagina (birth canal). Cells usually change from normal to precancer and then to cancer over a number of years, although some cases can happen more quickly. These changes are referred to by several terms, including cervical dysplasia (also known as cervical intraepithelial neoplasia). For some women, these changes may go away without any treatment, but more often they need to be treated to prevent them from becoming true cancers.

Cervical cancer is the focus of intense screening efforts using the Pap smear (also known as Pap test). The Pap smear is a diagnostic procedure that checks for changes in the cells of the cervix. In developed countries, the widespread use of cervical screening programs, such as Pap smear testing, has reduced the incidence of invasive cervical cancer by 50% or more. The causes of cervical cancer include the human papilloma virus (HPV).

Cervical cancer most commonly develops in women aged 40 years or older, and is the second most common cancer in women worldwide. Currently,

11% of U.S. women report that they do not have regular cervical cancer screenings.

Endometrial Cancer: Endometrial cancer, or carcinoma of the lining of the uterus, is the most common gynecological malignancy, comprising approximately 95% of all uterine cancers diagnosed. Approximately 40,000 American women receive a diagnosis of endometrial cancer each year, making it the fourth most common cancer found in women after breast cancer, lung cancer, and colon cancer. Endometrial cancer is most common after the reproductive years, between the ages of 60-70.

The uterus is part of a woman's reproductive system. It is the hollow, upside down, pear-shaped organ (womb) in which a baby grows. The uterus is in the pelvis between the bladder and the rectum. The narrow, lower portion of the uterus is the cervix. The broad, middle part of the uterus is the body or corpus. The dome-shaped top of the uterus is the fundus. The fallopian tubes extend from either side of the top of the uterus to the ovaries. The wall of the uterus has two layers of tissue. The inner layer, or lining, is the endometrium. The outer layer is muscle tissue called the myometrium. Uterine cancer originates in the myometrium and accounts for less than 10% of uterine cancer cases.

In women of childbearing age, the lining of the uterus grows and thickens each month to prepare for pregnancy. If a woman does not become pregnant, the thick, bloody lining flows out of the body through the vagina. This flow is called menstruation.

Endometrial cancer is often detected at an early stage because it frequently produces vaginal bleeding between menstrual periods or after menopause. If discovered early, this slow-growing cancer is likely to be confined to the uterus. Removing the uterus surgically often eliminates all of the cancer (see Treatment: hysterectomy). Unfortunately, not all endometrial cancer can be successfully treated. In these cases, the cancer has spread beyond the uterus by the time it is detected. About 7,000 American women die each year of endometrial cancer.

Ovarian Cancer: Women have two ovaries, one on each side of the uterus. The ovaries, each about the size of an almond, produce eggs (ova) as well as the female sex hormones estrogen and progesterone. Ovarian cancer is a disease in which normal ovarian cells begin to grow in an uncontrolled, abnormal manner and produce tumors in one or both ovaries.

According to the American Cancer Society, ovarian cancer ranks fifth in cancer deaths among women. Approximately 20,000 women in the United States develop ovarian cancer annually. About 15,000 deaths from ovarian cancer will occur in American women during that same time frame. The chances of surviving ovarian cancer are better if the cancer is found early. But because the disease is difficult to detect in its early stage, only about 20% of ovarian cancers are found before tumor growth has spread into adjacent tissues and organs beyond the ovaries. Most of the time, the disease has already advanced before it's diagnosed. Until recently, doctors thought that early-stage ovarian cancer rarely produced any symptoms. But new evidence has shown that most women may have signs and symptoms even in the early stages of the disease. Being aware of them may lead to earlier detection.

Vaginal Cancer: Cancer of the vagina, a rare type of gynecological cancer in women, is a disease in which cancer cells are found in the tissues of the vagina. The vagina is the passageway through which fluid passes out of the body during menstrual periods and through which a woman gives birth. It is also called the "birth canal." The vagina connects the cervix (the opening of the womb or uterus) and the vulva (the folds of skin around the opening to the vagina). There are two types of cancer of the vagina: squamous cell cancer (squamous carcinoma) and adenocarcinoma. Squamous carcinoma is usually found in women between the ages of 60 and 80. Adenocarcinoma is more often found in women between the ages of 12 and 30.

Individuals infected with HPV or certain subtypes of HPV may be also be at risk for vaginal cancer.

Vulvar Cancer: Cancer of the vulva, a rare kind of cancer in women, is a disease in which cancer cells are found in the vulva. The vulva is the outer part of a woman's vagina. The vagina is the passage between the uterus (the hollow, pear-shaped organ where a fetus grows) and the outside of the body. Approximately 4,000 women in the United States are diagnosed with vulvar cancer annually. Most women with cancer of the vulva are over age 50. However, it is becoming more common in women under age 40. Women who have constant itching and changes in the color and the way the vulva looks are at a high risk to get cancer of the vulva. A clinician should be seen if there is bleeding or discharge not related to menstruation (periods), severe burning/itching or pain in the vulva, or if the skin of the vulva looks white and feels rough. The chance of recovery and choice of treatment depend on whether the cancer in the vulva has spread to other places as well as the individual's general state of health.

CAUSES AND RISK FACTORS

Cervical Cancer

Human Papilloma Virus (HPV): For cervical cancer, the most important risk factor is infection with HPV. HPV is a group of more than 100 types of viruses that may cause genital warts or cancers of the cervix. If the viruses cause cervical cancer, they are known as high-risk HPVs. HPV is contracted during sexual intercourse. Having unprotected sex increases the risk of acquiring an HPV infection, and this occurs more often in the younger population. Women who have many sexual partners (or who have sex with men who have had many partners) have a greater chance of getting HPV and thereby developing cervical cancer.

Smoking: Women who smoke are twice as likely as to contract cervical cancer. Tobacco smoke can produce chemicals that may damage DNA in cells of the cervix, which makes the cancer more likely to occur.

Human Immunodeficiency Virus (HIV) Infection: HIV is the virus that causes AIDS and may also be a risk factor for cervical cancer. Being HIV positive makes a woman's immune system less able to fight both HPV and early cancers.

Many Sexual Partners: The larger the number of sexual partners, the greater the chances of acquiring HPV and possibly cervical cancer.

Early Sexual Activity: Having sex before the age of 18 may increase the risk of HPV infection. Immature cells are found in younger aged women and seem to be more susceptible to the precancerous changes that HPV can cause.

Chlamydia Infection: Chlamydia is a form of bacteria that can infect women's sex organs and spread during sexual intercourse. Many women are unaware that they have it unless samples are taken at the time of their Pap test. Some studies suggest that women who have this infection (or have had it in the past) are at greater risk for cervical cancer. While further studies are needed to determine if this is true, there are good reasons to avoid this infection or to have it treated. Long-term infections can cause other serious problems.

Dietary Choices: Diet can play a role in its development as well. Diets low in fruits and vegetables are linked to an increased risk of cancers, including cervical cancer. Women who are overweight have been reported to be at a higher risk.

Birth Control Pills: The long-term use of birth control pills increases the risk of cervical cancer. Some studies have shown a higher risk after five or more years of use.

Multiple Pregnancies: Women who have had more than one full-term pregnancy have an increased risk of cervical cancer. The cause is not well understood, but it has been proven to be true in large studies.

Low Income: Women who are poor are at greater risk for contracting cancer of the cervix. This may be due to their inability to afford good healthcare, such as Pap tests.

Diethylstilbestrol (DES): DES is a hormone that was used between 1940 and 1971 for women who were in danger of miscarriages. Daughters of women who took this drug have been reported to have a slightly higher risk of vaginal and cervical cancer.

Family History: Studies suggest that women whose family members have had cervical cancer are at an increased risk of getting the disease themselves. This may be because they are less able to fight HPV, or a number of other factors could be involved.

Age: Because full-blown cervical cancer typically takes years to develop, women between the ages of 35 and 50 years are the ones who are most frequently diagnosed. However, women older than 50 or who are postmenopausal are not protected from cervical cancer. Women aged 65 years and older account for 25% of cervical cancer cases and 41% of deaths.

Endometrial Cancer

When the balance of the hormones estrogen and progesterone shifts toward more estrogen (which stimulates growth of the endometrium), a woman's risk of developing endometrial cancer increases. Factors that increase levels of estrogen in the body include:

Long-Term Menstruation: Individuals who begin menstruating at an early age, such as before age 12, and continue to have periods into their 50s are at greater risk of endometrial cancer than a woman who has menstruated for fewer years. The more years the individual has had periods, the more exposure the endometrium has to estrogen.

Never Being Pregnant: Pregnancy seems to protect against endometrial cancer. The body produces more estrogen during pregnancy but also produces more progesterone. Increased progesterone production offsets the effects of the rise in estrogen levels. Women with excess exposure to estrogen that is not balanced by progesterone tend to be at an increased risk of endometrial cancer.

Irregular Ovulation: Ovulation, the monthly release of an egg from an ovary in menstruating women, is regulated by estrogen. Irregular ovulation or failure to ovulate can increase the individual's lifetime exposure to estrogen. Ovulation irregularities have many causes, including obesity and a condition known as polycystic ovary syndrome (PCOS). PCOS is a condition in which hormonal imbalances prevent ovulation and menstruation. Treating obesity and PCOS can help restore monthly ovulation and menstruation cycle, decreasing the risk of endometrial cancer.

Obesity: Fat tissue can alter estrogen levels. Being obese can increase levels of estrogen in the body by altering the metabolism of estrogen, putting the individual at a higher risk of endometrial cancer and other cancers. A high-fat diet and lack of exercise can also add to the risk by promoting obesity. Fatty foods (especially trans fats found in snacks and fried foods) may also directly affect estrogen metabolism, further increasing a woman's risk of endometrial cancer. Obesity may lead to diabetes and metabolic syndrome (including high cholesterol levels, blood sugar regulation problems, and inflammation).

Estrogen-Only Replacement Therapy (ERT): Replacing estrogen alone after menopause by using estrogen drug therapy may increase the risk of developing endometrial cancer. Taking synthetic progestin, a form of the hormone progesterone, with estrogen (combination hormone replacement therapy [HRT]) causes the lining of the uterus to shed and may actually lower the risk of endometrial cancer. Shedding is important because if the uterine lining becomes too thick and the endometrial glands too crowded, endometrial hyperplasia may occur, allowing for the development of cellular atypia and then possibly cancer. However, the combination of estrogen and progestin therapy may increase the risk of developing other health conditions, such as cardiovascular disease, breast cancer, and ovarian cancer.

Ovarian Tumors: Tumors in the ovaries may themselves be a source of estrogen, increasing estrogen levels.

Age: Most endometrial cancers develop over many years. Therefore, the older the individual, the greater the risk of developing gynecological cancers. Approximately 95% of endometrial cancer occurs in women older than 40.

History of Breast Cancer or Ovarian Cancer: A history of breast cancer or ovarian cancer can also increase the risk of endometrial cancer.

Tamoxifen Therapy: One in every 500 women whose breast cancer was treated with tamoxifen (Nolvadex) will develop endometrial cancer. Although tamoxifen acts mostly as an estrogen blocker, it does have some estrogen-like effects and can cause the uterine lining to grow. If the individual is being treated with tamoxifen, a doctor will recommend an annual pelvic examination and ask the individual to report any unusual vaginal bleeding.

Race: Caucasian women are more likely to develop endometrial cancer, but African-American women are much more likely to die of the disease. Although the reasons are not known for this increase in death rate among African-American women, socioeconomic, biological, and cultural factors increase their risks of death.

Hereditary Nonpolyposis Colorectal Cancer (HNPCC): HNPCC is an inherited disease caused by an abnormality in a gene important for DNA repair. Women with HNPCC also have a significantly higher risk of endometrial cancer as well as colon and other cancers.

Ovarian Cancer

Women who started menstruating at an early age (before age 12), have no children or had their first child after age 30, and/or experienced menopause after age 50 are at high risk of developing ovarian cancer. Women with a history of breast cancer also are at high risk for developing ovarian cancer. Menopause also increases the risk of developing ovarian cancer, especially if HRT is being used.

Inherited Gene Mutations: The most significant risk factor for ovarian cancer is having an inherited mutation in one of two genes called breast cancer gene 1 (*BRCA1*) and breast cancer gene 2 (*BRCA2*). These genes were originally identified in families with multiple cases of breast cancer, but they are also responsible for about 5-10% of ovarian cancers. Individuals are at particularly high risk of carrying these types of mutations if they are of Ashkenazi Jewish descent. Another known genetic link involves an inherited syndrome called HNPCC. Individuals in HNPCC families are at an increased risk of cancers of the uterine lining (endometrium), colon, ovary, stomach, and small intestine. Risk of ovarian cancer associated with HNPCC is lower than is that of ovarian cancer associated with BRCA mutations. Other hereditary risk factors include basal cell nevus syndrome, Lynch II syndrome (also known as HNPCC), multiple endocrine neoplasia I, and Peutz-Jeghers syndrome.

Family History: Ovarian cancer may occur in more than one family member, although it can occur in individuals who have no family members with the disease. If the individual has one first-degree relative (a mother, daughter, or sister) with ovarian cancer, the risk of developing the disease is 5% over a lifetime.

Age: Ovarian cancer most often develops after menopause. The risk of developing ovarian cancer increases with age through a woman's late 70s. Although most cases of ovarian cancer are diagnosed in postmenopausal women, the disease may also occur in premenopausal women.

Childbearing Status: Women who have had at least one pregnancy appear to have a lower risk of developing ovarian cancer unless the pregnancy was not carried to term.

Infertility: Studies indicate that infertility may increase the risk of ovarian cancer, even without the use of fertility drugs. The risk appears to be highest for women with unexplained infertility and for women with infertility who never conceive. In some studies, researchers have found that prolonged use of the fertility drug clomiphene citrate (Clomid), especially without achieving pregnancy, may increase the risk for developing ovarian tumors.

Ovarian Cysts: Cyst formation is a normal part of ovulation in premenopausal women. However, cysts that form after menopause have a greater chance of being cancerous. The likelihood of cancer increases with the size of the growth and with age. PCOS is a disorder where many fluid-filled cysts (sacs) are present and male hormones (androgens) are excessively high. PCOS can increase the risk of developing ovarian cancer.

HRT: Some research suggests that long-term use of HRT (10 years or more) increases the risk of ovarian cancer. In a study of more than 200,000 women, researchers from the American Cancer Society found that using ERT (estrogen without progestin) for 10 or more years increases the risk of death from ovarian cancer. While the chances of developing ovarian cancer doubles with prolonged estrogen use, the risk still appears to be small, estimated at approximately 2% over a lifetime. However, the study did not include data from women who used combination HRT (estrogen and progesterone), which is the most common regimen prescribed today. While researchers are not certain why estrogen therapy increases the risk of ovarian cancer, they do know that estrogen causes ovarian cells to produce at faster than normal rates.

Obesity in Early Adulthood: Studies have suggested that women who are obese at age 18 are at increased risk of developing ovarian cancer before menopause. Obesity may also be linked to more aggressive ovarian cancers, which can result in a shorter time to disease relapse and a decrease in the overall survival rate.

G

Talcum Powder: Some studies have shown a slight increase in the risk of ovarian cancer among women who used talcum powder (baby powder) on the genital area. Asbestos in the powder may explain the link, but these products have been free of asbestos for more than 20 years.

Smoking and Alcohol Use: Some studies have found smoking and alcohol use may increase the risk for developing one type of ovarian cancer called mucinous ovarian cancer.

Vaginal Cancer

Risk factors for developing vaginal cancer include being aged 60 or older and being exposed to DES while in the mother's womb. In the 1950s, the hormonal drug DES was given to some pregnant women to prevent miscarriage. Women who were exposed to DES before birth have an increased risk of developing vaginal cancer. Some of these women develop a rare form of cancer called clear cell adenocarcinoma. Having HPV infection and having a history of abnormal cells in the cervix or cervical cancer may also increase the risk of developing vaginal cancer.

Vulvar Cancer

Diabetes: Diabetes may be a risk factor for vulvar cancer. The reasons are not clear.

Age: Advancing age increases the risk for developing squamous cell carcinoma, the most common type of vulvar cancer. Many women diagnosed with this cancer are in their 70s or older.

HPV: HPV can cause genital warts or precancer of the cervix without visible warts. HPV may also increase the risk for vulvar cancer.

Smoking: Smoking increases the risk for vulvar cancer. If the individual smokes and also has genital warts or HPV infection in the genital tract, the risk is even greater for vulvar cancer.

Vulvar Intraepithelial Neoplasia (VIN): VIN is a precancerous condition that causes a change in the cells on the surface of the vulva. VIN may or may not be visible, but having it may increase the individual's risk for the most common type of vulvar cancer, squamous cell carcinoma.

Lichen Sclerosis: Lichen sclerosis, a condition that makes the vulvar skin itchy and thin, slightly increases the risk of developing vulvar cancer.

Melanoma: If a parent or sibling has had melanoma or atypical moles, an individual may have a higher risk of getting a melanoma of the vulva. Melanoma is a rare kind of vulvar cancer but one that can be quite aggressive. There is no known hereditary risk for other types of vulvar cancer. Any new mole, freckle, or dark spot on the vulva should be checked by a doctor.

Chronic Vulvar Infections or Irritations: Chronic infections or irritations of the skin of the vulva may also be a risk factor for vulvar cancer. Improving hygiene or managing infections will help to decrease the risk.

HIV: HIV infection increases the individual's risk for vulvar cancer due to a decrease in immunity.

SIGNS AND SYMPTOMS

Cervical Cancer: Early cervical cancer generally produces no signs or symptoms. Early signs may include abnormal vaginal bleeding, especially irregular heavy bleeding, bleeding after menopause, bleeding or spotting between periods, bleeding after sexual intercourse, pelvic (lower abdominal) pain, pain or pressure on the bladder or rectum, unexplained bladder irritation, and unexplained vaginal discharge (particularly when it is thick or foul smelling). As the cancer progresses, symptoms may include vaginal bleeding following intercourse, between periods, or after menopause; watery, bloody vaginal discharge that may be heavy and foul smelling; and pelvic pain or pain during intercourse. It is extremely important for women to have routine Pap tests to detect early, precancerous cellular changes. The American Cancer Society recommends that all women have a yearly Pap test starting at the age of 18 or the age they become sexually active. Some clinicians think that if the results are normal for three consecutive tests, then Pap tests can be performed every two to three years rather than annually. Older women should continue to have Pap tests because a large percentage of deaths from cervical cancer occur in women aged 65 and older.

Endometrial Cancer: Endometrial cancer often develops over a period of years. Abnormal vaginal bleeding may be one of the first signs of endometrial cancer. Most cases of endometrial cancer develop in postmenopausal women whose periods have stopped. However, a small percentage of cases affects women younger than 40. Signs and symptoms of endometrial cancer may include prolonged periods or bleeding between periods; more frequent vaginal bleeding or spotting during the years leading up to menopause (termed perimenopause); any bleeding after the time of menopause; a pink, watery, or white discharge from the vagina; pelvic pain, especially late in the disease; pain during intercourse; and weight loss. Rarely does endometrial cancer reach an advanced stage before any signs and symptoms are present.

Ovarian Cancer: Symptoms of ovarian cancer may mimic those of many other more common conditions, including digestive and bladder disorders. Symptoms include sensation of abdominal pressure, fullness, swelling, or bloating; urinary urgency; and pelvic discomfort or pain. These symptoms during ovarian cancer do not tend to subside. Additional signs and symptoms that women with ovarian cancer may experience include persistent indigestion, gas, or nausea; unexplained changes in bowel habits, including diarrhea or constipation; changes in bladder habits, including a frequent need to urinate; loss of appetite; unexplained weight loss or gain; increased abdominal girth or clothes fitting tighter around the waist; pain during intercourse (dyspareunia); lack of energy; and low back pain.

Vaginal Cancer: Signs and symptoms of vaginal cancer include vaginal bleeding after menopause, vaginal bleeding after intercourse, abnormal vaginal discharge, a mass in the vagina that can be felt, pain during sex, pain when urinating, constipation, and constant pain in the pelvis.

Vulvar Cancer: Signs and symptoms of vulvar cancer include vulvar itching that does not improve; a change in skin color around the vulva; a change in the feel of the skin around the vulva; and wartlike bump(s), cauliflower-like growths, or ulcers/sores on the vulva or clitoral area (the lump or sore can be red, gray, or white). Other symptoms include pain when urinating, burning or bleeding and discharge not related to the menstrual cycle, enlarged glands in the groin, a new mole on the vulva or a change in a mole that has been present for years, and an abnormal mole.

DIAGNOSIS

A gynecologist (a doctor who specializes in conditions affecting the female reproductive system) will conduct a complete medical history and perform a physical and pelvic examination. During the pelvic examination, the doctor feels for any lumps or changes in the shape of the uterus that may indicate a problem. Diagnosis of gynecological cancers may or may not involve these diagnostic tests:

Pap Test: Pap test, or Pap smear, involves the doctor taking a sample of cells from the cervix, the lower, narrower portion of the uterus that opens into the vagina. Doctors mainly use the Pap test to detect changes in cervical cells and to detect cervical cancer.

Endometrial Biopsy: Endometrial biopsy is usually performed in a doctor's office. Endometrial biopsy involves inserting a narrow tube into the uterus through the vagina and removing a small amount of tissue from the uterine wall. This tissue is tested

in a lab for cancerous or precancerous cells. The procedure usually takes just a few minutes and is painless.

Dilatation and Curettage (D&C): A dilatation and curettage (D&C) involves dilating (widening) the cervix (the opening of the uterus) and inserting an instrument to scrape or suction the uterine wall and collect tissue. D&C is also an outpatient procedure. It takes about an hour and usually requires general anesthesia.

Imaging Tests: Imaging tests are used in patients with certain medical conditions such as severe high blood pressure, obesity, diabetes, or cancer. These patients may not be able to safely have anesthesia. In these patients, imaging tests such as a magnetic resonance imagine (MRI) scan, computerized tomography (CT) scan, or ultrasound may help diagnose cancer of the uterus.

If gynecological cancer is found, more tests to determine if the cancer has spread (metastasized) to other parts of the body will be performed (termed "staging"). These tests may include a chest x-ray, a CT scan, and a blood test to measure cancer antigen 125, a substance that's released in the bloodstream by some endometrial and ovarian cancers.

COMPLICATIONS

Complications of gynecological cancers include metastasis (spreading) to other organs, including the pelvic and abdominal lymph nodes, the abdominal cavity (causing fluid buildup), the lungs and sac surrounding the lungs (pleura), bones, liver, and brain. Pain may be present, especially in the pelvic region and lower gastrointestinal system.

Women with certain gynecological cancers (such as endometrial cancer) may lose enough blood from vaginal bleeding to cause anemia—a condition in which the blood is low in red blood cells. Anemia causes fatigue and shortness of breath.

TREATMENT

The treatment of gynecological cancers is based on the stage of the disease, specifically the extent to which the cancer has spread to other parts of the body. Treatments include surgery, chemotherapy, radiation, and biological therapy.

Chemotherapy: Chemotherapy uses a combination of drugs to slow tumor growth and destroy cancer cells. Chemotherapy may be used in addition to surgery to treat gynecological cancer and to prevent recurrent disease. Drugs may be administered by mouth or intravenously (into the veins). Side effects of chemotherapy may be severe and include fatigue, fever, hair loss (alopecia), infection, low blood cell count (such as anemia, neutropenia, thrombocytopenia), and nausea.

Hormone Therapy: Some gynecological tumors, such as uterine tumors, contain certain proteins, called hormone receptors, that attract and bind to estrogen and use this hormone to grow. Hormone therapy is a treatment that uses progesterone to balance the effect of estrogen and slow tumor growth. Hormone therapy usually involves a synthetic type of progesterone (progestin) in pill form. Side effects include increased appetite, fluid retention, weight gain and, in premenopausal women, changes in the menstrual cycle.

Radiation Therapy: Radiation uses high-energy x-rays to destroy cancer cells and shrink tumors. This treatment may be used prior to surgery (called neoadjuvant therapy) or after surgery to destroy remaining cancer cells. Radiation also may be used in patients who are unable to undergo surgery.

External beam radiation is an outpatient treatment delivered by a machine outside the body. This treatment usually is administered five days a week for several weeks. Most individuals refrain from sexual intercourse during and for several weeks following radiation therapy because contact with the genitals and vagina may be painful.

Internal beam radiation may be administered for four to six weeks after surgery. In this procedure, which is usually performed in the radiation department of a hospital, a special applicator is used to insert pellets of radioactive material into the upper vagina. In some cases, both external and internal radiation therapies are used.

Side effects of radiation include diarrhea; dryness, itching, tightening, and burning in the skin of the vagina; fatigue; frequent, painful urination; hair loss; and changes in tastes and loss of appetite.

Surgery: Treatment for many gynecological cancers usually involves removal of the uterus, including the cervix (called total hysterectomy), and removal of the fallopian tubes and ovaries (called bilateral salpingo-oophorectomy). Surgery may be performed through an incision in the abdomen or through the vagina (called transvaginal hysterectomy). Postoperative pain, nausea, vomiting, and fatigue are common side effects of surgery. Individuals may remain hospitalized for a few days to one week and usually can resume normal activities in four to eight weeks. Complications include the following: adverse reaction to anesthesia; hemorrhage (bleeding) caused by injury to surrounding blood vessels, injury to surrounding organs (such as the large intestine), and

thromboembolism (blockage of an artery or vein by a blood clot).

Other Therapies: Biological therapies involve treatments to help improve the immune system. It uses such agents as interleukin-2, vaccine therapy, and anti-HER-2. Antiangiogenesis (the growth of new blood vessels to tumors) therapy decreases the amount of blood a tumor can get, thereby possibly killing or decreasing the tumor. Some drugs treat the side effects of chemotherapy. Anemia (low number of red blood cells) is a frequent side effect of chemotherapy and may cause symptoms such as extreme tiredness, dizziness, or shortness of breath. Epoetin alfa (Procrit, Epogen) is a synthetic hormone that is used for the treatment of chemotherapy-related anemia by stimulating red blood cell production. Immune system problems caused by chemotherapy may be treated with filgrastim (Neupogen), a human granulocyte colony stimulating factor (G-CSF). G-CSF helps stimulate the production of cells of the immune system, including granulocytes, macrophages, and stem cells.

INTEGRATIVE THERAPIES

Strong Scientific Evidence

Vitamin A: Vitamin A is a fat-soluble vitamin that is derived from two sources: preformed retinoids and provitamin carotenoids. Retinoids, such as retinal and retinoic acid, are found in animal sources such as livers, kidneys, eggs, and dairy produce. Carotenoids like beta-carotene (which has the highest vitamin A activity) are found in plants such as yellow vegetables and carrots. It is not clear if vitamin A or beta-carotene, taken by mouth or used on the skin with sunscreen, is beneficial in the prevention or treatment of skin cancers or wrinkles. At recommended doses, vitamin A is generally considered nontoxic.

Good Scientific Evidence

Psychotherapy: Psychotherapy is an interactive process between a person and a qualified mental health professional (psychiatrist, psychologist, clinical social worker, licensed counselor, or other trained practitioner). There is good evidence that psychotherapy can enhance cancer patients' quality of life by reducing emotional stress and challenges of cancer. Therapy may be supportive-expressive therapy, cognitive therapy, or group therapy. Studies conflict on whether therapy improves self-esteem, death anxiety, self-satisfaction, etc. While some patients seek psychotherapy in hopes of extending survival, there is no conclusive evidence of effects on medical prognosis.

Unclear or Conflicting Scientific Evidence

Acupuncture: Acupuncture, or the use of needles to manipulate the "chi" or body energy, originated in China more than 5,000 years ago. There has been limited research on acupuncture for cancer pain and the research that was done was shown to have mixed results. More studies are needed to determine potential benefits. Evidence from several small studies supports the use of acupuncture at a specific point on the wrist (P6), which helps reduce the nausea and vomiting associated with chemotherapy.

Aloe: Transparent gel from the pulp of the meaty leaves of *Aloe vera* has been used topically for thousands of years to treat wounds, skin infections, burns, and numerous other dermatological conditions. Preliminary research suggests that aloe may help prevent or aid in the regression of cancerous tumors. Additional research is needed in this area. Caution is advised when taking aloe supplements as numerous adverse effects, including a laxative effect, cramping, dehydration, and drug interactions, are possible. Aloe should not be used if the patient is pregnant or breastfeeding unless otherwise directed by a doctor.

American Pawpaw: Evidence supporting the use of the American pawpaw (*Asimina triloba*) tree for the treatment of cancer in humans is largely anecdotal and subjective. Use in humans has reported minimal side effects, and evidence from animal and in vitro studies suggests that American pawpaw extract does have some anticancer activity. Pawpaw standardized extract has been used for 18 months in patients with various forms of cancer. No well-designed studies on the long-term effects of pawpaw extracts have been conducted. Pawpaw should not be used if the patient is pregnant or breastfeeding unless otherwise directed by a doctor.

Antineoplastons: Antineoplastons comprise a group of naturally occurring peptide fractions, which were observed by Stanislaw Burzynski, MD, PhD, in the late 1970s and were found to be absent in the urine of cancer patients. There is inconclusive scientific evidence regarding the effectiveness of antineoplastons in the treatment of cancer. Several preliminary human studies (case series, phase I/II trials) have examined antineoplaston types A2, A5, A10, AS2-1, and AS2-5 for a variety of cancer types. It remains unclear if antineoplastons are effective or what doses may be safe. Until better research is available, no clear conclusion can be drawn.

Arabinoxylan: Arabinoxylan is made by altering the outer shell of rice bran using enzymes from *Hyphomycetes mycelia* mushroom extract. Arabinoxylan has been found to improve immune reactions in diabetes and cancer patients. Arabinoxylan products may contain high calcium and phosphorus levels, which may be harmful for patients with compromised renal (kidney) function.

Aromatherapy: Healing with fragrant oils has been used for thousands of years. Aromatherapy is often used in people with chronic illnesses (frequently in combination with massage), with the intention to improve quality of life or well-being. There is not enough scientific evidence in this area to form a firm conclusion about the effectiveness of aromatherapy. Essential oils are not for internal use.

Art Therapy: Art therapy involves the application of a variety of art modalities, including drawing, painting, clay, and sculpture. Art therapy enables the expression of inner thoughts or feelings when verbalization is difficult or not possible. Limited evidence suggests that family caregivers of cancer patients may benefit from art therapy to help them cope with the stress of care giving. Possible benefits include reduced stress, lowered anxiety, increased positive emotions, and increased positive communication with cancer patients and healthcare professionals. Art therapy may also reduce pain and other symptoms in cancer patients. More studies are needed to determine how best to use this form of intervention with this population.

Astragalus: Astragalus (*Astragalus membranaceus*) has been used in Chinese medicine for centuries for its immune-enhancing properties. Although early laboratory and animal studies report increased immune cell function and reduced cancer cell growth associated with the use of astragalus, there is no reliable human evidence in these areas. A recent study reports that astragalus-based Chinese herbal medicine may increase effectiveness of platinum-based chemotherapy when combined with chemotherapy. Astragalus is also sometimes used with the intention to reduce side effects of cancer treatments, such as fatigue and weight loss. Due to a lack of well-designed research, a firm conclusion cannot be drawn.

Bee Pollen: Bee pollen is considered a highly nutritious food because it contains a balance of vitamins, minerals, proteins, carbohydrates, fats, enzymes, and essential amino acids. Research has found that bee pollen may reduce some adverse effects of cancer treatment, but additional studies are needed before a firm recommendation can be made. Caution is advised when taking bee pollen supplements as allergic reactions may occur in sensitive individuals. Bee pollen should not be used if the patient is pregnant or breastfeeding unless otherwise directed by a doctor.

Avoid in individuals with a known allergy or hypersensitivity to bee pollen, especially pollen included in commercial preparations. Allergic reactions may include itching, swelling, shortness of breath, light-headedness, gastrointestinal upset, rash, asthma, hay fever, nausea, abdominal cramps, diarrhea, vomiting, and anaphylaxis.

Bitter Melon: Bitter melon (*Momordica charantia*) is used in the traditional Ayurvedic form of medicine from India for lowering blood sugar levels. Research has also found that bitter melon extracts may be beneficial in cancer therapies. MAP30, a protein isolated from bitter melon extract, is reported to possess anticancer effects in laboratory studies. Potential anticancer effects have not been studied appropriately in humans. Caution is advised when taking bitter melon supplements, as numerous adverse effects, including blood sugar lowering and drug interactions, are possible. Bitter melon should not be used if the patient is pregnant or breastfeeding unless otherwise directed by a doctor.

Black Tea: Black tea (*Camellia sinensis*) is from the same plant as green tea, but processed differently and containing more caffeine than green tea. Several studies have explored a possible association between regular consumption of black tea and rates of cancer in populations. This research has yielded conflicting results, with some studies suggesting benefits and others reporting no effects. Laboratory and animal studies report that components of tea, such as polyphenols, have antioxidant properties and effects against tumors. Effects in humans remain unclear, and these components may be more common in green tea rather than in black tea.

Bromelain: Bromelain is a sulfur-containing proteolytic digestive enzyme that is extracted from the stem and the fruit of the pineapple plant (*Ananas comosus*). There is not enough information to recommend for or against the use of bromelain in the treatment of cancer, either alone or in addition to other therapies. Caution is advised when taking bromelain supplements, as numerous adverse effects, including blood thinning and drug interactions, are possible.

Cat's Claw: Originally found in Peru, the use of cat's claw (*Uncaria tomentosa*) has been said to date back to the Inca civilization, possibly as far back as 2,000 years. Cat's claw has antiinflammatory properties, and several low-quality studies suggest it may slow tumor growth; however, this research is early and has not identified specific types of cancer that may benefit. A few studies suggest that cat's claw may also boost the immune system. Caution is advised when taking cat's claw supplements, as

numerous adverse effects, including blood thinning and drug interactions, are possible. Cat's claw should not be used if the patient is pregnant or breastfeeding unless otherwise directed by a doctor.

Copper: Copper is a mineral that occurs naturally in many foods, including vegetables, legumes, nuts, grains, and fruits, as well as shellfish and beef (organs such as liver). Preliminary research reports that lowering copper levels theoretically may arrest the progression of cancer by inhibiting blood vessel growth (angiogenesis). Copper intake has not been identified as a risk factor for the development or progression of cancer. Copper is potentially unsafe when used orally in higher doses than the recommended dietary allowance. Copper supplements should not be used if the patient is pregnant or breastfeeding unless otherwise directed by a doctor.

Cranberry: Several laboratory studies have reported positive effects of proanthocyanidins, flavonoid components of cranberry (*Vaccinium macrocarpon*) and other fruits such as blueberries, grape seed, and pomegranate, on health. Based on a small amount of laboratory research, cranberry has been proposed for cancer prevention, but studies are needed in humans before a recommendation can be made.

Echinacea: The evidence from a small number of randomized trials evaluating efficacy of echinacea in the treatment of radiation-induced leukopenia (decrease in white blood cells) is equivocal. Studies have used the combination product Esberitox, which includes extracts of echinacea (*Echinacea purpurea* and *pallida*) root, white cedar (*Thuja occidentalis*) leaf, and wild indigo (*Baptisia tinctoria*) root.

People with allergies to plants in the Asteraceae or Compositae family (ragweed, chrysanthemums, marigolds, daisies) are theoretically more likely to have allergic reactions to echinacea. Multiple cases of anaphylactic shock (severe allergic reactions) and allergic rash have been reported with echinacea taken by mouth. Allergic reactions including itching, rash, wheezing, facial swelling, and anaphylaxis may occur more commonly in people with asthma or other allergies.

Essiac: Essiac contains a combination of herbs, including burdock root (*Arctium lappa*), sheep sorrel (*Rumex acetosella*), slippery elm inner bark (*Ulmus fulva*), and Turkish rhubarb (*Rheum palmatum*). The original formula was developed by the Canadian nurse Rene Caisse (1888-1978) and is thought to be effective in cancer therapies, although there is currently no evidence for any type of cancer. Different brands may contain variable ingredients, and the comparative effectiveness of these formulas is not known. None of the individual herbs used in Essiac have been tested in rigorous human cancer trials, although some components have antitumor activity in laboratory studies. Caution is advised when taking Essiac supplements, as numerous adverse effects, including drug interactions, are possible. Essiac should not be used if the patient is pregnant or breastfeeding unless otherwise directed by a doctor.

Focusing: Focusing (experiential therapy) is a method of psychotherapy that involves being aware of one's feelings surrounding a particular issue and understanding the meaning behind words or images conveyed by those feelings. Early evidence suggests focusing may improve the mood and body attitude of cancer patients. Firm recommendations cannot be made until well-designed clinical trials are available.

Garlic: Preliminary human studies suggest that regular consumption of garlic (*Allium sativum,* particularly aged garlic) may reduce the risk of developing several types of cancer. Some studies use multi-ingredient products, so it is difficult to determine if garlic alone may play a beneficial role. Further well-designed human clinical trials are needed to conclude whether eating garlic or taking garlic supplements may prevent or treat cancer. Caution is advised when taking garlic supplements, as numerous adverse effects, including an increased risk of bleeding and drug interactions, are possible.

Ginseng: Several human studies suggest that Asian ginseng (*Panax ginseng*) may reduce the risk and progression of various organ cancers, especially if ginseng powder or extract is used. Results may have been affected by other lifestyle choices in people who use ginseng, such as exercise or dietary habits. Asian ginseng is also reported to help protect against radiation damage, to increase immunity and well-being, and to decrease fatigue. Additional trials are necessary before a clear conclusion can be reached. Caution is advised when taking ginseng supplements, as numerous adverse effects, including an increased risk of drug interactions, are possible. Ginseng should not be used if the patient is pregnant or breastfeeding unless otherwise directed by a doctor.

Green Tea: Green tea is made from the dried leaves of *Camellia sinensis,* a perennial evergreen shrub. Green tea has a long history of use in health and longevity, dating back to China approximately 5,000 years ago. Although used for centuries to help prevent diseases, the relationship of green tea consumption and human cancer remains inconclusive. Evidence from well-designed clinical trials is needed.

Healing Touch: Preliminary data suggest human touch may be of benefit in cancer patients for inducing relaxation and improving quality of life. However, due to weaknesses in design and the small number of studies, data are insufficient to make definitive recommendations. Studies with stronger designs are needed.

Hoxsey Formula: "Hoxsey formula" is a misleading name because it is not a single formula, but rather a therapeutic regimen consisting of an oral tonic and topical (on the skin) preparations. The tonic is individualized for cancer patients based on general condition, location of cancer, and previous history of treatment. An ingredient that usually remains constant for every patient is potassium iodide. Other ingredients are then added and may include licorice, red clover, burdock, stillingia root, berberis root, pokeroot, cascara, aromatic USP 14, prickly ash bark, and buckthorn bark. A red paste may be used, which tends to be caustic (irritating), and contains antimony trisulfide, zinc chloride, and bloodroot. A topical yellow powder may be used and contains arsenic sulfide, talc, sulfur, and a "yellow precipitate." A clear solution may also be administered and contains trichloroacetic acid. There are no well-designed human studies available evaluating the safety or effectiveness of Hoxsey formula. Caution is advised when taking the Hoxsey formula supplements, as numerous adverse effects, including an increased risk of drug interactions, are possible. Hoxsey formula should not be used if the patient is pregnant or breastfeeding unless otherwise directed by a doctor.

Hydrazine Sulfate: Hydrazine is an industrial chemical marketed as having the potential to repress weight loss and cachexia (muscle wasting) associated with cancer and to improve general appetite status. In large randomized, controlled trials, hydrazine has not been found effective for improving appetite, reducing weight loss, or improving survival in adults. The National Cancer Institute sponsored studies of hydrazine sulfate that claimed efficacy in improving survival for some patients with advanced cancer. Trial results showed that hydrazine sulfate did not prolong survival for cancer patients. The U.S. Food and Drug Administration (FDA) has received requests from individual physicians for approval to use hydrazine sulfate on a case-by-case "compassionate use" basis on the chance that patients with no other available effective therapy might benefit. The overall controversy in the use of hydrazine sulfate is ongoing, and relevance to clinical practice is unknown. The use of hydrazine sulfate needs to be evaluated further before any recommendations can be made. Side effects have been reported, including nausea, vomiting, stomach cramping, and diarrhea.

Lycopene: High levels of lycopene are found in tomatoes and in tomato-based products. Tomatoes are also sources of other nutrients such as vitamin C, folate, and potassium. Several laboratory and human studies examining tomato-based products and blood lycopene levels suggest that lycopene may be associated with a lower risk of developing cancer and may help stimulate the immune system. However, due to a lack of well-designed human research using lycopene supplements, this issue remains unclear.

Maitake Mushroom: Maitake is the Japanese name for the edible fungus *Grifola frondosa*. Maitake has been used traditionally both as a food and for medicinal purposes. Early studies in the laboratory as well as in humans suggest that beta-glucan extracts from maitake may increase the body's ability to fight cancer. These studies have not been well designed, and better research is needed before the use of maitake for cancer can be recommended.

Melatonin: There are several early-phase and controlled human trials of melatonin in patients with various advanced-stage malignancies, including brain, breast, colorectal, gastric, liver, lung, pancreatic, and testicular cancer, as well as lymphoma, melanoma, renal cell carcinoma, and soft-tissue sarcoma. Currently, no clear conclusion can be drawn in this area. There is not enough definitive scientific evidence to discern if melatonin is beneficial against any type of cancer, whether it increases (or decreases) the effectiveness of other cancer therapies, or if it safely reduces chemotherapy side effects. Caution is advised when taking melatonin supplements, as numerous adverse effects including drug interactions are possible.

Mistletoe: Mistletoe is one of the most widely used unconventional cancer treatments in Europe. Extracts have been studied for a variety of human cancers, including bladder, breast, cervical, central nervous system, colorectal, head and neck, liver, lung, lymphatic, ovarian, and renal (kidney) cancers as well as melanoma and leukemia. Efficacy has not been conclusively proven for any one condition, and in fact some studies have shown a lack of efficacy in certain preparations for a variety of cancers. Larger, well-designed clinical trials are needed. Caution is advised when taking mistletoe supplements, as numerous adverse effects, including nausea and vomiting and drug interactions, are possible. Mistletoe should not be used if the patient is pregnant or breastfeeding unless otherwise directed by a doctor.

Moxibustion: Moxibustion is a healing technique employed across the diverse traditions of acupuncture and oriental medicine for over 2,000 years. Moxibustion uses the principle of heat to stimulate circulation and break up congestion or stagnation of blood and chi. Moxibustion is more closely related to acupuncture as it is applied to specific acupuncture points. More studies are needed.

Omega-3 Fatty Acids: Omega-3 fatty acids are essential fatty acids found in some plants and fish. There should be a balance of omega-6 and omega-3 fatty acids for health. Randomized controlled trials are necessary before a clear conclusion can be drawn. Caution is advised when taking omega-3 supplements, as numerous adverse effects, including an increase in bleeding and drug interactions, are possible. Omega-3 supplements should not be used if the patient is pregnant or breastfeeding unless otherwise directed by a doctor.

Prayer: Initial studies in patients with cancer (such as leukemia) report variable effects on disease progression or death rates when intercessory prayer is used. Better-quality research is necessary before a firm conclusion can be drawn.

Reishi Mushroom: Reishi (*Ganoderma lucidum*) has been shown to have antineoplastic and immunomodulatory effects in animal studies. One clinical trial and two case reports exist on advanced cancer patients using Ganopoly, a Ganoderma lucidum polysaccharide extract. Results show improved quality of life and enhanced immune responses, which are typically reduced or damaged in cancer patients receiving chemotherapy and/or radiation therapy. The authors are closely related to the manufacturer of Ganopoly. Well-designed long-term studies are needed to confirm these results and potential side effects.

Seaweed: Bladderwrack (*Fucus vesiculosus*) is a brown seaweed that grows on the northern coasts of the Atlantic and Pacific oceans and the North and Baltic seas. Bladderwrack appears to suppress the growth of various cancer cells in animal and laboratory studies. Currently, there are no reliable human studies available to support a recommendation for use in cancer. Bladderwrack should not be used if the patient is pregnant or breastfeeding or has hyperthyroidism (increased thyroid hormone) unless otherwise directed by a doctor.

Selenium: Selenium is a trace mineral found in soil, water, and some foods, and it is an essential element in several metabolic pathways. Several studies suggest that low levels of selenium (measured in the blood or in tissues such as toenail clippings) may be a risk factor for developing cancer, particularly prostate cancer. Population studies suggest that people with cancer are more likely to have lower selenium levels than healthy matched individuals, but in most cases it is not clear if the low selenium levels are a cause or merely a consequence of disease. It remains unclear if selenium is beneficial in the treatment of any type of cancer.

Shark Cartilage: For several decades, shark cartilage has been proposed as a cancer treatment. Studies have shown shark cartilage or the shark cartilage product AE-941 (Neovastat) to block the growth of new blood vessels, a process called antiangiogenesis, which is believed to play a role in controlling the growth of some tumors. There have also been several reports of successful treatments of end-stage cancer patients with shark cartilage, but these have neither been well designed nor have they included reliable comparisons to accepted treatments. Many studies have been supported by shark cartilage product manufacturers, which may influence the results. In the United States, shark cartilage products cannot claim to cure cancer, and the FDA has sent warning letters to companies that promote products in this way. Without further evidence from well-designed human trials, it remains unclear if shark cartilage is of any benefit in cancer and patients are advised to check with their doctors and pharmacists before taking shark cartilage.

Shiitake Mushroom: Shiitake (*Lentinus edodes*) has been taken by mouth for boosting the immune system, decreasing cholesterol levels, and for antiaging. Lentinan, derived from shiitake, has been injected as an adjunct treatment for cancer and HIV infection. Laboratory, animal, and human studies of lentinan have shown positive results in cancer patients when used in addition to chemotherapy drugs. Further well-designed clinical trials on all types of cancer are required to confirm these results.

Soy: Soy (*Glycine max*) contains compounds that have been effective against tumors. Genistein, an isoflavone found in soy, has been found in laboratory and animal studies to possess anticancer effects, such as blocking new blood vessel growth (antiangiogenesis), acting as a tyrosine kinase inhibitor (a mechanism of many new cancer treatments), or causing cancer cell death (apoptosis). Until reliable human research is available, it remains unclear if dietary soy or soy isoflavone supplements are beneficial, harmful, or neutral in people with various types of cancer. Caution is advised when taking soy supplements, as numerous adverse effects including an increased risk of drug interactions are possible.

Soy can act as a food allergen similar to milk, eggs, peanuts, fish, and wheat.

The use of soy is often discouraged in patients with hormone-sensitive malignancies such as breast, ovarian, or uterine cancer due to concerns about possible estrogen-like effects (which theoretically may stimulate tumor growth). Other hormone-sensitive conditions such as endometriosis may also theoretically be worsened. In laboratory studies, it is not clear if isoflavones stimulate or block the effects of estrogen or both (acting as a receptor agonist/antagonist). Until additional research is available, patients with these conditions should be cautious and speak with a qualified healthcare practitioner before starting use.

It is not known if soy or soy isoflavones share the same side effects as estrogens, such as increased risk of blood clots. Preliminary studies suggest that soy isoflavones, unlike estrogens, do not cause the lining of the uterus (endometrium) to build up.

Transcutaneous Electrical Nerve Stimulation (TENS): TENS is a noninvasive technique in which a low-voltage electrical current is delivered through wires from a small power unit to electrodes located on the skin. Although TENS has been used with some success in pain associated with cancer, there is not enough reliable evidence to draw a firm conclusion in this area.

Thiamin (Vitamin B$_1$): Thiamin deficiency has been observed in some cancer patients, possibly due to increased metabolic needs. It is not clear if lowered levels of thiamin in such patients may actually be beneficial. Currently, it remains unclear if thiamin supplementation plays a role in the management of any particular type(s) of cancer.

Traditional Chinese Medicine (TCM): The ancient Chinese philosophy of Taoism provided the basis for the development of Chinese medical theory. TCM uses over 120 different herbs in cancer treatment depending upon the type and cause of the cancer. Studies have reported significant benefits, including reducing tumors, reducing treatment side effects, and improved response to treatment. More studies of stronger design are needed before TCM can be recommended with confidence as an adjunct to cancer treatment, although centuries of traditional use in cancer cannot be discounted.

Turmeric: Turmeric (*Curcuma longa*) is commonly used for its antiinflammatory properties. Several early animal and laboratory studies report anticancer (colon, skin, breast) properties of curcumin. Many mechanisms have been considered, including antioxidant activity, antiangiogenesis (prevention of new blood vessel growth), and direct effects on cancer cells. Currently, it remains unclear if turmeric or curcumin has a role in preventing or treating human cancers. There are several ongoing studies in this area. Caution is advised when taking turmeric supplements, as numerous adverse effects, including an increased risk of bleeding and drug interactions, are possible.

Vitamin C (Ascorbic Acid): Dietary intake of fruits and vegetables high in vitamin C has been associated with a reduced risk of various types of cancer in population studies (particularly cancers of the mouth, esophagus, stomach, colon, or lung). However, it is not clear that it is specifically the vitamin C in these foods that is beneficial, and vitamin C supplements have not been found to be associated with this protective effect. Experts have recommended increasing dietary consumption of fruits and vegetables high in vitamin C, such as apples, asparagus, berries, broccoli, cabbage, melon (cantaloupe, honeydew, watermelon), cauliflower, citrus fruits (lemons, oranges), fortified breads/grains/cereal, kale, kiwi, potatoes, spinach, and tomatoes. Vitamin C has a long history of adjunctive use in cancer therapy, and although there have not been any definitive studies using intravenous (or oral) vitamin C, there is evidence that it has benefit in some cases. Better-designed studies are needed. Large doses (greater than 2 grams) may cause diarrhea and gastrointestinal upset.

Vitamin E: There is no reliable scientific evidence that vitamin E is effective as a treatment for any specific type of cancer. Caution is merited in people undergoing treatment with chemotherapy or radiation because it has been proposed that the use of high-dose antioxidants may actually reduce the anticancer effects of these therapies. This remains an area of controversy and studies have produced variable results. Patients interested in using high-dose antioxidants such as vitamin E during chemotherapy or radiation should discuss this decision with their oncologists. Caution is advised when taking vitamin E supplements, as numerous adverse effects, including an increased risk of bleeding and drug interactions, are possible.

Yoga: Yoga is an ancient system of relaxation, exercise, and healing with origins in Indian philosophy. Several studies in cancer patients report enhanced quality of life, lower sleep disturbance, decreased stress symptoms, and changes in cancer-related immune cells after patients received relaxation, meditation, and gentle yoga therapy. Yoga is not recommended as a sole treatment for cancer but may be helpful as an adjunct therapy.

Fair Negative Scientific Evidence

Integrative therapies used in cancer therapies that have fair negative scientific evidence include apricot (*Prunus armeniaca*), beta-carotene, flaxseed and flaxseed oil (*Linum usitatissimum*), hypnotherapy, iridology, and protein-bound polysaccharide (PSK).

Traditional or Theoretical Uses Lacking Scientific Evidence

Integrative therapies with historical or theoretical uses in cancer but lacking sufficient clinical evidence include acerola (*Malpighia glabra, Malpighia punicifolia*), aconite (*Aconitum napellus*), African wild potato (*Hypoxis hemerocallidea*), alfalfa (*Medicago sativa*), andrographis (*Andrographis paniculata* Nees, Kan Jang, SHA-10), L-arginine, ashwagandha (*Withania somnifera*), asparagus (*Asparagus officinalis*), barley (*Hordeum vulgare*), bilberry (*Vaccinium myrtillus*), boron, bupleurum (*Bupleurum falcatum*), chicory (*Cichorium intybus*), DHEA, feverfew (*Tanacetum parthenium*), garcinia (*Garcinia cambogia*), hydroxycitric acid, holy basil (*Ocimum sanctum*), kava kava (*Piper methysticum*), licorice (*Glycyrrhiza glabra*), neem (*Azadirachta indica*), ozone therapy, PC-SPES, podophyllum (*Podophyllum peltatum*), Pycnogenol (*Pinus pinaster*), rehmannia (*Rehmannia glutinosa*), spiritual healing, sweet almond (*Prunus amygdalus dulcis*), thymus extract, watercress (*Nasturtium officinale*), and yew (Taxus spp.).

PREVENTION

Screening: Recently, the FDA approved Gardasil to protect against HPV in females nine to 26 years of age to prevent cervical cancer. The Centers for Disease Control and Prevention National Immunization Program and the federal Advisory Committee on Immunization Practices have recommended the use of the HPV vaccine. Although the vaccine could prevent up to 70% of cervical cancer cases, it can't prevent infection with every virus that causes cervical cancer. Routine Pap tests to screen for cervical cancer remain very important. Another vaccine against HPV that has been studied in clinical trials is Cervarix. Recommendations for prevention of cervical cancer include regular cervical cancer screening (Pap tests) for all women (within three years of when a woman begins sexual activity or at age 21) or HPV vaccination for girls and women aged nine to 26. The HPV vaccination for women aged

27 or older is not supported. All women receiving the HPV vaccine should continue to receive regular cervical cancer screenings (Pap tests) according to established screening recommendations.

Other Prevention Factors: Other factors recommended by healthcare professionals to prevent gynecological cancers include limiting the number of sexual partners, getting screened regularly with a Pap test, and following up any abnormal Pap test results as recommended by a healthcare provider.

Dietary Factors: Dietary factors that significantly reduce the risk of gynecological cancer include eating more antioxidant-containing fresh fruits and vegetables and decreasing the intake of red meats and foods high in animal fat (dairy products such as milk, cheese, sour cream). A study found the strongest link between dietary risk factors and ovarian cancer was meat and cheese intake. The same study found significantly reduced risk of all ovarian cancer with higher tomato consumption. Other studies have found no link between preventing ovarian cancer and dietary factors.

Exercise: An increase in physical activity has been reported to decrease the chances of developing cancer. High levels of sedentary behavior may increase the risk of ovarian cancer. A doctor can advise the patient as to what type of exercise would be best for that individual.

Oral Contraception: Studies have found a correlation between birth control pill use and a reduced risk of ovarian cancer. However, other studies have shown that oral contraception increases a woman's risk for breast cancer as well liver and cervical cancer.

Pregnancy and Breastfeeding: Having at least one child lowers the risk of developing ovarian cancer. Breastfeeding a child for a year or longer also may reduce the risk of ovarian cancer.

Tubal Ligation or Hysterectomy: The Nurses' Health Study, which followed thousands of women for 20 years, found a substantial reduction in ovarian cancer risk in women who had had tubal ligations. The procedure also has been shown to reduce ovarian cancer risk among women with mutations in the *BRCA1* gene, although how the procedure helps is uncertain. The Nurses' Health Study also indicated that having a hysterectomy may reduce ovarian cancer risk, but not by as much as tubal ligation. However, there are risks associated with tubal ligation and hysterectomy that should be discussed with a qualified healthcare professional. Studies conducted at the Alan Guttmacher Institute found that, depending on the sterilization technique used, up to 2% of women can expect a major complication at the time of operation. Patients may suffer from such complications as infection, injury to the bladder, bleeding from a major blood vessel, or burning of the bowel or other structures. A study in Britain followed 374 post-tubal patients and found that 43% had subsequent gynecological treatment for such conditions as heavy menstrual bleeding, menstrual disturbances requiring hormonal treatments, cervical erosion, ovarian tumors, and recanalization of the fallopian tubes requiring a second operation. The risk of cervical cancer among a study of 489 post-tubal women was 3.5 times the normal rate.

Weight Control: The incidence of obesity is increasing in the developed world such that it now contributes as much as smoking to overall cancer deaths. Women with a body mass index >40 have a 60% higher risk of dying from all cancers than women of normal weight. They are also at increased risk for gynecological cancer.

G

HEART ATTACK

BACKGROUND

A heart attack, or myocardial infarction (MI), occurs when the supply of blood and oxygen to an area of heart muscle is blocked. A clot (or thrombus) is the final product of the blood coagulation (thickening). Specifically, a thrombus is a blood clot in an intact blood vessel. A thrombus in a large blood vessel will decrease blood flow through that vessel. In a small blood vessel, blood flow may be completely cut off, resulting in the death of tissue supplied by that vessel (as in a heart attack). If a thrombus dislodges and becomes free-floating, it is an embolus. The clot can partially block the flow of blood in the arteries of the heart, causing a lack of oxygen to the heart muscle tissue (called ischemia). If the clot completely stops the blood flow in an artery in the heart (called coronary artery), then a heart attack develops. If treatment is not started quickly, the affected area of heart muscle begins to die. This injury to the heart muscle can lead to serious complications and can even be fatal. It is possible to survive a heart attack, but part of the heart muscle may be damaged, causing shortness of breath or chest pain on exertion or at rest, and increases the potential to have another heart attack. It is very important if an individual has had a heart attack in the past to follow a doctor's advice in preventing another one.

The survival rate for U.S. patients hospitalized with a heart attack is approximately 90-95%. This represents a significant improvement in survival and is related to improvements in emergency medical response and treatment strategies. In general, a heart attack can occur at any age, but its incidence rises with age and depends on predisposing risk factors. Approximately 50% of all heart attacks in the United States occur in people younger than 65 years of age, but as the baby boomers age, this percentage will probably lean toward over 65. Sudden death from a heart attack can occur due to an arrhythmia (irregular heartbeat or rhythm) called ventricular fibrillation. If an individual survives a heart attack, the injured area of the heart muscle is replaced by scar tissue. This weakens the pumping action of the heart and can lead to heart failure (inability of the heart to pump blood throughout the body) and other complications including fatigue (tiredness) and fluid buildup in the feet, ankles, or around the lungs (which makes it hard to breathe). Heart attack is the leading cause of death in the United States as well as in most industrialized nations throughout the world. Approximately 800,000 people in the U.S. are affected annually, and 250,000 die prior to arrival to a hospital. Approximately every 65 seconds, an American dies of a heart-related medical emergency. The World Health Organization (WHO) estimated that in 2002, 12.6% of deaths worldwide were from ischemic heart disease (lack of oxygen to the heart).

There are several types of heart attacks. Acute coronary syndrome is a name given to three types of coronary artery disease that are associated with sudden rupture of plaque inside the coronary artery: unstable angina, non-ST segment elevation MI (NSTEMI), and ST segment elevation MI (STEMI). The location of the blockage, the length of time that blood flow is blocked, and the amount of damage that occurs determine the type of acute coronary syndrome.

Unstable Angina: Unstable angina (chest pain) can occur more frequently, occur more easily at rest, feel more severe, or last longer than stable angina. Although this angina can often be relieved with oral medications, it is unstable and may progress to a heart attack. Usually more intense medical treatment or a procedure is required. Unstable angina is an acute coronary syndrome and should be treated as a medical emergency.

Non-ST segment elevation myocardial infarction (NSTEMI): This heart attack (MI) does not cause changes on an electrocardiogram (ECG). However, chemical markers in the blood indicate that damage has occurred to the heart muscle (including C-reactive protein, creatine kinase MB, and troponin). In NSTEMI, the blockage may be partial or temporary, and so the extent of the damage to the heart is relatively minimal.

ST segment elevation myocardial infarction (STEMI): This heart attack is caused by a prolonged period of blocked blood supply (ischemia). It affects a large area of the heart muscle and causes changes on the ECG as well as in blood levels of the key chemical markers.

Atherosclerosis: Atherosclerosis is the hardening and narrowing of the arteries. It is caused by the slow buildup of plaque on the inside of walls of the arteries. Arteries are blood vessels that carry oxygen-rich blood from the heart to other parts of the body. Plaque is made up of fat, cholesterol, calcium, and other substances found in the blood. As it grows, the buildup of plaque narrows the inside of the artery and, in time, may restrict blood flow.

Coronary Artery Disease (CAD): CAD, also known as coronary heart disease, occurs when the coronary arteries gradually become narrowed or blocked by plaque deposits. This can lead to a heart attack. Unfortunately, sometimes a heart attack is the first sign of CAD. According to the Framingham Heart Study, over 50% of men and 63% of women who died suddenly of CAD (mostly from heart attack) had no previous symptoms of this disease. Some individuals who have CAD and insufficient blood flow to the heart muscle (ischemia) do not have any symptoms. This is called silent ischemia. In rare instances a patient may have a "silent heart attack," which is a heart attack without symptoms.

Risk Factors

High Blood Cholesterol: Cholesterol is a major component of the atherosclerotic plaque (particles of blood, cholesterol, and protein that "clump") that leads to blocked arteries in the heart. These blockages may lead to a heart attack. An elevated level of total cholesterol is associated with an increased risk of coronary atherosclerosis (hardening of the arteries) and heart attack. Laboratory testing provides a measure of certain types of circulating fat particles. Elevated levels of low-density lipoprotein (LDL, or bad cholesterol) are also associated with an increased incidence of both atherosclerosis and heart attack. Total cholesterol levels should be below 200 mg/dL.

Diabetes Mellitus: Individuals with diabetes have a substantially greater risk of a heart attack because it adversely affects blood cholesterol levels and increases the rate of plaque buildup.

Hypertension: High blood pressure, or hypertension, has consistently been associated with an increased risk of heart attack.

Smoking: Certain chemicals present in tobacco, or that are inhaled after lighting tobacco, are known to damage blood vessel walls. The body's response to this type of injury elicits the formation of CAD. CAD causes less oxygen to get to heart muscle tissue (ischemia) and eventually will lead to a heart attack.

Male Gender: The incidence of CAD and heart attack is higher in men than women in all age groups. This gender difference in heart attack incidence, however, narrows with increasing age. Risks for heart attack increase in men over the age of 45 and women over the age of 55. The natural estrogen produced by the body protects women from heart disease before menopause. As levels of estrogen decline, the incidence of heart disease increases.

Family History: A family history of CAD increases an individual's risk of a heart attack.

Age: Age may also increase the risk of having a heart attack. Statistics point to the fact that 83% of people who die from heart disease are 65 years of age or older.

Previous History: Having a previous history of angina (chest pain), a previous heart attack, or a surgical procedure such as angioplasty (the insertion of a catheter into the blood vessels and to the heart) may increase the risk of having a heart attack.

Obesity: A high body mass index, or a high amount of body fat, increases the chances of developing high blood pressure, heart disease, atherosclerosis (hardening of the arteries), and diabetes, all of which increase risk factors associated with a heart attack.

Elevated Homocysteine and C-Reactive Protein: The amino acid homocysteine occurs naturally in the body, but elevated levels have been linked with a high risk of heart disease and heart attack. When atherosclerosis (hardening of the arteries) damages arteries around the heart, they become inflamed, which triggers C-reactive protein production.

Medications: Certain medications may increase the risk of developing a heart attack, such as hormone replacement therapy (HRT), which contains estrogen. For a long time it was thought that HRT reduced the risk of heart disease. However, research has found that women who have had a recent heart attack or a stroke are more likely to have a second heart attack or stroke (lack of blood supply to the brain) if they start taking HRT. For this reason, starting HRT is not recommended for women with cardiovascular disease. In addition, even healthy women who begin HRT (at least with Prempro, an estrogen/progesterone combination) may have a slightly increased risk of heart attack or stroke in the first year or two of therapy.

Causes

The WHO states that 49% of heart attacks worldwide are caused by high blood pressure.

Health Conditions: Underlying health conditions can contribute to the development of a heart attack. These include emotional stress, anger, exposure to cold, exertion from exercise or sex, anemia (low iron and oxygen in the blood), coronary heart disease, atherosclerosis (hardening of the arteries), coronary thrombosis (blood clots), embolus (blood clot that comes loose and travels in the bloodstream), arrhythmias (irregular heartbeat), Fabry's disease (genetic disease leading to blood vessel damage), hyperlipidemia (high levels of fat in the blood), electrolyte imbalance (minerals such as potassium and sodium are off balance), shock, severe injury,

H

sleep apnea (pauses in breathing during sleep), hemorrhage (blood loss), electrocution, anaphylactic shock (allergic reaction that affects the entire body), hypoxia (lack of oxygen such as in suffocation), and respiratory failure (not enough oxygen getting into the bloodstream from the lungs).

Medications: Certain medications may cause a heart attack, including high-dose oral contraceptives such as Necon 1/50, Norinyl 1/50, Ortho-Novum 1/50, and Yasmin (due to an increase of blood clots); short-acting nifedipine (Procardia), a calcium channel blocker for high blood pressure that was found to increase risk of heart attack for some patients on high doses; ribavirin (Copegus, Rebetol, Ribasphere, Vilona, Virazole, antiviral drugs); and Pegatron (combination of ribavirin and peginterferon alfa-2b, an immune system agent). Amphetamines, cocaine, methamphetamine, ecstasy, ephedra, and caffeine are stimulants and may also cause a heart attack.

SIGNS AND SYMPTOMS

Classical symptoms of a heart attack (MI) in men include chest pain or pressure (heaviness), jaw pain, or extension of pain into the arms or shoulder (especially the left arm), unexplained shortness of breath, unexplained sweating, heartburn or feeling of indigestion, nausea or vomiting, back pain or upper abdominal pain, general lethargy (tiredness), heart palpitations (irregular heartbeat), anxiety, and a sudden feeling of illness.

The most common symptoms of heart attack (MI) in women include shortness of breath, weakness, and fatigue. A study found that many women reported warning symptoms one month before having a heart attack. Only 30% of women reported chest pain, which the majority of men report. Although women may not have the classical symptoms of a heart attack, they should call 911 immediately if symptoms are present.

Unfortunately, sometimes a heart attack is the first sign of CAD. According to the Framingham Heart Study, over 50% of men and 63% of women who died suddenly of CAD (mostly from heart attack) had no previous symptoms of this disease.

Approximately one fourth of all MIs are silent, without chest pain or other symptoms. Silent heart attacks can occur more frequently in people with diabetes. Symptoms of a silent heart attack can include discomfort in the chest, arms, or jaw that seems to go away after resting; shortness of breath; and tiring easily. The most common complaints of visitors to the emergency room are chest pain (angina) and shortness of breath.

The symptoms of angina (chest pain) can be similar to the symptoms of a heart attack. Angina may lead to a heart attack.

A heart attack is a process that continues over several hours unless death occurs.

DIAGNOSIS

What to Do if a Heart Attack Is Happening: The most important thing to do if an individual thinks he or she is having heart attack symptoms is to call an ambulance (911) or get to a hospital emergency room as quickly as possible (someone other than the victim must drive). It is important to stop whatever is going on and sit or lie down. If nitroglycerin has been prescribed, place one tablet under the tongue as soon as possible. One tablet under the tongue every five minutes for three doses can be tried (if no relief with the first one). Also, crush or chew a full-strength aspirin (325 milligrams, swallow with a glass of water) to prevent further blood clotting.

Do not minimize the symptoms of a heart attack and do not delay calling for help (911). Waiting more than 15 minutes to see if the pain goes away can result in permanent damage to the heart and can even result in death. It is illegal for a hospital to refuse a person having a medical emergency, regardless of their ability to pay.

If a heart attack is in the middle of happening, the hospital staff will initiate medications described in the Treatment section.

Diagnosis of a heart attack includes ECG, echocardiogram, blood tests, nuclear scan, or coronary angiography.

Electrocardiogram (ECG): The ECG test detects the electrical activity of the heart and records each heartbeat (called waves) on a graph. It is safe and painless, and it takes only a few minutes. An ECG is performed by taping electrodes on the arms, legs, and chest. The electrodes pick up the electrical impulses of the heart from different points of view in the chest. ECG abnormalities diagnostic of heart attack are sometimes seen early in a heart attack, but the ECG may be normal at first and need to be repeated. Sometimes existing ECG abnormalities may make the diagnosis difficult.

Echocardiogram (Echo): This is an ultrasound examination of the heart. The ultrasound device uses sound waves to create a detailed "picture" of the heart, which is then transmitted to a video monitor. This test is safe, noninvasive, and very helpful. A wand is used that is rubbed over the heart area. The chest is lubricated with petroleum jelly so the wand slides easily over the area. Echo may show problems in the heart structure, such as abnormalities in the movements of the heart wall (a heart attack damages the heart wall). It can show abnormal enlargement or pouching of the heart wall (aneurysm). Echo may also visualize complications of heart attack, such as valve problems, rupture of the heart muscle, or accumulation of fluid in the cardiac sac (pericardial effusion). The most important information obtained from the echo is the ejection fraction. This is a measurement of the strength of heart muscle. This information may be used to help predict outcome and to decide on treatment after a heart attack.

Blood Tests: Blood tests include blood cell counts as well as measurements of electrolytes (sodium, potassium, calcium, magnesium, and other minerals), blood chemistry, homocysteine and/or C-reactive protein (both markers of inflammation), and coagulation (clotting) function (fibrinogen). A blood test will be done to check for enzymes (proteins that start chemical reactions in the body) or other proteins that are released when heart cells begin to die. These are "markers" of the amount of damage to the heart. The two most measured enzymes are creatine phosphokinase (CPK) and troponin.

CPK, or creatine kinase, is released from the heart muscle cells as they die and as their membranes dissolve. The level of the CPK enzyme (specifically the MB subform of the enzyme) takes a number of hours after the beginning of the heart attack to peak. It returns to normal by 24 hours after the beginning of the heart attack.

Troponin I and troponin T are also used to determine if a heart attack has occurred. The levels of these enzymes rise by 6-8 hours after the heart attack begins and remain elevated above normal for as long as a week. To some extent, the level of troponin can predict the likelihood of complications for an individual who has experienced a heart attack. The levels may also be helpful in deciding what treatments should be used.

Myoglobin test checks for the presence of myoglobin (a protein found in muscle tissue) in the blood. Myoglobin is released when the heart or other muscle is injured.

Cardiac Stress Test: A stress test determines how well the blood is flowing to the heart during exercise compared to resting. The patient either walks on a treadmill or is given intravenous (IV) medication that simulates exercise (usually dipyridamole [Persantine]) while connected to an ECG machine. The exercise stress test is about 60-70% accurate in predicting increased risk of future heart attacks.

Nuclear Scans: These tests shows areas of the heart that lack blood flow and are damaged. They also can reveal problems with the heart's pumping action. Radionuclide ventriculograms, also known as multiple gated acquisitions, are the radionuclear tests (tests using radioactive materials) normally performed. A small amount of radioactive material (usually technetium-99 m) attached to a carrier (a substance that will travel to a particular organ, such as the heart) is injected into a vein, usually in the arm. The radioactivity and carrier then travels to the heart, and a scanning camera positioned over the heart records whether the nuclear material is taken up by the heart muscle or not. This determines if there are blockages in blood flow within the heart muscle. Like the exercise stress test, pictures are obtained with exercise on the treadmill and then with rest. The camera also can evaluate how well the heart muscle pumps blood. This test can be done during both rest and exercise, enhancing the usefulness of its results. This test is quite accurate in diagnosing coronary artery blockage. The small amount of radioactivity used in the test is not considered to be harmful.

Coronary Angiography: A coronary angiography test is used to check blockages and narrowed areas inside coronary arteries. A fine tube is threaded through an artery of an arm or leg up into the heart. A dye that shows up on x-ray is then injected into the blood vessel, and the vessels and heart are filmed as the heart pumps. The picture is called an angiogram or arteriogram. It often is performed for people with persistent pain and those who have not received "clot-busting" drugs to re-open their blocked artery. Coronary angiography is an invasive test with potentially serious complications, but when performed by an experienced doctor, the risk of complications is relatively small. An angiogram is the best test to determine what treatment is most appropriate: medication, angioplasty (the mechanical widening of a narrowed or totally obstructed blood vessel), stent (a wire mesh that expands inside a blood vessel; may contain anticlotting drugs) placement, or bypass surgery.

COMPLICATIONS

The lack of blood flow to the heart can lead to irreversible damage to the heart muscle. Invasive surgery may be required (coronary artery bypass graft surgery). Death that occurs suddenly after the onset of a heart attack is most often due to unstable electrical rhythms, specifically ventricular tachycardia and ventricular fibrillation, which do not allow the pumping chamber of the heart (ventricle) to pump efficiently and use up its supply of oxygen. This event can be rapidly reversed with the use of medications or shocks from a defibrillator.

H

Other complications from a heart attack include heart blocks, congestive heart failure (the inability of the heart to fill with or pump a sufficient amount of blood to the body), cardiogenic shock (inadequate circulation of blood due to primary failure of the ventricles of the heart to function effectively), infarct extension (an increase of the amount of affected heart tissue), pericarditis (inflammation around the lining of the heart), pulmonary embolism (blood clot in the lungs), valve problems, rupture of the heart muscle, or accumulation of fluid in the cardiac sac (pericardial effusion).

TREATMENT

A heart attack is a medical emergency that demands immediate attention. The faster an individual is treated in the acute phase of a heart attack, the greater the ability to prevent further complications. As time passes, the risk of damage to the heart muscle increases. If an individual thinks he or she is having a heart attack based on the symptoms described, call 911 emergency immediately. Not seeking medical attention can cause serious damage to the heart muscle and even death.

First-Line Treatment: After a heart attack victim is brought to the hospital, oxygen will be started, 160-325 milligrams of aspirin will be given immediately, nitroglycerin (which dilates blood vessels and allows more oxygen to the tissue) will be given under the tongue or intravenously (in the veins), and analgesia (usually morphine) will be given intravenously. In many areas, first responders can be trained to administer these prior to arrival at the hospital.

Thrombolytic Therapy: Thrombolytic therapy, also known as clot busting, is indicated for the treatment of STEMI. Clot busting is used if the drug can be administered within 12 hours of the onset of symptoms, the patient is eligible based on exclusion criteria, and primary percutaneous coronary intervention (PCI) is not immediately available. The effectiveness of thrombolytic therapy is highest in the first two hours after a heart attack. Twelve hours after a heart attack, the risks associated with thrombolytic therapy, such as bleeding and stroke, outweigh any benefit. Because irreversible injury to the heart muscle occurs within two to four hours of the heart attack due to a lack of blood flow and oxygen, there is a limited window of time available for reperfusion to work.

Thrombolytic drugs are not used for the treatment of unstable angina, NSTEMI, and for the treatment of individuals with evidence of cardiogenic shock (primary failure of the ventricles of the heart to function effectively).

Currently available thrombolytic agents include streptokinase, urokinase, and tissue plasminogen activator (tPA [Alteplase]). More recently, thrombolytic agents similar in structure to tPA such as reteplase (Retavase) and tenecteplase (TNKase) have been used. These newer agents are easier to administer than tPA. However, all these agents are very expensive. If tPA and related agents are used, other anticoagulation (blood thinning) with heparin or low molecular weight heparin is needed to keep the coronary artery open. Because urokinase and streptokinase have anticoagulant activity, heparin use is less necessary when using these thrombolytic agents.

Thrombolytic therapy is not always successful and has a 10-20% failure rate. If the thrombolytic agent fails to open the infarct-related coronary artery, the patient is then either treated with anticoagulants or PCI is then performed. Complications, particularly bleeding, are significantly higher with rescue PCI than with primary PCI due to the increase bleeding associated with the thrombolytic agent.

Percutaneous Coronary Intervention (PCI): The use of PCI as a therapy to stop a MI (heart attack) is known as primary PCI. The goal of primary PCI is to open the artery as soon as possible, preferably within 90 minutes of the individual coming to the hospital. This time is referred to as the door-to-balloon time. Few hospitals can provide PCI within the 90-minute interval. The current guidelines in the United States restrict primary PCI to hospitals with available emergency bypass surgery as a backup, but this is not the case in other parts of the world. Primary PCI involves performing a coronary angiogram (injection of dye and then an x-ray to look at the blood vessels) to determine the location of the blocked vessel, followed by balloon angioplasty (the mechanical widening of a narrowed or totally obstructed blood vessel), and frequently deployment of a stent (an expandable wire mesh that is placed in a blocked coronary artery and opened; sometimes contains anticoagulant drugs). While the use of stents does not improve the short-term outcomes in primary PCI, the use of stents is widespread because of the decreased rates of procedures to treat restenosis (reclogging) compared to balloon angioplasty. Other therapies used during primary PCI include IV heparin, aspirin, or clopidogrel (Plavix).

Glycoprotein IIb/IIIa Inhibitors: Glycoprotein IIb/IIIa receptors on platelets (cells of the clotting system) bind to fibrinogen in the final common pathway of platelet aggregation. Antagonists (opposing) to glycoprotein IIb/IIIa receptors are potent inhibitors of platelet aggregation; drugs include abciximab

(ReoPro), eptifibatide (Integrilin), and tirofiban (Aggrastat). The use of IV glycoprotein IIb/IIIa inhibitors during PCI and in patients with heart attack or acute coronary syndromes has been reported to reduce death and reinfarction (re-blockage). Side effects include an increase in bleeding.

Angiotensin-Converting Enzyme Inhibitors (ACEIs): Oral angiotensin converting enzyme inhibitors (ACEIs, such as lisinopril (Prinivil, Zestril)) dilate blood vessels and increase oxygen to the heart. ACE inhibitor therapy should be started 24-48 hours after a heart attack, particularly in patients with a history of heart attacks, diabetes mellitus, hypertension, anterior (front) location of infarct (blockage), and/ or evidence of left ventricular dysfunction. ACEIs reduce mortality, the development of heart failure, and decrease ventricular remodeling (changes in size and shape of heart valves) after the heart attack. Contra-indications for ACEIs include hypotension (low blood pressure) and declining kidney function with ACEI use.

Coronary Artery Bypass Graft (CABG) Surgery: CABG surgery bypasses one or more blocked blood vessels by a blood vessel graft to restore normal blood flow to the heart. These grafts usually come from the patient's own arteries and veins located in the chest, leg, or arm. The graft goes around the clogged artery to create new pathways for oxygen-rich blood to flow to the heart. Some problems associated with CABG include a heart attack (occurs in 5% of patients), stroke (occurs in 5%, with the risk greatest in those over 70 years old), blood clots, death (occurs in 1-2% of individuals), and sternal wound infection (occurs in 1-4%). Infection is most often associated with obesity, diabetes, or having had a previous CABG. In about 30% of patients, post-pericardiotomy syndrome can occur anywhere from a few days to six months after surgery. The symptoms of this syndrome are fever and chest pain. This condition can be treated with medications. The incision in the chest or the graft site (if the graft was from the leg or arm) can be itchy, sore, numb, or bruised. Some individuals report memory loss and loss of mental clarity or "fuzzy thinking" following CABG.

Sometimes surgeons can perform open heart surgery without using a bypass pump and while the heart is beating (off-pump bypass surgery). The procedure causes fewer side effects than the standard procedure, but it is not practical in all situations. If just the front or right coronary arteries need bypass, a surgeon may replace the blocked artery with an artery from the chest via a small keyhole incision, without opening the chest, to detour the blockage (minimally invasive coronary bypass). This procedure also decreases the many problems associated with conventional CABG.

Monitoring for Arrhythmias: After a heart attack, monitoring for life-threatening arrhythmias (irregular heartbeat) or conduction disturbances is performed in a coronary care unit in the hospital. The patient will be given a type of drug called an antiarrhythmic agent such as amlodipine (Norvasc) or diltiazem (Cardizem) if arrhythmias are found.

Rehabilitation: Cardiac rehabilitation is a medically supervised program to help heart patients recover quickly and improve their overall physical and mental functioning. Cardiac rehabilitation is performed to optimize function and quality of life in those afflicted with a heart disease. This can be with the help of a physician or in the form of a cardiac rehabilitation program. Physical exercise may have beneficial effects on cholesterol, blood pressure, weight, and stress and is an important part of rehabilitation after a heart attack. An exercise program will be given to the patient by their health care provider. Some individuals are afraid to have sex after a heart attack. Most people can resume sexual activities after three to four weeks. The amount of activity needs to be determined by the patient's healthcare provider.

Secondary Prevention: The risk of a recurrent MI decreases with blood pressure management and lifestyle changes, including smoking cessation, regular exercise, a sensible diet (more fresh fruits and vegetables and a decrease in red meats, junk food, and saturated and trans fats), and limitation of alcohol intake (no more than two drinks daily). Medications including nitrates, antiplatelet drugs (aspirin), beta-blockers, ACEIs, and statins are used commonly after a heart attack.

Nitroglycerin: Sublingual (under the tongue, tablets or spray), oral, or topical (on the skin) nitrates are given to individuals after suffering a heart attack. Nitrates dilate (expand) blood vessels and allow more blood and oxygen to flow to heart tissue. When taken sublingually or intravenously, nitroglycerin works rapidly. Clinical trial data support the initial use of nitroglycerin for up to 48 hours in heart attack. There is little evidence that nitroglycerin provides substantive benefit as a long-term post-MI (after a heart attack) therapy except when severe pump dysfunction or residual ischemia (lack of blood flow and oxygen) is present. Nitrate tolerance (when nitrates no longer work as well) can be overcome either by increasing the dose or by providing a daily nitrate-free interval of eight to 12 hours. Side effects include hypotension (low blood pressure) and headache.

Antiplatelet Drug Therapy: Antiplatelet drugs such as aspirin and/or clopidogrel (Plavix) should be continued to reduce the risk of plaque rupture and recurrent MI. Aspirin is used for first-line (immediately) treatment owing to its low cost and comparable efficacy (effectiveness), with clopidogrel reserved for patients intolerant of aspirin. The combination of clopidogrel and aspirin may further reduce risk of heart attack; however, the risk of hemorrhage (bleeding) is increased. Side effects include many drug interactions and an increased risk of bleeding.

Beta-Blockers: Beta-blocker therapy such as metoprolol (Lopressor, Toprol) or atenolol (Tenormin) should be started. These have been particularly beneficial in high-risk patients such as those with left ventricular dysfunction and/or continuing cardiac ischemia (lack of blood flow and oxygen). They also improve symptoms of cardiac ischemia (lack of oxygen and blood flow to the heart) in NSTEMI (a type of arrhythmia). Side effects associated with beta-blockers include insomnia, loss of sexual drive, and tiredness (fatigue).

Statin Drugs: Statins (3-hydroxy-3-methylglutaryl coenzyme A [HMG-CoA] reductase inhibitors), such as atorvastatin (Lipitor) or lovastatin (Mevacor), help lower cholesterol levels and have been reported to reduce mortality and morbidity after a heart attack. Statin use may cause liver problems or muscle pain and can deplete coenzyme Q10 levels.

Other Medications: The aldosterone antagonist agent eplerenone (Inspra) has been reported to further reduce risk of cardiovascular death after a heart attack in patients with heart failure and left ventricular dysfunction when used in conjunction with standard therapies such as antiplatelet drugs and statins. Aldosterone is a hormone associated with sodium and potassium balance and fluid retention.

Fish Oil: Omega-3 fatty acids, commonly found in cold water fish (such as salmon and halibut), have been reported to reduce death after a heart attack. However, further studies have not shown a clear-cut decrease in potentially fatal arrhythmias (irregular heartbeat) due to omega-3 fatty acids. Fish oils may cause an increase in bleeding if taken with antiplatelet or anticoagulant medications.

Automated Implantable Cardiac Defibrillators (AICDs): Studies have found that AICDs in patients post-MI (after a heart attack) may be beneficial. A 31% risk reduction in all-cause mortality was found with the prophylactic (preventative) use of an AICD in patients post-MI with ejection fractions less than 30%. Cost therapy and benefits are weighed before a doctor uses this device.

Emerging Therapies: Therapies in development for patients suffering from a heart attack include stem cell treatment and tissue engineering (growing healthy heart tissue).

INTEGRATIVE THERAPIES

Integrative therapies for a heart attack include supplements that may lower cholesterol, decrease blood pressure, protect the heart, and decrease stress.

Strong Scientific Evidence

Beta-Glucan: Beta-glucan is a soluble fiber derived from the cell walls of algae, bacteria, fungi, yeast, and plants. It is commonly used for its cholesterol-lowering effects. Numerous trials have examined the effects of oral beta-glucan on cholesterol. Small reductions in total and LDL cholesterol ("bad cholesterol") have been reported. Little to no significant changes have been noted to occur on triglyceride levels or high-density lipoprotein (HDL, "good cholesterol") levels. The sum of existing evidence is suggestive and not definitive. Caution is advised when taking beta-glucan supplements, as numerous adverse effects including drug interactions are possible. Beta-glucan supplements are not generally used during pregnancy or breastfeeding unless otherwise advised by a doctor.

Beta-Sitosterol: Beta-sitosterol is one of the most common dietary plant sterols (chemical found in certain plants) found and synthesized exclusively by plants such as fruits, vegetables, soybeans, breads, peanuts, and peanut products. Many studies in humans and animals have demonstrated that eating more foods that contain beta-sitosterol decreases total serum cholesterol as well as LDL cholesterol. Caution is advised when taking beta-sitosterol supplements, as numerous adverse effects including drug interactions are possible. Beta-sitosterol supplements are not generally used during pregnancy or breastfeeding unless otherwise advised by a doctor.

Niacin: Niacin, also known as vitamin B_3 or nicotinic acid, is a well-accepted treatment for high cholesterol. Multiple studies show that niacin (not niacinamide) has significant benefits on levels of HDL ("good cholesterol"), with better results than prescription drugs such as statins (atorvastatin [Lipitor]). There are also benefits on levels LDL ("bad cholesterol"), although these effects are less dramatic. Adding niacin therapy as a second drug when using a statin may increase the effects on LDL. The use of niacin for the treatment of high blood cholesterol associated with type 2 diabetes has been controversial because of the possibility of worsening blood sugar control. Individuals should check with a physician and pharmacist before starting niacin.

Omega-3 Fatty Acids: Omega-3 fatty acids are essential fatty acids found in some plants and fish. There should be a balance of omega-6 and omega-3 fatty acids for health. There is strong scientific evidence from human trials that omega-3 fatty acids from fish or fish oil supplements significantly reduce blood triglyceride levels. Fish oil supplements also appear to cause small improvements in HDL ("good cholesterol"); however, increases (worsening) in LDL ("bad cholesterol") are also observed. Several well-conducted randomized, controlled trials report that in people with a history of heart attack, regular consumption of oily fish or fish oil/omega-3 supplements reduces the risk of nonfatal heart attack, fatal heart attack, sudden death, and all-cause mortality (death due to any cause). Most patients in these studies were also using conventional heart drugs, suggesting that the benefits of fish oils may add to the effects of other therapies. Preliminary studies also report reductions in angina associated with fish oil intake. Better research is necessary before a firm conclusion can be drawn. Caution is advised when taking omega-3 supplements as numerous adverse effects, including an increase in bleeding and drug interactions, are possible. Omega-3 supplements should not be used if pregnant or breastfeeding unless otherwise directed by a doctor.

Policosanol: Policosanol is a cholesterol-lowering natural mixture of higher aliphatic primary alcohols isolated and purified from sugar cane wax. Policosanol has been used to treat high cholesterol levels, and numerous studies have analyzed the effects of policosanol on cholesterol levels, including a number of well-designed trials. At this time, the evidence supporting the efficacy of this agent is compelling, although greater acceptance in the U.S. market may await completion of a large, well-conducted, randomized trial in the United States. Caution is advised when taking policosanol, as adverse effects including drug interactions are possible. Policosanol supplements should not be used if pregnant or breastfeeding unless otherwise directed by a doctor.

Psyllium: Psyllium (*Plantago ovata*), also referred to as ispaghula, is derived from the husks of the seeds of psyllium. Psyllium contains a high level of soluble dietary fiber and is the chief ingredient in many commonly used bulk laxatives, including products such as Metamucil and Serutan. Psyllium is well studied as a cholesterol-lowering agent, with generally modest reductions seen in blood levels of total cholesterol and LDL ("bad cholesterol"). Effects have been observed following eight weeks of regular use. Psyllium does not appear to have significant effects on HDL ("good cholesterol") or triglyceride levels. Because only small reductions have been observed, people with high cholesterol should discuss the use of more potent agents with their health care providers. Effects have been observed in adults and children, although long-term safety in children is not established. Psyllium can decrease the absorption of many prescription and nonprescription medications and dietary supplements.

Red Yeast Rice: Red yeast rice is the product of yeast (*Monascus purpureus*) grown on rice, and the resulting product is served as a dietary staple in some Asian countries. It contains several compounds collectively known as monacolins, substances known to inhibit cholesterol synthesis. One of these, monacolin K, is a potent inhibitor of HMG-CoA reductase and is also known as lovastatin (Mevacor). Preliminary evidence reports that taking red yeast rice by mouth may result in heart benefits and improve blood flow. Since the 1970s, human studies have reported that red yeast lowers blood levels of total cholesterol, LDL ("bad cholesterol"), and triglyceride levels. Caution is advised when taking red yeast rice supplements, as adverse effects including drug interactions are possible. Red yeast rice supplements should not be used if pregnant or breastfeeding unless otherwise directed by a doctor. Red yeast rice should not be used in people with liver problems or in heavy alcohol users.

Soy: Soy (*Glycine max*) is a member of the pea family and has been a dietary staple in Asian countries for at least 5,000 years. Numerous human studies report that adding soy protein to the diet can moderately decrease blood levels of total cholesterol and LDL ("bad cholesterol"). Small reductions in triglycerides may also occur, while HDL ("good cholesterol") does not seem to be significantly altered. Dietary soy protein has not been proven to affect long-term cardiovascular outcomes such as heart attack or stroke. Soy products such as tofu are high in protein and are an acceptable source of dietary protein. Caution is advised when taking soy supplements, as adverse effects including drug interactions are possible. Soy supplements should not be used if pregnant or breastfeeding unless otherwise directed by a doctor.

Good Scientific Evidence

Betaine: Betaine is found in most microorganisms, plants, and marine animals. Its main physiological functions are to protect cells under stress and to serve as a source of methyl groups needed for many biochemical pathways. Betaine is also found naturally in many foods and is most highly concentrated in beets, spinach, grain, and shellfish. Overall, betaine supplementation may produce significant reductions in homocysteine, a known risk factor of CAD. However, additional studies are needed. Betaine supplements should not be used if pregnant or breastfeeding unless otherwise directed by a doctor.

Cordyceps: *Cordyceps sinensis* is a fungus found mainly in China, Nepal, and Tibet. Cordyceps supplements may lower total cholesterol and triglyceride levels, although these changes may not be permanent or long lasting. Longer studies with follow-up are needed to determine the long-term effects of cordyceps on hyperlipidemia. Caution is advised when taking cordyceps supplements, as adverse effects including drug interactions are possible. Cordyceps supplements should not be used if pregnant or breastfeeding unless otherwise directed by a doctor.

Garlic: Garlic (*Allium sativum*) is traditionally used for heart health. Multiple studies in humans have reported small reductions in total blood cholesterol and LDL ("bad cholesterol") over short periods of time (4 to 12 weeks). It is not clear if there are benefits after this amount of time. Effects on HDL ("good cholesterol") are not clear. This remains an area of controversy. Well-designed and longer studies are needed in this area. Caution is advised when taking garlic supplements as adverse effects, including an increase in bleeding and drug interactions, are possible. Garlic supplements should not be used if pregnant or breastfeeding unless otherwise directed by a doctor.

L-Carnitine: L-carnitine, or acetyl-L-carnitine, is an amino acid found in the body. Evidence from clinical trials suggests that L-carnitine is effective in reducing symptoms of angina. Carnitine may not offer further benefit when patients continue conventional therapies. Additional study is needed to confirm these findings. L-carnitine is generally safe when used in recommended dosages.

Yoga: Yoga is an ancient system of relaxation, exercise, and healing with origins in Indian philosophy. Several human studies suggest that yoga is helpful in people with heart disease. However, it is not clear if yoga reduces the risk of heart attack or death, or if yoga is better than any other form of exercise therapy or lifestyle/dietary change. Therefore, yoga may be a useful addition to standard therapies (such as medications for blood pressure or cholesterol) in people at risk for heart attacks, but further research is necessary.

Unclear or Conflicting Scientific Evidence

Acupuncture: The practice of acupuncture, or the insertion of needles, originated in China 5,000 years ago. Some research has suggested that acupuncture might help reduce distress and symptoms of angina, but this has not been consistently shown in other studies.

L-Arginine: L-arginine, or arginine, is considered a semiessential amino acid because although it is normally synthesized in sufficient amounts by the body, supplementation is sometimes required. There is initial evidence from several studies that arginine taken by mouth or by injection improves exercise tolerance and blood flow in arteries of the heart. Benefits have been reported in some patients with CAD and angina. Studies also suggest that arginine supplementation after MI (heart attack) may decrease the heart damage. However, further research is needed to confirm these findings. L-arginine is generally safe in recommended dosages.

Astragalus: Astragalus products are derived from the roots of *Astragalus membranaceus* or related species, which are native to China. In Chinese medicine, herbal mixtures containing astragalus have been used to treat heart diseases. There are several human case reports of reduced symptoms and improved heart function, although these are not well described. High-quality human research is necessary before a conclusion can be drawn. Caution is advised when taking astragalus supplements, as adverse effects including drug interactions are possible. Astragalus supplements should not be used if pregnant or breastfeeding unless otherwise directed by a doctor.

Bilberry: Bilberry (*Vaccinium myrtillus*), also known as the European blueberry, is widely used as an antioxidant for general health. Bilberry has been used traditionally to treat heart disease and atherosclerosis. There is some laboratory research in this area, but there is no clear information in humans. Caution is advised when taking bilberry supplements as adverse effects, including an increase in bleeding and drug interactions, are possible. Bilberry supplements should not be used if pregnant or breastfeeding unless otherwise directed by a doctor.

Coenzyme Q10 (CoQ10): CoQ10 is produced by the human body and is necessary for the basic functioning of cells. Preliminary small human studies suggest that CoQ10 may reduce angina and improve exercise tolerance in people with clogged heart arteries. Several studies also suggest that the function of the heart may be improved after major heart surgeries such as CABG or valve replacement when CoQ10 is given to patients before or during surgery. Better studies are needed. CoQ10 is generally safe in recommended dosages.

Ginseng: Asian ginseng, or *Panax* ginseng, has been used for more than 2,000 years in Chinese medicine for various health conditions. Several studies from China report that ginseng in combination with various other herbs may reduce symptoms of CAD. Ginseng may also lower blood pressure. Caution is advised when taking ginseng supplements, as adverse effects including drug interactions are possible. Ginseng supplements should not be used if pregnant or breastfeeding unless otherwise directed by a doctor.

Green Tea: Green tea is made from the dried leaves of *Camellia sinensis,* a perennial evergreen shrub. Green tea has a long history of use, dating back to China approximately 5,000 years ago. Green tea, black tea, and oolong tea are all derived from the same plant, but the leaves are processed differently. There is evidence that regular intake of green tea may lower cholesterol levels and reduce the risk of heart attack or atherosclerosis (clogged arteries). Caution is advised when taking green tea supplements, as adverse effects including drug interactions are possible. Green tea supplements should not be used if pregnant or breastfeeding unless otherwise directed by a doctor.

Hawthorn: Hawthorn (*Crataegus* spp.), a flowering shrub of the rose family, has an extensive history of use in cardiovascular disease dating back to the first century. Increased blood flow to the heart and heart performance have been observed in animals when given hawthorn supplements, and one randomized clinical trial indicates that hawthorn may be effective in decreasing frequency or severity of anginal symptoms. Hawthorn has not been tested in the setting of concomitant drugs such as beta-blockers or ACEIs, which are often considered to be standard of care. At this time, there is insufficient evidence to recommend for or against hawthorn for CAD or angina. Caution is advised when taking hawthorn supplements, as adverse effects including drug interactions are possible. Hawthorn supplements should not be used if pregnant or breastfeeding unless otherwise directed by a doctor.

Kudzu: Kudzu (*Pueria lobota*) is well known to people in the Southeastern United States as an invasive weed, but it has been used in Chinese medicine for centuries. Kudzu has a long history of use in the treatment of cardiovascular disorders, including angina, acute MI, and heart failure. A small number of poorly designed trials found kudzu to reduce the frequency of angina events in human subjects. Overall, the studies have been methodologically weak. Caution is advised when taking kudzu supplements, as adverse effects including drug interactions are possible. Kudzu supplements should not be used if pregnant or breastfeeding unless otherwise directed by a doctor.

Kundalini Yoga: Kundalini yoga is one of many traditions of yoga that shares common roots in ancient Indian philosophy. It is comprehensive in that it combines physical poses with breath control exercises, chanting (mantras), meditations, prayer, visualizations, and guided relaxation. One case series report, but no formal clinical trials, suggests that breathing techniques used in Kundalini yoga may help people with angina pectoris reduce symptoms and need for medication. A specific breathing technique of Kundalini yoga reputed to help prevent heart attacks was examined in one study to determine its effects on heart function. The technique is a one breath per minute respiratory exercise with slow inspiration for 20 seconds, breath retention for 20 seconds, and slow expiration for 20 seconds, for 31 consecutive minutes. The technique was found to stabilize the heart's electrical wave patterns, which may have preventive value in heart health.

Prayer: Prayer has far-reaching healing effects that are hard to study. Initial studies in patients with heart disease report variable effects on severity of illness, complications during hospitalization, procedure outcome, and death rates when intercessory prayer is used. Results are found only when people know that others might be praying for them.

Psychotherapy: Psychotherapy is an interactive process between a person and a qualified mental health professional (psychiatrist, psychologist, clinical social worker, licensed counselor, or other trained practitioner). Its purpose is the exploration of thoughts, feelings, and behavior for the purpose of problem solving or achieving higher levels of functioning. Alexithymia, or the inability to express one's feelings, may influence the course of CAD. Educational sessions and group psychotherapy may decrease alexithymia and reduce cardiac events.

Quercetin: Quercetin is one of the almost 4,000 bioflavonoids (antioxidants) that occur in foods of plant origin, such as red wine, onions, green tea, apples, berries, and Brassica vegetables (cabbage, broccoli, cauliflower, turnips). Several of the effects of flavonoids that have been observed in laboratory and animal studies suggest that they might be effective in reducing cardiovascular disease risk. Studies in humans using polyphenolic compounds from red grapes showed improvement in endothelial function in patients with coronary heart disease. Antioxidant and cholesterol-lowering effects are proposed.

Reishi: Reishi (*Ganoderma lucidum*) is a mushroom that grows wild on decaying logs and tree stumps. Reishi has been used in traditional Chinese medicine for more than 4,000 years to treat liver disorders, high blood pressure, arthritis, and other ailments. A reishi supplement was reported to improve the major symptoms of coronary heart disease (e.g., angina [chest pain], palpitations, shortness of breath, blood pressure, and cholesterol) in patients. Long-term studies are needed to evaluate the efficacy and safety of reishi in coronary heart disease. Caution is advised when taking reishi supplements as adverse effects, including an increase in bleeding and drug interactions, are possible. Reishi supplements should not be used if pregnant or breastfeeding unless otherwise directed by a doctor.

Relaxation Therapy: Relaxation techniques include behavioral therapeutic approaches that differ widely in philosophy, methodology, and practice. The primary goal is usually nondirected relaxation. Most techniques share the components of repetitive focus (on a word, sound, prayer phrase, body sensation, or muscular activity), adoption of a passive attitude towards intruding thoughts, and return to the focus.

Resveratrol: Resveratrol is found in over 70 plant species, including nuts, grapes, pine trees, certain vines, and red wine. Resveratrol is used as an antioxidant in various health conditions, including heart disease prevention. Laboratory animal studies suggest resveratrol helps restore blood flow to the heart. Well-designed clinical trials in humans using resveratrol are needed. Caution is advised when taking resveratrol supplements as adverse effects, including an increase in bleeding and drug interactions, are possible. Resveratrol supplements should not be used if pregnant or breastfeeding unless otherwise directed by a doctor.

Tai Chi: Tai chi is a system of movements and positions believed to have developed in twelfth century China. Tai chi techniques aim to address the body and mind as an interconnected system and are traditionally believed to have mental and physical health benefits to improve posture, balance, flexibility, and strength. There is evidence that suggests tai chi decreases blood pressure and cholesterol as well as enhances quality of life in patients with chronic heart failure. Most studies have used elderly Chinese patients as their population. Additional research is needed before a firm conclusion can be drawn.

Vitamin B_{12}: Vitamin B_{12} (or cyanocobalamin) is an essential water-soluble vitamin that is commonly found in a variety of foods such as fish, shellfish, meats, and dairy products. Vitamin B_{12} is frequently used in combination with other B vitamins in a vitamin B–complex formulation. Folic acid, pyridoxine (vitamin B_6), and vitamin B_{12} supplementation can reduce total homocysteine levels (a known risk factor of CAD). However, this reduction does not seem to help with secondary prevention of death or cardiovascular events such as stroke or MI in people with prior stroke. More evidence is needed to fully explain the association of total homocysteine levels with vascular risk and the potential use of vitamin supplementation.

Vitamin B_6: Vitamin B_6, or pyridoxine, is found in cereal grains, legumes, vegetables (carrots, spinach, peas), potatoes, milk, cheese, eggs, fish, liver, meat, and flour. Mild deficiencies of this B vitamin are common. Vitamin B_6 may help lower homocysteine levels. Also, decreased vitamin B_6 concentrations are also associated with increased plasma levels of C-reactive protein. C-reactive protein is an indicator of inflammation that is associated with increased cardiovascular morbidity in epidemiological studies.

Vitamin E: Vitamin E is a fat-soluble vitamin with antioxidant properties. Vitamin E has been suggested and evaluated in patients with angina, although possible benefits remain unclear. Vitamin E has been proposed to have a role in preventing or reversing atherosclerosis by inhibiting oxidation of LDL ("bad cholesterol"). Several population studies have suggested that a high dietary intake of vitamin E and high blood concentrations of alpha-tocopherol are associated with lower rates of heart disease. However, while the Cambridge Heart Antioxidant Study supported this hypothesis, the more recent prospective Heart Outcomes Prevention Evaluation study did not. This area remains controversial.

Other: Other supplements that may have benefit in reducing the risk of developing CAD and heart attack include alfalfa (*Medicago sativa*), aortic acid, ashwagandha (*Withania somnifera*), astaxanthin, avocado (*Persea americana*), Ayurveda, barley (*Hordeum vulgare*), berberine, carob (*Ceratonia siliqua*), chamomile (*Matricaria recutita, Chamaemelum nobile*), chondroitin sulfate, coleus (*Coleus forskohlii*), copper, creatine, danshen (*Salvia miltiorrhiza*), dehydroepiandrosterone, dong quai (*Angelica sinensis*), elder (*Sambucus nigra*), fenugreek (*Trigonella foenum-graecum*), flaxseed and flaxseed oil (*Linum usitatissimum*), folate (folic acid), gamma oryzanol, globe artichoke (*Cynara scolymus*), goldenseal (*Hydrastis canadensis*), grapefruit (*Citrus paradisi*), guggul (*Commiphora mukul*), gymnema (*Gymnema sylvestre R. Br.*), honey, horny goat weed (*Epimedium grandiflorum*), *Lactobacillus acidophilus,* lemongrass (*Cymbopogon* spp.), lycopene, macrobiotic diet, meditation, milk thistle (*Silybum marianum*), nopal (*Opuntia* spp.), ozone therapy, pantethine (pantothenic acid), physical therapy, pomegranate (*Punica granatum*), probiotics, Pycnogenol (*Pinus pinaster* spp. *atlantica*), Red clover (*Trifolium pratense*), rhubarb (*Rheum officinale, Rheum palmatum*), safflower (*Carthamus tinctorius*), scotch broom (*Cytisus scoparius*), selenium, spirulina, squill (*Urginea maritima, Scilla maritima*), sweet almond (*Prunus amygdalus dulcis*), taurine, transcutaneous electrical nerve stimulation, traditional Chinese medicine, tribulus (*Tribulus terrestris*), turmeric (*Curcuma longa*), vitamin D, white horehound (*Marrubium vulgare*), wild yam (*Dioscoreaceae villosa*), and zinc.

PREVENTION

Control High Blood Pressure (Hypertension): One of the most important things that can be done for prevention of a heart attack is to reduce high blood pressure. Blood pressure should be a systolic reading of 120 and a diastolic reading of 80 (120/80 mm Hg). Exercising, managing stress, maintaining a healthy weight, and limiting sodium (salt) and alcohol intake are all ways to keep blood pressure in check. Medications to treat hypertension, such as diuretics, ACEIs, and angiotensin receptor blockers may be used.

Lower Cholesterol and Saturated Fat Intake: Eating less cholesterol and fat, especially saturated fat, may reduce the amount of plaque (deposits) in the arteries. Most people should aim for an LDL level below 130 mg/dL. If there are other risk factors for heart disease, the target LDL may be below 100 mg/dL. If the individuals are at very high risk for heart disease, such as having a previous heart attack, an LDL level below 70 mg/dL may be optimal. Statin drugs (HMG-CoA reductase inhibitors, such as lovastatin [Mevacor]) can be prescribed to help maintain healthy cholesterol levels.

Platelet Inhibitors: Platelet inhibitors keep platelets from clumping together. In otherwise healthy men older than 50 years, aspirin 325 mg every other day prevents MI (at a rate of two men per 1,000) but not stroke. In otherwise healthy women older than 45 years, aspirin 100 mg every other day prevents ischemic stroke (at a rate of three women per 1,000) but not MI. Aspirin may increase the risk of gastrointestinal bleeding. Other platelet inhibitors include dipyridamole (Persantine), ticlopidine (Ticlid), and clopidogrel (Plavix). A 15% relative risk reduction in vascular events (stroke, heart attack, and death) has been documented for aspirin compared with placebo.

Smoking Cessation: Smoking is a major risk factor for CAD and heart attack. Nicotine constricts blood vessels and forces the heart to pump harder. A buildup of carbon monoxide reduces oxygen in the blood and damages the lining of the blood vessels.

Control Diabetes: Managing diabetes with diet, exercise, weight control, and medication is essential. Strict control of blood sugar may reduce damage to the heart.

Flu Shots: Flu shots for patients with chronic cardiovascular disease are now used routinely.

Weight Control: Being overweight contributes to other risk factors of a heart attack, such as high blood pressure, cardiovascular disease, and diabetes. Weight loss of as little as 10 pounds may lower blood pressure and improve cholesterol levels.

Exercise: Exercise can lower blood pressure, increase the level of HDL cholesterol ("good cholesterol"), and improve the overall health of the blood vessels and heart. It also helps control weight, control diabetes, and reduce stress. Thirty minutes daily of exercise is normally recommended.

Manage Stress: Stress can cause an increase in blood pressure along with increasing the blood's tendency to clot. Managing stress can be vital to keeping a heart healthy.

Diet: Eat healthy foods. A brain-healthy diet should include five or more daily servings of fruits and vegetables, foods rich in soluble fiber (such as oatmeal and beans), foods rich in calcium (dairy products, spinach), soy products (such as tempeh, miso, tofu, and soy milk), and foods rich in omega-3 fatty acids, including cold water fish such as salmon, mackerel, and tuna. However, pregnant women and women who plan to become pregnant in the next several years should limit their weekly intake of cold water fish because of the potential for mercury contamination. The U.S. Food and Drug Administration has announced that whole grain barley and barley-containing products are allowed to claim that they reduce the risk of CAD.

H

HEPATITIS B

BACKGROUND

The liver is located on the right side of the abdomen, just below the lower ribs. The liver is primarily responsible for filtering most of the nutrients that are absorbed in the intestines as well as removing drugs, alcohol, and other harmful substances from the bloodstream. The liver also produces bile, a greenish fluid stored in the gallbladder that helps digest fats. In addition, the liver also produces cholesterol, blood-clotting factors, and other proteins.

The liver is able to regenerate or repair up to two-thirds of injured tissue, including hepatocytes, biliary epithelial cells, and endothelial cells. Healthy cells take over the function of damaged cells, either indefinitely or until the damage is repaired.

The hepatitis B virus (HBV) causes a serious liver infection. The infection can become chronic in some people and lead to liver failure, liver cancer, cirrhosis (a condition that causes permanent scarring and damage to the liver), or death.

HBV is transmitted through contact with bodily fluids, such as blood and semen, of someone who is infected. Even though HBV is transmitted the same way as the human immunodeficiency virus (HIV), the virus that causes acquired immunodeficiency syndrome (AIDS), HBV is nearly 100 times as infectious as HIV. Individuals of any age, race, nationality, gender, or sexual orientation can become infected with HBV. Also, women who have HBV can transmit the infection to their babies during childbirth. When the infection is passed from mother to fetus, it is called vertical transmission.

Certain individuals have an increased risk of developing the disease. Individuals who are more likely to become infected with HBV are those who use intravenous (IV) drugs, have unprotected sex, and are born in or travel to parts of the world where hepatitis B is prevalent (like sub-Saharan Africa, Southeast Asia, the Amazon Basin, the Pacific Islands, and the Middle East).

Most people who become infected as adults recover completely from HBV, even if their symptoms are severe. However, infants and children are more likely to develop chronic, long-term infections.

While there is no cure for HBV, the hepatitis B vaccine can prevent the disease. Also, infected individuals can take precautions to help prevent HBV from spreading to others by getting testing for the virus, using protection during sexual contact, and not sharing needles.

According to the U.S. Centers for Disease Control and Prevention (CDC), an estimated 1.25 million Americans have chronic hepatitis. About 20-30% of hepatitis patients acquired their infection during childhood. The incidence per year has declined from an average of 260,000 in the 1980s to about 60,000 in 2004. The most significant decline has occurred among children and adolescents as a result of the routine hepatitis B vaccination.

ACUTE AND CHRONIC FORMS

Acute: Acute hepatitis B lasts less than six months. If the infection is acute, the body's immune system is able to destroy the virus, and the patient should recover completely within a few months. Most patients who acquire HBV as adults are able to eradicate the infection.

Chronic: Chronic hepatitis B lasts six months or longer. The infection is chronic when the immune system is unable to fight off the virus. The infection may become lifelong and can potentially cause serious complications, such as cirrhosis, liver cancer, liver failure, and death. Infants and many children between the ages of one and five become chronically infected. Chronic infection may go undetected for years and possibly even decades. In most chronic cases, the individuals are unaware of the infection until a serious liver complication develops.

DIFFERENT STRAINS OF HEPATITIS

Hepatitis A: Hepatitis A is transmitted primarily through food or water contaminated by feces from an infected person. In rare cases, it may spread via infected blood. Hepatitis A usually resolves without treatment in several weeks. However, there is a hepatitis A vaccine.

Hepatitis C: Hepatitis C is primarily spread via blood. It may also be transmitted through sexual contact and childbirth, although this occurs less often. Currently, there is no vaccine for hepatitis C. The only way to prevent the disease is to reduce the risk of exposure to the virus. Individuals can minimize exposure to the virus by using protection during sexual contact and not sharing needles. According to the CDC, individuals who underwent hemodialysis or received blood clotting factors before 1987 are at a high risk of developing chronic hepatitis C because blood products were not tested for hepatitis C before then. Chronic hepatitis C is treated with the drug peginterferon or a combination treatment with peginterferon and ribavirin. Patients with acute hepatitis C should consult their healthcare providers if symptoms do not subside after two to three months.

Hepatitis D: Anyone who has chronic hepatitis B is also susceptible to infection with another strain of viral hepatitis known as hepatitis D (formerly called delta virus). Hepatitis D virus can only infect cells if HBV is present. Injection drug users with hepatitis B have the greatest risk of developing the infection. Individuals who are infected with both HBV and hepatitis D are more likely to develop cirrhosis or liver cancer than are patients who only have HBV.

Hepatitis E: Hepatitis E is uncommon in the United States. This disease is primarily spread through food or water that is contaminated by feces from an infected person. There is no vaccine for hepatitis E. The only way to prevent the disease is to reduce the risk of exposure to the virus. Hepatitis E usually resolves without treatment, within several weeks to months.

CAUSES

A virus that attacks the liver causes hepatitis B. The virus, known as HBV can cause a lifelong infection, cirrhosis (scarring) of the liver, liver cancer, liver failure, and death.

TRANSMISSION

General: HBV is transmitted via bodily fluids. Individuals become infected once an infected person's bodily fluids, including blood, semen, vaginal secretions, or saliva, enter their bodies. Sharing toothbrushes or nail clippers, for instance, can increase the chance of acquiring the infection.

HBV is not spread through casual contact, such as hugging or shaking hands. Also, the virus is not spread through sweat or tears.

Individuals who are 18 years and younger and adults who have an increased risk of developing HBV should be vaccinated.

Sexual Transmission: Individuals who engage in unprotected sex, including vaginal, anal, or oral sex, with an infected partner may acquire hepatitis B. The infection may also be transmitted if sexual devices are shared and not sterilized or covered with a condom.

Needle Sharing: HBV can be transmitted through needles and syringes that are contaminated with infected blood. Therefore, individuals who share IV drug paraphernalia have an increased risk of developing the infection.

Accidental Needle Sticks: Healthcare workers and anyone who comes into contact with human blood is at risk of acquiring HBV.

Pregnancy: Pregnant women who are infected with HBV can pass the virus to their babies. When the virus is transmitted from mother to fetus, it is called vertical transmission. Therefore, it is recommended that newborn babies of HBV-positive mothers receive hepatitis B immune globulin (HBIG) as well as the hepatitis vaccine, which includes a series of three injections. The vaccine will greatly reduce the baby's risk of acquiring the virus.

RISK FACTORS

Individuals who have unprotected sex with more than one partner.

Individuals who have unprotected sex with someone who is infected with HBV.

Individuals who have a sexually transmitted disease, such as gonorrhea or chlamydia.

Individuals who share needles during IV drug use.

Individuals who share a household with someone who has a chronic HBV infection. Close contact with an infected individual increases the likelihood of acquiring the viral infection.

Individuals who have a job that exposes them to human blood.

Individuals who have received a blood transfusion or blood products before 1970. It was not until after 1970 that the blood supply was routinely tested for HBV. Today, the risk of contracting HBV from donated blood is low.

Individuals who receive hemodialysis for end-stage renal disease.

Individuals who travel to regions of the world that have high infection rates of HBV, such as sub-Saharan Africa, Southeast Asia, the Amazon Basin, the Pacific Islands, and the Middle East.

Adolescents or young adults residing in a U.S. correctional facility.

Newborns whose mothers are infected with HBV.

Anyone can potentially become infected with HBV, even if he or she has no known risk factors for the disease.

SYMPTOMS

Hepatitis B is contagious even when symptoms do not appear. According to the CDC, about 30% of patients with chronic hepatitis show no signs or symptoms. Hepatitis B symptoms are less common in infants and children than adults.

Symptomatic patients usually experience the first symptoms four to six weeks after infection, which can range from mild to severe. Common symptoms include loss of appetite, nausea and vomiting, weakness and fatigue, abdominal pain (especially near the liver), dark urine, jaundice (yellowing of the skin and eyes), and joint pain.

COMPLICATIONS

Hepatitis D: Anyone who has chronic hepatitis B is also susceptible to infection with another strain of viral hepatitis known as hepatitis D (formerly called delta virus). Hepatitis D virus can only infect cells if the HBV is present. Injection drug users who have hepatitis B are at the greatest risk.

Liver Disease: Individuals with chronic HBV infection may develop serious liver diseases, such as cirrhosis (scarred, fibrous liver that is full of fat and not functioning properly) and liver cancer. Individuals who had HBV as an infant are at a greater risk of developing serious liver complications as an adult. Also, individuals who are infected with both hepatitis B and hepatitis D have an increased risk of developing cirrhosis or liver cancer, both of which can be fatal.

Liver Failure: Individuals diagnosed with HBV are at risk of acute liver failure, which occurs when all the vital functions of the liver shut down. Liver failure occurs if cirrhosis is present in more than two-thirds of the liver. Liver failure requires a liver transplant and can be fatal.

DIAGNOSIS

General

Pregnant women should be tested for HBV early in pregnancy. Individuals who are knowingly exposed to the virus should also be tested.

Individuals who adopt children from regions of the world where hepatitis B is prevalent are advised to have their children tested when they arrive in the United States. Tests performed in other countries may not always be reliable.

Tests are performed in a physician's office, a hospital, or public health clinic. Many public health clinics offer free testing for HBV and other sexually transmitted diseases.

Blood Tests

Hepatitis B Surface Antigens: The outer surface of the virus has hepatitis B surface antigens. Patients who test positive for this antigen can easily pass the virus to others. A negative test means the individual is probably not infected. However, a false-negative result may occur if the test was performed soon after the patient was initially exposed to the virus.

Antibody to Hepatitis B Surface Antigens: If individuals have antibodies to HBV, they will test positive for hepatitis B surface antigens. A positive result may indicate that the individual has previously been infected with HBV or the individual has been vaccinated. Patients who test positive cannot become infected.

Antibody to Hepatitis B Core Antigen: The blood test for antibodies to the hepatitis B core antigen identifies individuals who have a chronic infection. However, the results can sometimes be ambiguous. Individuals who test positive may have a chronic and contagious infection, or they may be recovering from an acute infection or have a slight immunity to HBV that cannot otherwise be detected. The interpretation of this test depends on the results of the other two blood tests.

Additional Tests

Once a patient is diagnosed with hepatitis B, a qualified healthcare provider may perform additional tests to determine the severity of the infection and condition of the liver.

E-Antigen Test: An E-antigen blood test is used to determine whether a protein that is secreted by HBV-infected cells is present. A positive result means that the patient has high levels of the virus in the blood, and it is very contagious. If the test is negative, the patient has lower levels of HBV in the blood and the virus is less contagious.

Liver Enzymes: Another blood test may be performed to check for elevated levels of liver enzymes, such as alanine aminotransferase and aspartate aminotransferase. These enzymes leak into the bloodstream when liver cells are injured.

Alpha-Fetoprotein Test: If the patient has high levels of the alpha-fetoprotein in the blood, it may be a sign of liver cancer. Healthy adult males and nonpregnant females typically have less than 40 micrograms of alpha-fetoprotein per liter of blood.

Liver Ultrasound or Computerized Tomography Scan: A liver ultrasound or computerized tomography scan may be performed to detect liver problems. The radiologist analyzes the detailed images of the liver for signs of complications like cirrhosis or liver cancer.

Liver Biopsy: A liver biopsy may be performed to determine the extent of liver damage and to determine the best treatment option for the patient. During the procedure, a needle is inserted into the liver and a small tissue sample is removed. The tissue is then analyzed under a microscope in a laboratory.

TREATMENT

General: Individuals who knowingly have been exposed to the HBV should consult their healthcare providers as soon as possible. Patients who receive an injection of HBIG within 24 hours of exposure to the virus may not develop HBV infection. Patients should also receive the first of three injections of the hepatitis B vaccine.

There are few treatment options for patients with chronic hepatitis B. In some cases, the doctor may suggest monitoring the patient's condition instead of treating it. In other instances, the doctor may recommend antiviral treatment. When liver damage is severe, a liver transplantation may be the only treatment option.

Alcohol Avoidance: Individuals who have been diagnosed with hepatitis should avoid drinking alcohol because it speeds the progression of liver disease.

Interferon: The body naturally produces interferon to fight against invading organisms, including viruses. Administering additional synthetic interferon may stimulate the body's immune response to HBV and help prevent the virus from spreading. Two interferon medications are available, including interferon alfa-2b (Intron A) and peginterferon alfa-2a (Pegasys). Intron A is administered by injection several times a week. Pegasys is given by injection once a week.

Not everyone is a candidate for interferon treatment. In a few cases, interferon has successfully eliminated the virus completely. However, the infection can return in the future. Several side effects are associated with interferon, including depression, fatigue, muscle pain, body aches, fever, and nausea. Interferon may also cause a decreased production of red blood cells. Symptoms are usually worse during the first two weeks of treatment and in the first four to six hours after receiving an injection of interferon.

Lamivudine (Epivir-HBV): Lamivudine (Epivir-HBV) is an antiviral medication that helps prevent HBV from replicating in the body's cells. The medication is usually taken in tablet form once daily. Side effects during treatment are generally mild, but some patients may experience a severe worsening of symptoms when they stop taking the medication. Patients should tell their healthcare providers if they have had any kidney problems or history of pancreatitis before starting this medication. Patients should call their healthcare providers immediately if they experience a worsening of jaundice (yellowing of the skin and eyes) or if they experience any unusual bruising, bleeding, or fatigue while taking the medication.

Adefovir Dipivoxil (Hepsera): Adefovir dipivoxil (Hepsera) is a tablet taken orally once a day to help prevent HBV from replicating inside the body's cells. This drug is effective in patients who are resistant to lamivudine. Like lamivudine, side effects are generally mild, but symptoms may worsen when treatment is stopped. Hepsera may cause kidney toxicity in patients with underlying kidney disease. A change in the amount of urine produced or blood in the urine may indicate kidney toxicity. Other side effects may include weakness, headache, fever, increased cough, nausea, vomiting, diarrhea, or gas.

Entecavir (Baraclude): Entecavir (Baraclude) is an antiviral medication that was approved by the U.S. Food and Drug Administration in March 2005. This medication is taken orally once a day. Studies comparing entecavir to lamivudine found that entecavir was more effective. Entecavir may cause symptoms of hepatitis to worsen once medication is discontinued.

Liver Transplant: When the liver has been severely damaged, a liver transplant may be the only treatment option. Liver transplants are increasingly successful. However, there are not enough donor organs available for every patient who needs a transplant, and not all patients are suitable transplant candidates.

INTEGRATIVE THERAPIES

Good Scientific Evidence

Cordyceps: Cordyceps may stimulate the immune system and improve serum gamma globulin levels in hepatitis B patients. Currently, there is insufficient evidence to recommend for or against the use of cordyceps for chronic hepatitis B. However, the results are promising. Additional research of cordyceps and current hepatitis treatments is needed.

Avoid if allergic or hypersensitive to cordyceps, mold, or fungi. Use cautiously with diabetes, bleeding disorders or anticoagulant medications, prostate conditions, immunosuppressive medications, or hormonal replacement therapy or oral contraceptives. Avoid with myelogenous-type cancers. Avoid if pregnant or breastfeeding.

Milk Thistle: Multiple studies from Europe suggest benefits of oral milk thistle for cirrhosis. In experiments up to five years long, milk thistle has improved liver function and decreased the number of deaths that occur in cirrhotic patients. Although these results are promising, most studies have been poorly designed. Further research is necessary before a strong recommendation can be made.

In addition, several studies of oral milk thistle for hepatitis caused by viruses or alcohol report improvements in liver tests. However, most studies have been small and poorly designed. More research is needed before a recommendation can be made.

H

Probiotics: Liver cirrhosis may be accompanied by an imbalance of intestinal bacteria flora. Probiotic supplementation in cirrhosis patients has been found to reduce the level of fecal acidity (pH) and fecal and blood ammonia, which are beneficial changes.

Probiotics are generally considered safe and well tolerated. Avoid if allergic or hypersensitive to probiotics. Use cautiously if lactose intolerant.

Unclear or Conflicting Scientific Evidence

Astragalus: Antiviral activity has been reported with the use of astragalus in laboratory and animal studies. Limited human research has examined the use of astragalus for viral infections in the lung, heart (pericarditis, myocarditis, endocarditis), liver (hepatitis B and C), and cervix (papilloma virus) and in HIV disease. Studies have included combinations of astragalus with the drug interferon or as a part of herbal mixtures. However, most studies have been small and poorly designed. Due to a lack of well-designed research, no firm conclusions can be drawn.

Also, several animal and human studies report that astragalus may protect the liver from damage related to toxins or hepatitis B and C. Overall, this research has been poorly designed and reported. Astragalus alone has not been well evaluated. Better-quality research is necessary before a conclusion can be drawn.

Ayurveda: Ayurveda is an integrated system of specific theories and techniques employing diet, herbs, exercise, meditation, yoga, and massage or bodywork. Evidence from one well-designed study suggests that the traditional herbal preparation Kamalahar may reduce clinical signs as well as indicators of liver damage in acute viral hepatitis. Kamalahar contains Tecoma undulata, *Phyllanthus urinaria, Embelia ribes, Taraxacum officinale, Nyctanthes arbor-tristis,* and *Terminalia arjuna.*

Another well-designed trial suggests that root powder from the herb *Picrorhiza kurroa* may improve levels of bilirubin, serum glutamic-oxaloacetic trans-aminase, and serum glutamic pyruvic transaminase in viral hepatitis. Further research is needed before a firm conclusion can be made.

Bupleurum: For more than 2,000 years, bupleurum has been used in Asia to treat hepatitis, cirrhosis, and other conditions associated with inflammation. A high-quality clinical trial and several small recent clinical reports suggest that bupleurum and/or herbal combination formulas containing bupleurum may be helpful in the treatment of chronic hepatitis. However, studies to date are small and not all well controlled. Further research is warranted to determine whether bupleurum can effectively treat hepatitis.

Chicory (*Cichorium intybus*): Chicory (*Cichorium intybus*) has been suggested as a possible treatment for chronic hepatitis. However, further research is needed before a definitive conclusion can be made.

Choline: Studies have assessed the use of choline for hepatitis, many of which have been poorly designed. There is insufficient evidence available to determine whether choline can effectively treat hepatitis.

Dandelion: One human study reports improved liver function in individuals with chronic hepatitis B after taking a combination herbal preparation containing dandelion root, called jiedu yanggan gao (also including *Artemisia capillaris, Taraxacum mongolicum,* Plantago seed, *Cephalanoplos segetum, Hedyotis diffusa, Flos chrysanthemi indici, Smilax glabra, Astragalus membranaceus, Salviae miltiorrhizae, Fructus polygoni orientalis, Radix paeoniae alba,* and *Polygonatum sibiricum*). Because multiple herbs were used, and this study was not well designed or reported, the effects of dandelion are unclear.

Danshen: Some studies suggest that danshen may provide benefits for treating liver diseases such as cirrhosis, fibrosis, and chronic hepatitis B. However, it is unclear whether there are any clinically significant effects of danshen in patients with liver disease.

Eyebright: Limited evidence from animal studies suggests that aucubin, a constituent of eyebright, may inhibit hepatic RNA and protein syntheses in vivo. These properties have been associated with protective effects in carbon tetrachloride and alpha-amanitin–induced hepatotoxicity in mice. Conversion of aucubin to its aglycone appears to be a prerequisite step for these hepatic effects to occur. The clinical relevance of these finding to humans is unclear, and there is currently insufficient evidence to determine whether eyebright is an effective hepatoprotective agent.

Germanium: There is limited evidence for the use of propagermanium (an organogermanium) in the treatment of hepatitis B. Additional research is warranted in this area.

Ginseng: There is a lack of sufficient evidence to recommend either American ginseng or *Panax ginseng* for or against hepatoprotection. One laboratory study investigated compound K, a ginseng metabolite that shows promise in protecting against liver injury. Additional human studies are warranted in this area.

L-Carnitine: Although early evidence suggests that L-carnitine may effectively treat liver cirrhosis, further research is needed to confirm these results.

Licorice: The licorice extracts DGL (deglycyrrhi-zinated licorice) and carbenoxolone have been proposed to be possible therapies for viral hepatitis. Further research is needed before a firm conclusion can be made.

Liver Extract: Liver extract seems to stimulate liver function. In two studies, liver extract did increase the liver function of patients with impaired liver function. More research is needed to compare liver extract to other hepatostimulatory treatments.

Mistletoe: In a preliminary description in 1997, some patients achieved complete elimination of the virus after treatment with *Viscum album,* although these studies were not well designed. A small exploratory trial investigated effects of mistletoe on liver function, reduction of viral load and inflammation, and maintaining quality of life by the immunomodulatory and/or cytotoxic actions of mistletoe extracts, but little effect was seen. Larger, well-designed clinical trials are needed to resolve these conflicting data.

Avoid if allergic to plants in the aster family (Compositeae, Asteraceae), daisies, artichoke, common thistle, or kiwi. Use cautiously with diabetes. Avoid if pregnant or breastfeeding.

Reishi Mushroom: Based on positive laboratory evidence, a clinical trial using Ganopoly or placebo was conducted in chronic hepatitis B patients. Ganopoly treatment decreased levels of HBV DNA. This virus is notoriously hard to clear from the body and recurrence after treatment is common. The authors are closely related to the manufacturer of Ganopoly. Further well-designed research is needed before a firm conclusion can be made.

Rhubarb: Two studies have been conducted on rhubarb and its effects on hepatitis. In the case series, high doses of rhubarb decreased the symptoms and serum levels associated with hepatitis. However, additional high-quality studies are needed to establish rhubarb's effects.

S-Adenosylmethionine (SAMe): Preliminary evidence from meta-analyses and randomized clinical trials suggests that SAMe may normalize levels of liver enzymes in individuals with liver disease. Well-designed clinical trials, with appropriate subject number in homogenous populations, are required before a definitive conclusion can be made in this field.

Selenium: Selenium supplementation has been studied in various liver disorders, including hepatitis, with mixed results. Further research is needed to establish selenium's effects.

Taurine: Early studies have found that taurine supplementation has the potential to modify the conjugation of bile acids, potentially modifying the disease. Furthermore, taurine has been examined as an adjunct to ursodeoxycholate in the treatment of liver disease. Results from these early studies suggest that conjugation of bile acids can be modified and that taurine as an adjunct to ursodeoxycholate does not offer more benefits. More recent studies are investigating the effect of tauroursodeoxycholate in liver disease treatment. As of yet, however, the evidence in support of taurine in liver disease is minimal, and well-designed clinical trials with positive results are needed before a firm conclusion can be made.

Fair Negative Scientific Evidence

Spirulina: Despite findings indicating potential hepatoprotective properties of spirulina, preliminary human study of spirulina for chronic viral hepatitis shows negative results. Additional high-quality study is needed to confirm these findings.

PREVENTION

Vaccination: Hepatitis B vaccination is the best way to prevent hepatitis B infection. A hepatitis B vaccine (Engerix-B) has been available since 1982. It is administered in a series of three immunizations and provides more than 90% protection for both adults and children. The vaccine generally protects against HBV for at least 15 years. Almost anyone can receive the vaccine, including infants, older adults, and those with immune deficiencies. Infants usually receive the vaccine during the first year of life, with injections administered at two, four, and nine months of age.

In the last decade, recombinant DNA technology has been used to produce the vaccine in the United States. Rather than using the blood of infected patients, the HBV antigen used in the vaccine is produced in a laboratory.

Side effects tend to be mild and may include weakness, fatigue, headache, nausea, and soreness or swelling at the injection site. Although concerns have been raised that the HBV vaccine may increase the risk of autoimmune disease and sudden infant death syndrome, studies have found no correlation.

Testing: Hepatitis B can be contagious even when the patient is asymptomatic (experiences no symptoms). Therefore, it is recommended that individuals who think they have been exposed to the virus get tested. Pregnant women who suspect they have been exposed to the virus should also get tested because they can pass HBV to their babies.

Protected Sex: Individuals should not engage in unprotected sex, especially if they do not know the health status of their partner. Avoid lambskin condoms because they do not prevent against STDs. Also, oil-based lubricants can weaken condoms and cause them to break.

Sterile Needle Use: While illicit drug use is illegal in the United States, individuals who use needles to inject drugs should use sterile needles and avoid sharing used needles with other people.

HERPES VIRUSES

BACKGROUND

Herpes is a group of viruses that infect humans. Types of herpes viruses include herpes simplex virus types 1 and 2 (HSV-1 and HSV-2, respectively), human herpesvirus type 3 (HHV-3, or varicella-zoster virus), human herpesvirus type 4 (including Epstein-Barr virus and lymphocryptovirus), human herpesvirus type 5 (cytomegalovirus), human herpesvirus type 6 (HHV-6, including human B-cell lymphotrophic virus and roseolovirus), human herpesvirus type 7 (HHV-7), and human herpesvirus type 8 (rhadinovirus and Kaposi's sarcoma–associated virus). The viruses fall into three categories: alpha herpes viruses (HSV-1, HSV-2, and varicella-zoster virus), beta herpes viruses (cytomegalovirus, HHV-6, and HHV-7), and gamma herpes viruses (Epstein-Barr virus, lymphocryptovirus, and HHV-8). The viruses are different and cause various conditions with many unique signs and symptoms. However, all herpes viruses share some common properties, including a pattern of active symptoms followed by latent (inactive) periods with no symptoms that can last for months, years, or even for a lifetime. Herpes symptoms may even never reappear. The severity of herpes symptoms depends on the type of virus with which the individual is infected.

HSV-1 is also known as a cold sore or fever blister. HSV-2 is also known as genital herpes. HHV-3 is also referred to as varicella-zoster virus (VZV). Herpes varicella is the primary infection that causes chickenpox, and herpes zoster is the reactivation of the varicella virus that causes shingles. HSV-1 and -2 infections are generally marked by painful, watery blisters on the skin or mucous membranes (such as the mouth or lips) or on the genitals. Lesions heal with a crust-forming scab, the hallmark of herpes. This is particularly likely during an outbreak, although individuals may shed virus between outbreaks. Although no cure is yet available, antiviral treatments exist that reduce the likelihood of viral shedding. An HSV infection on the lips, commonly known as a "cold sore" or "fever blister," should not to be confused with a canker sore; canker sores (painful sores on the tongue or oral membranes in the mouth) are not caused by the HSV virus. Herpes is a contagious infection that spreads when the carrier is producing and releasing ("shedding") virus. Herpes viruses are transmitted from human to human in different ways. With HSV-1, contact and infection can occur directly from another human (such as mouth-to-mouth, hand-to-mouth contact) or through the use of everyday objects that have come in contact with the virus, including razors, towels, dishes, and glasses. Genital herpes or HSV-2 can only be contracted through direct sexual contact (genital-to-genital, mouth-to-genital, or hand-to-genital; not kissing) with an infected partner. Occasionally, oral-genital contact can spread oral herpes to the genitals (and vice versa). Individuals with active herpes lesions on or around their mouths or on their genitals should avoid oral sex. VZV (chickenpox) spreads through the humidity in the air when inhaled and mainly spreads during the incubation period, which is just before an outbreak of symptoms. After an initial or primary infection, herpes viruses establish a period called latency, during which the virus is present in the cell bodies of nerves that innervate (attach) to the area of the original viral outbreak (such as genitals, mouth, and lips). At some point this latency ends, and the virus becomes active again. While active, the virus begins to multiply (called shedding), and becomes transmittable again. This shedding may or may not be accompanied by symptoms. During reactivation, virus is produced in the nerve cell and transported outwardly via the nerve to the skin. The ability of the herpes virus to become latent and reactive explains the chronic (long-term), recurring nature of a herpes infection. Recurrence of the viral symptoms is usually milder than the original infection. Recurrence may be triggered by menstruation, sun exposure, illness with fever, stress, immune system imbalances, and other unknown causes.

TYPES OF HERPES

HSV-1 and HSV-2

HSV: There are two types of HSV: HSV-1 and HSV-2. Although some symptoms of HSV-1 and HSV-2 are similar (such as lesions), they are usually transmitted differently and involve different areas of the body.

HSV-1: HSV-1 is the cause of herpes labialis (fever blisters, cold sores) and involves the lips and inflammation of the gums and mouth. Other conditions caused by HSV-1 include oropharyngeal, cutaneous, and ocular lesions, including HSV blepharitis, HSV conjunctivitis, HSV keratitis, HSV infectious epithelial keratitis, HSV anterior uveitis, HSV retinitis, and HSV neonatal infection. HSV-1 is a very common virus. It is thought that 90% of adults have been exposed to the virus during a lifetime, and most Americans are infected by the age of 20. After the first episode, the virus lies dormant in the nerves or skin around the original area until something sets the virus off into another eruption. Colds, flu, and even stress can cause an outbreak of cold sores. It is not well understood why an individual has an outbreak at one time of life and not another. Most people contract oral herpes when they are children by receiving a kiss from a friend or relative.

The first symptoms usually appear within one or two weeks and as late as three weeks after contact with an infected person. The lesions of herpes labialis usually last for seven to 10 days then begin to resolve. Following the active infection, the virus becomes latent (dormant), residing in the nerve cells and possibly reactivating later, causing a new outbreak at or near the original site. It should be noted that HSV-1 is becoming a major cause of genital herpes as well due to unprotected sex. In some studies, it is now a more important cause than HSV-2.

HSV-2: HSV-2 is considered the primary cause of genital herpes. In the United States, at least 45 million people ages 12 and older have had HSV-2 (or genital herpes) infection. According to researchers at the Centers for Disease Control and Prevention, HSV is present in as many as one in six teens and adults in the United States. HSV-2 is a sexually transmitted disease (STD), meaning an individual must engage in sexual activity (oral or manual sex or intercourse) in order to transmit or be infected with this virus. HSV-2 infection is more common in women (approximately one out of four women) than in men (almost one out of five). This may be because male-to-female transmissions are more likely than female-to-male transmission. Anyone who is sexually active can contract genital herpes. There are no documented cases of a person getting genital herpes from an inanimate object such as a toilet seat, bathtub, or towel. Herpes is a very fragile virus and does not live long on surfaces outside the body.

Most individuals infected with HSV-2 are not aware of their infection. However, if signs and symptoms occur during the first outbreak, they can be quite severe. The first outbreak usually occurs within two weeks after the virus is transmitted, and the sores typically heal within two to four weeks. Other signs and symptoms during the primary episode may include a second crop of sores and flulike symptoms, including fever and swollen glands. However, many individuals with HSV-2 infection may never have sores, or they may have very mild sores that they do not even notice or that they mistake for insect bites or another skin condition.

Most people diagnosed with a first episode of genital herpes can expect to have four to five outbreaks (called symptomatic recurrences) within a year. Over time these recurrences usually decrease in frequency. There is no cure for this recurrent (returning) infection, which may cause embarrassment and emotional distress. Having genital herpes does not preclude an individual from having a normal relationship. If the individual or his or her partner is infected with HSV-2, steps can be taken to manage the transmission of the virus (see Precautions). With HSV-2 (genital herpes), transmission of the virus can occur when the infected sexual partner does not have an active outbreak. Symptoms of an active outbreak include blisters or ulcers. Some individuals may never have any symptoms and may not know that they are infected with the herpes virus. However, they can still transmit the virus to others. Although HSV-2 is widely recognized as a cause of genital herpes, it can cause oral herpes as well. Moreover, HSV-1 can cause genital herpes, resulting in similar symptoms as infections caused by HSV-2 in the facial area as well as genital herpes (similar symptoms in the genital region). With genital infections, HSV-2 is more likely to shed than HSV-1, especially in women. It is possible that over half of the people infected with HSV-2 shed the virus at some time without having any symptoms or rash. It is also estimated that one-third of all HSV-2 infections are caused when a noninfected person comes in contact with someone who is shedding the virus without symptoms. HSV-2 can be passed in the urine or genital discharge of an infected person. The viruses become reactivated secondary to certain stimuli, including fever, physical, or emotional stress, ultraviolet light exposure (sunlight or tanning beds), and nerve injury.

HHV-3

VZV: Both shingles and chickenpox are caused by HHV-3, or VZV. HHV-3 is still referred as either herpes varicella (the primary infection that causes chickenpox) or herpes zoster (the reactivation of the virus that causes shingles). The human race is the only known carrier of HHV-3.

Chickenpox: Chickenpox is usually a childhood disease. Over 90% of cases occur in children aged 14 years and younger. Before widespread vaccination, the incidence of chickenpox in the United States approached the annual birth rate, averaging between 3.1-3.8 million cases per year. Chickenpox can occur at any time of year. Chickenpox is acquired by direct contact with infected blister fluid or by inhalation of respiratory droplets. When individuals with chickenpox cough or sneeze, they expel tiny droplets that carry the varicella virus. A person who has never been exposed to chickenpox inhales these droplets and the virus enters the lungs; it is then carried through the bloodstream to the skin, where it causes a rash. While the virus is in the bloodstream (before the rash begins), it causes typical viral symptoms such as fever, fatigue, joint pains, headache, and swollen glands. These symptoms usually resolve by the time the rash develops. The incubation period (time before the full-blown symptoms of the virus appear) of chickenpox averages 14 days, with a range of nine to 21 days.

The chickenpox rash usually begins on the trunk of the body and spreads to the face and extremities. The chickenpox lesion starts as a two- to four-millimeter red papule that develops an irregular outline (similar to a rose petal). A thin-walled, clear vesicle (a blister that looks like a dewdrop) develops on top of the area of redness. This lesion is unique to chickenpox. After about eight to 12 hours, the fluid in the vesicle gets cloudy and the vesicle breaks, leaving a crust. The fluid is highly contagious, but once the lesion crusts over it is not considered contagious. The crust usually falls off after seven days, sometimes leaving a craterlike scar. Although one lesion goes through this complete cycle in about seven days, another hallmark of chickenpox is the fact that new lesions can crop up every day for several days. Therefore, it may take about a week until new lesions stop appearing and existing lesions crust over. Children should not be sent back to school until all lesions have crusted over. The number of chickenpox lesions a person gets varies considerably. The usual range is 100-300 lesions. Usually, older children and adults develop more lesions than young children. Individuals who have previously traumatized skin, such as sunburn or eczema, may also develop more severe lesions. In addition to affecting the skin, chickenpox can also cause lesions on the mucous membranes in the eyes, mouth, throat, and vagina.

There is a varicella-zoster vaccine for use in individuals ages 12 months through 12 years. The chickenpox vaccine is a live attenuated vaccine, meaning the live, disease-producing virus was modified or weakened in the laboratory to produce an organism that can grow and produce immunity in the body without causing illness.

Shingles: Shingles (also called herpes zoster) is a disease caused by VZV, the same virus that causes chickenpox. After an individual contracts VZV, it remains dormant within the nerve roots (nerve tissue). Outbreaks are then termed shingles. Shingles affects an estimated two in every 10 people in their lifetime. More than 500,000 people in the United States develop shingles annually. It is most common in individuals over the age of 50 and those who have previously had chickenpox. Shingles is also more common in individuals with weakened immune systems, which can result from HIV infection, radiation treatment, certain medications (including steroids and chemotherapy), transplant operations, and high levels of or chronic (long-term) stress.

The first sign of shingles is often burning or tingling pain, or sometimes numbness or itch, in one particular location on only one side of the body. After several days or a week, a rash of fluid-filled blisters (similar to chickenpox) appears in the affected location. Shingles pain can be mild or severe. Some individuals experience only itching, while others feel pain from gentle touch or breeze. The most common location for shingles is a band, called a dermatome, spanning one side of the trunk around the waistline. Anyone who has had chickenpox is at risk for developing shingles at some point in life.

There is no cure for shingles. Early treatment with antiviral drugs that fight the virus may help. These medicines may also help prevent lingering pain. There is a vaccine now available that may prevent shingles or lessen its effects (Zostavax). The vaccine is for people 60 or over who have had chickenpox but who have not had shingles.

Postherpetic Neuralgia (PHN): Some individuals continue to feel pain long after the shingles rash and blisters heal. This condition is termed PHN. Not everyone who has had a recurrence of the virus develops PHN. But PHN is a common complication of shingles in older adults. The primary symptom of PHN is pain that can be debilitating. The pain associated with PHN may be aching, throbbing, stabbing, sharp, or piercing. Stress may intensify the severity of the pain. The intensity of the pain can vary, but pain-free intervals are rare. Some individuals who have had PHN describe the pain as the worst pain they have ever felt. The greater the age when the virus reactivates, the greater the chance the individual will develop PHN. In most individuals, the pain of PHN lessens over time. Treatments for PHN that may ease nerve-related pain include antidepressants (such as amitriptyline [Elavil]), anticonvulsants (such as gabapentin [Neurontin]), steroids (such as prednisone [Deltasone]), pain killers (such as opiates, including oxycodone [Percocet]), and topical anesthetic patches (such as lidocaine [Lidoderm]).

HHV-4

Epstein-Barr Virus (EBV): EBV is a herpes virus (HHV-4) that causes a viral syndrome referred to as mononucleosis. EBV has also been found to play a role in the development of Burkitt's lymphoma (a rare form of lymphoma, or cancer of the lymph system) and nasopharyngeal carcinoma (cancer of the nose and throat) in humans. The Epstein-Barr viral syndrome, mononucleosis (also known as mono, kissing disease, and Epstein-Barr viral syndrome), causes fever, a sore throat, swollen lymph glands (especially in the neck), and extreme fatigue or tiredness. Although typically caused by EBV, mononucleosis can also be caused by other herpes viruses, including cytomegalovirus. In the United States, as many as 95% of adults between 35-40 years of age have been infected with EBV. Infants become susceptible to EBV as soon as maternal protection present at birth disappears. Infection with EBV during adolescence or young adulthood results in mononucleosis in 35-50% of the cases. The incubation period for the mononucleosis is usually seven to 14 days in children and adolescents. The incubation period in adults is longer; at times it may be 30-50 days. If symptoms of mononuclcosis last morc than six months, it is frequently referred to as chronic EBV infection. EBV may be linked to chronic fatigue syndrome (CFS), a condition of chronic tiredness and exhaustion.

Mononucleosis spreads by contact with moisture from the mouth and throat of a person who is infected with the virus. Kissing; sharing drinking glasses, eating utensils, and toothbrushes; or touching anything that has been near the mouth of an infected person may result in transmission of the disease. The infection develops slowly, with such mild symptoms initially that it may be mistaken for a cold or the flu. As the condition progresses, the symptoms may include a sore throat that lasts two weeks or more, swollen lymph nodes (in the neck, armpits, and groin), a persistent fever, fatigue (tiredness), and malaise (a vague feeling of discomfort). These symptoms can be mild or so severe that throat pain impedes swallowing and fever reaches 105° F. Some people also experience a rash, eye pain, photophobia (discomfort with bright light), and a swollen spleen or liver. In most cases of mononucleosis, no specific treatment is necessary as the illness is usually self-limiting. Although the symptoms of infectious mononucleosis usually resolve in one or two months, EBV remains dormant in cells in the throat and blood for the rest of the person's life. Periodically, the virus can reactivate and can be found in the saliva of infected persons. This reactivation usually occurs without symptoms of illness, although it may be linked to symptoms of CFS. EBV also establishes a lifelong dormant infection in some cells of the body's immune system.

HHV-5

Cytomegalovirus (CMV): CMV is a herpes virus (HHV-5) found in body fluids, including urine, saliva (spit), breast milk, blood, tears, semen, and vaginal fluids. It is commonly transmitted from an infected pregnant woman to her unborn child. It is an opportunistic virus that does not usually cause disease in those with healthy immune systems. In people with weakened immune systems (such as those with HIV or AIDS), CMV can cause any number of infections, including retinitis (inflammation of the retina), pneumonia, colitis (inflammation of the colon), encephalitis (inflammation of the brain), mononucleosis, pneumonia, hepatitis, and uveitis. CMV syndrome and fever of unknown origin (known as pyrexia) are complications that may occur. CMV is a common a cause of serious disability, such as neural tube defects. Neural tube defects are serious birth defects with symptoms that range from mild to severe impairment. They are caused by incomplete development of the brain, spinal cord, and/or their protective coverings. Spina bifida is the most common neural tube defect. Spina bifida occurs when the spine fails to close properly during the first few weeks of pregnancy, causing damage to the nerves and spinal cord. It is estimated that more than 70,000 people in the United States are living with spina bifida.

Other Herpes Viruses

HHV-6: HHV-6 has been linked to two conditions, roseola and lymphotrophic virus. HHV-6 has also been considered as a possible cause of CFS, along with HHV-3 or varicella-zoster. CFS patients can have extremely high levels of antibodies to HHV-6, meaning there is an infection present. HHV-6 infection is a major cause of opportunistic viral infections in patients with compromised immune systems, especially due to AIDS or organ transplants. HHV-6 may cause rejection of transplanted organs and death. HHV-6 may also be a cause of multiple sclerosis, a chronic (long-term) inflammatory condition of the central nervous system resulting in changes in sensation, visual problems, muscle weakness, depression, difficulties with coordination and speech, severe fatigue, cognitive impairment, problems with balance, overheating, and pain. Multiple sclerosis will cause impaired mobility and disability in more severe cases. Roseola (also known as sixth disease, exanthem subitum, and roseola infantum) is a viral illness in young children, most commonly affecting those between the ages of six months and two years. It is typically marked by several days of high fever

H

(over 102° F), followed by a distinctive rash that occurs when the fever breaks.

There are two different types of HHV-6, the first type being responsible for roseola and the second responsible for infections in adults with weakened immune systems due to HIV/AIDS or cancer. This is the type that is thought to be associated with CFS.

HHV-7: HHV-7 is closely related to both HHV-6 and CMV. Of the three viruses, HHV-7 is the least pathogenic (disease causing). Like HHV-6, HHV-7 primarily causes roseola in infants and young children, which is a febrile (fever) illness that typically lasts for six days.

HHV-8: HHV-8 is a type of herpes virus responsible for diseases such as Kaposi's sarcoma (KS), lymphoproliferative disorders (condition of too many white blood cells produced), primary effusion lymphoma, and multicentric Castleman's disease. This virus only attacks immunocompromised individuals, such as those with HIV and AIDS. The virus has been identified in all types of KS, including classic, endemic, posttransplant, and AIDS-related KS, all of which have identical features under the microscope. Research suggest that HHV-8 infection is spread by mouth-to-mouth contact (kissing) or genital contact. Previous studies on KS have indicated that HHV-8 was more commonly found in saliva than in genital secretions.

RISK FACTORS AND CAUSES

HSV-1 (Herpes Labialis): Everyone is at risk for HSV-1 (herpes labialis or oral herpes). It is easily transmitted and is the most common form of HSV. Oral herpes (cold sores or fever blisters) affects between 15-30% of the entire population, and most people are infected when they are young, with the highest incidence first occurring between six months and three years old. HSV-1 can be spread by close contact with someone who has a cold sore or by using items contaminated with the virus. Kissing someone on the mouth will spread the virus, and sharing personal items such as razors, towels, or eating utensils with a person who has oral herpes will increase the risk of getting HSV-1. The virus can also be spread to the genital area of another individual by having oral sex. Individuals with oral herpes should not perform oral sex on their partners. They should also avoid kissing. Infants and young children (up to three years old) have an increased risk of being exposed to HSV-1 due to immune systems that are still not fully developed.

Exposure to sunlight or other ultraviolet light is a common trigger for the formation of cold sores.

Stress on the body due to illness or excessive exercise can weaken the body's immune system and lead to an outbreak of oral herpes. Common examples of stress or illness include infection, fever, a cold, physical injury, dental surgery, menstruation, medications (including steroids), or illnesses such as HIV that suppress the immune system, eczema, excessive exercise, and emotional stress. It should be noted that HSV-1 is becoming a major cause of genital herpes as well and in some studies it is now a more important cause.

HSV-2 (Genital Herpes): Anyone who is sexually active is at risk for genital herpes, and it is on the rise. Some reports estimate 31 million cases of HSV-2 or genital herpes occur in sexually active adults annually in the United States. The risk of HSV-2 infection is higher in women than in men. The largest increases in HSV-2 occur in women after their early twenties. Women have an 80-90% chance of contracting HSV-2 after unprotected sexual activity with an infected partner and are 1.7 times more likely to be infected than men. Men, however, have twice as many recurrent infections as women. Less than 1% of American children younger than 15 test positive for HSV-2; sexual abuse should be considered in children with HSV-2. Although African-Americans are more likely to test positively for HSV-2, Caucasians have a higher risk for active genital symptoms, and over the past few years the greatest increase in HSV-2 has been observed in white adolescents.

VZV (Chickenpox): Before the introduction of the vaccine, about four million cases of chickenpox were reported in the United States each year. Between 75-90% of chickenpox cases occur in children under 10 years of age. Since a varicella vaccine became available in the United States in 1995, however, the incidence of disease and hospitalizations due to chickenpox are showing a dramatic decrease. Experts expect the disease to become a rarity in the United States.

The risk of chickenpox is high in late winter and early spring months. Primary transmission of chickenpox includes direct contact with the individual carrying the virus or by inhaling the virus from the air. It can also be transmitted from direct contact with the open sores. However, clothing and bedding do not usually spread the disease. An individual with chickenpox can transmit the disease from about two days before the appearance of the spots to the end of the blister stage. This period lasts about five to seven days. Once dry scabs form, the disease is unlikely to spread. Most schools allow children with chickenpox back 10 days after onset to avoid the risk of spreading the infection. Some require children to stay home until the skin has completely cleared, although this measure is not necessary to prevent transmission.

Individuals at a higher risk for developing chickenpox include individuals of any age who have neither had chickenpox in the past nor been immunized against chickenpox, newborns, individuals with weakened immune systems, and individuals who are taking immunosuppressant drugs. Also at risk are individuals who are moderately or severely ill and are not yet fully recovered; individuals who have disorders affecting the blood, bone marrow, or lymphatic system; the elderly; and pregnant women. If an individual is not immune to chickenpox, traveling abroad can increase the risk of contracting the condition. Males (both boys and men) have a higher risk for a severe case of chickenpox than females. The older the child, the higher the risk for a more severe case. But even in such circumstances chickenpox is rarely serious in children.

VZV (Shingles): About 500,000 cases of shingles occur each year in the United States. Anyone who has had chickenpox has a risk for shingles later in life, which means that 90% of U.S. adults are at risk for shingles. Shingles occurs in about 10-20% of adults who have had chickenpox. The risk for herpes zoster increases as people age, so the overall number of cases will undoubtedly increase as the baby-boomer generation gets older. One study estimated that an individual who reaches 85 has a 50% chance of having herpes zoster. The risk for PHN (pain that persists after the outbreak has healed) is also highest in older people with the infection, increasing dramatically after age 50. Individuals whose immune systems are impaired from diseases, such as those with HIV, AIDS, or childhood cancer, have a risk for herpes zoster that is much higher than those with healthy immune systems. In fact, herpes zoster in people who are HIV positive may be a sign of full-blown AIDS. Current drugs used for HIV, called protease inhibitors, may also increase the risk for herpes zoster. Cancer places people at high risk for herpes zoster. At highest risk are those with Hodgkin's disease (13-15% of these patients develop shingles). About 7-9% of patients with lymphomas and between 1-3% of patients with other cancers have herpes zoster. Individuals who take certain drugs that suppress the immune system are at risk for shingles (as well as other infections), including azathioprine (Imuran), chlorambucil (Leukeran), cyclophosphamide (Cytoxan), and cyclosporine (Sandimmune, Neoral). These drugs are used in patients who have undergone organ transplantation,

but they are also often used for severe autoimmune diseases caused by the inflammatory process. Such disorders include rheumatoid arthritis, systemic lupus erythematosus, diabetes, multiple sclerosis, Crohn's disease, and ulcerative colitis.

Interestingly, one study suggested that previously infected adults who are exposed to children with chickenpox may receive an extra boost in antibody production that can actually help them fight off herpes zoster. This means that as more children are vaccinated against chickenpox, more adults may be at risk for herpes zoster. There is a vaccine now available that may prevent shingles or lessen its effects (Zostavax). The vaccine is for people 60 or older who have had chickenpox but who have not had shingles. Although most common in adults, shingles can also develop in children. One study reported that only 5% of shingles cases occur in those under age 15. Children with immune deficiencies are at highest risk. Children with no immune problems and those who had chickenpox before they were one year old are at higher risk for shingles. It is still uncommon, however.

SIGNS AND SYMPTOMS

HSV-1 (Oral Herpes): Symptoms of cold sores are blisters on or around the lips and the edge of the mouth. The first symptom that may appear during an outbreak of oral herpes or cold sores may include tingling, burning, or itching in the area around the mouth or nose. This first portion of the outbreak is known as the prodromal stage or period. Within a few hours to days, the area may become reddened and develop small fluid-filled blisters called vesicles. Several of these small blisters may even come together and form one large blister. Cold sore blisters usually break open, weep clear fluid, and then crust over and disappear after a few days. The patient may experience symptoms including a sore mouth that makes eating, drinking, and sleeping uncomfortable. Other symptoms include fever, sore throat, and swollen lymph nodes in the neck. Symptoms usually last seven to 10 days.

HSV-2 (Genital Herpes): Signs of genital herpes (HSV-2) tend to develop within three to seven days of skin-to-skin contact with an infected person. Genital herpes infections look like small blisters or ulcers (round areas of broken skin) on the genitals. Each blister or ulcer is typically only one to three millimeters in size, and the blisters or ulcers tend to occur in groups. The blisters usually form first, then soon open to form ulcers. Herpes infections may be painless or slightly tender. In some individuals, however, the blisters or ulcers can be very tender and painful. In men, genital herpes (sores or lesions) usually appear on or around the penis. In women, the lesions may be visible outside the vagina, but they commonly occur inside the vagina. Lesions inside the vagina may cause discomfort or vaginal discharge and may be difficult to see, except during a doctor's examination. In any individual, ulcers or blisters may be found anywhere around the genitals (the perineum) and in and around the anus. The first herpes outbreak is usually the most painful, and the initial episode may last longer than later outbreaks. Some individuals develop other signs of herpes infection, particularly with the first episode, including fever, muscle aches, headaches (may be severe), vaginal discharge, painful urination, and swollen and tender lymph glands in the groin (glands swell as the body tries to fight the infection). If the disease returns, later outbreaks generally have much less severe symptoms. Many individuals with recurrent disease develop pain in the area of the infection even before any blisters or ulcers can be seen. This pain is due to irritation and inflammation of the nerves leading to the infected area of skin. These are signs that an outbreak is about to start. An individual is particularly contagious during this period, even though the skin still appears normal.

VZV (Chickenpox): Individuals with chickenpox may notice several symptoms before the typical chickenpox rash appears. Known as prodromal, or early symptoms, they include fever, a vague feeling of sickness, or decreased appetite. Within a few days, a rash appears as small red pimples or blisters. The rash appears in batches over the next two to four days. It usually starts on the trunk and then spreads to the head, face, arms, and legs. Blisters may also be found in the mouth or the genital areas because the virus can affect mucous membranes. Although some individuals may have only a few blisters, some have 100-300 blisters present. The pimples will progress to red teardrop blisters about five to 10 millimeters (¼-½ inch) wide. The blisters mature, break open, form a sore, and then crust over. Most of the blisters will heal within 10-14 days and usually do not cause scarring unless the blisters become infected.

VZV (Shingles): Shingles usually begins with an unpleasant itching, burning, tingling, or painful sensation in a bandlike area. The period of time when these sensations occur without a skin rash is called the prodromal period. During this time, the individual may have symptoms including fever, muscle aches, fatigue, anxiety (nervousness), and discomfort in the skin (usually on one side of the face, torso, trunk, back, or buttocks). The discomfort may feel

like numbness, itching, burning, stinging, tingling, shooting pain, electric shock, sharp pain, and extreme sensitivity to even light touch. Symptoms of active shingles includes a rash that begins as a reddish band or individual bumps running in a line and bumps developing with fluid-filled centers. Over the course of seven to 10 days, the bumps begin to dry and crust over. The individual may continue to have pain and/ or itching in the area of the rash. The pain may be severe. If the rash develops on the side of the nose or elsewhere on the face, the individual should contact his or her healthcare provider immediately. This can signal that the eyes may be infected. Although the rash of active shingles usually subsides within a week to a month, some individuals continue to have pain and discomfort well after the rash has healed. This syndrome of pain in the area of the previously infected nerve is called post herpetic neuralgia (PHN), and it can be quite severe and debilitating.

EBV: EBV can cause fever, a sore throat, swollen lymph glands (especially in the neck), and extreme fatigue or tiredness. Although typically caused by the EBV, mononucleosis can also be caused by other herpes viruses, including CMV. Infection with EBV during adolescence or young adulthood results in mononucleosis in 35-50% of the cases. The incubation period for the mononucleosis is usually seven to 14 days in children and adolescents. The incubation period in adults is longer; at times it may be 30-50 days. If symptoms of mononucleosis last more than six months, it is frequently referred to as chronic EBV infection. EBV may be linked to CFS, a condition of chronic tiredness and exhaustion.

Symptoms of mononucleosis develop slowly, with such mild symptoms initially that it may be mistaken for a cold or the flu. As the condition progresses the symptoms may include a sore throat that lasts two weeks or more, swollen lymph nodes (in the neck, armpits, and groin), a persistent fever, fatigue (tiredness), and malaise (a vague feeling of discomfort). These symptoms can be mild or so severe that throat pain impedes swallowing and fever reaches 105° F. Some individuals also experience a rash, eye pain, photophobia (discomfort with bright light), and a swollen spleen or liver. In most cases of mononucleosis, no specific treatment is necessary as the illness is usually self-limiting. Although the symptoms of infectious mononucleosis usually resolve in one or two months, EBV remains dormant in cells in the throat and blood for the rest of the person's life. Periodically, the virus can reactivate and can be found in the saliva of infected persons. This reactivation usually occurs without symptoms of illness, although it may be linked to symptoms of CFS. EBV also establishes a lifelong dormant infection in some cells of the body's immune system.

CMV: In people with weakened immune systems (such as those with HIV or AIDS), CMV can cause any number of infections, including retinitis (inflammation of the retina), pneumonia, colitis (inflammation of the colon), encephalitis (inflammation of the brain), mononucleosis, pneumonia, hepatitis, and uveitis. CMV syndrome and fever of unknown origin (known as pyrexia) are complications that may occur. CMV is a common a cause of serious disability such as neural tube defects. Neural tube defects are serious birth defects with symptoms that range from mild to severe impairment. They are caused by incomplete development of the brain, spinal cord, and/or their protective coverings.

DIAGNOSIS

Physical Exam: Signs and symptoms associated with herpes viral infections in humans can vary greatly depending upon the specific virus infecting the individual. Healthcare providers diagnose this group of infections by visual inspection and by taking a sample from the sore(s) for testing in a laboratory. Between outbreaks, these herpes infections can be difficult to diagnose. Viral diagnostic tests can also be performed to determine what type of herpes virus is infecting the individual.

Herpes viral infections may be confused with other conditions. VZV (chickenpox), particularly in early stages, may be confused with herpes simplex, impetigo (bacterial skin infection), insect bites, or scabies (skin infection by mites). The early prodromal stage of shingles can cause severe pain on one side of the lower back, chest, or abdomen before the rash appears. It therefore may be mistaken for disorders, such as gallstones, that cause acute pain in internal organs. In the active rash stage, shingles may be confused with HSV, particularly in young adults and if the blisters occur on the buttocks or around the mouth. Herpes simplex does not usually generate severe or chronic pain. A diagnosis may be difficult if herpes zoster takes an atypical course, such as with Bell's palsy (a neurological condition involving facial paralysis) or Ramsay Hunt syndrome (a neurological disorder caused by VZV that infects certain nerves in the head) or if it affects the eye or causes fever and delirium.

Viral Culture: A viral culture uses specimens taken from the blister, fluid in the blister, or sometimes spinal fluid. The samples are sent to a laboratory where they are analyzed. It takes between one and 14 days to detect the virus in the preparation made from the specimen. A viral culture is also sometimes used in vaccinated patients to determine if a varicella-like infection is caused by a natural virus or by the vaccine. This test is useful, but it is sometimes difficult to detect the virus in the samples.

Immunofluorescence Assay: Immunofluorescence is a diagnostic technique used to identify antibodies to a specific virus. In the case of herpes zoster, the technique uses ultraviolet rays applied to a preparation composed of cells taken from the patient's zoster blisters. The specific characteristics of the light, as seen through a microscope, will identify the presence of the antibodies. This test is less expensive, more accurate, and faster than a viral culture.

Polymerase Chain Reaction: Polymerase chain reaction uses a piece of the DNA of the virus, which is then replicated millions of times until the virus is detectable. A sample of the individual's tissue from a sore is prepared and analyzed in a complicated laboratory test. This technique is expensive but is useful for unusual cases, such as identifying infection in the brain and spinal cord. This type of testing would be used to detect the presence of HSV in those who have genital sores or encephalitis (inflammation of the brain) and in newborns suspected of having neonatal herpes (a rare but serious condition where herpes is contracted during birth). A pregnant woman who has been diagnosed with herpes may be monitored regularly prior to delivery to identify a reactivation of her infection (which would indicate the necessity for a caesarean section to avoid infecting the baby). The primary methods of testing for the virus are the herpes culture and HSV DNA testing. A positive herpes simplex culture or HSV DNA test from a vesicle scraping indicates an active HSV-1 or HSV-2 infection. A negative test result does not definitely rule out the presence of virus; for instance, the test may not be accurate if the HSV was not isolated from the vesicle scraping.

COMPLICATIONS

HSV: Although genital herpes usually causes mild symptoms, some people may experience recurrent painful genital ulcers, which can be especially severe in people with suppressed immune systems. Like other STDs, herpes may also increase the risk for transmitting or acquiring HIV.

All herpes viruses can be passed from mother to baby. The chance of giving herpes to the baby is highest if the first infection occurs near the time of delivery. The virus can be transmitted to the fetus while in utero (inside the womb) or during passage through

H

an infected vagina at birth. First-time infection during pregnancy leads to an increased risk of miscarriage, decreased fetal growth, and preterm labor. About 30-50% of infants who are born vaginally to a mother with first-time infection become infected with the herpes virus. Of babies born to women experiencing recurrent herpes at the time of birth, 1-4% become infected with HSV.

If a woman is having an active outbreak of genital herpes at the time of delivery, the baby will usually be delivered by cesarean section to prevent transmission of herpes. Of infants infected with herpes at birth, 30-60% die within the first month. Survivors may have long-term complications such as mental retardation and seizures. To prevent transmission of herpes to their babies, pregnant women should discuss any past history of herpes with their healthcare providers and take adequate measures to prevent infection during pregnancy. The risk of herpes can be reduced during pregnancy by avoiding sexual intercourse (vaginal, anal, and oral) during the last three months of pregnancy if the partner is known to have or suspected of having genital herpes and avoiding receptive oral sex during the last three months of pregnancy if the partner is known to have or suspected of having herpes sores on the mouth, tongue, gum, or lips. Infidelity plays an important role in genital herpes transmission.

HSVs can also cause several ocular (eye) lesions, including HSV blepharitis, HSV conjunctivitis, HSV keratitis, HSV infectious epithelial keratitis, HSV anterior uveitis, and HSV retinitis.

VZV: Pregnant women and anyone with immune system problems should not be near a person with chickenpox. If a pregnant woman who has not had chickenpox in the past contracts the virus (especially in the first 20 weeks of pregnancy), the fetus is at risk for birth defects. The mother is at risk for more health complications than if she had been infected when she was not pregnant. If the mother develops chickenpox just before or after the child is born, the newborn is at risk for serious health complications. There is no risk to the developing baby if the woman develops shingles during the pregnancy. If a pregnant woman has had chickenpox before the pregnancy, the baby will be protected from infection for the first few months of life since the mother's immunity gets passed on to the baby through the placenta and breast milk. Those at risk for severe disease or serious complications may be given varicella-zoster immune globulin (a vaccine for VZV) after exposure to chickenpox to reduce its severity. This group of people includes newborns whose mothers had chickenpox at the time of delivery, individuals

with leukemia or immune deficiencies, and children receiving drugs that suppress the immune system.

Chickenpox rarely causes complications, but it is not always harmless. Five out of every 1,000 children who have the infection require hospitalization and, in rare cases, chickenpox can be fatal. Chickenpox has caused about 11,000 hospitalizations each year and 100 deaths per year in the United States. Widespread vaccination, however, has produced a dramatic decline in these numbers.

The most common complications of chickenpox include itching, infections (usually from *Staphylococcus aureus* or *Streptococcus pyogenes*), scarring (complicated by scratching), ear infections, pneumonia, and encephalitis (inflammation of the brain). Other extremely rare complications of chickenpox include problems in blood clotting and inflammation of the nerves in the hands and feet. Inflammation in other parts of the body, including the heart, testicles, liver, joints, or kidney, may also occur. Such cases of inflammation are almost always temporary in otherwise healthy patients.

Complications of shingles (herpes zoster) include PHN pain, which can either be continuous burning or aching pain, periodic piercing pain, or spasm similar to electric shock. The pain tends to be more severe at night. Temperature changes can also affect pain. The pain may extend beyond the areas of the initial zoster attack, and some areas have no feeling at all. In most cases, it does not affect daily life. Rarely, however, the pain of herpes zoster affects sleep, mood, work, and overall quality of life. This can lead to fatigue, loss of appetite, depression, social withdrawal, and impaired daily functioning. Itching is also common in individuals with shingles. Infections may occur in the blisters associated with shingles.

Shingles may lead to meningitis (inflammation of the membrane around the brain) or encephalitis (inflammation of the brain). The encephalitis is generally mild and resolves in a short period. In rare cases, particularly in patients with impaired immune systems, these inflammations can be severe and even life threatening. Also, in rare situations herpes zoster can infect the urinary tract and cause difficult urination. The condition is temporary but may require a catheter to eliminate urine in some patients who have prolonged difficulty urinating. If shingles occurs in the face, the eyes are at risk, particularly if the path of the infection follows the side of the nose. If the eyes become involved, severe infections, called herpes zoster ophthalmicus, can occur that are difficult to treat and can threaten vision. AIDS patients may be at particular risk for a chronic infection in the cornea of the eye. Herpes zoster can also cause a devastating infection in the retina called imminent acute retinal necrosis syndrome. In such cases, visual changes develop within weeks or months after herpes zoster outbreak has resolved. It should be noted that this complication does not always follow a herpes outbreak in the face but can occur after an outbreak in any part of the body. Prompt treatment with a drug called acyclovir (Zovirax) can often halt the progress of vision loss, at least in people with healthy immune systems. In very rare cases, herpes zoster has been associated with Stevens-Johnson syndrome, an extensive and serious condition in which blisters cover most mucous membranes along with large areas of the body.

Ramsay Hunt Syndrome: Ramsay Hunt syndrome is a condition of facial paralysis and rash on the ear or mouth that occurs during a herpes zoster viral infection. Symptoms include severe ear pain and hearing loss, ringing in the ear(s), loss of taste, nausea, vomiting, and dizziness. Ramsay Hunt syndrome may also cause a mild inflammation in the brain. The dizziness may last for a few days or even for weeks, but usually resolves. Severity of hearing loss varies from partial to total. However, this hearing loss almost always goes away. Facial paralysis, on the other hand, may be permanent.

Bell's Palsy: Bell's palsy is partial paralysis of the face. In some cases, it is difficult to distinguish between Bell's palsy and Ramsay Hunt syndrome, particularly in the early stages. Ramsay Hunt syndrome tends to be more severe than Bell's palsy. Some healthcare providers recommend oral prednisone (a corticosteroid) along with an antiviral drug (such as acyclovir [Zovirax]) within seven days after symptoms appear.

TREATMENT

HSV

Genital Herpes: There are three antiviral medications that the U.S. Food and Drug Administration (FDA) has approved for the treatment of genital herpes. Approved antiviral drugs include acyclovir (Zovirax), valacyclovir (Valtrex), and famciclovir (Famvir). Antiviral medication is commonly prescribed for patients having a first episode of genital herpes, but they can be used for recurrent episodes as well. There are two kinds of treatment regimens: episodic therapy and suppressive therapy. With episodic therapy, the patient begins taking the medication at the first sign of recurrence. The medication is then taken for several days to hasten the recovery or healing or to prevent a full outbreak from fully occurring. All three of the antiviral treatments mentioned above have been proven to help shorten the amount of time that a

person may experience symptoms of herpes. However, results may vary from person to person. Side effects of antiviral medicines include stomach upset, loss of appetite, nausea, vomiting, diarrhea, headache, dizziness, and/or weakness.

Suppressive therapy is used in individuals with genital herpes who want to eliminate (suppress) outbreaks altogether. Suppressive therapy is usually given to patients who have six or more recurrences per year. For these individuals, studies have reported that suppressive therapy may reduce the number of outbreaks by at least 75% while the medication is being taken. Also, for some, taking an antiviral on a daily basis can prevent outbreaks altogether. Suppressive therapy may completely prevent outbreaks in some patients. Side effects include nausea and vomiting. Suppressive therapy may need to be taken for life.

Oral Herpes: Medications that are swallowed to treat oral herpes include the antiviral medications acyclovir (Zovirax), valacyclovir (Valtrex), and famciclovir (Famvir). There are two topical antiviral medications prescribed for the treatment of oral HSV: topical acyclovir ointment (Zovirax) and topical penciclovir cream (Denavir). Both of these drugs work to speed up the healing process and reduce the viral activity. These drugs are put directly on the lesions themselves but can also be used at the onset of prodrome (early symptoms of itching and burning lasting up to one to two days).

Other topical treatments for oral herpes are available over the counter (OTC) but are not antiviral compounds like acyclovir and penciclovir. Some also contain anesthetic ingredients (such as lidocaine or benzocaine) that numb the area and induce temporary relief from the discomfort of an outbreak. Unfortunately, some OTC treatments may actually delay the healing time of symptoms because they can further irritate the area with repeated applications. There is only one FDA-approved cream, docosanol (Abreva), the only OTC drug that has been clinically proven to help speed the healing process.

Infected individuals can also prevent recurring outbreaks by avoiding some of the known causes. During an outbreak, symptomatic relief may be obtained by keeping the area clean and dry or by taking pain relievers (such as aspirin, acetaminophen, or ibuprofen). Some patients with genital herpes find relief by taking a bath where a person simply sits in a tub with warm water up to the hips.

VZV (Chickenpox)

Pain Medications: Treatment for chickenpox includes pain medicines such as acetaminophen

(Tylenol) or ibuprofen (Motrin, Advil). Do not give children less than 18 years of age aspirin, as a dangerous condition called Reye's syndrome can develop.

Soothing Baths: Frequent baths are particularly helpful in relieving itching, especially when used with preparations of finely ground (colloidal) oatmeal. Commercial preparations of oatmeal, such as Aveeno, are available in drugstores, or one can be made at home by grinding or blending dry oatmeal into a fine powder. Use about two cups per bath. The oatmeal will not dissolve, and the water will have a scum. One-half to one cup of baking soda in a bath may also be helpful.

Lotions: Calamine lotion and similar OTC preparations can be applied to soothe the skin and help dry out blisters.

Antihistamines: For severe itching, a type of OTC medication called an antihistamine (such as diphenhydramine [Benadryl]) is useful; it also helps children sleep.

Antiviral Drugs: Acyclovir is an antiviral drug that may be used in adult varicella-zoster patients or those of any age with a high risk for complications and severe forms of chickenpox. The drug may also benefit smokers with chickenpox, who are at higher than normal risk for pneumonia. Some experts recommend its use for children who catch chickenpox from other family members because such patients are at risk for more serious cases. To be effective, oral acyclovir must be taken within 24 hours of the first signs of the rash. Early intravenous administration of acyclovir is also treatment for chickenpox pneumonia. Foscavir (Foscarnet) is an injectable antiviral agent commonly used in treating CMV (an infection caused by HHV-5). It is used in cases of varicella-zoster strains that have become resistant to acyclovir (Zovirax) and similar drugs. Administered intravenously (into the veins), the drug can have toxic effects such as kidney damage (which is reversible) and seizures. Fever, nausea, and vomiting are common side effects. It can also cause ulcers on the genitals organs. As with other drugs, it does not cure shingles. Antiviral drugs require a prescription.

VZV (Shingles)

The treatment goals for an acute (immediate) attack of shingles (herpes zoster) include reduce pain, reduce discomfort, hasten healing of blisters, and prevent the disease from spreading. OTC remedies are often effective in reducing the pain of an attack.

Antiviral Drugs: Antiviral agents (acyclovir [Zovirax]), corticosteroids (prednisone [Delatasone])

are sometimes given to patients with severe symptoms, particularly if they are older and at risk for PHN.

Antihistamines: In general, to prevent or reduce itching, home treatments are similar to those used for chickenpox. Patients can try antihistamines, particularly diphenhydramine (Benadryl, either orally or topically), oatmeal baths, and calamine lotion.

Oral Corticosteroids: Drugs called oral corticosteroids, including methylprednisolone (Medrol) and prednisone (Deltasone), are used for inflammation associated with shingles. They have some benefit for reducing pain and accelerating healing in acute attacks of shingles when used with acyclovir (Zovirax). However, they are not recommended without acyclovir. They also may be helpful for improving symptoms of Bell's palsy and Ramsay Hunt syndrome. Corticosteroids do not appear to prevent a further attack or reduce the risk for PHN. Side effects of corticosteroids, including weight gain and lowered immunity, can be severe, and oral steroids should be taken at as low a dose and for as short a time as possible.

Epidural Blocks: Epidural blocks are injections of local anesthetics, pain medications, or steroids outside the tough membrane surrounding the spinal cord (the dura matter). The injected substances block the nerves and offer relief from acute herpes zoster pain for some people. Some studies, but not all, have indicated that if they are given early enough (within two months), they may prevent nerve damage that leads to PHN. Combinations of anesthetics with steroids in the epidural blockade may be particularly beneficial. This procedure is invasive, however, and is not widely used.

OTC Pain Relievers: For an acute (immediate) shingles attack, individuals may take OTC pain relievers, including acetaminophen (Tylenol) or ibuprofen (Motrin, Advil). Children should take acetaminophen, not aspirin. Adults may take aspirin. Such remedies, however, are not very effective for PHN.

PHN

PHN is difficult to treat. Once PHN develops, a multidisciplinary approach that involves a pain specialist, psychiatrist, primary care physician, and other healthcare professionals may provide the best means to relieve the pain and distress associated with this condition.

Anesthetic Patches: Topical (on the skin) preparations, including a skin patch containing the anesthetic drug lidocaine (Lidoderm), are generally used. They are effective in many people without producing any known severe side effects. The patch appears to reduce pain and improve quality of life for many patients. One to four patches can be applied over the course of 24 hours. Another patch (EMLA) contains both the anesthetic drugs lidocaine and prilocaine. These patches are expensive and require a prescription. The most common side effects are skin redness or rash.

Topical Creams: Capsaicin (Zostrix) is prepared from the active ingredient in hot chili peppers. An ointment form has been approved for PHN and is available OTC. Its benefits are limited, however, and it is uncertain whether they are meaningful for most patients. A new patch form that uses a higher than standard dose may be more effective than current options. In one study, it reduced pain by 33% in nearly half of patients. Capsaicin should not be used until the blisters have completely dried out and are falling off the skin. Capsaicin ointment should be handled using a glove and applied to affected areas three or four times daily. The patient will usually experience a burning sensation when the drug is first applied, but this sensation diminishes with use. It may take up to six weeks for the patient to experience its full effect, however, and about a third cannot tolerate the burning sensation. Many find no benefit.

Topical aspirin, known chemically as triethanolamine salicylate (Aspercreme), may bring relief. Also, menthol-containing creams such as Ben Gay and Flexall 454 may be helpful.

Oral Medicines: Low-dose tricyclic antidepressants, preferably nortriptyline (Pamelor, Aventyl), are also used. Side effects include drowsiness, fatigue (tiredness), dry mouth, and constipation. If that does not work, gabapentin (Neurontin), an antiseizure drug, can be used. Doctors usually start with a low dose and slowly increase the amount given until relief or severe side effects occur. Side effects include drowsiness and nausea or vomiting. Painkilling drugs known as opiates, including oxycodone (OxyContin) or hydrocodone (Vicodin, Lortab), may be used. These drugs cause drowsiness and may cause physical dependence, even in short-term use (two weeks or less).

Investigative Agents: Cannabinoids are compounds in marijuana (cannabis) that may have properties that protect nerve cells. They are being studied for a number of nerve disorders, including chronic nerve-related pain. In one study, they were effective in reducing pain and had no major side effects.

Mexiletine (Mexitil) is a calcium channel–blocking agent that alters nerve impulse transmission. It is normally used for heart rhythm disorders but is being used in some cases for PHN in patients who do not respond to standard agents. The agent can have adverse effects, including serious allergic reactions, nausea, vomiting, flushing, and arrhythmias (irregular heartbeat).

Psychological Approaches: A number of relaxation and stress-reduction techniques are helpful in managing chronic pain. They include meditation, deep-breathing exercises, biofeedback, and muscle relaxation. Such techniques may apply to those with severe pain from acute infection and from persistent long-term PHN. Cognitive behavioral therapy is showing benefit in enhancing patients' beliefs in their own abilities for dealing with pain. Using specific tasks and self-observation, patients gradually shift their fixed ideas that they are helpless against the pain that dominates their lives to the perception that it is only one negative and, to a degree, a manageable experience among many positive ones.

INTEGRATIVE THERAPIES
Good Scientific Evidence

Aloe: The transparent gel from the pulp of the meaty leaves of aloe (*Aloe vera*) has been used topically (on the skin) for thousands of years to treat wounds, skin infections, burns, and numerous other dermatological conditions. Limited evidence suggests that *A. vera* in a cream preparation is an effective treatment for genital herpes in men. Additional research is warranted in this area.

Guided Imagery: Therapeutic guided imagery may be used to help patients relax and focus on images associated with personal issues they are confronting. Experienced guided imagery practitioners may use an interactive, objective guiding style to encourage patients to find solutions to problems by exploring their existing inner resources. Although not clinically proven to work in herpes infections, guided imagery does seem to help lower pain in individuals in several clinical studies.

Lemon Balm: Several clinical studies have reported that a topical preparation of lemon balm (*Melissa officinalis*) heals sores associated with oral herpes (HSV-1). More studies are needed in this area.

Lysine: Lysine is an amino acid that has been reported in several clinical studies to decrease the recurrence of herpes labialis (oral herpes, HSV-1). However, this use remains controversial and more scientific studies should be performed.

Therapeutic Touch: Therapeutic touch may reduce pain associated with many conditions, including herpes viruses, although no clinical studies have been performed in this area. However, most studies of therapeutic touch have not been well designed, and therapeutic touch has not been clearly compared to common pain treatments such as pain-relieving drugs. Further research is needed before a firm conclusion can be drawn.

H

Zinc: Proper nutrition, including vitamins and minerals, has been reported to help in decreasing recurrent herpes infections. Lesser quality studies have been conducted to assess the effects of zinc (topical or taken by mouth) in HSV-1 or HSV-2. A small study found that oral zinc sulfate appeared to reduce both the number of episodes and the time to recovery of herpes labialis. Several of these studies used combination treatments or permitted the continued use of other medications, so the exact role of zinc in those studies is unclear. However, the positive results obtained in most trials suggest that zinc may represent a safe and effective alternative or adjunct treatment for HSV-1 and HSV-2 and should encourage further research into the topic using well-designed studies.

Unclear or Conflicting Scientific Evidence

Acupuncture: Several clinical studies have reported that acupuncture therapy is effective in reducing the pain associated with PHN. More studies need to be performed before a firm conclusion can be drawn.

Chlorophyll: Oral consumption of chlorophyll liquid was reported in one clinical study to be effective in both herpes simplex and varicella-zoster infections. More clinical research is needed.

Dimethylsulfoxide (DMSO): Topical use of DMSO has been reported effective in the treatment of herpes zoster (shingles). One study reported that benefits may be more effective when DMSO is combined with the drug idoxuridine. Further research is necessary.

Honey: Honey is a sweet, viscid fluid produced by honeybees (*Apis mellifera*) from the nectar of flowers. It has been used for thousands of years as a healing agent. One small controlled trial found topical honey effective in treating labial but not genital herpes. More research is needed in this area to draw a conclusion. Honey should not be used in diabetic individuals.

Hypnosis: Hypnosis is associated with a deep state of relaxation. A small study showed potential benefit of a hypnotherapeutic treatment program for patients suffering from recurrent orofacial herpes infections. Further research is needed to confirm these results.

Licorice: Licorice (*Glycyrrhiza glabra*) has been found in laboratory studies to hinder the spread and infection of HSV. Clinical studies need to be performed. Licorice may increase blood pressure in sensitive individuals.

Peppermint Oil: The essential oil from peppermint (*Mentha piperita*) has been reported effective in decreasing recurrent herpes infection. One case report found that topical peppermint oil was effecting in reducing the pain of PHN. More clinical studies are needed. Peppermint oil may burn the skin if undiluted.

Propolis: Propolis is a natural flavonoid-rich resin created by bees, used in the construction of hives. Propolis is produced from the buds of conifer and poplar trees, in combination with beeswax and other bee secretions. A limited number of laboratory studies have demonstrated effectiveness of propolis and its constituents against HSV-1 and HSV-2. Preliminary results from human trials suggest some degree of efficacy of topical propolis for resolving the lesions associated with genital herpes virus infections. More clinical research is needed.

Reishi: Reishi mushroom (*Ganoderma lucidum*) has been reported to improve immune system function in humans. Reishi extract was effective in decreasing postherpetic pain in one case series. However, there are insufficient data to make any conclusion.

Rhubarb: One double-blind, controlled trial indicates that topically applied rhubarb-sage extract cream may reduce the symptoms of herpes. It was compared to acyclovir (Zovirax) cream and was equally effective in relieving the symptoms. More high-quality studies using rhubarb as a monotherapy are needed to discern rhubarb's effect on herpes symptoms.

Tai Chi: Tai chi is a system of movements and positions believed to have developed in twelfth century China. Tai chi techniques aim to address the body and mind as an interconnected system and are traditionally believed to have mental and physical health benefits to improve posture, balance, flexibility, and strength. A small trial showed that treatment with tai chi might increase immunity to the virus that causes shingles. This may suggest the use of tai chi in the prevention of chickenpox and shingles, but further well-designed, large studies should be performed. Tai chi can also help with physical fitness, which is important with individuals with weakened immune systems.

Tea Tree Oil: Tea tree oil, from the *Melaleuca alternifolia* tree, has been proposed as a potential topical therapy for genital HSV infections based on in vitro findings of antiviral activity. However, at this time there is insufficient human evidence to recommend either for or against this use of tea tree oil. Tea tree oil should not be taken internally, although vaginal and rectal use is recommended by some healthcare providers. Apply tea tree oil with a cotton ball. If sensitivity develops, such as rash or irritation, diluting the oil with water may help. If the rash or irritation continues, discontinue use.

Transcutaneous Electrical Nerve Stimulation (TENS): TENS is a noninvasive technique in which a low-voltage electrical current is delivered through wires from a small power unit to electrodes located on the skin or using acupuncture-like needles. TENS helps stimulate the chi, or energy of the body. TENS has been effectively used in treating pain associated with PHN in several clinical studies. However, more studies are needed.

Historical or Theoretical Uses Lacking Sufficient Evidence

Arabinoxylan: Arabinoxylan is produced from *Hyphomycetes mycelia* mushroom extract. Arabinoxylan has been used traditionally for herpes zoster infection and to treat PHN. Arabinoxylan increases immune function and may help the body fight off infection. Clinical studies are needed to support these uses.

Astragalus: Astragalus (*Astragalus membranaceous*) has been used for centuries in traditional Chinese medicine as a restorative tonic for the aged and debilitated, according to secondary sources. Astragalus is used traditionally for immune support and may be used for viral infections such as herpes. Several laboratory studies report that astragalus is effective against HSV-1. Clinical studies need to be performed to support these findings.

Other integrative therapies that may have benefit in the treatment of herpes infections or the prevention of herpes recurrence include bitter melon (*Momordica charantia*), bromelain (from *Ananas comosus*), topical calendula (*Calendula officinalis*), cat's claw (*Uncaria tomentosa*), topical clove (*Eugenia aromatica*) and clove oil (eugenol), topical eucalyptus oil (*Eucalyptus globulus*), ginseng (*Panax ginseng*), goldenseal (*Hydrastis canadensis*), gotu kola (*Centella asiatica*), olive leaf (*Olea europaea*), raspberry (*Rubus idaeus*), reflexology, and shiitake (*Lentinus edodes*).

PREVENTION

HSV-1 (Herpes Labialis, Oral Herpes)

Taking steps to guard against the development of cold sores, to prevent spreading them to other parts of the body, or to avoid passing them along to another person is important when dealing with oral herpes.

Contact with Infected Individuals: The virus can spread easily as long as there are moist secretions from blisters. In individuals with depressed immune systems, the virus can be spread even after the skin appears to be healed. Also, not kissing others on the mouth if a herpes viral infection is present is important.

Sharing Common Items: Utensils, towels, water glasses, and other commonly used items can spread the virus when blisters are present.

Clean Hands: Washing the hands carefully before touching another person when a cold sore is present is very important. The eyes and genital area may be particularly susceptible to spread of the virus.

Triggers: Avoiding or preventing conditions that stress the body, such as poor diet, not getting enough sleep, or staying in the sun for long periods of time without applying sun block is very important in preventing oral herpes outbreaks.

HSV-2 (Genital Herpes)

Measures for preventing genital herpes are the same as those for preventing other STDs. HSV-2 is highly contagious while lesions are present. The best way to prevent infection is to abstain from sexual activity or to limit sexual contact to only one person who is infection free. Individuals should use, or have their partners use, a latex condom during each sexual contact; limit the number of sex partners; avoid any contact with a partner who has sores until the sores are completely healed or use a male or female condom during anal, oral, or vaginal sex (however, transmission can still occur if the condom does not cover the sores); avoid having sex just before or during an outbreak since the risk for transmission is highest at that time; and ask the sexual partners if they have ever had a herpes outbreak or been exposed to the herpes virus. Also, getting tested for HSVs is important if the individual is sexually active outside of a monogamous relationship.

If an individual is pregnant, it is important to tell the doctor that HSV is present. If the individual has had unprotected sex and is unsure, testing for HSV is recommended by healthcare professionals. Watch for signs and symptoms of HSV during pregnancy. A doctor may recommend that individual start taking herpes antiviral medications when she is about 36 weeks pregnant to try to prevent an outbreak from occurring around the time of delivery. If the individual is having an outbreak when she goes into labor, the doctor will probably suggest a cesarean section to reduce the risk of passing the virus to the baby.

A vaccine in clinical trials is being tested in women who have not been infected with HSV. The vaccine is HerpeVac and may become available for prevention of genital and oral herpes infections.

HHV-3 (VZV, Chickenpox)

Varivax: A vaccine for varicella-zoster infections is now used to prevent chickenpox. Varivax, a live virus vaccine, produces persistent immunity against chickenpox. Data show that the vaccine can prevent chickenpox or reduce the severity of the illness even if it is used within three days, and possibly up to five days, after exposure to the infection. The vaccine against chickenpox is now recommended in the United States for all children between the ages of 18 months and adolescence who have not yet had chickenpox. Children are given one dose of the vaccine. Two doses one to two months apart are given to people over 13 years of age. To date, more than 75% of children have been vaccinated.

Some experts suggest that every healthy adult without a known history of chickenpox be vaccinated. Adults without such a history of infection by varicella-zoster should strongly consider vaccination if they are adults who are at high risk of exposure or transmission (hospital or day care workers, parents of young children), individuals who live or work in environments in which viral transmission is likely, individuals who are in contact with people who have compromised immune systems, nonpregnant women of childbearing age, adolescents and adults living in households with children, and international travelers.

Women who are trying to become pregnant should postpone conception until three months after the vaccine.

Side effects of Varivax include discomfort at the injection site. About 20% of vaccine recipients have pain, swelling, or redness at the injection site. Only about 5% of adverse reactions are serious. Adverse events may include seizures, pneumonia, anaphylactic reaction (a life-threatening allergic reaction), encephalitis (inflammation of the brain), Stevens-Johnson syndrome, neuropathy (nerve damage), herpes zoster, and blood abnormalities. The vaccine may also produce a mild rash within about a month of the vaccination that has been known to transmit chickenpox to others. Individuals who have recently been vaccinated should avoid close contact with anyone who might be susceptible to severe complications from chickenpox until the risk for a rash has passed. Months or even years after the vaccination, some people develop a mild infection termed modified varicella-like syndrome. The condition appears to be less contagious and has fewer complications than naturally acquired chickenpox.

There is currently intense debate over the long-term protection of the vaccine. Studies have reported that more than 15% of vaccinated children still develop chickenpox (called breakthrough infections). The long-term protective effect for adults is even less clear. Between 1979 and 1999, it was reported that although 9% developed chickenpox months to years after their last vaccination, in all cases infection was mild, with none of the serious complications of adult chickenpox. A 2003 study on booster shots in older adults suggests that revaccination with the live virus is safe and effective.

Varicella-Zoster Immune Globulin (VZIG): VZIG is a substance that triggers an immune response against VZV. It is used to protect high-risk patients who are exposed to chickenpox or those who cannot receive a vaccination of the live virus. Such groups include pregnant women with no history of chickenpox, newborns under four weeks who are exposed to chickenpox or shingles, premature infants, children with weakened immune systems, adults with no immunity to VZV, and recipients of bone marrow transplants (even if they have had chickenpox). VZIG should be given within 96 hours and no later than 10 days after exposure to someone with chickenpox.

HHV-3 (VZV, Shingles)

Zostavax: Zostavax is a live vaccine made from the herpes zoster virus that causes shingles. Zostavax has been reported to reduce the incidence of herpes zoster by 51.3% in adults aged 60 and older who received the vaccine. The vaccine also reduced by 66.5% the number of cases of PHN and reduced the severity and duration of pain and discomfort associated with shingles by 61.1%. Zostavax was approved by the FDA in May 2006. The FDA recommended it only for adults aged 60 and older who meet requirements. These requirements include not having a life-threatening allergy to gelatin or a life-threatening allergy to the antibiotic neomycin or other component of the herpes zoster vaccine. Individuals should not have a weakened immune system due to HIV/AIDS or any other disease. Patients should also not be on other disease medications, such as steroids, radiation, or chemotherapy, which affect the immune system. There should be no history of cancer of the bone marrow or lymphatic system, such as leukemia or lymphoma, and also no active or untreated tuberculosis. Side effects include headache, itching, and tenderness or redness at site of injection.

Zostavax is not a substitute for Varivax in children.

HIGH BLOOD PRESSURE

BACKGROUND

Blood pressure is the force of blood pushing against the walls of arteries (blood vessels). Each time the heart beats, it pumps blood through blood vessels, supplying the body's muscles, organs, and tissues with the oxygen and nutrients that they need to function. Over the course of a day, an individual's blood pressure rises and falls transiently many times in response to various stimuli. Elevated blood pressure over a sustained period of time is a condition referred to as hypertension. Nearly one in three American adults has high blood pressure. Approximately two-thirds of people over the age of 65 have high blood pressure. Of those people with high blood pressure, 71.8% are aware of their condition. Of all people with high blood pressure, 61.4% are under current treatment, 35.1% have it under control, and 64.9% do not have it controlled.

The cause of 90-95% of the cases of high blood pressure is not known; however, high blood pressure is easily detected and usually controllable. From 1994-2004 the death rate from high blood pressure increased 15.5% and the actual number of deaths rose 41.8%. Non-Hispanic blacks are more likely to suffer from high blood pressure than are non-Hispanic whites. Within the African-American community, those with the highest rates of hypertension are more likely to be middle aged or older, less educated, overweight or obese, physically inactive, and diabetic. In 2004 the death rates per 100,000 population from high blood pressure were 15.6 for white males, 49.9 for black males, 14.3 for white females, and 40.6 for black females.

The World Health Organization estimates that the prevalence of hypertension exceeds 10% in developed nations. High blood pressure increases the risk of coronary heart disease (CHD) and stroke (lack of blood and oxygen to the brain), which are the leading causes of death among Americans.

CLASSIFYING HYPERTENSION

Hypertension (high blood pressure) can be mild, moderate, or severe. The National Heart, Lung, and Blood Institute classifies blood pressure as normal, prehypertension, hypertension stage 1, and hypertension stage 2. Normal blood pressure is a systolic pressure of less than 120 mm Hg and a diastolic pressure less than 80 mm Hg (120/80 mm Hg).

Prehypertension is when the systolic and diastolic blood pressure is higher than normal (120/80 mm Hg) but not high enough to be considered high blood pressure (140/90 mm Hg). Prehypertension is a systolic (top number) between 120-139 or a diastolic (bottom number) between 80-89. For example, blood pressure readings of 138/82, 128/70, and 115/86 are all in the prehypertension range.

Stage 1 hypertension is a systolic pressure between 140-159 mm Hg and a diastolic pressure between 90-99 mm Hg or higher. Stage 2 hypertension is a systolic pressure of 160 mm Hg or higher and a diastolic pressure of 100 mm Hg or higher.

Both increased systolic and diastolic blood pressures can increase the risk for congestive heart failure (CHF, or problems with the heart pumping blood to the body), heart attack, kidney disease, stroke (neurological damage to the brain due to a lack of oxygen), erectile dysfunction (inability of males to get an erection), amputation of the legs, and blindness.

As people become older, the diastolic pressure will begin to decrease and the systolic blood pressure will begin to increase, which may lead to high blood pressure. This disorder is called isolated systolic hypertension.

RELATED CONDITIONS

Hypertensive Emergency: Hypertensive emergency is a life-threatening form of high blood pressure, also known as malignant or accelerated hypertension, and is extremely rare. Uncontrolled blood pressures lead to progressive target organ dysfunction, or organ damage. Kidneys, brain, and heart can be damaged. Hypertensive emergency affects less than 1% of individuals with high blood pressure. Unlike the more common form of high blood pressure that usually develops over a number of years, this condition is marked by a rapid rise in blood pressure (called a hypertensive emergency), with the diastolic pressure shooting to 120 mm Hg or higher. Hypertensive emergencies must be treated immediately. Hypertensive emergencies can be caused by a history of kidney disorders, pheochromocytoma (tumor of the adrenal glands), and spinal cord disorders. Hypertensive urgency is a severe elevation of blood pressure without evidence of organ damage.

Medications that may cause a hypertensive emergency include cocaine, monoamine oxidase inhibitors (used in depression), dopamine (an injectable blood pressure–raising drug), and oral contraceptives. The withdrawal of beta-blockers (including propranolol, metoprolol, and amlodipine) and alpha-stimulants (including clonidine), or alcohol may also

H

cause a hypertensive emergency. An intravenous (into the veins) drug called sodium nitroprusside (Nipride) is used in hypertensive emergencies.

Preeclampsia: Preeclampsia is a condition characterized by high blood pressure during pregnancy along with protein in the urine. It can cause serious complications for the mother and baby. Preeclampsia can decrease the supply of blood and oxygen available to the mother and developing child. This may result in conditions such as a lower birth weight and neurological (nervous system) damage. The mother is at risk for kidney problems, seizures, strokes, breathing problems, and even death in rare instances. The cause of preeclampsia is not known. Preeclampsia usually occurs during the second half of the pregnancy and affects about 5% of pregnant women.

Pulmonary Hypertension: When pressure in the pulmonary circulation (blood flow to and from the lungs) becomes abnormally elevated, it is referred to as pulmonary hypertension. Pulmonary hypertension results from constriction, or tightening of the blood vessels that supply blood to the lungs. As a result, it becomes difficult for blood to pass through the lungs, making it harder for the heart to pump blood forward. This stress on the heart leads to enlargement of the heart and eventually fluid can build up in the liver and tissues, such as in the legs. Affected patients can sometimes notice increasing shortness of breath and dizziness. Pulmonary hypertension can be caused by diseases of the heart and the lungs, such as chronic obstructive pulmonary disease or emphysema, sleep apnea (a sleeping disorder characterized by pauses in breathing), failure of the left heart ventricle, recurrent pulmonary embolism (blood clots traveling from the legs or pelvic veins obstructing the pulmonary arteries), or underlying diseases such as scleroderma (scar tissue in the organs).

RISK FACTORS

Obesity: Individuals with a body mass index (BMI, or body fat content) of 30.0 or higher are more likely to develop high blood pressure. Individuals are considered underweight if their BMI is less than 18.5. A BMI of 18.5-24.9 is considered a "normal" weight. A BMI of 25-29.9 is considered overweight. Individuals who fall into the BMI range of 25-34.9 begin having some health risk concerns, such as the development of diabetes, hypertension (high blood pressure), and heart disease. Specifically, those who have a waist size of more than 40 inches for men or 35 inches for women have a higher risk for obesity-related health problems. A BMI of 30 or more qualifies an individual as obese. A BMI over 40 indicates that a person is morbidly obese. The greater the number, the greater the chances of developing health concerns.

Salt Sensitivity: Salt (or sodium chloride) contains sodium, which may cause fluid retention and thereby cause pressure around the blood vessels, which can lead to hypertension. It is noted that approximately 60% of the essential hypertension population may decrease their blood pressure by decreasing sodium (salt) intake.

Drinking Too Much Alcohol: Chronic (long-term) use of alcohol can increase blood pressure dramatically by placing stress on the heart and blood vessels.

Lack of Physical Activity: An inactive lifestyle makes it easier to become overweight and increases the chance of high blood pressure. Physical inactivity increases the risk of hypertension by 30%.

Smoking: Cigarette smoking can repeatedly produce a temporary rise in blood pressure of approximately 5-10 mm Hg. This effect may be most prominent with the first cigarette of the day in habitual smokers. However, research indicates that habitual or chronic (regular) smokers in general have lower blood pressure than nonsmokers, possibly due to weight loss associated with smoking. Experts agree that smoking should be avoided in any person with high blood pressure because it can substantially increase the risk of secondary cardiovascular complications such as atherosclerosis (hardening of the arteries) and appears to enhance the progression of kidney disease. Cigarette smoking also increases the chances of men having erectile dysfunction, or the inability to get or maintain and erection.

Stress: Stress is a normal part of everyday life. Responses to stress vary from person to person, but chronic (regular) stress can lead to an increase in the release of the stress hormone cortisol from the adrenal glands (above the kidneys). Cushing's disease can also cause too much cortisol to be released. Scientists think that excess cortisol can lead to an increase in blood pressure, an inability of insulin to control blood sugar (insulin sensitivity), inflammation, and weight gain.

Ethnicity (Race): African Americans develop high blood pressure more often than Caucasians, and it tends to occur earlier and be more severe. Compared to other groups, African-Americans tend to get high blood pressure earlier in life, usually have more severe high blood pressure, and have a higher death rate from stroke (lack of blood and oxygen to the brain), CHD (the lack of blood and oxygen to the heart), and kidney failure.

Heredity: Having a parent or other close blood relatives with high blood pressure increases the chances of developing it.

Age: In general, blood pressure increases with age, occurring most often in people over age 35. Men seem to develop it most often between age 35 and 55. Women are more likely to develop it after menopause. Over half of all Americans aged 60 and older have high blood pressure.

Diet: A diet poor in fruits, vegetables, and whole grains and high in sodium (salt), high-fat foods such as dairy (milk, cheese, sour cream), animal fat, and fried foods (potato chips, French fries, fried chicken) can lead to high cholesterol levels in the blood, which can lead to high blood pressure.

CAUSES

Essential, or Primary, Hypertension: There is no known cause of essential hypertension. However, there are risk factors that contribute to developing high blood pressure. A number of environmental factors have been implicated in the development of high blood pressure, including salt intake, obesity, race, physical activity level, heredity, diet, and stress level.

Secondary Hypertension: Secondary hypertension accounts for approximately 5-10% of all cases of high blood pressure, with the remaining being essential or primary hypertension. Secondary hypertension has an identifiable cause, unlike essential hypertension. There are many known conditions that can cause secondary hypertension. Regardless of the cause, pressure in the arteries becomes elevated either due to an increase in how much blood the heart pumps to the body (cardiac output), an increase in the resistance of the blood vessels in the body, or both. Individuals with secondary hypertension are best treated by controlling or removing the underlying disease or cause, although they may still require antihypertensive (blood pressure–lowering) drugs. Causes of secondary hypertension can be broken down into renal (kidney related), endocrine (hormonally related), neurological (of the nervous system), and miscellaneous.

Renal: The kidneys regulate fluid (water) and electrolyte (including sodium, potassium, and chloride) levels in the body. Renal causes (related to the kidneys) of high blood pressure include radiation damage, renal artery stenosis (the narrowing of the main artery to the kidneys), and chronic renal disease such as diabetic neuropathy (damage to nerves cause by high blood sugar levels) and polycystic kidney disease (many cysts or closed sacs).

Endocrine: Hormonal (estrogen, progesterone, testosterone) changes or imbalances can cause increases in blood pressure. Oral contraceptives (birth control pills) can also cause hypertension. Diseases of the adrenal glands (located on top of the kidneys) can also cause high blood pressure, including pheochromocytoma (tumor of the adrenal gland), acromegaly (a disease caused by the secretion of excessive amounts of growth hormone), hyperthyroidism or hypothyroidism (high or low thyroid hormone), hyperparathyroidism (too much calcium in the blood, which raises blood pressure), Cushing's disease (release of excess stress hormone from the adrenal glands), insulin resistance (inability of insulin to control blood sugar levels), and primary hyperaldosteronism (an increased release of adrenal hormones that control fluid and electrolyte balance).

Neurological: Some disorders of mental or emotional origin, including anxiety (nervousness) and mania (hyperactivity), may cause high blood pressure. Damage to the central nervous system, such as damage to the spinal cord, increased intracranial pressure (pressure around the brain), or nervous system tumors may also cause hypertension.

Medications: Medications such as amphetamines (including cocaine, dextroamphetamine [Dexedrine], and mixed amphetamine [Adderall]), nasal decongestants (pseudoephedrine), nonsteroidal antiinflammatory drugs (NSAIDs, including ibuprofen [Motrin, Advil]), monoamine oxidase inhibitors (including phenelzine [Nardil]), adrenergic stimulants (including clonidine [Catapres]), and birth control pills (in about 5% of users) can cause hypertension with use.

Alcohol Use: Chronic (long-term) alcohol use can also lead to hypertension.

Other Causes: Other causes of high blood pressure include aortic coarctation (genetic narrowing of the aorta, the largest artery of the body leading from the heart to the body), sleep apnea (disorder where people stop breathing for short periods of time in their sleep), licorice (when consumed in excessive amounts, can cause hyperaldosteronism), scleroderma (formation of scar tissue in organs), neurofibromatosis (genetic disorder that causes tumors to grow along the nerves), pregnancy (causing preeclampsia), and cancers (tumors can interfere with blood flow).

SIGNS AND SYMPTOMS

Hypertension is called the silent killer because an individual can have it for years without knowing it. Hypertension rarely causes symptoms at first but is a risk factor for many other conditions including kidney disease and CHD, which may lead to heart attack and/or stroke (lack of blood and oxygen to the tissues). Although it rarely happens, hypertension occasionally

H

causes symptoms, such as vertigo (dizziness), tinnitus (ringing in the ears), dimmed vision, fatigue (tiredness), palpitations (irregular heartbeat), impotence (inability of males to achieve or maintain erection), and fainting. Extremely elevated blood pressure can cause a headache upon awakening or, even more rarely, nosebleed, nausea, or vomiting.

Malignant hypertension can be life threatening and has recognizable symptoms that require immediate treatment. Symptoms include blurred vision, headache, confusion, anxiety, drowsiness, fatigue (tiredness), nausea, vomiting, chest pain (angina), shortness of breath, cough, decreased urinary output, and weakness or numbness in the arms, legs, face, or other areas. If symptoms of malignant hypertension are noticed, call 911 emergency immediately.

DIAGNOSIS

Blood pressure is measured with a stethoscope (device used to listen to internal sounds), an inflatable arm cuff, and a pressure-measuring gauge called a sphygmomanometer. A blood pressure reading, given in millimeters of mercury (mm Hg), has two numbers. The first, or upper, number measures the pressure in the arteries when the heart beats (systolic pressure). The second, or lower, number measures the pressure in the arteries between beats when the chambers of the heart are filling with blood (diastolic pressure). In general, lower is better. However, very low blood pressure (hypotension) can sometimes be a cause for concern and should be checked out by a doctor.

The latest blood pressure guidelines, issued in 2003 by the National Heart, Lung, and Blood Institute, divide blood pressure measurements into four general categories: normal (below 120/80 mm Hg), prehypertension (120-139 systolic and 80-89 diastolic), stage 1 hypertension (140-159 systolic and 90-99 diastolic), and stage 2 hypertension (160 or higher systolic and 100 or higher diastolic). To get an accurate blood pressure reading, a healthcare professional should evaluate the readings based on the average of two or more blood pressure readings.

In a doctor's office, blood pressure readings are usually taken when the individual is sitting or lying down and relaxed. Healthcare professionals recommend to not drink coffee or smoke cigarettes 30 minutes before having blood pressure taken, wear short sleeves, and go to the bathroom before the blood pressure reading. Having a full bladder can change the blood pressure reading. Also sit for five minutes before the test.

Physical Examination and Blood Tests: If hypertension is found, the doctor may ask questions regarding medical history and diet and lifestyle. The doctor may also order various routine tests. Risk factors of high blood pressure are evaluated, including electrolyte levels (sodium, potassium, and chloride), high cholesterol levels (total cholesterol, low-density lipoprotein, high-density lipoprotein [HDL], and triglycerides), calcium levels, diabetes (blood sugar levels), medications and supplements the individual is currently taking, and obesity (BMI) measurement.

COMPLICATIONS

Excessive and uncontrolled pressure on the artery walls can damage vital organs. The higher the blood pressure and the longer it goes uncontrolled, the greater the damage.

Damage to the Arteries: This can result in hardening and thickening of the arteries (atherosclerosis), which can lead to a heart attack or other complications. An enlarged, bulging blood vessel (aneurysm) also is possible.

Heart Failure: The heart muscle can have a hard time pumping blood against the higher pressure in the vessels, leading to increasing heart muscle thickness. Eventually, the thickened muscle may have a hard time pumping enough blood to meet the body's needs, which can lead to chronic heart failure.

Stroke: Excessive blood pressure can lead to a blocked or ruptured blood vessel in the brain, leading to a lack of blood flow and oxygen to the brain (stroke).

Metabolic Syndrome: This syndrome is a cluster of disorders of the body's metabolism, including increase waist circumference, high triglycerides, low HDL ("good" cholesterol), high blood pressure, and high insulin levels. The more components an individual has, the greater the risk of developing diabetes, heart disease, or stroke.

Hypertensive Nephropathy: Weakened and narrowed blood vessels in the kidneys can develop, leading to the inability of these organs to function normally.

Hypertensive Retinopathy: Thickened, narrowed, or torn blood vessels in the eyes can develop that may result in vision loss.

Cognitive Impairment: Chronic (long-term) or acute (immediate) high blood pressure can impair the ability to think, remember, and learn.

Preeclampsia: Preeclampsia, or high blood pressure and protein in the urine during pregnancy, is diagnosed through blood pressure checks, which are routine at prenatal visits. A doctor will also order a test to determine whether protein is in the urine (albumin test). A rapid increase in blood pressure is a sign that the individual may be developing preeclampsia.

Endothelial Dysfunction: Endothelial dysfunction is a malfunction of the endothelium, the cells that line the inner surface of all blood vessels, including arteries and veins. Normal functions of endothelial cells include helping with coagulation (blood clotting), platelet adhesion (also involved in clotting), immune function, and control of fluid and electrolyte content in and out of the cells. Endothelial dysfunction can result from high blood pressure. High blood pressure causes the blood vessels to become stiff and less able to constrict (narrow) and dilate (expand). Other causes include septic shock (inability of the tissues to get blood and oxygen), hypercholesterolemia (high cholesterol), diabetes, and environmental factors such as cigarette smoking. Endothelial dysfunction is thought to be a key event in the development of atherosclerosis (hardening of the arteries), leading to heart attacks.

TREATMENT

Treating high blood pressure can help prevent serious and life-threatening complications. A doctor also may suggest steps to control conditions that can contribute to high blood pressure, such as diabetes and high cholesterol. Evidence suggests that reduction of the blood pressure by 5 to 6 mm Hg can decrease the risk of stroke by 40% and CHD by 15-20% and reduces the likelihood of dementia, heart failure, and mortality from vascular disease. Blood pressure goals are not the same for everyone. Although everyone should strive for blood pressure readings below 140/90 mm Hg, doctors recommend lower readings for people with certain conditions. The goal is 130/80 mm Hg if the patient has or has had chronic kidney disease or diabetes.

Lifestyle Changes: Lifestyle changes can help control and prevent high blood pressure. Even if the individual is diagnosed with high blood pressure, lifestyle changes can still help prevent further damage to blood vessels and the heart.

Healthy Foods: Experts recommend using the Dietary Approaches to Stop Hypertension (DASH) diet, which emphasizes fruits, vegetables, whole grains, and low-fat dairy foods. Get plenty of potassium (as in bananas and green leafy vegetables such as spinach), which can help prevent and control high blood pressure. Eat less saturated fat (animal fat) and total fat. Limit the amount of sodium (salt) in the diet. Although 2,400 milligrams of sodium a day is the current limit for otherwise healthy adults, limiting sodium intake to 1,500 milligrams a day will have a more dramatic effect on blood pressure. Look at the food labels to determine sodium content.

If cooking at home, use less salt or a salt substitute (contains potassium iodide, which does not increase blood pressure).

Healthy Body Weight: If an individual is overweight, losing even five pounds can lower blood pressure. Eating healthy and exercising regularly can help lower weight. No eating between meals and late at night also helps decrease weight gain.

Physical Activity: Regular physical activity can help lower blood pressure and keep weight under control. Individuals should strive for at least 30 minutes of moderate physical activity a day.

Alcohol Consumption: Alcohol can raise the blood pressure even in a healthy person. If individuals choose to drink alcohol, they should do so in moderation. One drink a day for women and two drinks a day for men should not be exceeded. Consumption of red wine, which has heart-healthy components, is better than other types of spirits.

Smoking Cessation: Tobacco injures blood vessel walls and speeds up the process of hardening of the arteries. A doctor can help an individual choose the right method of smoking cessation (stopping).

Stress Management: Reduce stress as much as possible. Practice healthy coping techniques, such as muscle relaxation and deep breathing. Getting plenty of sleep can help, too. Practice slow, deep breathing. In various clinical trials, regular use of RESPeRATE (InterCure Inc., New York), an over-the-counter device approved by the U.S. Food and Drug Administration to analyze breathing patterns and help guide inhalation and exhalation, significantly lowered blood pressure. It is used for 15 minutes daily several times a week. Changing the lifestyle can help control high blood pressure. But sometimes lifestyle changes are not enough. In addition to diet and exercise, a doctor may recommend medication to lower blood pressure. Which category of medication the doctor prescribes depends on the stage of high blood pressure and whether there are other medical conditions.

Diuretics: These medications act on the kidneys to help the body eliminate sodium and water, thereby reducing blood volume. Thiazide diuretics, including hydrochlorothiazide (HCTZ, HydroDIURIL), is often the first choice of medicine in treating high blood pressure. In a 2006 study, diuretics were a key factor in preventing heart failure associated with high blood pressure. Adverse effects of thiazide diuretics include sexual dysfunction, glucose intolerance, gout, elevated potassium level, and low sodium level (hyponatremia). Other diuretics include loop diuretics such as furosemide (Lasix) and bumetanide (Bumex) and potassium-sparing diuretics (keep potassium from being depleted from the body), including amiloride (Midamor) and triamterene (Maxzide).

Beta-Blockers: These medications reduce the workload on the heart, causing the heart to beat slower and with less force. When prescribed alone, beta blockers do not work as well in African-Americans, but they are effective when combined with a thiazide diuretic in these individuals. Beta-blockers include propranolol (Inderal), metoprolol (Lopressor, Toprol) or atenolol (Tenormin). Side effects associated with the use of beta-blockers include nausea, diarrhea, bronchospasm (spasm of the bronchial tubes), dyspnea (difficulty breathing), cold extremities (fingers, toes), bradycardia (slow heat rate), hypotension (low blood pressure), fatigue (tiredness), dizziness, abnormal vision, decreased concentration, hallucinations, insomnia (difficulty sleeping), nightmares, depression, sexual dysfunction (lack of interest in sex), erectile dysfunction (inability to achieve or maintain an erection in men), and/or alteration of glucose and cholesterol metabolism. These drugs may worsen blood glucose control, elevate triglyceride levels, and lower HDL ("good" cholesterol).

Angiotensin-Converting Enzyme (ACE) Inhibitors: Oral ACE inhibitors, including lisinopril (Prinivil, Zestril), benazepril (Lotensin), captopril (Capoten), and enalapril (Vasotec), dilate blood vessels and increase oxygen to the heart. Angiotensin is made when the kidneys receive a signal to raise blood pressure. ACE inhibitors prevent or reduce the production of angiotensin, which keeps vessels from narrowing and helps them relax. This relaxation lowers blood pressure and increases the supply of blood and oxygen to the heart. ACE inhibitors may be especially important in treating high blood pressure in people with coronary artery disease, heart failure, or kidney failure. Like beta-blockers, ACE inhibitors do not work as well in African-Americans when prescribed alone but seem to be more effective when combined with a thiazide diuretic such as hydrochlorothiazide. Contraindications to ACE inhibitor use include hypotension (low blood pressure) and declining kidney function with ACE inhibitor use. The use of an ACE inhibitor four to six weeks after a heart attack is recommended for patients with CHF, left ventricular dysfunction, hypertension (high blood pressure), or diabetes.

Angiotensin II Receptor Blockers (ARBs): ARBs work similarly to ACE inhibitors. However, instead of inhibiting the production of the angiotensin enzyme in the kidneys, they block the effects of angiotensin on cell receptor membranes. They are more effective than ACE inhibitors in treating some

people who have high blood pressure. They are particularly useful for treating high blood pressure in individuals who cannot tolerate ACE inhibitors well. ARBs include irbesartan (Avapro), candesartan (Atacand), and losartan (Cozaar). Adverse effects of ARBs can include headache, drowsiness, diarrhea, and a metallic or salty taste in the mouth.

Calcium Channel Blockers (CCBs): CCBs affect the transport of calcium into the cells of the heart and blood vessels, causing blood vessels to relax. This relaxation increases the blood and oxygen supply to the heart, lowers blood pressure, and reduces the heart's workload. CCBs include amlodipine (Norvasc), felodipine (Plendil), nicardipine (Cardene, Carden SR), and nifedipine (Procardia, Adalat). Physicians often recommend CCBs to treat high blood pressure in women who have pregnancy-induced high blood pressure, elderly patients, patients who have a history of angina (chest pain), or patients of African or Caribbean descent. CCBs are not a good choice for patients who have had a heart attack or who have CHF. Adverse effects of CCBs include constipation, swelling of the lower part of the legs, flushing, or headache.

Alpha-Blockers: Alpha-blockers (also called alpha-adrenergic blocking agents) block alpha receptors in vascular smooth muscle (including blood vessels), preventing the uptake of catecholamines (brain hormones such as epinephrine), which are produced in response to stress. This blocking mechanism permits blood vessel dilation (relaxing) and allows blood to flow more freely. Alpha-blockers are not advised for those who have a history of (or are at risk for) CHF. Alpha-blockers include doxazosin (Cardura), prazosin (Minipress), and terazosin (Hytrin). Alpha-blockers tend to interfere with the blood pressure–regulating adjustments the body has to make when a person goes from sitting or lying down to standing. Individuals using alpha-blockers may experience a drop in blood pressure (called orthostatic hypotension) when they go from sitting or lying down to standing. Other common adverse effects include stuffy nose and dizziness.

Alpha-Beta Blockers: In addition to reducing nerve impulses to blood vessels, alpha-beta blockers slow the heartbeat to reduce the amount of blood that must be pumped through the vessels (acting like both alpha-blockers and beta-blockers). Alpha-beta blockers include carvedilol (Coreg) and labetalol (Normodyne, Trandate). Side effects include those similar to both alpha- and beta-blockers.

Centrally Acting Agents: Central alpha-agonists lower blood pressure by stimulating alpha receptors in the brain that open peripheral arteries, easing blood flow. Central alpha-agonists include clonidine (Catapres), guanabenz (Wytensin), and methyldopa (Aldomet). Adrenergic neuron blockers decrease the amount of brain neurochemicals (epinephrine, dopamine) available and include reserpine (Serpasil) and guanethidine (Ismelin). Both centrally acting drugs are usually prescribed when all other antihypertensive medications have failed.

Vasodilators: These medications work directly on the muscles in the walls of the arteries, preventing the muscles from tightening and the arteries from narrowing. Oral vasodilators include hydralazine (Apresoline). The vasodilators only used in medical emergency hypertension include sodium nitroprusside (Nipride) and nitroglycerin. Once the blood pressure is under control, a doctor may add low-dose aspirin (81 milligrams) to the therapy to reduce the risk of CHD. Aspirin is a platelet inhibitor and helps platelets from "clumping" together and blocking blood vessels, which could increase blood pressure.

To reduce the number of doses needed a day, which can reduce side effects, a doctor may prescribe a combination of low-dose medications rather than larger doses of one single drug. These are commonly used antihypertensive drugs (such as ACE inhibitor and beta-blockers) combined with the thiazide diuretic hydrochlorothiazide. Companies manufacture drugs that combine hydrochlorothiazide and ACE inhibitors, including Prinizide (lisinopril plus hydrochlorothiazide) and Capozide (captopril plus hydrochlorothiazide). Studies report that using an antihypertensive drugs combined with a thiazide diuretic reduces costs and may increase effectiveness against high blood pressure.

INTEGRATIVE THERAPIES

Strong Scientific Evidence

Omega-3 Fatty Acids: Omega-3 fatty acids are essential fatty acids found in some plants and fish. There should be a balance of omega-6 and omega-3 fatty acids for health. Multiple human trials report small reductions in blood pressure with intake of omega-3 fatty acids. Docosahexaenoic acid may have greater benefits than eicosapentaenoic acid. However, high intakes of omega-3 fatty acids per day may be necessary to obtain clinically relevant effects and, at this dose level, there is an increased risk of bleeding. There is strong scientific evidence from human trials that omega-3 fatty acids from fish or fish oil supplements significantly reduce cholesterol levels, which may also help in reducing blood pressure. Omega-3 supplements can cause an increase in bleeding in susceptible individuals, including those taking blood-thinning medications such as warfarin (Coumadin).

Good Scientific Evidence

Coenzyme Q10 (CoQ10): CoQ10 is produced by the human body and is necessary for the basic functioning of cells. CoQ10 levels are reported to decrease with age and to be low in patients with some chronic diseases such as heart conditions, muscular dystrophy, Parkinson's disease, cancer, diabetes, and HIV/AIDS. Some prescription drugs may also deplete CoQ10 levels, such as 3-hydroxy-3-methylglutaryl coenzyme A inhibitors, or statin drugs, for high cholesterol. Preliminary research suggests that CoQ10 causes small decreases in blood pressure (systolic and possibly diastolic). Low blood levels of CoQ10 have been found in people with hypertension, although it is not clear if CoQ10 "deficiency" is a cause of high blood pressure. Well-designed long-term research is needed.

Hibiscus: Hibiscus (*Hibiscus* spp.) has been used for centuries by Ayurvedic (Hindu) and Chinese medical practitioners. Two human studies have shown that extracts of hibiscus may lower systolic and diastolic pressure. In one study, hibiscus standardized extract worked as well as captopril (Capoten), a commonly used ACE inhibitor, in lowering blood pressure. Additional high-quality studies comparing hibiscus to placebo are needed to confirm these results, although the use of hibiscus for lowering blood pressure looks promising. Caution is advised when taking hibiscus, as numerous adverse effects including diuresis (increased excretion of fluid) can occur.

Qi Gong: Qi gong is a type of traditional Chinese medicine that is thought to be at least 4,000 years old. There are two main types of qi gong practice: internal and external. Internal qi gong is a self-directed technique that involves the use of sounds, movements, and meditation. Internal qi gong actively engages people in their own health and well-being and can be performed with or without the presence of a master instructor. It may be practiced daily to promote health maintenance and disease prevention. Several human trials suggest benefits of qi gong in the treatment of high blood pressure, particularly when added to conventional treatments such as prescription drugs. There is early evidence that there may be lower death rates in people with high blood pressure who practice qi gong. Some studies report that high blood pressure associated with pregnancy may be partially controlled through internal qi gong relaxation exercises. Although this research is promising, a major problem is that the way qi gong is practiced is not always clear in these studies and may not be similar to the way qi gong is practiced in the community.

Stevia: Stevia (*Stevia rebaudiana*) standardized extracts are used as natural sweeteners and dietary supplements. Stevioside is a natural plant component isolated from stevia that has demonstrated blood pressure–lowering effects. Despite evidence of benefits in some human studies and support from laboratory and animal studies, more research is warranted to compare stevia's effectiveness with the current standard of care. Caution is advised when taking stevia, as numerous adverse effects, including blood sugar lowering, have been observed. Stevia should not be used if pregnant or breastfeeding unless otherwise directed by a doctor.

Yoga: Yoga is an ancient system of relaxation, exercise, and healing with origins in Indian philosophy over 2,000 years ago. Several human studies support the use of yoga in the treatment of high blood pressure when practiced for up to one year. It is not clear if yoga is better than other forms of exercise for blood pressure control. Better research is needed in this area. Yoga practitioners sometimes recommend that patients with high blood pressure should avoid certain positions, such as headstands or shoulder stands, which may increase blood pressure.

Unclear or Conflicting Scientific Evidence

Acupressure, Shiatsu: The practice of applying finger pressure to specific acupoints throughout the body has been used in China since 2000 BC, prior to the use of acupuncture. Acupressure techniques are widely practiced internationally for relaxation, wellness promotion, and the treatment of various health conditions. Small studies in men and women report that acupressure may reduce blood pressure. Study results on the effect of acupressure on heart rate have yielded mixed results. Large, well-designed studies are needed.

Acupuncture: The practice of acupuncture originated in China 5,000 years ago. Today it is widely used throughout the world and is one of the main pillars of Chinese medicine. It involves the insertion of needles in various points of the body to help move the "chi," or energy. Although used for centuries to lower blood pressure, human trials are lacking.

Acustimulation: Acustimulation is the mild electrical stimulation of acupuncture points to control symptoms such as nausea and vomiting. A low-intensity electrical current is used to penetrate just slightly below the surface of the skin. It may be delivered by acupuncture needles attached to electrodes or, more commonly, by battery-powered appliances that can be worn on the body (touching the surface of the skin). Acustimulation has been examined in the treatment of high blood pressure in one small study of patients diagnosed with diastolic hypertension. A set of four different acupuncture points was used, with results showing an immediate reduction of diastolic blood pressure. At this time, the evidence is insufficient for use of acustimulation in high blood pressure.

L-Arginine: L-arginine, or arginine, is considered a semiessential amino acid, because although it is normally synthesized in sufficient amounts by the body, supplementation is sometimes required. A small study suggests that arginine taken by mouth may dilate the arteries and temporarily reduce blood pressure in hypertensive patients with type 2 diabetes. Larger, high-quality studies are needed. L-arginine is generally safe in recommended dosages.

Beta-Glucan: Beta-glucan is a soluble fiber derived from the cell walls of algae, bacteria, fungi, yeast, and plants. It is commonly used for its cholesterol-lowering effects. A study found that the addition of oat cereals to the normal diet of patients with hypertension significantly reduces both systolic and diastolic blood pressure. Soluble fiber-rich whole oats may be an effective dietary therapy in the prevention and adjunct treatment of hypertension.

Chiropractic: Chiropractic is a healthcare discipline that focuses on the relationship between musculoskeletal structure (primarily the spine) and body function (as coordinated by the nervous system) and how this relationship affects the preservation and restoration of health. Manipulation involves the hands-on application of a physical therapy. The effects of spinal manipulative techniques on blood pressure remain controversial. It has been hypothesized that nervous system effects of spinal manipulation can lower both systolic and diastolic pressure. Numerous trials, reviews, and commentaries have been published in this area. Although some studies are suggestive, overall the existing evidence remains debatable. Better research is necessary before a firm conclusion can be drawn.

Flaxseed Oil: Flaxseed (*Linum usitatissimum*) and its derivative flaxseed oil/linseed oil are rich sources of the essential fatty acid alpha-linolenic acid, which makes omega-3 essential fatty acids in the body. Omega-3 fatty acids have been associated with a decreased risk of heart disease. In animals, diets high in flaxseed have mixed effects on blood pressure. One study in humans suggests that flaxseed might lower blood pressure. The evidence in this area is not clear, and more research is needed. Caution is advised when taking flaxseed supplements, as numerous adverse effects, including an increased risk of bleeding and drug interactions, are possible.

Garlic: Garlic (*Allium sativum*) is traditionally used for heart health. Numerous human studies report that garlic can lower blood pressure by a small amount, but larger, well-designed studies are needed to confirm this possible effect. Garlic supplements can cause an increase in bleeding in susceptible individuals, including those taking blood-thinning medications such as warfarin (Coumadin).

Ginseng: Asian ginseng, or *Panax ginseng,* has been used for more than 2,000 years in Chinese medicine for various health conditions. Several studies from China report that ginseng in combination with various other herbs may reduce symptoms of coronary artery disease. Preliminary research suggests that ginseng may lower blood pressure (systolic and diastolic). It is not clear what doses may be safe or effective. Well-conducted studies are needed to confirm these early results. Caution is advised when taking ginseng supplements, as adverse effects including drug interactions are possible. Ginseng supplements should not be used if pregnant or breastfeeding unless otherwise directed by a doctor.

Green Tea: Green tea is made from the dried leaves of *Camellia sinensis,* a perennial evergreen shrub. Green tea has a long history of use, dating back to China approximately 5,000 years ago. Green tea, black tea, and oolong tea are all derived from the same plant, just processed differently. Green tea helps protect blood vessels from injury and has been reported in laboratory studies to lower blood pressure. Green tea is considered cardioprotective, or helping protect the heart from disease. Healthcare professionals recommend using caffeine-free supplements when using in people with hypertension (high blood pressure).

Iridology: Iridology is the study of the iris (colored part of the eye) with the intention of gaining information about underlying diseases. Iridologists believe that the degrees of light and darkness in the iris give clues to the body's general health. Preliminary studies by a South Korean team of researchers using a computerized approach suggest that iridology may assist in the identification of individual predispositions for vascular diseases such as hypertension. Further research is needed to confirm these findings, and further teams of researchers would need to conduct parallel work in order for these methods to become validated.

Lycopene: Lycopene is a carotenoid, which is a naturally occurring class of fat-soluble pigments (coloring) found mainly in plants and algae, where they play a critical role in the photosynthetic process. Photosynthesis is the making of glucose (energy) from sunlight, carbon dioxide, and water, with oxygen as a waste product. Lycopene is present in human serum, liver, adrenal glands, lungs, prostate, colon, and skin at higher levels than other carotenoids. Based on early study, lycopene may reduce the development of preeclampsia and intrauterine growth retardation in women having their first child. Further research is needed to confirm these results.

Massage: Various forms of therapeutic superficial tissue manipulation have been practiced for thousands of years across cultures. Chinese use of massage dates to 1600 BC, and Hippocrates made reference to the importance of physicians being experienced with "rubbing" as early as 400 BC. Based on early study, massage may decrease blood pressure in hypertensive patients. More high-quality studies are needed.

Meditation: Various forms of meditation have been practiced for thousands of years throughout the world, with many techniques originating in Eastern religious practices. Meditation may involve breathing exercises or repeating phrases or words over and over to "clear" the mind. Several studies of transcendental meditation (repeating phrases or words) report small decreases in blood pressure levels over short periods of time and that its long-term effects may improve mortality. However, the available research has not been well designed or reported and cannot be considered conclusive.

Melatonin: Melatonin is a hormone produced in the brain by the pineal gland from the amino acid tryptophan. The synthesis and release of melatonin are stimulated by darkness and suppressed by light, suggesting the involvement of melatonin in circadian rhythm and regulation of diverse body functions. Levels of melatonin in the blood are highest prior to bedtime. Synthetic melatonin supplements have been used for a variety of medical conditions, most notably for disorders related to sleep and as an antioxidant. Antioxidants help stop free radical (reactive oxygen) damage to vessels. Several controlled studies in patients with high blood pressure report small reductions blood pressure when taking melatonin by mouth (orally) or inhaled through the nose (intranasally). Better-designed research is necessary before a firm conclusion can be reached. Caution is advised when taking melatonin, as adverse effects, including drowsiness and drug interactions, are possible. Melatonin should not be used if pregnant or breastfeeding unless otherwise directed by a doctor. Melatonin is for short-term use only (one to two weeks).

Pet Therapy: Animal companionship has been used as an informal source of comfort and relief of suffering across cultures throughout history. There is evidence from one well-designed trial that pet ownership may have additive value in patients with hypertension who are taking conventional blood pressure medication.

Psychotherapy: Psychotherapy is an interactive process between a person and a qualified mental health professional (psychiatrist, psychologist, clinical social worker, licensed counselor, or other trained practitioner). Its purpose is the exploration of thoughts, feelings, and behavior for the purpose of problem solving or achieving higher levels of functioning. Relaxation techniques have been associated with reduced pulse rate, systolic blood pressure, and diastolic blood pressure; lower perception of stress; and enhanced perception of health. Further research is needed to confirm these results.

Pycnogenol: Pycnogenol (Horphag Research, Berlin) is the patented trade name for a water extract of the bark of the French maritime pine (*Pinus pinaster* spp. *atlantica*), which is grown in coastal southwest France. Use of Pycnogenol may reduce the need for nifedipine (Procardia) and decrease systolic blood pressure in patients with high blood pressure. Further research is needed to confirm these results.

Reishi: Reishi (*Ganoderma lucidum*) is a fungus (mushroom) that grows wild on decaying logs and tree stumps. Reishi has been used in traditional Chinese medicine for more than 4,000 years to treat liver disorders, high blood pressure, arthritis, and other ailments. Ancient Chinese monks utilized the reishi mushroom to calm their mind for meditation. Theory would lead one to believe that the physiological effects of decreasing blood pressure may have lead to the calming effect after ingested reishi. Preliminary data suggest that reishi may exert a blood pressure–lowering effect; however, the currently available evidence in this area is weak. Future studies are warranted to validate the results of these small studies and to provide clinical usefulness of reishi as a possible treatment for high blood pressure. Caution is advised when taking reishi supplements, as adverse effects, including an increase in bleeding and drug interactions, are possible. Reishi supplements should not be used if pregnant or breastfeeding unless otherwise directed by a doctor.

Relaxation Therapy: Relaxation techniques include behavioral therapeutic approaches that differ widely in philosophy, methodology, and practice. The primary goal is usually nondirected relaxation. Most techniques share the components of repetitive focus (on a word, sound, prayer phrase, body sensation, or muscular activity), adoption of a passive attitude towards intruding thoughts, and return to the focus.

Rhubarb: Chinese herbalists have relied on rhubarb (*Rheum palmatum*) for thousands of years. The rhizomes and roots contain powerful anthraquinones (laxatives) and tannins, which tone tissue. Two studies on rhubarb's effect on preeclampsia indicate that it may be a helpful treatment to decrease blood pressure. More high-quality trials are needed to confirm this hypothesis. Caution is advised when taking rhubarb, as adverse effects, including dehydration (loss of fluid) and drug interactions, are possible. Rhubarb should not be used if pregnant or breastfeeding unless otherwise directed by a doctor.

Riboflavin: Riboflavin, or vitamin B_2, is a water-soluble vitamin that is involved in vital metabolic processes in the body and is necessary for normal cell function, growth, and energy production. Limited study has reported an association between low riboflavin levels and an increased risk of preeclampsia (high blood pressure in pregnancy). However, it is not clear if low riboflavin levels are a cause or consequence of this condition or if additional supplementation is warranted in pregnant women at risk of preeclampsia/eclampsia beyond the routine use of prenatal vitamins. Riboflavin is safe in recommended dosages.

Rutin: Rutin is an antioxidant that naturally occurs in various plants (apple peels, black tea, rue, tobacco, and buckwheat). Quercetin (a flavonoid found in rutin) and rutin are used as vasoprotectants (blood vessel protective) and are ingredients of numerous multivitamin preparations and herbal remedies. The flavonoids found in rutin have documented effects on capillary permeability (leakage) and edema (swelling) and have been used for the treatment of disorders of the venous and microcirculatory (capillary) systems. Overall the results of clinical studies suggest a benefit of rutin for venous hypertension. Well-designed studies are required. Rutin is safe in recommended dosages. Nausea and stomach upset may occur.

Soy: Soy (*Glycine max*) has been a dietary staple in Asian countries for at least 5,000 years. Large-scale soybean cultivation began in the United States during World War II, and currently, midwestern U.S. growers produce approximately half of the world's supply of soybeans. Soy and components of soy called isoflavones have been studied scientifically for numerous health conditions. Although soy products have not been proven to be effective in lowering blood pressure in humans, laboratory and some human studies do support the use of soy in reducing the risk of developing coronary artery disease. Caution is advised when taking soy, as adverse effects including drug interactions are possible. Soy supplements should not be used if pregnant or breastfeeding unless otherwise directed by a doctor. Experts recommend that individuals with breast cancer not use soy products unless under the supervision of a doctor.

Taurine: Taurine is a nonessential amino acid (building blocks of protein) and is important in several metabolic processes of the body, including stabilizing cell membranes in electrically active tissues, such as the brain and heart. It also has functions in the gallbladder, eyes, and blood vessels, and may have some antioxidant and detoxifying effects. In animal studies, taurine has been reported to result in decreased blood pressure in hypertension. Preliminary results from a randomized, controlled trial and a case series suggest that taurine may be beneficial in blood pressure lowering in individuals with borderline hypertension. Well-designed and reported clinical trials are still needed. Caution is advised when taking taurine supplements, as adverse effects, including an increase in bleeding and drug interactions, are possible. Taurine supplements should not be used if pregnant or breastfeeding unless otherwise directed by a doctor.

Vitamin D: Vitamin D is found in numerous dietary sources such as fish, eggs, fortified milk, and cod liver oil. The sun is also a significant contributor to our daily production of vitamin D, and as little as 10 minutes of exposure is thought to be enough to prevent deficiencies. The term "vitamin D" refers to several different forms of this vitamin. Two forms are important in humans: ergocalciferol (vitamin D_2) and cholecalciferol (vitamin D_3). Vitamin D_2 is made by plants. Vitamin D_3 is made by humans in the skin when it is exposed to ultraviolet B rays from sunlight or the diet. Low levels of vitamin D may play a role in the development of high blood pressure. It has been noted that blood pressure is often elevated during the winter season, at further distance from the equator, and in dark skin pigmentation (color), all of which are associated with lower exposure to vitamin D via sunlight. However, evidence is not clear and comparison with more proven methods to reduce blood pressure has not been conducted.

PREVENTION

Blood pressure should be a systolic reading of 120 and a diastolic reading of 80 (120/80 millimeters of mercury). Exercising, managing stress, maintaining a healthy weight, and limiting sodium and alcohol intake are all ways to keep blood pressure in check.

Medications to treat hypertension, such as diuretics, angiotensin-converting enzyme (ACE) inhibitors, and angiotensin receptor blockers, may also be used.

Cholesterol and Saturated Fat Intake Reduction: A diet rich in high fat foods such as dairy (milk, cheese, sour cream), animal fat, and fried foods (potato chips, French fries, fried chicken) can lead to high cholesterol levels in the blood, which can lead to high blood pressure. Eating less cholesterol and fat, especially saturated fat, may reduce the amount of plaque in the arteries. Most people should aim for a low density lipoprotein (LDL) level below 130 milligrams per deciliter of blood. If there are other risk factors for heart disease, the target LDL may be below 100 milligrams per deciliter of blood. If the individual is at a very high risk for heart disease, such as having a previous heart attack, an LDL level below 70 milligrams per deciliter of blood may be optimal.

Smoking Cessation: Cigarette smoking can repeatedly produce a temporary rise in blood pressure (BP) of approximately 5-10mmHg, and is a major risk factor for coronary artery disease. Nicotine constricts blood vessels and forces the heart to pump harder. A buildup of carbon monoxide (CO) reduces oxygen in the blood and damages the lining of the blood vessels. Experts agree that smoking should be avoided in any person with high blood pressure because it can substantially increase the risk of secondary cardiovascular complications such as atherosclerosis (hardening of the arteries).

Weight Control: Being overweight contributes to several risk factors for stroke, high blood pressure, cardiovascular disease, and diabetes. Individuals with a body mass index (BMI, or body fat content) of 30.0 or higher are more likely to develop high blood pressure. Weight loss of as little as 10 pounds may lower blood pressure and improve cholesterol levels.

Exercise: An inactive lifestyle makes it easier to become overweight and increases the chance of high blood pressure. It has been found that physical inactivity increases the risk of hypertension by 30%. Exercise can lower blood pressure, increase the level of HDL cholesterol (good cholesterol), and improve the overall health of blood vessels and the heart. It also helps control weight, control diabetes and reduce stress. Thirty minutes of daily exercise is normally recommended.

Stress Management: Stress can cause an increase in blood pressure along with increasing the blood's tendency to clot. Chronic stress can lead to an increase in the release of the stress hormone cortisol from the adrenal glands. Researchers believe that this increase in cortisol leads to increased blood pressure. Managing stress can be vital to keeping a heart healthy.

Sodium Reduction: Salt (or sodium chloride) contains sodium, which may cause fluid retention and thereby cause pressure around the blood vessels which can lead to hypertension. It is noted that approximately 60% of the essential hypertension population may decrease blood pressure (BP) by decreasing sodium (salt) intake.

Limiting Alcohol Consumption: In some studies, moderate use of alcohol (particularly red wine) has been linked with increasing levels of HDL cholesterol. However, excessive drinking can have a negative impact on cholesterol levels, actually raising triglyceride levels and increasing blood pressure. It has been found that chronic (long-term) use of alcohol can increase blood pressure dramatically by placing stress on the heart and blood vessels.

HIGH CHOLESTEROL

BACKGROUND

High cholesterol, or hypercholesterolemia, is a condition in which there are unhealthy high levels of cholesterol in the blood. It is also called dyslipidemia, hyperlipidemia, and lipid disorder. Too much cholesterol in the blood is a major risk for heart disease, which may lead to a heart attack, heart failure (cannot pump enough blood to the body), and death. High cholesterol levels are also a risk factor for stroke (lack of blood and oxygen to the brain), causing nerve damage. Cholesterol is a soft, waxy, fatlike substance found within the bloodstream and cells of the body. Cholesterol synthesis is a naturally occurring process that functions to produce membranes for all cells in the body, including those in the brain, nerves, muscles, skin, liver, intestines, and heart. Cholesterol is also converted into steroid hormones, such as the male and female sex hormones (androgens and estrogens) and the adrenal hormones (cortisol, corticosterone, and aldosterone). In the liver, cholesterol is the precursor to bile acids that aid in the digestion of food, especially fats. Cholesterol is also used in making vitamin D. The body obtains cholesterol in two ways, producing the majority of it in the body and consuming the rest in the diet in the form of animal products such as meats, poultry, fish, eggs, butter, cheese, and whole milk. Plant foods, like fruits, vegetables, and grains, do not contain cholesterol. Fat that occurs naturally contains varying amounts of saturated and unsaturated fat.

High cholesterol can cause the formation and accumulation of plaque deposits in the arteries. Plaque is composed of cholesterol, other fatty substances, fibrous tissue, and calcium, normal substances in the blood that become deposited on the artery walls if the blood does not flow properly. When plaque builds up in the arteries, it results in atherosclerosis (hardening of the arteries), or coronary heart disease (CHD). Atherosclerosis can lead to plaque ruptures and blockages in the arteries, which increase the risk for heart attack, stroke, and death as well as circulation problems such as Raynaud's disease and high blood pressure. The development of plaques and blockages in the arteries involves several steps. When the innermost lining of the arteries (endothelium) is damaged by oxidation, cholesterol particles, proteins, and other substances deposit into the damaged wall and form plaques. More cholesterol and other substances incorporate into the plaque and the plaque grows, narrowing the artery. Over time, plaque deposits may grow large enough to interfere with blood flow through the artery (called a blockage). When the arteries supplying the heart with blood (coronary arteries) are blocked, chest pain (angina) may occur; when arteries in the legs are blocked, leg pain or cramping may occur; and when arteries supplying the brain with blood are blocked, stroke may occur.

The platelets collecting on the plaque deposit are forming a clot as they try to rush by and get caught because the lining of the artery is rough and the platelets are sticky. Then the clot can break off and travel through the body, getting lodged in vessels of the leg, brain or, less commonly, the lungs. If a plaque ruptures or tears, a blood clot (thrombus) may develop. If a blood clot completely blocks blood flow through a coronary artery, heart attack (myocardial infarction) occurs; if an artery supplying blood to the brain is completely blocked, stroke occurs. Blood clots can break loose and travel through the bloodstream (called an embolus) and lodge in blood vessels in other parts of the body, including the lungs, heart, brain, and legs. A thromboembolus is when the blood clot lodges in vessels. According to current estimates, 71.3 million people in America have one or more forms of heart disease. High cholesterol affects about 20% of adults over the age of 20 in the United States. The highest prevalence occurs in women between the ages of 65-74. The World Health Organization reports that high cholesterol contributes to 56% of cases of CHD worldwide and causes about 4.4 million deaths each year. Generally, people who live in countries where blood cholesterol levels are lower, such as Japan, have lower rates of heart disease. Countries with very high cholesterol levels, such as Finland, have very high rates of CHD. However, some populations with similar total cholesterol levels have very different heart disease rates, suggesting that other factors (such as diet, heredity, and smoking) also influence risk for CHD.

Evidence is accumulating that eating more carbohydrates, especially simpler, more refined carbohydrates such as white breads, sugar, and pasta, may increase levels of triglycerides in the blood, lower high-density lipoprotein (HDL, or "good" cholesterol), and may increase low-density lipoprotein (LDL, or "bad" cholesterol). Thus, a low-fat diet, which often means a higher carbohydrate intake, may actually be an unhealthy change.

TYPES OF CHOLESTEROL

Saturated Fats: Saturated fats are solid at room temperature. Foods that contain a high proportion of saturated fat are butter, lard, coconut oil, cottonseed oil and palm oil, dairy products (such as cream and cheese), meat, skin, and some prepared foods. People with diets high in saturated fat are reported to have an increased incidence of atherosclerosis (hardening of the arteries) and CHD. Saturated fats are popular with manufacturers of processed foods because they are less vulnerable to rancidity and are generally more solid at room temperature than unsaturated fats.

Unsaturated Fats: Unsaturated fats are liquid at room temperature. Unsaturated fats include monounsaturated and polyunsaturated fats. Monounsaturated fat remains liquid at room temperature but may start to solidify in the refrigerator. Foods high in monounsaturated fat include olive, peanut, and canola oils. Avocados and most nuts also have high amounts of monounsaturated fat. Polyunsaturated fat is usually liquid at room temperature and in the refrigerator. Foods high in polyunsaturated fats include vegetable oils, such as safflower, corn, sunflower, soy, and cottonseed oils. The use of monounsaturated and polyunsaturated fats instead of saturated fat can help to lower blood cholesterol levels.

Trans Fats: Trans fatty acids (trans fats) are a type of unsaturated fat. Trans fat is formed when liquid vegetable oils go through a chemical process called hydrogenation, in which hydrogen is added to make the oils more solid. Hydrogenated vegetable fats are utilized in food production because they allow longer shelf life and give food desirable taste, shape, and texture. Trans fat can be found in shortenings (Crisco), margarine, cookies, crackers, snack foods, fried foods (including fried fast food), doughnuts, pastries, baked goods, and other foods processed with partially hydrogenated oils. Some trans fat is found naturally in small amounts in dairy products and some meats. The primary health risk associated with trans fat consumption is an increased risk of CHD. Effective January 1, 2006, the U.S. Food and Drug Administration required food companies to list trans fat content separately on the Nutrition Facts panel of all packaged foods.

Lipoproteins: Cholesterol and other fats cannot dissolve in the blood. They have to be transported to and from the cells by special carriers called lipoproteins. There are two main types of lipoproteins: LDL ("bad cholesterol") and HDL ("good cholesterol"). Another type, very-low-density lipoprotein (VLDL) is converted to LDL in the bloodstream. Each form of lipoprotein contains a specific combination of cholesterol, protein, and triglyceride (a blood fat). VLDL cholesterol contains the highest amount of triglyceride. Too much LDL cholesterol can block

the arteries, increasing the risk of heart attack and stroke. LDL takes cholesterol into the bloodstream and HDL takes it back to the liver for storage. It is also believed that HDL removes excess cholesterol from plaque in arteries, thus slowing the buildup. Studies suggest that high levels of HDL cholesterol reduce the risk of heart attack.

Lipoprotein(a) [Lp(a)] Cholesterol: Lp(a) is a lipoprotein (fat/protein molecule) found in the body that is a genetic variation of LDL cholesterol. A high level of Lp(a) is an important risk factor for developing fatty deposits in arteries. The way an increased Lp(a) contributes to disease is not understood, but Lp(a) may attract substances that increase inflammation, such as interleukins (IL) (IL-1, IL-6, tumor necrosis factor-alpha) and prostaglandins (PG2), leading to the buildup of fatty deposits.

Triglycerides: Triglycerides are the body's storage form for fat. Most triglycerides are found in adipose (fat) tissue. Some triglycerides circulate in the blood to provide fuel for muscles to work. Extra triglycerides are found in the blood after eating a meal when fat is being sent from the intestines to fat tissue for storage. People with high triglycerides often have high LDL cholesterol and low HDL cholesterol levels. Many people with heart disease also have high triglyceride levels. People with diabetes or who are overweight are also likely to have high triglycerides.

RISK FACTORS AND CAUSES

Diet: Saturated fat and cholesterol in foods makes total cholesterol and LDL levels rise. Cholesterol is consumed in the diet in the form of animal products, such as meats, poultry, fish, eggs, butter, cheese, and whole milk. Plant foods, like fruits, vegetables, and grains, do not contain cholesterol. Fat that occurs naturally contains varying amounts of saturated and unsaturated fat.

Weight: Being overweight may increase "bad" cholesterol levels and is a risk factor for heart disease. Losing weight may help lower LDL, triglyceride, and total cholesterol levels as well as raise HDL. Individuals with a large waist measurement (more than 40 inches for men and more than 35 inches for women) are at high risk for heart disease.

Physical Activity: A lack of physical activity is a risk factor for heart disease. Exercise helps strengthen the heart and blood vessels. Exercising regularly can help lower LDL ("bad cholesterol") and raise HDL ("good cholesterol") levels. Being physically active for at least 30 minutes on most, if not all, days may help with reducing the risk of developing high cholesterol and CHD.

Age and Gender: Cholesterol levels rise with age due to various factors, including hormonal changes, diet, and general health. Before the age of menopause, women have lower total cholesterol levels than men of the same age. After the age of menopause, women's LDL levels tend to rise due to hormonal imbalances. As a rule, women have higher HDL cholesterol levels than men do. The female sex hormone estrogen tends to raise HDL cholesterol, which may help explain why premenopausal women are usually protected from developing heart disease. Estrogen production is highest during the childbearing years (20s to 40s). Women also tend to have higher triglyceride levels. As people get older and/or gain weight, their triglyceride and cholesterol levels tend to rise. Evidence reports that the atherosclerotic process (buildup of fatty plaque in arteries) begins in childhood and progresses slowly into adulthood. Then it often leads to CHD, the single leading cause of death in the United States. Eating patterns and genetics affect blood cholesterol levels in children and increase the risk of developing heart disease later in life.

Heredity: Genetics partially determine how much cholesterol is produced endogenously. High blood cholesterol can run in families. If a parent or sibling developed heart disease before age 55, high cholesterol levels place an individual at a greater than average risk of developing heart disease.

Smoking: Cigarette smoking damages the walls of blood vessels through a process called oxidation, making them prone to build up fatty deposits. Smoking may also lower levels of HDL cholesterol.

High Blood Pressure: Increased pressure on the blood vessel walls damages arteries, which can speed the accumulation of plaque.

Diabetes: High blood sugar contributes to high LDL cholesterol and low HDL cholesterol. High blood sugar can also damage the lining of the arteries, making it easier for plaque (protein, fat, and cholesterol) to deposit.

Others: Kidney disease (nephrotic syndrome), hypothyroidism (low thyroid levels), anorexia nervosa (eating disorder), and Zieve's syndrome (a condition that causes high cholesterol during withdrawal from long-term alcohol abuse) can all contribute to high cholesterol.

SIGNS AND SYMPTOMS

High cholesterol does not lead to specific symptoms unless it has been chronic (long term). High cholesterol levels may lead to specific physical findings such as xanthoma (thickening of tendons due to accumulation of cholesterol), xanthelasma (yellowish patches around the eyelids), and arcus senilis (white discoloration of the outer edges of the cornea due to cholesterol deposits).

A high level of blood cholesterol causes the arteries to narrow and can slow, or even block, blood flow to the heart. This reduced blood supply prevents the heart from receiving enough oxygen. Chronic (long-term) high cholesterol can lead to atherosclerosis (hardening of the arteries), angina (chest pain), heart attack, transient ischemic attacks (temporary lack of blood flow and oxygen to the brain), cerebrovascular accidents/strokes (lack of blood and oxygen in the brain), and peripheral artery disease.

DIAGNOSIS AND SCREENING

Recommendations for cholesterol screening and treatment have been provided by the National Institutes of Health and are summarized in the National Cholesterol Education Program. The guidelines recommend that all adults have their cholesterol levels checked at least once every five years. Patients with CHD or other forms of atherosclerosis are at the highest risk for heart attack and stroke (lack of blood and oxygen to the brain). These patients may benefit the most from cholesterol-reduction therapy and should have a full lipid profile (lipid panel) performed annually. This includes measuring total cholesterol, LDL, HDL, and triglycerides. VLDL and Lp(a) levels can also be taken. For the most accurate measurements, there is no eating or drinking anything (other than water) for nine to 12 hours before the blood sample is taken.

There is no formula to determine what cholesterol level is considered "safe" and what cholesterol level requires treatment for each individual. General recommendations are based on ongoing research regarding future risk for heart attack. In a person with established CHD, the risk for heart attack (or subsequent heart attack) and death is much higher, so even mildly elevated cholesterol levels must be treated aggressively.

Total Cholesterol Levels: The total blood cholesterol will fall into one of three categories, including desirable (less than 200 mg/dL, or milligrams per deciliter), borderline high risk (200-239 mg/dL), and high risk (240 mg/dL and above). If the total cholesterol is less than 200 mg/dL, the risk of heart attack risk is relatively low unless there are other risk factors, such as smoking, a previous heart attack, or high blood pressure. If the total cholesterol level is from 200-239 mg/dL, individuals are classified as borderline high risk. About one-third of American adults are in this group, whereas almost one-half of adults have total cholesterol levels below 200 mg/dL. Not every person whose cholesterol level is in the 200-239 range is at increased risk. If the total cholesterol level is 240 mg/dL or more, an individual is at high risk of heart attack and stroke. In general, people who have a total cholesterol level of 240 mg/dL have twice the risk of CHD as people whose cholesterol level is 200 mg/dL. About 20% of the U.S. population has high blood cholesterol levels.

Lipoprotein Levels: LDL, or "bad" cholesterol, is a major risk factor for developing atherosclerosis (hardening of the arteries) and coronary artery disease (CAD). LDL levels are reported in several categories. An LDL level below 100 mg/dL is best for people at risk for heart disease. If an individual is at very high risk for heart disease, such as having had a previous heart attack, an LDL level less than 70 mg/dL is optimal. LDL levels can also be near optimal (100-129 mg/dL), borderline high (130-159 mg/dL), high (160-189 mg/dL), and very high (190 mg/dL and above). HDL ("good cholesterol") protects against heart disease, so for HDL higher numbers are better. A level less than 40 mg/dL is low and is considered a major risk factor for developing heart disease. HDL levels of 60 mg/dL or more help to lower the risk for developing heart disease.

Triglyceride Levels: High levels of triglycerides can increase heart disease risk. Levels that are borderline high (150-199 mg/dL) or high (200 mg/dL or more) may need treatment.

Children: Total cholesterol levels in children and adolescents (2-19 years old) are acceptable (less than 170 mg/dL), borderline (170-199 mg/dL, and high (200 mg/dL and greater). LDL cholesterol levels for children include acceptable (less than 110 mg/dL, borderline (110-129 mg/dL), and high (130 mg/dL or greater).

COMPLICATIONS

Possible complications of high cholesterol include atherosclerosis (hardening of the arteries), CAD or CHD, stroke (lack of blood flow to the brain), heart attack, and death. As discussed, high cholesterol levels can lead to plaque deposits in blood vessels. Plaque is composed of cholesterol, other fatty substances, fibrous tissue, and calcium, normal substances in the blood that become deposited on the artery walls if the blood does not flow properly. Over time, plaque deposits may grow large enough to interfere with blood flow through the artery (called a blockage). When the arteries supplying the heart with blood (coronary arteries) are blocked, chest pain (angina) may occur; when arteries in the legs are blocked,

leg pain or cramping may occur; and when arteries supplying the brain with blood are blocked, stroke may occur.

TREATMENT

The main goal of cholesterol-lowering treatment is to lower LDL levels enough to reduce the risk of developing heart disease or having a heart attack. The higher the risk, the lower the LDL goal should be. There are two main ways to lower cholesterol, including therapeutic lifestyle changes (TLC) and drug therapy. TLC includes a cholesterol-lowering diet (called the TLC diet), physical activity, and weight management. TLC is for individuals whose LDL is above their target number and goal. Drug treatment with cholesterol-lowering drugs can be used together with TLC treatment to help lower LDL. Prevention of elevated cholesterol is started if the individual is at risk for high cholesterol levels or heart disease or a previous heart attack or stroke has occurred.

Category I, Highest Risk: In those with highest risk, the LDL goal is less than 100 mg/dL. They will begin the TLC diet to reduce high risk even if the LDL is below 100 mg/dL. If the LDL is 100 or above, drug treatment will be started at the same time as the TLC diet. If the LDL is below 100 mg/dL, drug treatment may also be started together with the TLC diet if the doctor finds the risk is very high, for example, if the individuals has had a recent heart attack or has both heart disease and diabetes.

Category II, Next Highest Risk: The LDL goal is less than 130 mg/dL. If the LDL is 130 mg/dL or above, treatment with the TLC diet should be started. If the LDL is 130 mg/dL or more after 3 months on the TLC diet, drug treatment is started along with the TLC diet. If the LDL is less than 130 mg/dL, individuals should follow the heart-healthy diet for all Americans, which allows a little more saturated fat and cholesterol than the TLC diet.

Category III, Moderate Risk: The LDL goal is less than 130 mg/dL. If the LDL is 130 mg/dL or above, the TLC diet is started. If the LDL is 160 mg/dL or more after having tried the TLC diet for 3 months, drug treatment may be started along with the TLC diet. If the LDL is less than 130 mg/dL, the heart-healthy diet for all Americans (low saturated fat and cholesterol) is used.

Category IV, Low-to-Moderate Risk: The LDL goal is less than 160 mg/dL. If the LDL is 160 mg/dL or above, the TLC diet is started. If the LDL is still 160 mg/dL or more after three months on the TLC diet, drug treatment may be started along with the TLC diet to lower LDL, especially if the LDL is

190 mg/dL or more. If the LDL is less than 160 mg/dL, the heart-healthy diet for all Americans is used.

Diet: Individuals with high risk associated with developing heart disease will be started on the TLC diet. The TLC diet is a low saturated fat, low-cholesterol eating plan that calls for less than 7% of calories to come from saturated fat (such as in animal products) and less than 200 milligrams of dietary cholesterol daily. The TLC diet recommends only enough calories to maintain a desirable weight and avoid weight gain. If the LDL is not lowered enough by reducing saturated fat and cholesterol intakes, the amount of soluble fiber, such as psyllium, oat bran, and beta-glucan, in the diet can be increased (found in cereals, breads, and supplements), thereby helping to raise HDL and lower LDL. Certain food products that contain plant sterols (a cholesterol-lowering component in many plants) can also be added to the TLC diet to boost its LDL-lowering power. Examples include cholesterol-lowering margarines (containing Benecol, a plant sterol) and sterol supplements in capsule and tablet form. Plant sterols are found naturally in fruits, vegetables, nuts, seeds, cereals, legumes (beans), and vegetable oils (particularly soybean oil).

Weight Management: When the body mass index (BMI, or fat content) is greater than 25, an individual is considered overweight. BMI uses an equation based on height and weight to determine the level of obesity. Losing weight can help lower LDL and is especially important for those with a cluster of risk factors that includes high triglyceride and/or low HDL levels.

Physical Activity: Regular physical activity (at least 30 minutes on most, if not all, days) is recommended for those who can tolerate exercise. Taking a brisk 30-minute walk three to four times a week can positively impact cholesterol levels. Patients with chest pain and/or known or suspected heart disease should talk to their doctors before beginning any exercise program. Exercise can help raise HDL and lower LDL and is especially important for those with high triglyceride and/or low HDL levels who are overweight with a large waist measurement. Individuals with a large waist measurement (more than 40 inches for men and more than 35 inches for women) are at high risk for heart disease.

Medication Therapy: There are several medications that may help lower cholesterol, including total cholesterol, lipoproteins, and triglycerides. Medications can reduce LDL cholesterol levels by 20-40%. They also can modestly increase HDL ("good") cholesterol levels, usually by about 5-10%. Available drugs include 5-hydroxy-3-methylglutaryl-coenzyme A reductase inhibitors (HMG-CoA reductase inhibitors), bile acid–binding resins, cholesterol absorption inhibitors, fibrates, and niacin.

HMG-CoA Reductase Inhibitors, or Statins: Statins have significantly advanced the treatment of high cholesterol. Statins block a substance (HMG-CoA reductase) that the liver needs to make cholesterol. This decreases cholesterol in liver cells (hepatocytes), which causes the liver to remove cholesterol from the blood, thereby lowering cholesterol levels. Statins may also help the body reabsorb cholesterol from accumulated deposits on artery walls, potentially reversing CAD. Commonly prescribed statins include atorvastatin (Lipitor), fluvastatin (Lescol), lovastatin (Mevacol), pravastatin (Pravachol), rosuvastatin calcium (Crestor), and simvastatin (Zocor). Statins may also be added to blood pressure–lowering drugs for use in protection from CHD (Caduet, a combination of atorvastatin [Lipitor] and amlodipine [Norvasc]). Results from statin treatment should be seen after several weeks, with a maximum effect in four to six weeks. After about six to eight weeks, a doctor will check the LDL cholesterol levels while the individual is on the statin. Serious side effects are rare and include liver problems and muscle soreness, pain, and weakness. If this happens, or if there is brown urine present, contact a doctor immediately. Although rare, muscle breakdown, known as rhabdomyolysis, can occur. This is a medical emergency and a doctor should be contacted immediately.

Bile Acid–Binding Resins (Sequestrants): The liver uses cholesterol to make bile acids, a substance needed for digestion. The medications cholestyramine (Prevalite, Questran), colesevelam (WelChol), and colestipol (Colestid) lower cholesterol indirectly by binding to bile acids (called sequestrant therapy). This causes the liver to use excess cholesterol to make more bile acids, which reduces the level of cholesterol in the blood. Bile acid sequestrant powders must be mixed with water or fruit juice and must be taken once or twice (rarely, three times) daily with meals. Tablets must be taken with large amounts of fluids to avoid stomach and intestinal problems. Sequestrant therapy may produce a variety of symptoms, including constipation, bloating, nausea, and gas. Although sequestrants are not absorbed, they may interfere with the absorption of other medicines if taken at the same time. Other medications should be taken at least one hour before or four to six hours after taking the sequestrant.

Cholesterol Absorption Inhibitors: The small intestine absorbs the cholesterol from the diet and releases it into the bloodstream. The drug ezetimibe (Zetia) helps reduce blood cholesterol by limiting the absorption of dietary cholesterol. Zetia can cause headaches, nausea, fever, and muscle weakness. Zetia by itself lowers LDL cholesterol levels similar to statins, but when combined with a statin, Zetia works better to control elevated LDL levels. There is a combination of ezetimibe and simvastatin on the market (Vytorin).

Fibrates: The medications fenofibrate (Lofibra, Tricor) and gemfibrozil (Lopid) decrease triglycerides by reducing the liver's production of VLDL cholesterol and by speeding up the removal of triglycerides from the blood. VLDL cholesterol contains mostly triglycerides. Some people taking fibrates may have side effects such as stomach or intestinal discomfort. Fibrates may increase the likelihood of developing gallstones and can increase the effect of medications that thin the blood. The dose of fibrates should be reduced if kidney function declines.

Niacin: Niacin, also known as nicotinic acid or vitamin B_3, decreases triglycerides by limiting the liver's ability to produce LDL and VLDL cholesterol. There are two types of niacin: immediate release and extended (or slow) release. Niacin can reduce LDL cholesterol levels by 10-20%, reduce triglycerides by 20-50%, and raise HDL cholesterol by 15-35%. A common and troublesome side effect of immediate-release niacin is flushing or hot flashes, which are the result of blood vessels opening wide. The causes of this flushing are not well known. Most people develop a tolerance to flushing, which can sometimes be decreased by taking the drug during or after meals or by the use of aspirin 30 minutes prior to taking niacin; a doctor will guide the individual. The extended-release form may cause less flushing than the other forms (Niaspan). Individuals will be started on regular niacin therapy to see how well it is tolerated, then the individual can be started on the extended-release products if needed. Blood pressure may also be reduced while taking niacin. Niacin can cause a variety of gastrointestinal symptoms, including nausea, indigestion, gas, vomiting, diarrhea, and the irritation of peptic ulcers.

Other: If there are other symptoms of CHD besides high cholesterol, other medications may be used to decrease the risk of stroke (lack of blood and oxygen to the brain) and heart attack. These include platelet inhibitors ("thin" the blood) such as aspirin (81-325 mg daily, may cause bleeding) or Plavix (clopidogrel), beta-blockers (decrease the heart rate and blood pressure, reducing the heart's demand for oxygen; may cause fatigue) such as metoprolol (Lopressor, Toprol), nitroglycerin (increases the oxygen available to the heart by dilating coronary arteries; may cause headache), calcium channel blockers (slow heart rate and dilate coronary blood vessels; may cause slow heart rate) such as amlodipine (Norvasc) or diltiazem (Cardizem), angiotensin-inhibiting drugs or ACE inhibitors (dilate blood vessels and increase oxygen to the heart; may cause cough) such as lisinopril (Prinivil, Zestril) or ramipril (Altace), and statins or HMG-CoA reductase inhibitors (help lower cholesterol levels; may cause liver problems or muscle pain) such as atorvastatin (Lipitor) or lovastatin (Mevacor). Interventional procedures may also be used to treat CHD, including balloon angioplasty (percutaneous transluminal coronary angioplasty) and stent (a wire mesh that opens blocked blood vessels) placement. CABG surgery may be required to restore normal blood flow to the heart. CABG is a serious surgery, with complications including infection, lowered immunity, memory loss, "fuzzy" thinking, and even death.

INTEGRATIVE THERAPIES
Strong Scientific Evidence

Beta-Glucan: Beta-glucan is a soluble fiber derived from the cell walls of algae, bacteria, fungi, yeast, and plants. It is commonly used for its cholesterol-lowering effects. Numerous trials have examined the effects of oral beta-glucan on cholesterol. Small reductions in total and LDL cholesterol ("bad cholesterol") have been reported. Little to no significant changes have been noted to occur in triglyceride levels or HDL ("good cholesterol") levels. The sum of existing positive evidence is suggestive and not definitive.

Beta-Sitosterol: Beta-sitosterol is one of the most common dietary phytosterols (plant sterols) found and synthesized exclusively by plants such as fruits, vegetables, soybeans, breads, peanuts, and peanut products. Many studies in humans and animals have demonstrated that supplementation of beta-sitosterol into the diet decreases total serum cholesterol as well as LDL cholesterol.

Niacin: Niacin, also known as vitamin B_3 or nicotinic acid, is a well-accepted treatment for high cholesterol. Multiple studies show that niacin (not niacinamide) has significant benefits on levels of HDL ("good cholesterol"), with better results than prescription drugs such as statins like atorvastatin (Lipitor). There are also benefits on levels of LDL ("bad cholesterol"), although these effects are less dramatic. Adding niacin to a second drug such as a statin may increase the effects on LDL. The use of niacin for the treatment of dyslipidemia associated with type 2 diabetes has been controversial because of the possibility of worsening glycemic control.

Niacin is available as an OTC drug in a lower strength that the prescription medicine.

Omega-3 Fatty Acids: Omega-3 fatty acids are essential fatty acids found in some plants and fish. There should be a balance of omega-6 and omega-3 fatty acids for health. There is strong scientific evidence from human trials that omega-3 fatty acids from fish or fish oil supplements significantly reduce blood triglyceride levels. Fish oil supplements also appear to cause small improvements in HDL ("good cholesterol"); however, increases (worsening) in LDL levels ("bad cholesterol") are also observed. Several well-conducted, randomized, controlled trials report that in people with a history of heart attack, regular consumption of oily fish or fish oil/ omega-3 supplements reduces the risk of nonfatal heart attack, fatal heart attack, sudden death, and all-cause mortality (death due to any cause). Most patients in these studies were also using conventional heart drugs, suggesting that the benefits of fish oils may add to the effects of other therapies. Preliminary studies also report reductions in angina (chest pain) associated with fish oil intake. Better research is necessary before a firm conclusion can be drawn. Caution is advised when taking omega-3 supplements, as an increase in bleeding is possible, especially if taken with medications for bleeding disorders.

Policosanol: Policosanol is a cholesterol-lowering natural mixture of higher aliphatic primary alcohols, isolated and purified from sugar cane wax. Policosanol has been used to treat hypercholesterolemia (high cholesterol levels), and numerous studies have analyzed the effects of policosanol on cholesterol levels, including a number of well-designed trials. There is a plausible, well-described mechanism supporting this use. Notably, most human studies have been conducted in Cuba, and many have been conducted by the same author(s). At this time, the evidence supporting the efficacy of this agent is compelling, although greater acceptance in the U.S. market may await conduct of a large, well-conducted randomized trial in the U.S. Caution is advised when taking policosanol, as adverse effects including drug interactions are possible. Policosanol supplements should not be used if pregnant or breastfeeding unless otherwise directed by a doctor.

Psyllium: Psyllium, also referred to as ispaghula, is derived from the husks of the seeds of *Plantago ovata*. Psyllium contains a high level of soluble dietary fiber and is the chief ingredient in many commonly used bulk laxatives, including products such as Metamucil and Serutan. Psyllium is well studied as a cholesterol-lowering agent with generally modest reductions seen in blood levels of total cholesterol and LDL ("bad cholesterol"). Effects have been observed following eight weeks of regular use. Psyllium does not appear to have significant effects on HDL ("good cholesterol") or triglyceride levels. Because only small reductions have been observed, people with high cholesterol should discuss the use of more potent agents with their healthcare provider. Effects have been observed in adults and children, although long-term safety in children is not established. Psyllium can decrease the absorption of many prescription and nonprescription medications and dietary supplements. Psyllium should be taken either one half hour before or two hours after taking prescription and nonprescription medications and dietary supplements.

Red Yeast Rice: Red yeast rice is the product of yeast (*Monascus purpureus*) grown on rice and is served as a dietary staple in some Asian countries. It contains several compounds collectively known as monacolins, substances known to inhibit cholesterol synthesis. One of these, monacolin K, is a potent inhibitor of HMG-CoA reductase and is also known as lovastatin (Mevacor). Preliminary evidence reports that taking red yeast rice by mouth may result in cardiovascular benefits and improve blood flow. Since the 1970s, human studies have reported that red yeast lowers blood levels of total cholesterol, LDL ("bad cholesterol"), and triglyceride levels. Adverse effects including drug interactions are possible when using red yeast rice supplements. Red yeast rice supplements should not be used if pregnant or breastfeeding unless otherwise directed by a doctor. Red yeast rice should not be used in people with liver problems or in heavy alcohol users due to the potential for an increase in liver damage.

Soy: Soy (*Glycine max*) is a member of the pea family and has been a dietary staple in Asian countries for at least 5,000 years. Numerous human studies report that adding soy protein to the diet can moderately decrease blood levels of total cholesterol and LDL ("bad cholesterol"). Small reductions in triglycerides may also occur, while HDL ("good cholesterol") does not seem to be significantly altered. Dietary soy protein has not been proven to affect long-term cardiovascular outcomes such as heart attack or stroke. Soy products such as tofu are high in protein and are an acceptable source of dietary protein. Soy supplements should not be used if pregnant or breastfeeding unless otherwise directed by a doctor. It is not known if soy products increase the risk of developing breast cancer, so healthcare professionals recommend not using soy if there is a history of breast cancer or risk factors, such as taking hormonal replacement therapy (including estrogen and progesterone).

Good Scientific Evidence

Betaine: Betaine is found in most microorganisms, plants, and marine animals. Its main physiological functions are to protect cells under stress and to function as a source of methyl groups needed for many biochemical pathways. Betaine is also found naturally in many foods and is most highly concentrated in beets, spinach, grain, and shellfish. Overall, betaine supplementation may produce significant reductions in homocysteine, a known risk factor of CAD. However, additional studies are needed.

Cordyceps: Cordyceps sinensis is a fungus found mainly in China, Nepal, and Tibet. Cordyceps supplements may lower total cholesterol and triglyceride levels, although these changes may not be permanent or long lasting. Longer studies with follow up are needed to determine the long-term effects of cordyceps on hyperlipidemia.

Garlic: Garlic (*Allium sativum*) is traditionally used for heart health. Multiple studies in humans have reported small reductions in total blood cholesterol and LDL ("bad cholesterol") over short periods of time (four to 12 weeks). It is not clear if there are benefits after this amount of time. Effects on HDL ("good cholesterol") are not clear. This remains an area of controversy. Well-designed and longer studies are needed in this area. Caution is advised when taking garlic supplements, as adverse effects including an increase in bleeding are possible, especially if taking drugs for bleeding disorders such as warfarin (Coumadin). Garlic supplements should not be used if pregnant or breastfeeding unless otherwise directed by a doctor.

L-Carnitine: L-carnitine, or acetyl-L-carnitine, is an amino acid found in the body. Evidence from clinical trials suggests that L-carnitine is effective in reducing symptoms of angina. Carnitine may not offer further benefit when patients continue conventional therapies. Additional study is needed to confirm these findings. L-carnitine is generally safe when used in the recommended dosage.

Yoga: Yoga is an ancient system of relaxation, exercise, and healing with origins in Indian philosophy. Several human studies suggest that yoga is helpful in people with heart disease. However, it is not clear if yoga reduces the risk of heart attack or death, or if yoga is better than any other form of exercise therapy or lifestyle/dietary change. Therefore, yoga may be a useful addition to standard

therapies (such as medications for blood pressure or cholesterol) in people at risk for heart attacks, but further research is necessary.

Unclear or Conflicting Scientific Evidence

Acupuncture: The practice of acupuncture, or the insertion of needles into the body at various energy points, originated in China 5,000 years ago. Some research has suggested that acupuncture might help reduce distress and symptoms of angina, but this has not been consistently shown in other studies.

L-Arginine: L-arginine, or arginine, is considered a semiessential amino acid because although it is normally synthesized in sufficient amounts by the body, supplementation is sometimes required. There is initial evidence from several studies that arginine taken by mouth or by injection improves exercise tolerance and blood flow in arteries of the heart. Benefits have been reported in some patients with CAD and angina. Studies also suggest that arginine supplementation after myocardial infarction (heart attack) may decrease heart damage. However, further research is needed to confirm these findings. L-arginine is generally safe in the recommended dosage.

Astragalus: Astragalus products are derived from the roots of *Astragalus membranaceus* or related species, which are native to China. In Chinese medicine, herbal mixtures containing astragalus have been used to treat heart diseases. There are several human case reports of reduced symptoms and improved heart function, although these are not well described. High-quality human research is necessary before a conclusion can be drawn.

Astaxanthin: Astaxanthin is classified as a xanthophyll, which is a carotenoid (naturally occurring pigment or coloring), and can be found in microalgae, yeast, salmon, trout, krill, shrimp, crayfish, crustaceans, and the feathers of some birds. There is insufficient evidence to recommend for or against the use of astaxanthin for LDL oxidation prevention. More research is needed to make a firm recommendation. Caution is advised when taking astaxanthin, as adverse effects including an increase in bleeding and drug interactions are possible.

Bilberry: Bilberry (*Vaccinium myrtillus*), also known as the European blueberry, is widely used as an antioxidant for general health. Bilberry has been used traditionally to treat heart disease and atherosclerosis. There is some laboratory research in this area, but there is no clear information in humans. Caution is advised when taking bilberry supplements, as adverse effects, including an increase in bleeding and drug interactions, are possible.

Coenzyme Q10 (CoQ10): CoQ10 is a vitamin-like substance produced by the human body and is necessary for the basic functioning of cells. Preliminary small human studies suggest that CoQ10 may reduce angina and improve exercise tolerance in people with clogged heart arteries. Several studies also suggest that the function of the heart may be improved after major heart surgeries such as CABG or valve replacement when CoQ10 is given to patients before or during surgery. Better studies are needed. CoQ10 is considered safe in recommended dosages.

Ginseng: Asian ginseng, or *Panax ginseng,* has been used for more than 2,000 years in Chinese medicine for various health conditions. Several studies from China report that ginseng in combination with various other herbs may reduce symptoms of CAD. Ginseng may also lower blood pressure. Caution is advised when taking ginseng supplements, as adverse effects including drug interactions are possible.

Green Tea: Green tea is made from the dried leaves of *Camellia sinensis,* a perennial evergreen shrub. Green tea has a long history of use, dating back to China approximately 5,000 years ago. Green tea, black tea, and oolong tea are all derived from the same plant but are processed differently. There is evidence that regular intake of green tea may lower cholesterol levels and reduce the risk of heart attack or atherosclerosis (clogged arteries).

Hawthorn: Hawthorn (*Crataegus* spp.), a flowering shrub of the rose family, has an extensive history of use in cardiovascular disease dating back to the first century. Increased blood flow to the heart and heart performance have been observed in animals when given hawthorn supplements, and one randomized clinical trial indicates that hawthorn may be effective in decreasing frequency or severity of anginal symptoms. Hawthorn has not been tested in the setting of concomitant drugs such as beta-blockers or ACE inhibitors, which are often considered to be standard of care. At this time, there is insufficient evidence to recommend for or against hawthorn for CAD or angina.

Kudzu: Kudzu (*Pueria lobota*) is well known to people in the southeastern United States as an invasive weed, but it has been used in Chinese medicine for centuries. Kudzu has a long history of use in the treatment of cardiovascular disorders, including angina, acute myocardial infarction, and heart failure. A small number of poorly designed trials found kudzu to reduce the frequency of angina events in human subjects. Overall, the studies have been methodologically weak.

Kundalini Yoga: Kundalini yoga is one of many traditions of yoga that share common roots in ancient Indian philosophy. It is comprehensive in that it combines physical poses with breath control exercises, chanting (mantras), meditations, prayer, visualizations, and guided relaxation. One case series report, but no formal clinical trials, suggests that breathing techniques used in Kundalini yoga may help people with angina pectoris (chest pain) reduce symptoms and need for medication.

Prayer: Prayer has far-reaching healing effects that are hard to study. Initial studies in patients with heart disease report variable effects on severity of illness, complications during hospitalization, procedure outcome, or death rates when intercessory prayer is used.

Psychotherapy: Psychotherapy is an interactive process between a person and a qualified mental health professional (psychiatrist, psychologist, clinical social worker, licensed counselor, or other trained practitioner). Its purpose is the exploration of thoughts, feelings and behavior for the purpose of problem solving or achieving higher levels of functioning. Alexithymia, or the inability to express one's feelings, may influence the course of CHD. Educational sessions and group psychotherapy may decrease alexithymia and reduce cardiac events.

Quercetin: Quercetin is one of the almost 4,000 bioflavonoids (antioxidants) that occur in foods of plant origin, such as red wine, onions, green tea, apples, berries, and *Brassica* vegetables (cabbage, broccoli, cauliflower, turnips). Several of the effects of flavonoids that have been observed in laboratory and animal studies suggest that they might be effective in reducing cardiovascular disease risk. Studies in humans using polyphenolic compounds from red grapes showed improvement in endothelial function in patients with CHD. Antioxidant and cholesterol-lowering effects are proposed.

Reishi: Reishi (*Ganoderma lucidum*) is a fungus (mushroom) that grows wild on decaying logs and tree stumps. Reishi has been used in traditional Chinese medicine for more than 4,000 years to treat liver disorders, high blood pressure, arthritis and other ailments. A reishi supplement was reported to improve the major symptoms of CHD (angina, palpitations, shortness of breath, elevated blood pressure, and high cholesterol) in patients. Long-term studies are needed to evaluate the efficacy and safety of reishi in CHD. Caution is advised when taking reishi supplements, as adverse effects, including an increase in bleeding, and drug interactions, are possible.

Relaxation Therapy: Relaxation techniques include behavioral therapeutic approaches that differ widely in philosophy, methodology, and practice. The primary goal is usually nondirected relaxation. Most techniques share the components of repetitive focus (on a word, sound, prayer phrase, body sensation, or muscular activity), adoption of a passive attitude towards intruding thoughts, and return to the focus.

Resveratrol: Resveratrol is found in over 70 plant species, including nuts, grapes, pine trees, certain vines, and red wine. Resveratrol is used as an antioxidant in various health conditions, including heart disease prevention. Laboratory animal studies suggest resveratrol helps restore blood flow to the heart. Well-designed clinical trials in humans using resveratrol are needed.

Tai Chi: Tai chi is a system of movements and positions believed to have developed in twelfth century China. Tai chi techniques aim to address the body and mind as an interconnected system and are traditionally believed to have mental and physical health benefits to improve posture, balance, flexibility, and strength. There is evidence that suggests tai chi decreases blood pressure and cholesterol as well as enhances quality of life in patients with chronic heart failure. Most studies have used elderly Chinese patients as their population. Additional research is needed before a firm conclusion can be drawn.

Vitamin B$_{12}$: Vitamin B$_{12}$ (or cyanocobalamin) is an essential water soluble vitamin that is commonly found in a variety of foods such as fish, shellfish, meats, and dairy products. Vitamin B$_{12}$ is frequently used in combination with other B vitamins in a vitamin B–complex formulation. Folic acid, pyridoxine (vitamin B$_6$), and vitamin B$_{12}$ supplementation can reduce total homocysteine levels (a known risk factor of CAD). However, this reduction does not seem to help with secondary prevention of death or cardiovascular events such as stroke or myocardial infarction in people with prior stroke. More evidence is needed to fully explain the association of total homocysteine levels with vascular risk and the potential use of vitamin supplementation.

Vitamin B$_6$: Vitamin B$_6$ or pyridoxine is found in cereal grains, legumes, vegetables (carrots, spinach, peas), potatoes, milk, cheese, eggs, fish, liver, meat, and flour. Mild deficiencies of this B vitamin are common. Vitamin B$_6$ may help lower homocysteine levels. Also, decreased vitamin B$_6$ concentrations are also associated with increased plasma levels of C-reactive protein. CRP is an indicator of inflammation that is associated with increased cardiovascular morbidity in epidemiological studies.

Vitamin E: Vitamin E is a fat-soluble vitamin with antioxidant properties. Vitamin E has been suggested and evaluated in patients with angina, although possible benefits remain unclear. Vitamin E has been proposed to have a role in preventing or reversing atherosclerosis by inhibiting oxidation of LDL ("bad cholesterol"). Several population studies have suggested that a high dietary intake of vitamin E and high blood concentrations of alpha-tocopherol are associated with lower rates of heart disease. However, while the Cambridge Heart Antioxidant Study supported this hypothesis, the more recent prospective Heart Outcomes Prevention Evaluation study did not. This area remains controversial.

Others: Other integrative therapies that may have benefit in reducing the risk of developing or in treating high cholesterol levels include alfalfa (*Medicago sativa L.*), aortic acid, ashwagandha (*Withania somnifera L.*), avocado (*Persea americana*), Ayurveda, barley (*Hordeum vulgare*), berberine, carob (*Ceratonia siliqua*), chamomile (*Matricaria recutita, Chamaemelum nobile*), chondroitin sulfate, coleus (*Coleus forskohlii*), copper, creatine, danshen (*Salvia miltiorrhiza*), dehydroepiandrosterone, dong quai (*Angelica sinensis*), elder (*Sambucas nigra L.*), fenugreek (*Trigonella foenum-graecum*), flaxseed and flaxseed oil (*Linum usitatissimum*), folate (folic acid), gamma-oryzanol, globe artichoke (*Cynara scolymus L.*), goldenseal (*Hydrastis canadensis L.*), grapefruit (*Citrus paradisi*), guggul (*Commiphora mukul*), gymnema (*Gymnema sylvestre R.Br.*), honey, horny goat weed (*Epimedium grandiflorum*), *Lactobacillus acidophilus,* lemongrass (*Cymbopogon* spp.), lycopene, macrobiotic diet, meditation, milk thistle (*Silybum marianum*), nopal (*Opuntia* spp.), ozone therapy, pantethine (pantothenic acid), physical therapy, pomegranate (*Punica granatum*), probiotics, Pycnogenol (*Pinus pinaster* spp. *atlantica*), red clover (*Trifolium pratense*), rhubarb (*Rheum officinale, Rheum palmatum*), safflower (*Carthamus tinctorius*), scotch broom (*Cytisus scoparius Linn.*), selenium, spirulina, squill (*Urginea maritima, Scilla maritima*), sweet almond (*Prunus amygdalus dulcis*), taurine, transcutaneous electrical nerve stimulation, traditional Chinese medicine, tribulus (*Tribulus terrestris*), turmeric (*Curcuma longa Linn.*), vitamin D, white horehound (*Marrubium vulgare*), wild yam (*Dioscoreaceae villosa*), and zinc.

PREVENTION

Dietary Modification: Minimize cholesterol and fat intake, especially saturated fat, which raises cholesterol levels more than any other substance. Cholesterol and saturated fats are found primarily in foods derived from animals, such as meats and dairy products. Dietary guidelines for reducing cholesterol and fat consumption include eating lean fish, poultry, and meat (remove the skin from chicken and trim the fat from beef before cooking); avoiding commercially prepared and processed food (cakes, cookies, doughnuts) and breaded fried foods; increasing the intake of fruits, vegetables, breads, cereals, rice, and legumes (beans, peas); using skim or 1% milk; and using cooking oils that are high in unsaturated fat (corn, olive, canola, safflower oils). Healthcare professionals recommend eating fish, including salmon, tuna, and herring, which are high in omega-3 fatty acids and therefore proposed to have a heart-protective action. Eggs do contain cholesterol but may be eaten without negative effects on cholesterol levels.

Weight Loss: Excess weight contributes to high cholesterol. Losing 5% of the total body weight can have a significant impact on lowering total cholesterol levels. Fad diets such as the Atkins diet may not give a person the balance of nutrients needed for a healthy heart and body. Exercising and eating the right foods in moderation help to increase weight loss.

Smoking Cessation: Quitting smoking can improve HDL cholesterol levels, decrease blood pressure, and reduce the risk of a heart attack. Within one year after stopping, the risk of heart disease is half that of a smoker. Within 15 years of stopping, the risk of heart disease is similar to that of someone who has never smoked.

Alcohol Consumption: In some studies, moderate use of alcohol (particularly red wine) has been linked with increasing levels of HDL cholesterol. No more than two glasses of red wine (four ounces each) should be consumed daily for heart protection. Excessive drinking can have a negative impact on cholesterol levels, actually raising triglyceride levels and increasing blood pressure.

Cholesterol Screenings: Everyone age 20 and older should have their cholesterol measured at least once every five years.

HIV/AIDS

BACKGROUND

The human immunodeficiency virus (HIV) is the virus that potentially causes acquired immune deficiency syndrome (AIDS). HIV primarily attacks the immune defense system, making the patient extremely vulnerable to opportunistic infections. HIV primarily infects and destroys immune cells with the CD4 receptor protein on their cell surfaces (also called CD4-positive or CD4+ T cells). Healthy individuals have a CD4 cell count between 600 and 1,200 cells per microliter of blood. HIV patients have less than 600 CD4 cells per microliter of blood. Patients progress to AIDS when/if their CD4 cell counts drop to lower than 200 cells per microliter (one-one millionth of a liter) of blood. This may happen if a person does not receive adequate treatment or if he/she develops a serious infection or illness. Individuals with a CD4 cell counts lower than 200 have the greatest risk of developing potentially fatal opportunistic infections, such as *Mycobacterium avium* complex (MAC) infections, because their immune systems are very weak.

HIV is transmitted from person to person via bodily fluids, including blood, semen, vaginal secretions, and breast milk. Therefore, it can be transmitted through sexual contact with an infected person, by sharing needles/syringes with someone who is infected, through breastfeeding, during vaginal birth or, less commonly, through transfusions with infected blood. However, in countries where blood is screened for HIV antibodies, HIV infection is rarely transmitted through blood transfusions. Very low amounts of HIV have been found in saliva and tears in some AIDS patients. However, contact with saliva, tears, or sweat has not been shown to result in HIV transmission. The most common type of HIV worldwide is called HIV-1. It is easily transmitted and is the cause of most HIV/AIDS infections around the world. HIV-1 has several subtypes (A through H and O), which are more common in certain parts of the world but produce AIDS similarly. The second type, called HIV-2, is much less common and less virulent or infectious. Since 1981, when the first case of AIDS was reported in the United States, the disease has become a global pandemic, causing an estimated 65 million infections and 25 million deaths worldwide. According to the U.S. Centers for Disease Control and Prevention (CDC), an estimated 2.8 million patients died from AIDS, 4.1 million people became infected with HIV, and 38.6 million were living with HIV worldwide in 2005. According to the Joint United Nations Programme on HIV/AIDS and World Health Organization 2006 AIDS Epidemic Update, an estimated 39.5 million people are currently living with HIV worldwide. It is also estimated that 4.3 million people became newly infected in 2006, with 2.8 million (65%) of these cases occurring in Sub-Saharan Africa. In 2006, 2.9 million people died from AIDS-related illnesses. Certain geographic regions, such as Sub-Saharan Africa and the Caribbean, have much higher rates of infection than others. Certain populations, such as Sub-Saharan women, men who have sex with men, prostitutes, and injection drug users, are also at increased risk for HIV infection.

Currently, there is no cure for HIV/AIDS. However, treatment with anti-HIV drugs, called antiretrovirals, may suppress the virus, which subsequently helps boost the immune system. Although these drugs may help patients live longer lives, they do not reduce the risk of transmitting the disease to someone else.

PATHOLOGY

General: HIV is transmitted from person to person via bodily fluids, including blood, semen, vaginal secretions, and breast milk. Individuals who have other sexually transmitted diseases (STDs) are more susceptible to the virus. This is because some STDs, such as syphilis, cause breaks in the skin or sores that make it easy for HIV to enter the body.

HIV is particularly difficult to treat because it reproduces very quickly and has a high mutation rate. When HIV reproduces, different strains (types) of the virus emerge. Mutations (changes in genetic information) occur almost every time a new copy of the virus is produced. Therefore, many types of HIV can be produced in a single person in one day. For this reason, HIV patients receive different combinations of antiretrovirals to suppress the virus.

HIV primary targets immune cells called CD4 T-cells. The CD4 T-cells are white blood cells that help coordinate the immune system's response to infection and disease. These cells have a molecule called CD4 on their surfaces, which allows the cells to detect foreign substances, including viruses that enter the body. This process then triggers the immune system to destroy the foreign substance. When HIV enters the body, the virus recognizes this protein, binds to the receptors on the CD4 cell wall, and enters the cell. Once inside the cell, HIV replicates and eventually kills the cell.

Primary, or Acute, Infection: Patients can transmit the virus to others during all stages of infection. The first stage of HIV, known as the primary or acute infection, is the most infectious stage of the disease, and it typically lasts several weeks. During this phase, the virus replicates rapidly, which leads to an abundance of the virus in the bloodstream and a drastic decline in the number of CD4 T-cells. The CD8 T-cells, which kill abnormal or infected body cells, are then activated to destroy HIV-infected body cells and antibodies are produced.

Clinical Latency: The next stage, called clinical latency, may last anywhere from two weeks to 20 years. During this phase, HIV is not considered dormant. Instead, it is active in the lymph nodes, where large amounts of the virus become trapped. The surrounding tissues, which contain high levels of CD4 T-cells, may also become infected. The virus accumulates in infected cells and in the blood as free virus. Patients generally do not experience symptoms during this stage until the CD4 cell count drops to 600 microliters of blood or lower.

Symptomatic Stage: As the virus continues to weaken the immune system, patients eventually become more susceptible to infections. The next stage is the symptomatic stage, in which the person experiences symptoms associated with a weakened immune system.

AIDS: The term AIDS refers to the most advanced stage of HIV infection. This stage happens when HIV multiplies rapidly and severely affects the immune system. Individuals have AIDS when they have fewer than 200 CD4 T-cells per microliter of blood. This low CD4 T-cell count makes them extremely vulnerable to potentially fatal opportunistic infections such as pneumonia or tuberculosis. Several infections, including *Pneumocystis jiroveci* pneumonia (formerly called *Pneumocystis carinii* pneumonia) and Kaposi's sarcoma, are considered AIDS-defining illnesses. This means that once patients develop one of these infections, their condition has progressed to AIDS.

TRENDS

The spread of HIV and AIDS in the United States is tracked by the CDC. During the mid-to-late 1990s, advances in HIV treatment slowed the progression of HIV infection to AIDS. This consequently led to decreases in AIDS-related deaths. According to the CDC, the number of AIDS-related deaths continues to decline, with an 8% decrease from 2000 through 2004. However, the number of AIDS diagnoses increased 8% during that period as well. From 2000 to 2004, the estimated number of people living with

AIDS increased from 320,177 to 415,193, according to the CDC. This 30% increase can partially be attributed to advanced treatments that have helped HIV/AIDS patients to live longer lives as well as increased access to testing and information about the disease.

DEMOGRAPHICS

General: Race and ethnicity by themselves do not increase or decrease a person's risk of acquiring HIV infection. However, certain people are more likely to face challenges associated with the risk for HIV infection, such as lack of awareness of HIV status, substance abuse, or socioeconomic issues.

African-Americans: In 2004, African-Americans accounted for 20,965 (49%) of the 42,514 estimated AIDS cases (not HIV) diagnosed in the United States. The rate of AIDS diagnoses among African-American adults and adolescents was 10 times higher than the rate of Caucasians and almost three times higher than the rate of Latinos. In addition, 23 times more African-American women were diagnosed with AIDS than Caucasian women. Eight times more African-American men were diagnosed with AIDS than Caucasian men, according to the CDC.

Latinos: In 2004, Latinos accounted for 20% (8,672) of the 42,514 new diagnoses in the United States, according to the CDC. The top causes of infection in most Latino men were infections after HIV exposure through sexual contact with other men, injection drug use, and heterosexual contact. The top causes of infection in Latino women were HIV exposure through heterosexual contact and injection drug use. Latinos were shown to get tested for HIV more often than any other race or ethnicity except African-Americans. According to the CDC, in 2004, about 50% of Hispanics between the ages of 15-44 were tested, and 18% had been tested during the past year.

Women: After the initial outbreak of HIV, few women were diagnosed with the virus. Today, women account for more than 25% of all new HIV/AIDS diagnoses in the United States. In 2004, an estimated 93,566 women were living with AIDS, making up 23% of the estimated 415,193 people living with AIDS in the United States.

Youth (13-24 Years Old): In the United States, it is estimated that 50% of the 40,000 new HIV infections each year occur in people younger than age 25, and 25% of infections occur in people younger than 21. HIV/AIDS ranks as the sixth-leading cause of death among individuals ages 15-24 in the United States, with the number of AIDS cases reported each year in that age group increasing by 417% from 1981 through 1994.

Injection Drug Users: Since the AIDS epidemic began, injection drug use with illegal drugs has directly and indirectly (drug use clouds judgment, leading people to engage in high-risk behaviors) accounted for more than one-third of AIDS cases in the United States. In the year 2000, out of the 42,156 new cases of AIDS reported, 11,635 were linked to injection drug use. Injection drug use is more common among racial and ethnic minorities in the United States, which makes them more likely to acquire HIV through injection drug use. In 2000, injection drug use accounted for 26% of all AIDS cases among African-American adults and 31% among Hispanic adults and adolescents compared to 19% of all cases among Caucasian adults and adolescents.

Homosexuals: Men who have sex with men accounted for 70% of all estimated HIV infections among male adults and adolescents in 2004 in the United States, according to the CDC. Although the number of HIV diagnoses for men who have sex with men decreased during the 1980s and 1990s, the number increased by 8% from 2003 through 2004. According to the CDC, it is unknown whether this increase is because more people are getting tested for HIV or because more patients are becoming infected with HIV.

Healthcare Workers: Although healthcare workers are exposed to the virus at work, it is unlikely that they will acquire the virus from a patient, especially if they follow universal precautions, which should be taken with all patients. For healthcare workers, HIV transmission is most likely to occur through accidental injuries from needles or other sharp medical instruments that may be contaminated with the virus. However, this risk is small. Researchers estimate that about 0.3-1% of healthcare workers exposed to the virus by an accidental needle stick or puncture develop HIV.

Since December 2001, there have been 57 documented reports of healthcare workers acquiring HIV from a patient. To prevent transmission of HIV to healthcare personnel in the workplace, the CDC offers precautionary guidelines.

EARLY SYMPTOMS

Many patients are asymptomatic (experience no symptoms) when they first become infected with HIV. After one or two months, an estimated 80-90% of HIV patients develops flulike symptoms, including headache, fever, fatigue, and enlarged lymph nodes. These symptoms usually last about one week to one month and are often mistaken for another viral infection, such as the flu. Despite having minimal or no symptoms during this stage, individuals are very infectious because the virus is present in large quantities in bodily fluids. The most obvious sign of HIV infection is a decrease in the number of CD4 cells in the blood. These cells help fight against infection. HIV slowly kills these cells without causing symptoms. Even when the infected individual is asymptomatic, the virus is multiplying, infecting, and destroying cells in the immune system.

CLINICAL LATENCY SYMPTOMS

After the initial infection with HIV, more serious symptoms develop. This next stage of infection is called clinical latency. Once infected with HIV, it may take 10 or more years for more severe symptoms to appear in adults or up to two years in children who are born with HIV infection. The length of this asymptomatic period varies among individuals. Some people may start to experience more serious symptoms within a few weeks, while others may have no symptoms for several years. The virus can also hide within infected cells. Patients can transmit the virus to others during all stages of the disease.

As the immune system continues to weaken, many symptoms appear, including inflamed lymph nodes (swollen glands) that may be enlarged for longer than three months. Other symptoms may include fatigue, weight loss, frequent fevers and sweats, persistent or frequent yeast infections (oral or vaginal), persistent skin rashes or flaky skin, pelvic inflammatory disease in women that does not respond well to treatment, and short-term memory loss. In addition, some individuals develop a painful nerve disease called shingles or frequent and severe herpes infections that cause sores to develop on the mouth, genitals, or anus. Infected children may be sick often or grow slowly (failure to thrive) because their immune systems are still developing.

AIDS SYMPTOMS

Once the patient's CD4 T-cell count is less than 200 cells per microliter of blood, their condition has progressed to AIDS, the final stage of the disease. The first symptoms often include moderate and unexplained weight loss, frequent lung infections, and oral ulcerations (sores). Patients are vulnerable to opportunistic infections and tumors. Opportunistic infections and tumors may include tuberculosis, thrush, herpes viruses, shingles, Epstein-Barr virus, pneumonia, and a type of cancer called Kaposi's sarcoma. In the last stages of AIDS, it is common for individuals to have cytomegalovirus or MAC infections.

OPPORTUNISTIC INFECTIONS

General: Opportunistic infections are conditions that occur in individuals who have weakened immune systems. The organisms (bacteria, fungi, or viruses) that cause these infections do not cause illnesses in patients who have healthy immune systems because they are able to fight off the infection. The most common opportunistic infections associated with HIV and AIDS are *Pneumocystis jiroveci* pneumonia, MAC, toxoplasmosis, and tuberculosis. Patients at risk of developing these infections typically receive medication to prevent infections.

***Pneumocystis Jiroveci* Pneumonia:** *Pneumocystis jiroveci* pneumonia (formerly called *Pneumocystis carinii* or PCP) is the most common opportunistic infection among HIV patients. Before antiretroviral therapy and preventative treatment was available, about 70-80% of people with HIV developed PCP. However, this number has been declining significantly over the years. Originally, researchers thought a one-cell organism called *Pneumocystis carinii* caused the infection. However, recent research suggests that a fungus called *Pneumocystis jiroveci* is the cause. The condition is still commonly referred to as PCP pneumonia.

According to the CDC, PCP is classified as an AIDS-defining illness. This means that when HIV-infected patients develop PCP, their condition has progressed to AIDS. Individuals with a CD4 cell (helper T-cells that help fight against disease and infection) count lower than 200 cells per microliter of blood have the greatest risk of developing PCP. In addition, people who have CD4 cell counts lower than 300 who have already had another opportunistic infection have an increased risk of developing PCP. This infection almost always affects the lungs, causing a type of pneumonia. The first signs of PCP are difficulty breathing, fever, and a dry cough. Other common symptoms include chest discomfort, weight loss, chills, tachypnea (rapid breathing), tachycardia (fast heart rate), mild crackles (bubbling or rattling sounds that occur when air moves through fluid-filled airways), cyanosis (bluish discoloration of the skin), nasal flaring, and intercostal retractions (visible use of muscles between the ribs, which indicates labored breathing). The patient may also cough up blood, although this is considered a rare symptom.

Historically, mortality ranged from 20-40%, depending on the severity of the disease when it was diagnosed. Today, however, mortality rates range between 10-20%. Today, PCP is almost entirely preventable, and it can be treated effectively with medications. Unfortunately, PCP is still common in patients who are infected with HIV for a long time before they begin antiretroviral therapy. In fact, 30-40% of HIV patients develop PCP if they begin treatment when their CD4 cell counts are very low (around 50 cells per microliter of blood).

***Mycobacterium Avium* Complex (MAC):** MAC, or *Mycobacterium avium intracellulare,* is a bacterial infection that is caused by either *Mycobacterium avium* or *Mycobacterium avium* subspecies *intracellulare*. These bacteria are commonly found in water, soil, dust, and food. In fact, these bacteria are present in almost every human. However, a healthy immune system prevents the bacteria from causing an infection. HIV/AIDS patients are at risk of developing MAC. According to the CDC, MAC is considered an AIDS-defining illness. It is estimated that up to 50% of individuals with HIV/AIDS develop MAC, especially if their CD4 count is lower than 50 cells per microliter of blood. MAC rarely causes infections in patients who have CD4 cell counts higher than 100 cells per microliter of blood.

MAC infections may be localized (limited to one part of the body) or disseminated (spread throughout the entire body, sometimes called DMAC). MAC infection often occurs in the lungs, intestines, bone marrow, liver, and spleen. Common symptoms of MAC include weight loss, fever, chills, night sweats, swollen glands, abdominal pain, diarrhea, inflammation, and an overall feeling of weakness. MAC usually affects the intestines and inner organs first. The most common complication of DMAC is anemia (low levels of red blood cells), which may require a blood transfusion. If the infection involves many organs, it may lead to respiratory failure and death. Patients who have localized infections that have not spread to other parts of the body have a low mortality rate because they are easier to treat.

Toxoplasmosis: Toxoplasmosis is a parasitic infection that is caused by a single-celled parasite called *Toxoplasma gondii.*

Toxoplasma gondii is one of the most common parasites found all over the world. Individuals may be exposed to the parasite in soil, cat feces, or in raw or undercooked meat (especially lamb, pork, or venison). There have also been rare reports of toxoplasmosis infection as a result of organ transplantation or blood transfusion. It is estimated that more than 60 million Americans carry the parasite. However, 80-90% of infected patients are carriers (experience no symptoms) because the body's immune system prevents the parasite from causing illness. Toxoplasmosis is considered

H

an AIDS-defining illness, according to the CDC. HIV patients often experience symptoms such as headache, confusion, poor coordination, seizures, and ocular toxoplasmosis (severe inflammation of the retina) as well as lung problems that are similar to tuberculosis or pneumocystis pneumonia.

Tuberculosis (TB): TB is a bacterial infection of the lungs that is caused by the bacteria *Mycobacterium tuberculosis*. Symptoms may include cough, shortness of breath, pleurisy (pain with breathing or coughing), fever, weight loss, night sweats, chills, and loss of appetite. The disease can cause serious breathing problems, which can be life threatening, especially if left untreated. TB is highly contagious. The disease is transmitted through airborne droplets when a person with the infection coughs, talks, or sneezes. About 10-15 million Americans have latent TB infection, which means they are not sick, but they carry the bacteria that causes the disease. Only 10% of individuals with latent TB ever develop the infection.

While TB is not considered an AIDS-defining illness, HIV patients have an increased risk of developing TB because they have weakened immune systems. The risk of developing active TB increases 7-10% in HIV patients who have latent TB. HIV patients are more likely to experience symptoms in areas of the body other than the lungs. This is called extrapulmonary TB. The disease may affect the bones, joints, nervous system, or urinary tract. Also, TB appears to make HIV infection worse; researchers have observed faster HIV replication when TB is also present.

TRANSMISSION

Bodily Fluids: HIV is transmitted from person to person via bodily fluids because the virus is present in varying concentrations in the blood, semen, vaginal fluid, and breast milk. It can be spread by sexual contact with an infected person, by sharing needles/syringes with someone who is infected or, less commonly, through transfusions with infected blood. HIV infection through blood transfusion is extremely rare in countries where blood is screened for HIV antibodies.

Environment: HIV does not survive well in the environment outside of the body. According to studies performed by the CDC, drying HIV reduces the amount of viral particles by 90-99% within several hours. The virus also cannot reproduce when it is outside of the body. Therefore, it is highly unlikely that the disease can be transmitted through contact with the environment, such as public toilet seats.

Kissing: Casual contact through closed-mouth or "social" kissing does not put an individual at risk for

HIV. However, there is the potential for blood contact with open-mouth kissing. The risk for acquiring the virus from open-mouth kissing is low, and the CDC has only investigated one case in which HIV transmission may have been caused by blood contact during open-mouth kissing. The CDC recommends that individuals avoid open-mouth kissing with an infected person.

Biting: There have been medical reports that found that HIV transmission resulted after a human bite. Severe trauma and extensive tissue tearing were reported in each of these cases. However, biting is not a common way of transmitting the disease.

Saliva, Tears, and Sweat: Very low amounts of HIV have been found in the saliva and tears of some AIDS patients. However, a small amount of HIV in body fluid does not necessarily mean that the fluid can transmit the virus. Contact with saliva, tears, or sweat has not been shown to result in transmission of HIV.

Insects: According to numerous studies, there is no evidence to suggest that HIV has been transmitted through insects, even in areas such as Africa that have high numbers of AIDS patients and mosquito populations. HIV can only live for a short time inside an insect and does not reproduce inside insects.

Effectiveness of Condoms: If a condom is used properly during sexual intercourse, an individual may reduce the risk of acquiring or transmitting STDs, including HIV. Several studies show that using condoms correctly and consistently may reduce the breakage rates of latex condoms to less than 2%. There are many types and brands of condoms, but only latex or polyurethane condoms have been shown to effectively prevent HIV transmission when used appropriately. According to the CDC, natural membrane condoms, such as those made with lambskin, have natural pores that can possibly transmit diseases. Therefore, lambskin condoms are not considered to be effective in preventing HIV transmission.

Recent evidence has suggested that condom use by high-risk populations increases, rather than decreases, the infection rate. According to the latest studies, condom promotion is only effective in lowering the rate of AIDS in concentrated, high-risk groups; condoms have never been shown to reduce HIV infection rates and AIDS deaths in general-population epidemics like those in Sub-Saharan Africa. In one study, researchers asserted that of the three interventions scientifically shown to prevent AIDS—abstinence, being faithful, and using condoms—they argue that the use of condoms clearly comes last and should be promoted as a first-line defense only to those in extremely high-risk groups, such as commercial sex workers. One prospective study showed that for "receptive" men during anal sex, it made little or no difference whether their partners used a condom or not. Researchers suggested that condoms are less effective in anal sex than in vaginal sex.

HIV AND PREGNANCY

Babies born to HIV-infected mothers may become infected during pregnancy, delivery, or breastfeeding. Therefore, the CDC recommends that all pregnant women get tested for HIV.

Antiretroviral therapy can significantly reduce the likelihood of an HIV-infected pregnant mother passing the virus to her baby. Patients who were taking antiretroviral medication before becoming pregnant should talk to their healthcare providers to determine the safest and most effective treatment option. In general, efavirenz (Sustiva), stavudine (Zerit), hydroxyurea (Droxia, Hydrea), and the oral liquid formulation of amprenavir (Agenerase) should not be taken during pregnancy because they may cause harm to the fetus.

Because a baby may become infected though exposure to the mother's blood and vaginal secretions during delivery, the risk of infection increases with delivery time. Mothers with high levels of the virus in their blood might reduce their risk if they deliver their babies by cesarean section (surgical delivery of an infant), also called c-section. While c-sections may reduce the risk of transmission during birth, it is not typically necessary in patients taking antiretroviral therapy. HIV infection rates of babies shortly before or after birth have been shown to drop to as low as 1-2% if their mothers take combination antiretroviral therapy during pregnancy as well as zidovudine or nevirapine (Viramune) preventative therapy during labor and after birth.

HIV-infected mothers should not breastfeed their babies because the virus may be transmitted via the breast milk. Instead, baby formulas should be used.

DIAGNOSIS

General: HIV is diagnosed after HIV antibodies or HIV itself is detected in the patient's body. As soon as the virus enters the body, the immune system produces antibodies, which are proteins that detect foreign substances in the body, including infectious agents like HIV. The presence of HIV antibodies in the blood, oral fluid, or urine can be used to determine whether HIV is in the body. Blood tests are the most commonly used HIV tests. It may take some time for the immune system to produce enough antibodies for the antibody test to detect them. This time period, known as the "window period," varies among patients. Most people will develop detectable antibodies two to eight weeks after exposure, with the average being 25 days. However, some individuals might take longer to develop detectable antibodies. Of those infected with HIV, 97% develop antibodies within the first three months of infection. In very rare cases, it can take up to six months to develop antibodies to HIV. Therefore, if a patient tests negative for HIV in the first three months after possible exposure, repeat testing should be considered at least three months after the exposure. In the United States, the test results must remain confidential. Individuals who are younger than 18 years old can consent to or refuse to be tested for HIV without the involvement of their legal guardians. Test results may not be released to the patient's legal guardian(s) without his/her consent.

Pretest Counseling: According to the CDC's new guidelines for HIV testing, HIV prevention counseling is not required to accompany HIV screening. However, the CDC still recommends that patients receive information about HIV infection, transmission, and prevention. Patients should receive information about HIV testing and the meaning of test results. Healthcare providers should also tell the patient when to expect results and that confirmatory testing is necessary if the test result is positive. This is because it is possible for a false-positive test result. The patient may receive information through a pamphlet, brochure, video, or a one-on-one meeting with a certified counselor. Patients who are tested with a rapid HIV test should have equal access to the same types of information.

Prevention Counseling: Prevention counseling is not mandatory, but it should be offered to all patients when they receive their test results. Counseling focuses on reducing the risks of HIV infection or transmission. The counselor makes a personalized, detailed risk assessment of the patient. The counselor should also suggest behavior changes that may help reduce the patient's risk of developing or transmitting HIV. The counseling session is a chance to clear up any misconceptions or questions the patient may have about the disease.

Enzyme-Linked Immunosorbent Assay (ELISA): The most common HIV tests use blood to detect HIV infection. ELISA tests a patient's blood sample for antibodies. Oral fluid (not saliva), collected from the cheeks and gums, may also be used to perform an ELISA. Oral fluid ELISA tests are considered as sensitive as a blood test. A urine sample may also be used during an ELISA, but this is considered less accurate than a blood or oral fluid test. A positive (reactive) ELISA for all samples must be used with a follow-up (confirmatory) test, such as the Western blot test, to make a positive diagnosis. Although false-negative or false-positive results are extremely rare, they may occur if the patient has not yet developed antibodies to HIV or if a mistake was made at the laboratory. When used in combination with the confirmatory Western blot test, ELISA tests are 99.9% accurate.

Western Blot Test: A Western blot test is typically used to confirm a positive HIV diagnosis. During the test, a small sample of blood is taken and it is used to detect HIV antibodies, not the HIV virus itself. The Western blot test separates the blood proteins and detects the specific proteins (called HIV antibodies) that indicate an HIV infection. The Western blot is used to confirm a positive ELISA, and the combined tests are 99.9% accurate.

Polymerase Chain Reaction (PCR): PCR tests are used to detect HIV's genetic material (RNA). These tests can be used to screen the donated blood supply and to detect very early infections before antibodies have been developed. This test may be performed just days or weeks after exposure to HIV. Although these tests are the most accurate, they are not performed as often as the other HIV tests because they are expensive and also time and labor intensive.

Rapid Test: A rapid test produces results in about 20 minutes. Rapid tests use a sample of blood or oral fluid to detect HIV antibodies. The patient's sample is placed on a test strip that contains HIV antigens. If the patient has developed HIV antibodies, the strip will change colors, indicating a positive result. A positive HIV test should be confirmed with a follow-up confirmatory test before a final HIV diagnosis can be made. These tests have similar accuracy rates as traditional ELISA screening tests.

Home-Testing Kit: Consumer-controlled test kits, also called home-testing kits, were first licensed in 1997. The Home Access HIV-1 Test System (Home Access Health, Hoffman Estates, Ill.) is the only home kit that is approved by the U.S. Food and Drug Administration (FDA). The Home Access HIV-1 Test System is available at most local pharmacies. The individual pricks a finger with a special device and places drops of blood on a specially treated card. The card is then mailed to a licensed laboratory for testing. Home testing kits are confidential, and patients do not need to

provide any personal information (such as name or address) when submitting samples. Instead, they call for results using a personal identification number. Callers may speak to a counselor any time before, during, or after the test. All individuals with positive test results are given referrals for follow-up confirmatory tests, as well as information and resources on treatment and support services. FDA-approved tests are equally as accurate as the tests performed in a doctor's office when performed correctly.

WHO SHOULD GET TESTED

The U.S. Centers for Disease Control (CDC) recommends that the following individuals get tested for HIV: individuals who have injected illegal drugs; individuals who have had unprotected vaginal, anal, or oral sex; individuals who have multiple or anonymous sexual partners; individuals who have exchanged sex for drugs or money; individuals who have been diagnosed with or treated for hepatitis, tuberculosis (TB), or a sexually transmitted disease (STD), such as syphilis, gonorrhea, or chlamydia; individuals who have come in direct contact with an HIV-infected person's blood; individuals who have had unprotected sex with someone who meets any of the above stipulations. Individuals between the ages of 13 and 64 should be tested annually. Pregnant women should be screened for HIV as part of regular prenatal tests.

TREATMENT

General: Although current antiretroviral drugs cannot cure HIV/AIDS, they may suppress the virus, even to undetectable levels. The guidelines for antiretroviral treatment are the same for adolescents and adults.

In emergency situations, or if parental involvement is impossible or could cause harm, and if the patient can adhere to treatment regimens, a minor can consent to treatment without parental involvement. However, communication with legal guardians should be encouraged in all patients who are younger than 18 years old and need to make healthcare decisions.

Patients who were taking antiretroviral medication before becoming pregnant should talk to their healthcare providers to determine the safest and most effective treatment options. In general, efavirenz (Sustiva), stavudine (Zerit), hydroxyurea (Droxia, Hydrea), and the oral liquid formulation of amprenavir (Agenerase) should not be taken during pregnancy because they may cause harm to the fetus.

Highly Active Antiretroviral Therapy (HAART): HIV patients typically receive a combination of antiretroviral drugs because a single patient may have several different strains (types) of the virus circulating in the blood. The different strains of the virus may respond differently to specific types of drugs. Therefore, HAART, which is a combination of drugs from at least two different drug classes, is recommended. There are five major classes of antiretrovirals: fusion inhibitors, nucleoside/nucleotide reverse transcriptase inhibitors (NRTIs/NtRTIs), nonnucleoside reverse transcriptase inhibitors (NNRTIs), protease inhibitors, and integrase inhibitors. Each drug class disrupts different stages of HIV's life cycle.

Fusion inhibitors prevent the virus from entering and infecting human cells. Currently, the FDA has approved one fusion inhibitor, enfuvirtide (Fuzeon), also called T-20. Clinical trials have demonstrated that enfuvirtide-based therapy is an effective treatment for patients who have taken other types of antiretrovirals in the past. Enfuvirtide should not be taken in patients who have never received antiretroviral drugs before because it is only recommended when other drugs have not worked.

NRTIs and NtRTIs, also called "nukes," inhibit HIV replication. HIV replicates by converting the viral RNA into complementary DNA (cDNA), which then integrates into the host DNA. A viral enzyme called reverse transcriptase converts the viral RNA into cDNA using host nucleotides, which are the building blocks of DNA. NRTIs are nucleoside analogs, or fake versions of nucleosides (which are the precursors to nucleotides), and the resulting DNA cannot be incorporated into the host DNA. NtRTIs are nucleotide analogs and do not need to be converted. Therefore, NtRTIs may have fewer side effects than NRTIs. The FDA has approved the following NRTIs: lamivudine/zidovudine (Combivir), emtricitabine (Emtriva), lamivudine (Epivir), abacavir sulfate/lamivudine (Epzicom), zalcitabine (Hivid), zidovudine (Retrovir), abacavir sulfate/lamivudine/zidovudine (Trizivir), emtricitabine/tenofovir disoproxil fumarate (Truvada), didanosine (Videx, Videx EC), stavudine (Zerit), and abacavir sulfate (Ziagen). Tenofovir disoproxil fumarate (Viread) is the only FDA-approved NtRTI at this time.

NNRTIs, also called nonnucleoside analogs, interfere with viral replication. HIV replication requires the enzyme reverse transcriptase, which is targeted by NNRTIs. When patients take NNRTIs, the drug attaches to HIV's enzyme before it can use the patient's nucleic acid to multiply. NNRTIs

significantly reduce the ability of HIV to multiply and infect new cells. Currently, the FDA has approved three NNRTIs: delavirdine (Rescriptor), efavirenz (Sustiva), and nevirapine (Viramune). Also, in July 2006, the FDA approved the multiclass combination drug efavirenz/emtricitabine/tenofovir disoproxil fumarate (Atripla), which includes one NNRTI and two NRTIs.

Protease inhibitors also interfere with HIV replication; they prevent the production of viral proteins that require an enzyme called protease. When protease is blocked, the new copies of HIV do not form properly and cannot infect new cells. The FDA has approved 10 protease inhibitors: amprenavir (Agenerase), tipranavir (Aptivus), indinavir (Crixivan), saquinavir mesylate (Invirase), lopinavir/ritonavir (Kaletra), fosamprenavir calcium (Lexiva), ritonavir (Norvir), darunavir (Prezista), atazanavir sulfate (Reyataz), and nelfinavir mesylate (Viracept).

In October 2007, the FDA approved an integrase inhibitor, called raltegravir (Isentress), for the treatment of HIV in combination with other antiretrovirals. Integrase inhibitors are a new class of antiretrovirals that block the integrase enzyme that HIV uses to incorporate cDNA into host DNA.

Antiretroviral Side Effects: Individuals taking antiretroviral drugs often find it difficult to follow complicated drug plans. Current treatments involve taking at least two different classes of antiretroviral drugs daily. Also, some of the drugs may cause nausea or vomiting, some pills should be taken on an empty stomach, and others should be taken with food. Specific side effects depend on the specific drugs. In general, common side effects include changes in body fat distribution and blood lipid levels. Glucose metabolism (the breakdown of carbohydrates to produce energy) is also affected, which may lead to the onset or worsening of diabetes. It is estimated that about 2-10% of people taking antiretrovirals have diabetes. The National Institute of Allergy and Infectious Diseases is among many research organizations that is investigating simpler, less toxic, and more effective drug plans.

Synergistic Enhancers: Another group of medications, called synergistic enhancers, may also be used in combination with other antiretroviral drugs to treat HIV, although this use is not FDA approved. These medications do not act as antiretrovirals when taken alone, but they have been shown to improve the antiretrovirals effects of other drugs, including ritonavir. Very small doses of synergistic enhancers may also be used to reduce the liver metabolism of other antiretroviral drugs.

Surgery: Patients infected with HIV may require surgery to treat infections and diseases associated with the condition. With the introduction of HAART, HIV patients are able to live longer lives. As a result, it is possible that surgical interventions may be needed to diagnoses and/or treat long-term conditions. For example, lung infections, which may be caused by PCP, MAC, or TB, often require invasive diagnostic procedures such as bronchoalveolar lavage or an open lung biopsy. Like any surgical procedure, there are potential health risks. It remains unclear whether HIV patients are more likely to develop complications than HIV-negative patients.

Common complications of surgery include bleeding, infections, and nerve damage. It has been suggested that HIV patients may have an increased risk of surgical complications (especially infections) because they have weakened immune systems. However, there are currently no scientific data on the prevalence of surgical complications among HIV patients compared to noninfected patients.

Researchers believe that the risks of surgical complications for HIV patients can be predicted in a way similar to the method used in HIV-negative patients. Prior to surgery, healthcare providers should perform a physical examination, detailed medical history, and laboratory testing to determine the patient's overall health. Healthcare providers must also consider possible interactions between the patient's anti-HIV drugs (antiretrovirals) and medications, such as pain relievers, that are used before, during, and after surgical procedures.

It remains unclear whether a patient's CD4 cell count influences their risk of surgical complications. Healthy individuals have a CD4 cell count between 600-1,200 cells per microliter of blood. The lower the CD4 count, the weaker the patient's immune system. Some studies have found no correlation between low CD4 cell counts and surgical complications, while others have found an increase in complications with lower CD4 counts. Further research is needed before a firm conclusion can be made.

Organ Transplants: As mentioned above, HAART enables HIV/AIDS patients to live longer lives. Today, most patients with HIV/AIDS are dying from end-stage organ disease and organ failure rather than AIDS-associated opportunistic infections. Since HAART prolongs the lives of HIV patients, it is possible for chronic conditions to progress to organ failure. For instance, HIV patients may experience end-stage liver disease as a complication of chronic hepatitis C virus. Glomeruli diseases are also common among HIV patients, and they may lead to kidney failure. In advanced stages of liver or kidney damage, organ transplants may be the patient's only chance of survival.

Until recently, people who had HIV were not considered good candidates for organ transplantations. Many patients were denied transplants under the assumption that they had shorter life expectancies and less favorable survival rates than other patients in need of transplants. However, now that patients are living longer lives, many groups are reconsidering whether HIV patients should be transplant candidates. Although the United Network for Organ Sharing does not consider HIV infection a contraindication for organ transplantation, individual transplant centers are in charge of deciding whether or not to perform surgery in an HIV-positive patient. Some centers will not provide organ transplants to HIV-positive patients, even if they are good candidates based on their physical and mental health.

Some health insurance companies are reluctant to cover transplantation in HIV-positive candidates because they consider it to be an experimental procedure. Currently, only a few medical centers worldwide perform organ transplants in HIV-positive patients. However, health insurance companies and doctors consider organ transplantations in HIV-negative patients to be a well-established, reimbursable procedure. Recent legislation in California and a ruling in Arizona may help increase HIV patients' access to transplant surgery. In October 2005, an administrative law judge declared that Medicaid had to pay for a liver transplant for an Arizona woman who was HIV positive. In the same month, California Governor Arnold Schwarzenegger signed a law that prohibits health insurance companies from denying coverage for organ transplants in HIV patients solely on the basis of their HIV status. The law is the first of its kind to target such denials.

The limited number of transplants that have been performed in HIV patients have produced encouraging results. However, organ transplants for people with HIV/AIDS have not gained widespread medical support, and there are still concerns regarding the long-term prognosis for HIV-positive transplant recipients.

TREATMENT ADHERENCE

In order for anti-HIV drugs to work correctly, they must be taken exactly as prescribed. Skipping doses or not taking the medications correctly can cause the amount of an antiretroviral drug to decrease in the bloodstream. If the drug level becomes too low, HIV can begin reproducing more quickly. The faster HIV reproduces, the more mutations occur, including those that may be resistant to drugs. When a patient becomes resistant to a drug, the medication is no longer effective, even if it is taken in the future. As a result, patients have fewer treatment options.

According to several studies, HIV patients must be more than 95% adherent to their treatment plans in order for them to remain effective. This means that missing more than one dose per month may reduce the drugs' effectiveness.

Healthcare providers evaluate treatment effectiveness by measuring CD4 cell counts in the patient's blood. These immune cells are the primary targets of HIV. If the CD4 cell count is maintained, the likelihood of the virus mutating into resistant strains is decreased. HIV patients who are otherwise healthy and symptom free should have their CD4 cell count and viral load tested about two to four times a year. However, symptomatic patients should be tested more frequently to evaluate both the risk of opportunistic infections and the response to HIV drug treatments.

INTEGRATIVE THERAPIES

Integrative therapies should not replace antiretroviral therapy in HIV patients. Patients should consult their healthcare providers before taking any herbs or supplements because they may interact with treatment. In particular, patients should not take St. John's wort because it may interact with HIV treatment.

Unclear or Conflicting Scientific Evidence

Aloe Vera: Clear gel from the pulp of *Aloe vera* leaves has been used on the skin for thousands of years to treat wounds, skin infections, minor burns, and other skin conditions. Although aloe has been suggested as a possible treatment for HIV, further research is needed before a firm conclusion can be made.

Avoid if allergic to aloe or other plants of the Lilaceae family (garlic, onions, and tulips). Avoid injecting aloe. Do not apply to open skin, surgical wounds, or pressure ulcers. Avoid taking by mouth with diarrhea, bowel blockage, intestinal diseases, bloody stools, or hepatitis. Avoid with a history of irregular heartbeat (arrhythmia), electrolyte imbalances, diabetes, heart disease, or kidney disease. Avoid taking by mouth if pregnant or breastfeeding.

Antineoplastons: Antineoplastons are substances found in human blood and urine. A small preliminary study reported increased energy and weight in patients with HIV as well as a decreased number of opportunistic infections and increased CD4 cell counts. These patients were treated with antineoplaston AS2-1. However, this evidence cannot be considered conclusive. Currently, there are drug therapy regimens available for HIV with clearly demonstrated effects (HAART), and patients with HIV are recommended to consult with their physicians about treatment options.

Avoid if allergic or hypersensitive to antineoplastons. Use cautiously with high medical or psychiatric risk. Use cautiously with an active infection due to a possible decrease in white blood cells. Use cautiously with high blood pressure, heart conditions, chronic obstructive pulmonary disease, liver disease/damage, or kidney disease/damage. Avoid if pregnant or breastfeeding.

Beta-Sitosterol: Beta-sitosterol is found in plant-based foods, such as fruits, vegetables, soybeans, breads, peanuts, and peanut products. It is also found in bourbon and oils (such as olive oil, flaxseed, and tuna). Due to data that suggest immune-modulating effects of beta-sitosterol and beta-sitosterol glucoside, these sterols have been studied in combination in the treatment of HIV. Larger populations of patients with HIV should be evaluated in randomized, controlled trials to draw any conclusions.

Avoid if allergic or hypersensitive to beta-sitosterol, beta-sitosterol glucoside, or pine. Use cautiously with asthma or breathing disorders, diabetes, primary biliary cirrhosis (destruction of the small bile duct in the liver), ileostomy, neurodegenerative disorders (like Parkinson's disease or Alzheimer's disease), diverticular disease (bulging of the colon), short-bowel syndrome, celiac disease, and sitosterolemia. Use cautiously with a history of gallstones. Avoid if pregnant or breastfeeding.

Bitter Melon: Laboratory studies have shown that a protein in bitter melon called MAP30 may have antiviral activity. However, this has not been studied in humans. Further research is needed before a firm conclusion can be made.

Avoid if allergic to bitter melon or members of the Curcurbitaceae (gourd or melon) family. Avoid ingesting bitter melon seeds. Avoid with glucose-6-phosphate dehydrogenase deficiency. Use cautiously with diabetes, glucose intolerance, or with hypoglycemic agents due to the risk of hypoglycemia (low blood sugar). Avoid if pregnant or breastfeeding.

Chiropractic: Chiropractic care focuses on how the relationship between musculoskeletal structure (mainly the spine) and bodily function (mainly nervous system) affects health. There is not enough reliable scientific evidence to conclude the effects of chiropractic techniques on CD4 cell count or quality of life in patients with HIV/AIDS.

Use extra caution during cervical adjustments. Use cautiously with acute arthritis, conditions that cause decreased bone mineralization, brittle bone disease, bone-softening conditions, bleeding disorders, or migraines. Use cautiously if at risk of tumors or cancer. Avoid with symptoms of vertebrobasilar vascular insufficiency, aneurysms, unstable spondylolisthesis, or arthritis. Avoid with agents that increase the risk of bleeding. Avoid in areas of paraspinal tissue after surgery. Avoid if pregnant or breastfeeding due to a lack of scientific data.

Coenzyme Q10 (CoQ10): CoQ10 is produced by the body and is necessary for basic functioning of cells. CoQ10 levels decrease with age. There is limited evidence that natural levels of CoQ10 in the body may be reduced in people with HIV/AIDS. There is no reliable scientific research showing that CoQ10 supplements have any effect on this disease.

There are currently no documented cases of allergy associated with CoQ10 supplements, although rash and itching have rarely been reported. Stop use two weeks before and immediately after surgery/dental/diagnostic procedures with bleeding risks. Use cautiously with a history of blood clots, diabetes, high blood pressure, heart attack, or stroke. Use cautiously with anticoagulants (blood thinners), antiplatelet drugs, blood pressure drugs, blood sugar drugs, cholesterol drugs, or thyroid drugs. Avoid if pregnant or breastfeeding.

Dehydroepiandrosterone (DHEA): DHEA is a hormone that is secreted by the adrenal glands. Although some studies suggest that DHEA supplementation may be beneficial in patents with HIV, results from different studies do not agree with each other. There is currently not enough scientific evidence to recommend DHEA for this condition, and other therapies are more proven in this area.

Avoid if allergic to DHEA. Avoid with a history of seizures. Use cautiously with adrenal or thyroid disorders. Use cautiously if taking anticoagulants or drugs, herbs, or supplements used to treat diabetes, heart disease, seizures, or stroke. Stop use two weeks before and immediately after surgery/dental/diagnostic procedures with bleeding risks. Avoid if pregnant or breastfeeding.

Flaxseed: Flaxseed and flaxseed oil/linseed oil are rich sources of the essential fatty acid alpha-linolenic acid (omega-6). While flaxseed has been used to treat HIV, no strong evidence supports its use and no recommendation can be made without further research.

Flaxseed has been well tolerated in studies for up to four months. Avoid if allergic to flaxseed, flaxseed oil, or other plants of the Linaceae family. Avoid with prostate cancer, breast cancer, uterine cancer, or endometriosis. Avoid ingestion of immature flaxseed pods. Avoid large amounts of flaxseed by mouth and mix with plenty of water or liquid. Avoid flaxseed (not flaxseed oil) with a history of esophageal stricture, ileus, gastrointestinal stricture, or bowel obstruction. Avoid with a history of acute or chronic diarrhea, irritable bowel syndrome, diverticulitis (inflammation of the diverticula, small sacs in the intestine's inner lining), or inflammatory bowel disease. Avoid topical flaxseed in open wounds or abraded skin surfaces. Use cautiously with a history of a bleeding disorder or with drugs that increase the risk of bleeding (such as anticoagulants and nonsteroidal antiinflammatories). Use cautiously with high triglyceride levels, diabetes, mania, seizures, or asthma. Avoid if pregnant or breastfeeding.

Healing Touch: Healing touch is a combination of hands-on and off-body techniques that influence the flow of energy through a person's biofield. Data from small preliminary studies are insufficient to support any recommendations for or against the use of healing touch in HIV/AIDS patients. Studies of better design are needed before any conclusions can be reached.

HT should not be regarded as a substitute for established medical treatments. Use cautiously if pregnant or breastfeeding.

L-Carnitine: L-carnitine may be beneficial in AIDS treatment by increasing proliferation of mononuclear cells and increasing CD4 counts. Additional study is needed to make a firm recommendation.

Avoid if allergic or hypersensitive to carnitine. Use cautiously with peripheral vascular disease, high blood pressure, alcohol-induced liver cirrhosis, and diabetes. Use cautiously in low birth weight infants and individuals on hemodialysis. Use cautiously if taking anticoagulants (blood thinners), beta-blockers, or calcium channel blockers. Avoid if pregnant or breastfeeding.

Meditation: Various forms of meditation have been practiced for thousands of years throughout the world, with many techniques originating in Eastern religious practices. A common goal is to attain a state of "thoughtless awareness" of sensations and mental activities occurring at the present moment. More studies are needed to establish how meditation may be useful as an adjunctive therapy in HIV/AIDS patients.

Use cautiously with underlying mental illnesses. People with psychiatric disorders should consult with their primary mental healthcare professionals before starting a program of meditation, and they should explore how meditation may or may not fit in with their current treatment plans. Avoid with risk of seizures. The practice of meditation should not delay the time to diagnosis or treatment with more proven techniques or therapies, and it should not be used as the sole approach to illnesses.

Melatonin: Melatonin is a neurohormone produced in the brain. There is a lack of well-designed scientific evidence to recommend for or against the use of melatonin as a treatment for AIDS. Melatonin should not be used in place of more proven therapies, and patients with HIV/AIDS should be treated under the supervision of their healthcare professionals.

Based on available studies and clinical use, melatonin is generally regarded as safe in recommended doses for short-term use. There are rare reports of allergic skin reactions after taking melatonin by mouth. Use cautiously with bleeding disorders, seizure disorders, or drugs that increase the risk of bleeding.

Mistletoe: Once considered a sacred herb in Celtic tradition, mistletoe has been used for centuries for high blood pressure, epilepsy, exhaustion, anxiety, arthritis, vertigo (dizziness), and degenerative inflammation of the joints. Treatment of HIV patients with mistletoe has been done in Europe since the beginning of the AIDS epidemic. Treatment seems to be tolerable, with minimal side effects reported. Mistletoe may assist in inhibiting disease progression. However, not all mistletoe preparations have shown equal effects. Further study is needed before a firm conclusion can be made.

Avoid if allergic or hypersensitive to mistletoe or to any of its constituents. Anaphylactic reactions (life-threatening shock) have been described after injections of mistletoe. Avoid with acute, highly febrile, inflammatory disease; thyroid disorders; seizure disorders; or heart disease. Use cautiously with diabetes, glaucoma, or with cholinergics.

Prayer: Prayer can be defined as a "reverent petition," the act of asking for something while aiming to connect with God or another object of worship. Limited study of prayer in patients with AIDS reports fewer new AIDS-related illnesses and hospitalizations. However, due to methodological problems, these results cannot be considered conclusive.

Prayer is not recommended as the sole treatment approach for potentially serious medical conditions, and it should not delay the time it takes to consult with a healthcare professional or receive established therapies. Sometimes religious beliefs come into conflict with standard medical approaches and require an open dialog between patients and caregivers.

Psychotherapy: Psychotherapy is an interactive process between a person and a qualified mental health professional. The patient will explore thoughts, feelings, and behaviors to help with problem solving. Psychotherapy, especially supportive psychotherapy, may reduce depression in HIV-positive patients. It may also help treat substance abuse when used in combination with prescription medicine. Supportive-expressive group therapy may also have concomitant improvements in CD4 cell count and viral load. More research is needed in this area, especially to determine the best type of psychotherapy.

Psychotherapy cannot always fix mental or emotional conditions. Psychiatric drugs are sometimes needed. In some cases, symptoms may get worse if the proper medication is not taken. Not all therapists are qualified to work with all problems. Use cautiously with serious mental illness or some medical conditions because some forms of psychotherapy may stir up strong emotional feelings and expression.

Relaxation Therapy: Relaxation techniques include behavioral therapeutic approaches that differ widely in philosophy, methodology, and practice. Mental health and quality-of-life improvements have been seen in preliminary studies of HIV/AIDS patients. These findings suggest the need for further, well-controlled research.

Avoid with psychiatric disorders like schizophrenia/psychosis. Jacobson relaxation (flexing specific muscles, holding that position, then relaxing the muscles) should be used cautiously with illnesses like heart disease, high blood pressure, or musculoskeletal injury. Relaxation therapy is not recommended as the sole treatment approach for potentially serious medical conditions, and it should not delay the time to diagnosis or treatment with more proven techniques.

Selenium: Selenium is a mineral found in soil, water, and some foods. Selenium supplementation has been studied in HIV/AIDS patients, and some reports associate low selenium levels with complications such as cardiomyopathy. It remains unclear if selenium supplementation is beneficial in patients with HIV, particularly during antiretroviral therapy.

Avoid if allergic or sensitive to products containing selenium. Avoid with a history of nonmelanoma skin cancer. Selenium is generally regarded as safe for pregnant or breastfeeding women. However, animal research reports that large doses of selenium may lead to birth defects.

Shiitake: Shiitake mushrooms were originally grown on natural oak logs found in Japan. Today, they are available in the United States. These mushrooms are large, black-brown, and have an

H

earthy, rich flavor. Based on preliminary studies, lentinan may increase CD4 counts and may qualify in future multidrug studies in HIV patients. Further well-designed studies are needed to confirm these results. Side effects have been reported, and more proven therapies are recommended at this time.

Avoid if allergic or hypersensitive to shiitake mushrooms. Avoid if pregnant or breastfeeding.

Thymus Extract: Thymus extracts for nutritional supplements are usually derived from young calves. Preliminary evidence found no improvement in HIV progression to AIDS or immunostimulation, although some immunological activity was noted in a nonrandomized, controlled trial. Additional study is needed in this area.

Avoid if allergic or hypersensitive to thymus extracts. Use bovine thymus extract supplements cautiously due to potential for exposure to the virus that causes "mad cow disease." Avoid use with an organ transplant or other forms of allografts or xenografts. Avoid if receiving immunosuppressive therapy or hormone therapy. Avoid with thymic tumors, myasthenia gravis (neuromuscular disorder), or untreated hypothyroidism. Avoid if pregnant or breastfeeding. Thymic extract increases human sperm motility and progression.

Traditional Chinese Medicine (TCM): TCM is a broad term that refers to many different treatments and traditions of healing. They share a common heritage of technique or theory rooted in ancient Chinese philosophy (Taoism) that dates back over 5,000 years. TCM herbs are a popular complementary therapy in HIV/AIDS. However, study results conflict. More studies are needed before the potential benefits of TCM herbs in HIV/AIDS can be established.

Chinese herbs can be potent and may interact with other herbs, foods, or drugs. Consult a qualified healthcare professional before taking. There have been reports of manufactured or processed Chinese herbal products being tainted with toxins or heavy metal or not containing the listed ingredients. Herbal products should be purchased from reliable sources. Avoid ephedra and ma huang, which is the active ingredient in ephedra. Avoid ginseng if pregnant or breastfeeding.

Turmeric: Turmeric is a perennial plant native to India and Indonesia, and it is often used as a spice in cooking. Several laboratory studies suggest that curcumin, a component of turmeric, may have activity against HIV. However, reliable human studies are lacking in this area.

Avoid if allergic or hypersensitive to turmeric (curcumin), yellow food colorings, or plants belonging to the Curcuma or Zingiberaceae (ginger)

families. Use cautiously with a history of bleeding disorders, immune system deficiencies, liver disease, or gallstones. Use cautiously with blood thinners (e.g., warfarin). Use cautiously if pregnant or breastfeeding.

Vitamin A: Vitamin A is a fat-soluble vitamin that is derived from two sources: retinoids and carotenoids. Retinoids are found in animal sources (such as the liver, kidney, eggs, and dairy products). Carotenoids are found in plants like dark-green or yellow vegetables and carrots. The role of vitamin A in the prevention, transmission, or treatment of HIV is controversial and not well established. A clear conclusion cannot be formed based on the available scientific research.

Avoid if allergic or hypersensitive to vitamin A. Vitamin A toxicity can occur if taken at high dosages. Use cautiously with liver disease or alcoholism. Smokers who consume alcohol and beta-carotene may have an increased risk for lung cancer or heart disease. Vitamin A appears safe in pregnant women if taken at recommended doses. Use cautiously if breastfeeding because the benefits or dangers to nursing infants are not clearly established.

Zinc: Zinc formulations have been used since ancient Egyptian times to enhance wound healing. Patients with HIV/AIDS, especially those with low zinc levels, may benefit from zinc supplementation. Some low-quality studies cite reduction in infections, increased weight gain, and enhanced immune system function, including increased CD4 and CD8 cell counts. However, other low-quality studies conflict with these findings. Further research is needed before a conclusion can be drawn.

Zinc is generally considered safe when taken at the recommended dosages. Avoid zinc chloride since studies have not been done on its safety or effectiveness. While zinc appears safe during pregnancy in amounts lower than the established upper intake level, caution should be used since studies cannot rule out the possibility of harm to the fetus.

Fair Negative Scientific Evidence

Ozone Therapy: Ozone molecules are composed of three oxygen atoms. Ozone exists high in the earth's atmosphere and absorbs radiation from the sun. Reports of using ozone for medicinal purposes date to the late nineteenth century. Laboratory studies have shown HIV to be sensitive to ozone, but no high-quality human studies exist. A preliminary study measured the safety and effectiveness of ozone-treated blood in the treatment of HIV infection and immune disease. Ozone therapy was not shown to enhance immune activation or diminish the HIV virus.

Autohemotherapy (a therapy in which blood is withdrawn from the body, infused with ozone, and then replaced into the body) has been associated with the transmission of viral hepatitis and with a possible case of dangerously lowered blood cell counts. Insufflation of the ear carries a risk of tympanic membrane (eardrum) damage, and colon insufflation may increase the risk of bowel rupture. Consult a qualified health professional before undergoing any ozone-related treatment.

St John's Wort: St. John's wort is a perennial herb that grows up to 32 inches tall and is commonly found in many parts of the world, including eastern North America and the Pacific coast. Antiviral effects of St. John's wort have been observed in laboratory studies but were not found in one human study. Multiple reports of significant adverse effects and interactions with drugs used for HIV/AIDS, including protease inhibitors and NNRTIs, suggest that patients being treated for HIV/AIDS should avoid this herb. Therefore, there is evidence to recommend against using St. John's wort in the treatment of patients with HIV/AIDS.

Avoid if allergic or hypersensitive to plants in the Hypericaceae family. Rare allergic skin reactions like itchy rash have been reported. Avoid with immunosuppressant drugs (such as cyclosporine, tacrolimus). Avoid with NNRTIs or protease inhibitors. Avoid with organ transplants, suicidal symptoms, or before surgery. Use cautiously with a history of thyroid disorders. Use cautiously with drugs that are broken down by the liver, with monoamine oxidase inhibitors or selective serotonin reuptake inhibitors, digoxin, or birth control pills. Use cautiously with diabetes or with a history of mania, hypomania, or seasonal affective disorder. Avoid if pregnant or breastfeeding.

Traditional or Theoretical Uses Lacking Sufficient Evidence

Eucalyptus Oil: Eucalyptus oil is found in numerous over-the-counter cough and cold lozenges as well as in inhalation vapors or topical ointments. Early laboratory research suggests that globoidnan A from eucalyptus oil may help inhibit the reproduction of HIV. However, additional well-designed trials are needed to determine if eucalyptus oil is an effective treatment for HIV patients.

Avoid if allergic to eucalyptus oil. Avoid in infants and young children. Use cautiously with asthma or other lung diseases, dyspnea, tachypnea, seizure disorders, low blood pressure, liver disease, kidney disease, or inflammation of the bile duct and gastrointestinal tract. Avoid if pregnant or breastfeeding due to a lack of available safety evidence.

Green Tea: Green tea is made from the dried leaves of *Camellia sinensis,* an evergreen shrub. It has been suggested that epigallocatechin gallate, derived from green tea, may disrupt the replication cycle of HIV. However, until research is performed in this area, it remains unknown if this is a safe and effective treatment.

Avoid if allergic or hypersensitive to caffeine or tannin. Use cautiously with diabetes or liver disease.

PREVENTION

Ways to Prevent Acquiring and/or Transmitting HIV: Individuals who are either at risk for acquiring HIV or are 13-64 should be tested for HIV annually. This is because this age group is most likely to be sexually active.

Needles or syringes should be avoided.

Unprotected sexual contact, including vaginal, anal, or oral sex, should be avoided with an infected person. Unprotected sexual contact with someone with unknown HIV status should also be avoided.

Behavioral modification may help prevent HIV/AIDS infection. In Uganda, there has been a dramatic decline in HIV prevalence as well as a decline in multipartner sexual behavior. The decrease in HIV/AIDS infection came after the launch of behavior change programs largely developed by the Ugandan government and local nongovernmental organizations. The "ABC" initiative (Abstain, Be faithful, or for those who refuse to do either, use Condoms) resulted in a significant decrease in HIV infections in generalized epidemics. Researchers explained that once the ABC program was launched, rates of 13- to 16-year-olds having sex in one district of Uganda dropped from nearly 60% in 1994 to less than 5% in 2001. Uganda's message for the majority of the population focused on mutual fidelity; the reduction in casual sex, not the elimination of all sex, seems to have led to Uganda's falling HIV rates. Uganda has shown a 70% decline in HIV prevalence since the early 1990s, linked to a 60% reduction in casual sex.

Gloves should be worn when in contact with blood or other body fluids that could possibly contain blood, such as urine, feces, or vomit.

Cuts, scrapes, sores, or breaks on the exposed skin of both the caregiver and patient should be covered with bandages.

Any body area that comes into contact with blood or other body fluids should be thoroughly washed.

Surfaces that have been tainted with blood should be disinfected with antibacterial soap.

Practices that increase the likelihood of blood contact, such as the sharing of razors, toothbrushes, and nail clippers, should be avoided.

Needles and other sharp instruments should be used only when medically necessary and handled appropriately.

In 1985, the CDC issued a list of routine precautions for all personal service workers, such as hairdressers, barbers, cosmetologists, and massage therapists, to take. Instruments that penetrate the skin, such as tattoo and acupuncture needles or ear-piercing guns, should either be used once and disposed of or thoroughly sterilized. Instruments that are not meant to penetrate the skin but may come in contact with blood (such as razors) should not be shared unless thoroughly sterilized.

Antiviral therapy during pregnancy can significantly lower the chance that the virus will be passed to the infant before, during, or after birth. The treatment is most effective if it is started as early as possible during pregnancy. However, there are still health benefits if treatment is begun during labor or shortly after the baby is born.

Delivering the baby by cesarean section has been shown to reduce the risk of transmission to the newborn. However, this is not the standard preventative care for HIV-infected pregnant women. It should only be considered in certain clinical circumstances (such as for patients who have a very high viral load or for patients who do not adhere to antiretroviral therapy).

Infected mothers should not breastfeed their newborn(s).

Preventing/Delaying the Onset of AIDS: HIV patients should receive HAART, which suppresses the virus and helps restore the body's immune system. Research has shown that HAART dramatically slows the progression of opportunistic infections in HIV/AIDS patients.

Preventing Opportunistic Infections: HIV patients may receive medications to help prevent infections from developing. Specific preventative treatment, such as antibiotics, is administered when HIV-infected patients are at risk of developing opportunistic infections or to prevent recurrence of a recent opportunistic infection. Treatment is typically given to patients who have *Pneumocystis jiroveci* pneumonia, MAC, toxoplasmosis, or latent TB.

In addition, HIV patients typically receive HAART, which suppresses the virus and helps restore and maintain the immune system. Patients with a healthy or near-healthy immune system are less likely to develop opportunistic infections.

NEW RESEARCH

The Pharmaceutical Research and Manufacturers Association of America has a database of new HIV drugs that are in the developmental stage. Researchers are currently testing new protease inhibitors and more potent, less toxic reverse transcriptase inhibitors as well as drugs that interfere with different steps in the HIV life cycle.

Cellular Metabolism Modulators: Cellular metabolism modulators are undergoing research. These drugs disrupt the cellular processes involved in HIV replication.

Gene Therapy: Gene therapy may be a beneficial treatment in the future. The process involves inserting modified genes (DNA) directly into the body's cells in order to slow or stop HIV from multiplying. Scientists are trying to insert genes that provide the body with instructions on how to produce T-cells that are genetically resistant to the virus.

Immune Modulators: Scientists are also learning how immune modulators, or drugs that alter the immune system, help enhance the immune system's response to HIV in order to potentially make current anti-HIV drugs more effective.

Maturation Inhibitors: Researchers are studying maturation inhibitors as a potential new class of antiretrovirals. These drugs disrupt the final stage of the HIV life cycle, when new virus particles are released into the blood. Currently, Bevirimat (PA-457) is the only maturation inhibitor undergoing clinical testing. This drug is derived from a Chinese herb called *Syzigium claviflorum*.

Portmanteau Inhibitors: Portmanteau inhibitors are also being investigated as a possible drug treatment for HIV patients. These inhibitors are a combination of one reverse transcriptase inhibitor and one integrase inhibitor.

Synergistic Enhancers: Another group of medications, called synergistic enhancers, may also be used in combination with other antiretroviral drugs to treat HIV, although this use is not FDA approved. These medications do not act as antiretrovirals when taken alone, but they have been shown to improve the antiretroviral effects of other drugs, including ritonavir (Norvir). Very small doses of synergistic enhancers may also be used to reduce the liver metabolism of other antiretroviral drugs. For instance, grapefruit juice is considered a synergistic enhancer that may be beneficial for patients taking antiretrovirals.

Vaccines: Therapeutic vaccines are also being tested as a way to prevent HIV infection.

CLINICAL TRIALS

General: HIV/AIDS clinical trials are performed to develop and test more effective and safer ways to diagnose, treat, and prevent HIV/AIDS. A clinical trial is a research study in volunteer human subjects to determine the safety and efficacy of new treatments, screening methods, preventive techniques, or diagnostic methods for a disease. New devices, drugs, procedures, and medical innovations must be thoroughly tested to ensure that they are safe and effective for human patients. Human trials are only conducted after both laboratory and animal studies show promising results.

Phases of Trials: There are four phases of trials. In phase I clinical trials, researchers test a new drug or treatment in a small group of 20-80 patients for the first time. The goal is to evaluate the drug or treatment's safety, determine a safe dosage range, and identify side effects. Phase II clinical trials study the effects of a drug or treatment in a larger group of 100-300 patients. During this phase, researchers aim to determine the drug or treatment's efficacy and further assess its safety. During phase III trials, researchers study the effect of a drug or treatment in large groups of 1,000-3,000 patients. This type of trial is used to confirm the drug or treatment's effectiveness and monitor side effects. The drug or treatment is also compared to commonly used treatments, and researchers collect information that will help ensure that the drug or treatment is used safely. Phase IV clinical trials are performed after the drug or treatment has been marketed to the general public. These studies are conducted to collect information on the drug or treatment's long-term effects and side effects in various patient populations.

Who Can Participate: All HIV patients can volunteer to participate in clinical trials. However, each clinical trial has unique guidelines for who can participate in the study, called criteria. Patients interested in enrolling in a particular study must meet the criteria. This helps ensure the patient's safety and helps ensure that researchers are able to accurately prove or disprove their hypotheses. Factors that allow a patient to enroll in a clinical trial are called inclusion criteria, and factors that prevent a patient from enrolling are called exclusion criteria. Criteria may include or exclude patients based on factors such as age, medical history, gender, current medications, coexisting illnesses, and overall health.

Weighing the Pros and Cons: Participation in clinical trials is completely voluntarily, and the decision should only be made after the patient has carefully considered the potential health benefits and risks. These risks and benefits will be different for each trial and each individual patient. It is important for patients to consult their personal healthcare providers and family members before deciding whether or not to participate in a clinical trial.

Patients will meet with the researchers before being enrolled in the study. This allows patients to ask any questions and address any concerns about participating. Patients should consider writing down questions ahead of time, asking a friend or family member to join them for support, and/or recording the discussion.

Participating in a clinical trial allows patients to take an active role in their healthcare. Participants gain access to new treatments that are not available to the public, and participants help others by contributing to medical research. However, risks of participating in a trial may include side effects or adverse reactions, the treatment may not be effective, the trial may take up a lot of the patient's time, and participation may require hospital visits or involve complex treatment plans.

Safety: The federal government has guidelines and safeguards to protect participants in clinical trials. All clinical trials in the United States must be approved and monitored by an Institutional Review Board (IRB) to ensure that the risks are minimal and worth the potential benefits. An IRB is an independent committee that consists of physicians, statisticians, community advocates, and other professionals.

During the Trial: The process of each clinical trial is different. The research team generally includes doctors, nurses, and other healthcare professionals. Participants should closely follow the trial's protocol to ensure their safety. Participants are evaluated at the beginning and end of the trial, and their health is monitored continually throughout the trial. Some researchers will stay in touch with participants after the study to perform follow-up tests and/or questionnaires. While enrolled in the trial, patients should continue to regularly visit their primary healthcare providers. This helps ensure that the clinical trial protocol is not interfering with the patient's regular medications or treatments.

Leaving Early: Participants can choose to leave a clinical trial at any time. Patients who want to stop participating should let the researcher(s) know why they are leaving the trial.

Payment: Some clinical trials pay participants to enroll in the study, while others do not. Some trials will reimburse participants for expenses associated with the trial, such as transportation costs,

H

accommodations, meals, or childcare. Potential study participants can discuss whether payment is offered when they meet with the researcher(s). Payment is often not offered if a patient leaves the trial early or does not adhere to protocol.

SUPPORT GROUPS

AIDSinfo, sponsored by the National Institutes of Health, provides the latest information about government and industry sponsored HIV/AIDS treatment and prevention clinical trials. AIDSinfo also provides the most current, federally approved guidelines for treating and preventing HIV/AIDS in adults and children. It provides information about AIDS-related illnesses, how to manage occupational exposure to HIV, and how to prevent HIV transmission from mother to child during pregnancy.

The Elizabeth Glaser Pediatric AIDS Foundation provides treatment to HIV/AIDS patients. The organization promotes the discovery of new treatments for other serious and life-threatening pediatric illnesses.

The American Foundation for AIDS Research is one of the world's leading nonprofit organizations dedicated to the support of HIV/AIDS research, prevention, treatment education, and the advocacy of AIDS-related public policies.

The National AIDS hotline is available in English and Spanish, 24 hours a day, seven days a week. The number is: 1-800-CDC-INFO (1-800-232-4636).

INFLAMMATORY BOWEL DISEASE (IBD)

BACKGROUND

Inflammatory bowel disease (IBD) refers to two chronic diseases that cause inflammation of the intestines: ulcerative colitis and Crohn's disease. The symptoms of these two illnesses are very similar, which often makes it difficult to distinguish between the two. In fact, about 10% of colitis (inflamed colon) cases cannot be diagnosed as either ulcerative colitis or Crohn's disease. When physicians cannot diagnose the specific IBD, the condition is called indeterminate colitis.

IBD is not the same as irritable bowel syndrome. Irritable bowel syndrome is characterized by cramping, abdominal pain, bloating, constipation, and diarrhea. IBS causes discomfort and distress, but it does not permanently damage the intestines and it does not cause serious diseases, such as cancer. IBD, on the other hand, causes chronic inflammation in the gastrointestinal tract and may lead to complications like colon cancer.

Researchers estimate that about one million Americans have IBD. While IBD can develop at any age, it is most prevalent among individuals aged 15 to 30.

CROHN'S DISEASE

Dr. Burill B. Crohn and two of his colleagues, Dr. Leon Ginzburg and Dr. Gordon D. Oppenheimer, discovered Crohn's disease in 1932. Crohn's disease is a chronic disorder that causes inflammation of the gastrointestinal tract.

Although it can cause inflammation in any area of the gastrointestinal tract from the mouth to the anus, it most commonly affects the ileum (small intestine) and/or colon.

Unlike ulcerative colitis, Crohn's disease may affect any layer of the intestine, and it often spreads deep into the layers of affected tissues. Also unlike ulcerative colitis, the inflammation is not consistent throughout the bowel. There may be healthy bowel (tissue/mucosa) in between areas of diseased bowel.

An estimated 500,000 Americans have Crohn's disease, which may develop at any age.

ULCERATIVE COLITIS

Ulcerative colitis is different from Crohn's disease because inflammation is limited to only the colon. Also, ulcerative colitis only affects the superficial layers (the mucosa) of the colon. With more than 500,000 Americans living with ulcerative colitis, the condition is slightly more prevalent than Crohn's disease. However, it is sometimes difficult to differentiate between the two diseases. Also, the early stages of Crohn's disease may be mistaken for ulcerative colitis because the disease starts in the colon and progresses throughout the gastrointestinal tract.

Ulcerative colitis may develop at any age.

CAUSES

The cause of IBD remains unknown. However, current research indicates that the inflammation in IBD patients involves a complex interaction of factors, including heredity, the immune system, and antigens in the environment.

Environment: Since IBD occurs more often among people who live in cities and industrialized nations, it is possible that environmental factors, including a diet high in fat or refined foods, may play a role.

Heredity: Individuals are more likely to develop IBD if there is a family history of the disease. Therefore, researchers believe that an individual's genetic makeup may be a contributing factor to development of the disease.

Immune System: Some evidence suggests that a virus or bacteria may cause IBD. When the immune system attacks the invading substance, the gastrointestinal tract becomes inflamed. Other researchers speculate that the inflammation may stem from the virus or bacteria directly.

Mycobacterium avium subspecies *paratuberculosis* (MAP) may be involved the development of Crohn's disease and ulcerative colitis. This microorganism is known to cause intestinal diseases in cattle. In addition, researchers have found MAP in the blood and intestinal tissue of individuals diagnosed with Crohn's disease, but rarely in individuals with ulcerative colitis.

SYMPTOMS

The severity of IBD symptoms varies among patients, and they may develop gradually or come on suddenly. Some individuals will experience long periods with no symptoms, while others may experience chronic or recurrent symptoms.

The most common symptoms of both ulcerative colitis and Crohn's disease are diarrhea (ranging from mild to severe), abdominal pain, decreased appetite, and weight loss. If the diarrhea is extreme, it may lead to dehydration, increased heartbeat, and decreased blood pressure. As food moves through inflamed areas of the gastrointestinal tract, it may cause bleeding. Continued loss of blood in the stool may result in anemia. In addition, Crohn's disease may also cause intestinal ulcers, fever, fatigue, arthritis, eye inflammation, skin disorders, and inflammation of the liver or bile ducts.

COMPLICATIONS

Anal Fissure: An anal fissure is a cleft in the anus or in the skin around the anus where infection may occur. This is commonly associated with painful bowel movements.

Fistulas: Ulcers may extend through the intestinal wall, creating a fistula (an abnormal opening). If an internal fistula develops, food may not reach the area of the intestine involved in absorption. External fistulas may result in continuous bowel drainage onto the skin. Fistulas may also become infected, a condition that can be life threatening if left untreated.

Malnutrition: Diarrhea, abdominal pain, and cramping may make it difficult to eat. The body may not be able to consume a sufficient amount of nutrients.

Obstruction: Individual's who have Crohn's disease may experience blockage in the intestine. Food contents may become lodged in areas of the intestine that are inflamed. Some cases may require surgery to remove the diseased portion of the gastrointestinal tract.

Toxic Megacolon: Toxic megacolon is a rare but potentially life-threatening complication of severe IBD. Toxic megacolon is characterized by a dilated colon (megacolon), abdominal distension (bloating), and occasionally fever, abdominal pain, or shock. In severe cases, the condition may cause the colon to become paralyzed. Toxic megacolon prevents the individual from having bowel movements. If the condition is not treated, the colon may rupture, resulting in peritonitis, a life-threatening condition that requires emergency surgery.

Ulcers: Ulcers (open sores) may develop anywhere there is chronic inflammation in the gastrointestinal tract, including the mouth or anus.

Other: Many individuals who have had long-standing Crohn's disease may develop osteoporosis (weak, brittle bones). Researchers speculate that this may be related to low levels of vitamin K, which is involved in binding calcium to bone.

IBD AND COLON CANCER

Individuals who have IBD are more likely to develop colon cancer, even if the condition is managed with treatment. The risk of colon cancer is related to the extent and duration of disease, not its activity. The risk is the greatest among individuals who have had IBD for more than eight years and if it has spread throughout the entire colon. Despite the increased risk, more than 90% of individuals with IBD do not develop cancer.

Individuals who have had IBD for more than eight years should visit a gastroenterologist at least once a year. Regular colonoscopies may also be recommended.

DIAGNOSIS

General: The diagnosis of IBD is based on a combination of exams. A colonoscopy is the standard diagnostic test for IBD. In order to determine whether the IBD is ulcerative colitis or Crohn's disease, tests such as capsule endoscopy, upper endoscopy, barium study, or computerized tomographic scan may be conducted. These tests help the gastroenterologist determine whether there is inflammation in gastrointestinal areas other than the colon. If there is inflammation in areas other than the colon, the patient is diagnosed with Crohn's disease.

Colonoscopy: A qualified healthcare provider may observe the colon with an endoscope. The endoscope is a thin tube that is inserted through the anus and attached to a television monitor. The physician looks for inflammation, bleeding, or ulcers on the colon wall.

Capsule Endoscopy: Capsule endoscopy may be performed if an individual experiences symptoms of Crohn's disease but other diagnostic tests are negative for the disease. The patient swallows a capsule that has a camera inside. The camera photographs the gastrointestinal tract. The pictures are then subsequently transmitted to a computer screen. The healthcare provider will then look for abnormalities in the gastrointestinal tract, including inflammation and ulcers. Once the device has traveled through the digestive tract, it will pass painlessly in the stool.

Barium Study: During a barium study, the patient drinks a barium solution before x-rays of the intestines are taken. The barium will appear white on the x-ray film, which allows the physician to see possible problems, such as inflammation.

Computerized Tomography (CT) Scan: A CT scan, which provides more detail than a standard x-ray, may also be performed. This test shows the entire gastrointestinal tract and tissues outside of the bowel. This test may help the healthcare provider detect complications such as blockages, abscesses, or fistulas.

Flexible Sigmoidoscopy: A qualified healthcare provider may perform a sigmoidoscopy. During this procedure, the physician uses a slender, flexible tube to examine the last two feet of the colon, known as the sigmoid. The test is usually completed in a few minutes. However, it is slightly uncomfortable, and there is a slight risk that the colon wall may become perforated. In addition, this test may not detect problems higher in the colon or small intestine.

Upper Endoscopy: An upper endoscopy may be performed to check the esophagus, stomach, and upper small intestine for bleeding, inflammation, or ulcers associated with Crohn's disease.

TREATMENT
Antiinflammatories

There is no known cure for IBD. However, many medications may help to relieve the symptoms.

Sulfasalazine (Azulfidine): Sulfasalazine (Azulfidine) has been used to treat the symptoms of Crohn's disease. Adverse effects include nausea, vomiting, heartburn, and headache. Individuals should avoid this medication if they are allergic to sulfa medications.

Mesalamine and Olsalazine: Mesalamine (Asacol, Rowasa) and olsalazine (Dipentum) have been used to decrease inflammation in the gastrointestinal tract caused by IBD. They are typically taken orally or rectally in the form of enemas or suppositories. Olsalazine may cause or worsen existing diarrhea in some people.

Balsalazide (Colazal): Balsalazide (Colazal) has also been used to decrease inflammation in the gastrointestinal tract caused by IBD.

Corticosteroids: Corticosteroids have shown to effectively reduce inflammation of the gastrointestinal tract in IBD patients. They may also be used in conjunction with other forms of medications. For instance, in some cases, a physician may prescribe steroid enemas to treat symptoms in the lower colon or rectum. Corticosteroids should only be used as short-term medication. Treatment generally lasts about two weeks.

Immunosuppressive Medications

Azathioprine and Mercaptopurine: Azathioprine (Imuran) and mercaptopurine (Purinethol) have been used for years to treat Crohn's disease. However, their efficacy for ulcerative colitis is still being researched. Since these medications are slow acting, they are occasionally combined with a corticosteroid.

Cyclosporine: Cyclosporine (Neoral, Sandimmune) is usually only prescribed to individuals who are not responding to other medications. Cyclosporine begins working within one to two weeks. However, severe side effects may include kidney and liver damage, fatal infections, and an increased risk of lymphoma.

Infliximab (Remicade): The U.S. Food and Drug Administration approved infliximab (Remicade) in September 2005 for the treatment of ulcerative colitis. The drug neutralizes a protein produced by the immune system known as tumor necrosis factor. Infliximab removes tumor necrosis factor from the bloodstream before it can cause inflammation in the gastrointestinal tract.

Other Medications

Antidiarrheals: A fiber supplement like psyllium powder (Metamucil) or methylcellulose (Citrucel) may help relieve symptoms of mild to moderate diarrhea. For more severe diarrhea, loperamide (Imodium) may be effective.

Laxatives: Inflammation may cause the intestines to narrow, resulting in constipation. Laxatives may be taken to relieve symptoms of constipation. Oral laxatives like Correctol and sigmoidoscopy have been used.

Pain Relievers: A qualified healthcare provider may recommend acetaminophen (Tylenol) for mild pain. Avoid nonsteroidal antiinflammatories (NSAIDs) like aspirin, ibuprofen (Advil, Motrin), or naproxen (Aleve). Researchers have found a strong relationship between NSAIDs and IBD flare-ups. Therefore, NSAIDs should not be taken.

Surgery: If all other treatments fail to relieve symptoms, a qualified healthcare provider may recommend surgery. Surgery is more commonly performed in ulcerative colitis patients because inflammation is limited to the colon.

During the procedure, the entire colon and rectum are removed (proctocolectomy). A new procedure, known as ileoanal anastomosis, eliminates the need for recovered patients to wear a bag to collect stool. This new procedure involves attaching a pouch directly to the anus, allowing the patient to expel waste normally. However, the patient may have as many as five to seven watery bowel movements a day because there is no longer a colon to absorb water. Between 25-40% of patients with ulcerative colitis eventually need surgery.

Some Crohn's patients may experience blockages in the intestine that require surgery to remove the diseased portion of the gastrointestinal tract.

INTEGRATIVE THERAPIES
Good Scientific Evidence

Probiotics: *Escherichia coli Nissle 1917* appears to be as effective as the drug mesalamine in the treatment of ulcerative colitis. However, it is not currently available in the United States. A variety of Bifidophilus preparations have shown effects of preventing relapse or maintaining remission. These include Bifidophilus alone, Bifidophilus in fermented milk products, and a synbiotic preparation. A probiotic combination consisting of VSL#3 plus balsalazide may be more effective than balsalazide or mesalamine alone. More studies are needed to more clearly determine what outcomes can be expected. Probiotics are generally regarded as safe for human consumption. Long-term consumption of probiotics is considered safe and well tolerated.

Unclear or Conflicting Scientific Evidence

Acupuncture: Acupuncture appears to be safe when used in decreasing inflammation and pain associated with IBD, although scientific evidence is inconclusive about its effectiveness. Avoid acupuncture in patients who have valvular heart disease, infections, or bleeding disorders; drugs that increase the risk of bleeding (anticoagulants); medical conditions of unknown origin; and neurological disorders. Avoid on areas that have received radiation therapy and during pregnancy. Use cautiously with pulmonary disease (like asthma or emphysema). Use cautiously in the elderly or medically compromised patients, diabetics, or individuals with a history of seizures.

Acustimulation: Acustimulation is the mild electrical stimulation of acupuncture points to control symptoms such as nausea and vomiting. One small study suggests that acustimulation may help reduce inflammation and pain caused by IBD. The only known side effect of acustimulation devices is slight skin irritation under the electrodes when the wristband is used. Switch wrists to avoid. Acustimulation devices should only be used on the designated area. Use cautiously with pacemakers. Avoid if the cause of medical symptoms is unknown. Keep acustimulation devices out of the reach of children.

Aloe: There is limited but promising research of the use of oral aloe vera in ulcerative colitis compared to placebo. It is not clear how aloe vera compares to other treatments used for ulcerative colitis. People with known allergy to garlic, onions, tulips, or other plants of the Lilaceae family may have allergic reactions to aloe. Individuals using aloe gel for prolonged times have developed allergic reactions, including hives and eczema-like rash. Although topical (skin) use of aloe is unlikely to be harmful during pregnancy or breastfeeding, oral (by mouth) use is not recommended due to theoretical stimulation of uterine contractions. It is not known whether active ingredients of aloe may be present in breast milk. Breastfeeding mothers should not consume the dried juice of aloe leaves.

Barley: Germinated barley foodstuff comes from maturing barley and has been suggested as possibly helpful in patients with ulcerative colitis. Scientific evidence in this area is preliminary, and further research is needed before germinated barley foodstuff can be recommended for ulcerative colitis. Patients who are allergic to barley flour or beer should avoid barley products. Severe allergic reactions (anaphylaxis) and skin rashes have been reported from drinking beer made with malted barley. Patients with allergy/hypersensitivity to grass pollens, rice, rye, oats, or wheat may also react to barley. Barley appears to be well tolerated in nonallergic, healthy adults in recommended doses for short periods of time as a cereal or in the form of beer. Avoid consuming large amounts of barley sprouts if pregnant. Avoid if breastfeeding.

Boswellia: Boswellia has been noted in animal and laboratory studies to possess antiinflammatory properties. Based on these observations, boswellia has been suggested as a potential treatment for ulcerative colitis. At this time, however, only a limited number of poor-quality human trials have evaluated this use of boswellia, with inconclusive results. Therefore, there is inadequate evidence for or against this use of boswellia. Avoid if allergic to boswellia or other herbs in the Burseraceae family (like myrrh or *Garuga*). Boswellia is generally believed to be safe when used as directed, although safety and toxicity have not been well studied in humans. Indian literature suggests that boswellia may promote menstruation and induce abortion. However, there is insufficient scientific evidence regarding the safety of boswellia. Therefore, pregnant or breastfeeding women should avoid boswellia.

Dehydroepiandrosterone (DHEA): Initial research reports have shown that DHEA supplements are safe for short-term use in patients with Crohn's disease. Preliminary research suggests possible beneficial effects, although further research is necessary before a clear conclusion can be drawn. Avoid if allergic to DHEA products. Avoid if pregnant or breastfeeding because DHEA is a hormone.

Gamma-Linolenic Acid (GLA): One double-blind, randomized clinical trial suggests that a combination of GLA plus eicosapentaenoic acid and docosahexaenoic acid does not prolong the period of disease remission in ulcerative colitis. Further well-designed clinical trials are required in this area before recommendations can be made. GLA is generally considered nontoxic and well tolerated for up to 18 months. Avoid if pregnant or breastfeeding due to insufficient evidence.

Glucosamine: Preliminary research reports improvements with *N*-acetylglucosamine as an added therapy in IBD. Further scientific evidence is necessary before a recommendation can be made. Avoid if allergic to shellfish or iodine. In most human studies, glucosamine sulfate has been well tolerated for 30 to 90 days. Avoid if pregnant or breastfeeding.

Moxibustion: One study suggests acupuncture combined with moxibustion (burning dried herbs, sometimes with glass cups or bowls, on the surface of the skin) may benefit symptoms in Crohn's disease. Well-designed studies are needed to verify this finding before concrete recommendations can be made.

Omega-3 Fatty Acids: It has been suggested that effects of omega-3 fatty acids on inflammation may be beneficial in patients with ulcerative colitis when added to standard therapy, and several studies have been conducted in this area. Better research is necessary before a clear conclusion can be drawn.

It has also been suggested that effects of omega-3 fatty acids on inflammation may be beneficial in patients with Crohn's disease when added to standard therapy, and several studies have been conducted in this area. Results are conflicting, and no clear conclusion can be drawn at this time. Avoid if allergic to fish. The U.S. Food and Drug Administration classifies low intake of omega-3 fatty acids from fish as generally regarded as safe. Caution may be warranted, however, in diabetic patients due to potential (albeit unlikely) increases in blood sugar levels, patients at risk of bleeding, or in those with high levels of low-density lipoprotein. Fish meat may contain methylmercury, and caution is warranted in young children and pregnant/breastfeeding women.

Psychotherapy: Psychotherapy may not improve the course of Crohn's disease, although patients undergoing psychotherapy tended to have fewer operations and relapses. More research in this area is needed.

Psyllium: There is limited and unclear evidence regarding the use of psyllium in patients with IBD. Serious allergic reactions, including anaphylaxis, difficulty breathing/wheezing, skin rash, and hives, have been reported after ingestion of psyllium products. Less-severe hypersensitivity reactions have also been noted. Cross-sensitivity may occur in people with allergy to English plantain pollen (*Plantago lanceolata*), grass pollen, or melon. Psyllium appears to be safe during pregnancy and breastfeeding.

Reflexology: Reflexology involves the application of manual pressure to specific points or areas of the feet that are believed to correspond to other parts of the body. Reflexology is often used with the intention to relieve stress or prevent/treat physical disorders. Reflexology may help relieve IBD symptoms. However, more research is necessary before recommendations can be made. Avoid with recent or healing foot fractures, unhealed wounds, or active gout flares affecting the foot. Use cautiously and seek prior medical consultation with osteoarthritis affecting the foot or ankle or severe vascular disease of the legs or feet. Use cautiously with diabetes, heart disease or the presence of a pacemaker, unstable blood pressure, cancer, active infections, past episodes of fainting (syncope), mental illness, gallstones, or kidney stones. Use cautiously if pregnant or breastfeeding. Reflexology should not delay diagnosis or treatment with more proven techniques or therapies.

Saccharomyces boulardii: Evidence supports mild improvement of symptoms and quality of life in patients with Crohn's disease who use *Saccharomyces boulardii*, although studies have been small. The pathogenesis of Crohn's disease may involve genetically influenced dysregulation of the mucosal immune response to antigens present in normal bacterial flora. Probiotics may change the enteric microenvironment, thereby alleviating the misguided immune response. More clinical trials are required before recommendations can be made in this field. Avoid if allergic to yeast, *Saccharomyces boulardii, Saccharomyces cerevisiae,* or other species in the Saccharomycetaceae family. *Saccharomyces boulardii* has been generally well tolerated in human studies for up to 15 months. However, *Saccharomyces boulardii* fungemia does occur. Multiple case reports describe fungemia in patients taking *Saccharomyces boulardii*. Avoid if pregnant or breastfeeding.

Soy: Due to limited human study, there is not enough evidence to recommend for or against the use of soy as a therapy in preventing Crohn's disease. Further research is needed before a recommendation can be made. Soy can act as a food allergen similar to milk, eggs, peanuts, fish, and wheat. Soy has been a dietary staple in many countries for over 5,000 years and is generally regarded as not having significant long-term toxicity. Limited side effects have been reported in infants, children, and adults aside from allergic reactions. Soy as a part of the regular diet is traditionally considered to be safe during pregnancy and breastfeeding, although scientific research is limited in these areas.

Thiamin (Vitamin B$_1$): Decreased serum thiamine levels have been reported in patients with Crohn's disease. It is not clear if routine thiamin supplementation is beneficial in such patients generally. Allergic reactions to thiamin supplements are rare. A small number of life-threatening anaphylactic reactions have been observed with large parenteral (intravenous, intramuscular, subcutaneous) doses of thiamin, generally after multiple doses. Thiamin is generally considered safe and relatively nontoxic, even at high doses. Thiamin appears to be safe at recommended doses during pregnancy and breastfeeding.

Wheatgrass: One well-designed study reported potential benefits of wheatgrass in the treatment of ulcerative colitis. However, further research is needed to confirm these findings. Wheatgrass is generally considered safe but should be avoided in patients who are allergic to it. Because it is grown in soils or water and consumed raw, wheatgrass may be contaminated with bacteria, molds, or other substances. Theoretically, women who are pregnant or breastfeeding should use wheatgrass cautiously.

Zinc: Preliminary research of zinc supplements in patients with Crohn's disease has yielded positive results. However, one small study found that zinc supplementation does not seem to improve IBD. Well-designed clinical trials are needed to confirm these results. Zinc is regarded as a relatively safe and generally well tolerated when taken at recommended doses, and few studies report side effects. Occasionally, adverse affects such as nausea, vomiting, or diarrhea have been observed. Zinc acetate should only be used during pregnancy if clearly needed. Zinc appears to be safe in amounts that do not exceed the established tolerable upper intake level. Zinc chloride should be given to a pregnant woman only if clearly needed under medical supervision.

Traditional or Theoretical Uses Lacking Sufficient Evidence

Homeopathy: Homeopathy may be helpful for helping balance immune function and decreasing symptoms of IBD. Further research is needed before recommendations can be made. Safety and effectiveness are not well studied, although most homeopathic practitioners regard these approaches as safe. Aside from rare adulteration of commercial products, there are no published reports of serious adverse effects. Severe or chronic health conditions may require additional medical attention beyond homeopathy.

PREVENTION

Since the cause of IBD is unknown, there is currently no known method of prevention.

Individuals who are diagnosed with IBD should consult their qualified healthcare providers before becoming pregnant or fathering a child. Some IBD medications have the potential to cause birth defects or may be passed to the infant during breastfeeding. Active IBD increases the risk of fetal death or premature labor.

Individuals who are diagnosed with IBD should consult their gastroenterologists regularly to monitor the condition and prevent complications.

BACKGROUND

Influenza, commonly referred to as the flu, is a contagious (able to be spread) infection of the respiratory system that is caused by viruses, including influenza types A, B, and C. Influenza viruses are transmitted through the air in tiny droplets when someone with the infection coughs, sneezes, or talks. Individuals are then exposed to the virus through inhalation or by contact with objects such as telephones, door handles, railings, or computer keyboards. An infection may occur when the virus is then transferred to the eyes, nose, or mouth. In general, the flu is more debilitating than the common cold, and symptoms such as fever, body ache, extreme fatigue (tiredness), and dry cough are seen more in the flu and are more severe. Some influenza viruses can even cause death in otherwise healthy individuals.

Although many individuals confuse common colds with influenza because they both affect the upper respiratory system and present with similar symptoms, they are actually caused by different viruses. The upper respiratory system includes the nose, trachea (windpipe), throat, sinuses (air-filled spaces in the skull), bronchial tubes (lead from the trachea to the lungs), and larynx (voice box). Every year in the United States an average of 5-20% of the population gets the flu and more than 200,000 people are hospitalized from flu complications, such as dehydration (loss of water), high fever (over 102° F), and extreme fatigue. About 36,000 people die from flu every year. Some patients, such as older people, young children, and people with certain health conditions that lower immunity, including cancer, human immunodeficiency virus (HIV), and acquired immunodeficiency syndrome (AIDS), are at high risk for serious flu complications. Children are two to three times more likely than adults to get sick with the flu. Also, children frequently spread the virus to others due to bad hygiene, such as sneezing without covering the nose. Treatment for the flu includes bed rest and plenty of fluids along with symptomatic treatment such as drugs to fight viral infections, reduce fever, and help with sore throat and cough. Prevention includes an influenza vaccine.

Flu Epidemics: When a flu epidemic occurs, specific populations are infected with a type of influenza virus that has not been encountered before.

The immune system of most of the general population cannot respond to the viral infection, and widespread illness and even death can occur. Some individuals, for reasons unknown, may be immune. Epidemics may be restricted to one locale (an outbreak), more general (an epidemic), or even global (pandemic).

Bird Flu: An emerging type of virus infecting humans is the avian influenza virus, or bird flu. Several cases of human infection with bird flu viruses have occurred since 1997, mostly in Asia. No human infections with avian influenza A virus have been identified in the United States. The death rate for these reported cases has been about 50% in infected humans and 100% in birds. This virus is mainly transmitted to humans through direct contact with live or dead poultry; however, it is thought that a few cases of human-to-human spread have occurred.

RISK FACTORS

Current Health Condition: Those individuals who are at high risk and are most susceptible to infection by influenza viruses include those with chronic lung diseases such as asthma, emphysema (lung disease), chronic (long-term) bronchitis (inflammation of the bronchial tubes), bronchiectasis (chronic opening of bronchial tubes), tuberculosis (an infection of the lungs), and cystic fibrosis (scar tissue formation in the lungs). Heart conditions such as coronary heart disease (which includes high blood pressure, high cholesterol, and heart attack), chronic kidney disease, diabetes, severe anemia (decrease in red blood cells that carry oxygen), and diseases that depress immunity, such as cancer, HIV, and AIDS, are risk factors for infection with an influenza virus. Drugs such as chemotherapy and steroids lower immune function and can increase susceptibility to developing the flu.

Social Exposure: Individuals exposed to large volumes of people during the day are also exposed to many viruses, including influenza. Children attending school or playing with their peers are at increased risk of influenza infection and transmission. Individuals working for the public and for large businesses with many workers are at an increased risk. Traveling in airplanes or buses also increases the risk of exposure to influenza viruses.

Age: Children and the elderly are especially susceptible to the flu. Children's immune systems have not adjusted to as many viruses as have those of adults, and their bodies are still developing resistance to most microorganisms. Children may not be as careful about cleanliness, such as handwashing, and they also tend to spend an increased amount of time with other children, making it easy for viruses to be transmitted from person to person. Individuals residing in nursing homes or long-term care facilities are also at high risk of contracting influenza due to increased chances of exposure. Elderly individuals are at an increased risk for influenza infection due to a decrease in immunity seen in these individuals usually caused by chronic (long-term) health conditions such as heart, lung, and kidney diseases.

Flu Season: Both children and adults seem to be most susceptible to the flu in the winter months. In cold months when the air is very dry, people turn on their heating systems, drying the air even more. The dry air tends to dry out the mucous membranes in the nose and throat, the first line of defense against the viruses, allowing the viruses to attack the tissue in the nose and throat. Flu season in the United States starts to peak in November and continues to peak through April.

Other Risk Factors Affecting Immunity: Stress can lower the resistance to infection by depressing the immune system. Stress during premenstrual syndrome or menopause may increase the chances of developing the flu. Low vitamin and mineral levels, such as vitamins A, C, E, and the B vitamins as well as selenium and zinc, may decrease immunity and increase the chances of getting the flu. Very-low-fat diets also appear to lower the immune system. Sleep helps the body recharge. Proper sleep (eight hours of uninterrupted sleep for an adult) can help keep the body's immune system healthy, helping it to fight off the flu. Bad hygiene, such as not washing the hands before they are placed near the mouth or nose, can contribute to influenza infection and transmission.

CAUSES

Influenza Virus: Influenza is an infection caused by the influenza virus. There are three major types of influenza viruses that cause the flu: types A, B, and C. These types are further divided into virus subtypes and then into strains. There are limitless numbers of strains for the influenza viruses that infect humans because the influenza virus can evolve and change to escape the immune system's recognition of the virus. When the influenza virus is no longer recognized by the body's immunity, the virus can reinfect the individual.

Type A viruses most commonly affect adults and are the most severe, while type B viruses typically affect children and may also be severe. Type C causes either a very mild illness (usually in children)

or no symptoms at all. It does not cause epidemics and does not have the severe public health impact that influenza types A and B do. The bird flu is a type of A virus.

Every 10 years or so, an influenza virus strain appears that is dramatically different from the other members of its family. When this major change occurs, a pandemic (worldwide epidemic) can occur. Very few people have immune systems that are prepared to deal with this radically new virus, so most of the public is very susceptible to becoming ill.

SIGNS AND SYMPTOMS

Adults: Mild cases of the flu present with symptoms very similar to the common cold (sneezing, nasal drainage, stuffy nose, sore throat, and low fever). Symptoms usually appear suddenly and may include fevers of 101° F or above, cough, muscle aches and pains, headache, sore throat, chills and sweats, loss of appetite, fatigue (tiredness), and malaise (general bad feeling). The fever and body aches can last three to five days, and the cough and lack of energy may last for two weeks or more. Most adults recover from the flu within one or two weeks, but others, especially the elderly and those with compromised immune systems (such as HIV/AIDS or cancer patients), may feel weak and debilitated for several weeks after the infection has gone.

Children: Flu symptoms in school-age children and adolescents are similar to those in adults. However, children may experience vomiting and diarrhea with the flu, which are rare in adults. Influenza infection in preschool children and infants is difficult to diagnose since its symptoms are so similar to infections caused by other viruses.

DIAGNOSIS

Physical Exam: The flu is usually diagnosed using the typical symptoms, which include coldlike symptoms (runny nose, sore throat, or stuffy nose), a fever of 101° F or above, cough, muscle ache and pains, headache, sore throat, chills and sweats, loss of appetite, fatigue (tiredness), and malaise (general bad feeling). Those individuals infected by the influenza virus who are otherwise healthy may not need diagnosis by a doctor unless symptoms persist for more than a few weeks or are severe.

Laboratory Tests: A doctor may do a throat culture, sputum (phlegm from lungs), or blood test to rule out a secondary infection from a bacterium such as *Streptococcus* (strep throat) or pneumonia. The most common method for diagnosing the flu is an antigen detection test, which is done by swabbing the nose and throat, then sending a sample to the laboratory for testing. Results are usually available within 30 minutes. This test can determine if an influenza virus is present and what type of virus it is. The results of these tests are helpful in deciding whether pharmacological (drug) treatment is appropriate.

COMPLICATIONS

If an individual is healthy with a properly functioning immune system, influenza usually is not serious. Although the individual may feel tired and sick, the flu usually goes away within a few days to a few weeks with no lasting effects.

Complications of flu arise when the individual's immune system cannot fight off the viral infection. Complications can include bacterial pneumonia, ear infections, bronchitis (inflammation of the bronchial tubes), sinus infections, dehydration (loss of fluids), and worsening of chronic medical conditions, such as congestive heart failure, asthma, or diabetes. These complications can be long term.

TREATMENT

Healthcare professionals recommend bed rest, adequate liquids, and good nutrition for rapid recovery and to prevent dehydration (fluid loss). Those individuals infected by the influenza virus who are otherwise healthy may not need treatment by a doctor unless symptoms persist for more than a few weeks or are severe. There are effective treatments available that can reduce the duration of the symptoms caused by the flu. Over-the-counter (OTC) medications can be purchased without a prescription and may help relieve symptoms associated with the flu, including body aches and pains, stuffy and/or runny nose, and cough. Many products in pharmacies and other retailers contain these medicines separately or in various combination products. Specific formulations are chosen based upon the patient's symptoms.

Pain Relievers and Fever Reducers: For fever, sore throat, body aches, and headache, acetaminophen (Tylenol) or ibuprofen (Advil, Motrin) may be used OTC. Acetaminophen can cause liver damage, especially if taken chronically, or in doses that exceed four grams daily. Healthcare professionals recommend to carefully follow dosing guidelines when giving acetaminophen to children, as dosing can be confusing. Ibuprofen in prolonged and large doses can cause kidney and liver damage. Also, it is recommended to never give aspirin to children until they reach the age of 18. Aspirin may play a role in causing Reye's syndrome, a rare but potentially fatal illness in children.

Nasal Decongestants: Nasal decongestants are useful medications for nasal symptoms, such as "stuffy" nasal passages, associated with the flu. Nasal decongestants help dilate (open) swollen mucous membranes of the nasal passages so the individual can breathe easier. Nasal decongestants include tablets, sprays, inhalers, and nose drops. Nasal decongestants include the oral decongestant pseudo-ephedrine (Sudafed), nasal sprays oxymetolazone (Afrin) and phenylephrine (Neo-Synephrine), and the nasal inhalers propylhexedrine (Benzedrex) or levmetamfetamine (Vicks Vapor Inhaler). They are safe for most patients, but they do have many side effects and conditions in which they should not be used, including in people with heart disease, high blood pressure, thyroid disease, glaucoma (increased pressure in the eyes), diabetes, seizure disorders, or enlarged prostate or by individuals using a monoamine oxidase inhibitor (type of a rarely prescribed antidepressant). Stinging, burning, sneezing, increased nasal discharge, drying of the nostrils, and altered taste may occur. If these effects continue or become bothersome, inform a doctor. Other side effects include rapid or pounding heartbeat, dizziness, trouble sleeping, shaking of the hands, and tremors. Healthcare professionals recommend not using decongestants while pregnant or breastfeeding. Over time, decongestant nose drops, inhalers, and sprays can actually cause rebound congestion, which means the nasal passages are not able to function normally without using these medications. Prolonged use can also cause chronic inflammation of the mucous membranes. Decongestant nasal drops and sprays are not used for more than three days, which helps to stop the potential of nasal rebound.

There is widespread national abuse of pseudo-ephedrine tablets as a drug to make methamphetamine (crystal meth or meth), an illegal drug. Methamphetamine is a highly addictive, synthetically produced central nervous system stimulant with effects similar to cocaine. Meth is the most prevalent synthetic drug manufactured in the United States and is easily produced in home laboratories using common store-bought chemicals. The ease of manufacturing meth and its highly addictive potential has caused the use of the drug to increase throughout the nation. Its use has reached epidemic levels in many parts of the country. National and state laws have attempted to stem this criminal activity by establishing limits on sales of pseudoephedrine. The pharmacist or pharmacy representative may ask for a name and address in many states to prove that the pseudoephedrine is purchased legitimately as a decongestant. There may also be limits on the how much pseudoephedrine can be purchased in one transaction as well as over a certain time period. Pseudoephedrine products may not be available in all states OTC and may need to be purchased from behind the pharmacy counter. Also, a new oral nasal decongestant formulation (Sudafed PE) is available that decreases the potential for abuse. Sudafed PE contains the nasal decongestant phenylephrine and not pseudoephedrine.

Antihistamines: Antihistamines dry up excess nasal secretions (mucus) and in this way help to temporarily stop a runny nose. But they can also cause side effects such as dry mouth, constipation, and drowsiness as well as confusion and increased risk of falls if administered to elderly patients. Nonsedating antihistamines include fexofenadine (Allegra) and cetirizine (Zyrtec). Antihistamines that cause sedation include diphenhydramine (Benadryl), clemastine (Tavist), chlorpheniramine (Chlor-Trimeton), and brompheniramine (Dimetane).

Cough Syrups: Nonprescription cough syrups containing various combinations of antihistamines, decongestants, and cough suppressants are available OTC for symptomatic relief of cough associated with the flu. Many doctors strongly discourage the use of these combination medications for any child younger than age two, in whom accidental overdoses could be fatal. Coughs associated with the flu usually last less than two to three weeks. If a cough lasts longer than three weeks, a doctor should be seen. If the cough is productive (brings up mucus), the ingredient guaifenesin can help break up the chest congestion (water intake is also important). If the cough is dry and hacking, a cough suppressant (dextromethorphan) can stop the cough.

Lozenges: Sore throat caused by the flu may be self-treated if the pain is minor. Healthcare professionals recommend not self-treating sore throat for more than two days. Lozenges for sore throat contain active ingredients such as the anesthetics benzocaine, menthol, dyclonine, phenol/sodium phenolate, and hexylresorcinol. Phenol/sodium phenolate and hexylresorcinol also have antibacterial properties.

Antiviral Drugs: Antiviral medications, including amantadine (Symmetrel), rimantadine (Flumadine), zanamavir (Relenza, inhaled), and oseltamivir (Tamiflu), have been approved by the United States Food and Drug Administration (FDA) for the treatment and prevention of influenza. When used prophylactically, they are about 70-90% effective in preventing illness in healthy adults. These medications are not used preventatively due to the potential for influenza viral strains to mutate

and become resistant to the drugs. When used as a treatment, it is necessary to begin taking the medication within two days after becoming sick. When used in this manner, these medications can reduce influenza symptoms and may shorten the time an individual is sick by one or two days. They also may make the person less contagious. All of these medications must be prescribed by a doctor and taken for three to five days in a row (five days for oseltamivir and zanamivir). The four antiviral medications are effective against influenza viruses only; they will not help symptoms associated with the common cold or many other unrelated illnesses caused by viruses that circulate in the winter.

All of the antiviral medications may be effective for influenza A viruses. However, only zanamavir (Relenza) and oseltamivir (Tamiflu) are effective for influenza B viruses. These two also can reduce the symptoms associated with the flu, including fever, body aches and pains, and chills. Recent evidence indicates that a high proportion of currently circulating influenza A viruses in the United States have developed resistance to amantadine (Symmetrel) and rimantadine (Flumadine). Antiviral drugs require a prescription.

In November 2006, the FDA required the maker of oseltamivir (Tamiflu) to include a warning that people with the flu, particularly children, may be at increased risk of self-injury and confusion after taking oseltamivir (Tamiflu). The FDA recommends that individuals with the flu who take oseltamivir (Tamiflu) be closely monitored for signs of unusual behavior.

Antiviral medications can cause side effects, including lightheadedness, nausea, vomiting, loss of appetite, and trouble breathing. If symptoms of the flu (such as fever, aches) get worse, individuals should consult with a doctor.

INTEGRATIVE THERAPIES

Unclear or Conflicting Scientific Evidence

Andrographis: Andrographis (*Andrographis paniculata*) has been widely used in Indian (Hindu) folk medicine and the Ayurvedic form of medicine. A combination of andrographis with Siberian ginseng or eleuthero (*Eleutherococcus senticosus*) called Kan Jang has been reported effective as part of a regimen to treat influenza in Asian medical systems. The one clinical trial to date of a standardized andrographis preparation does report a significant reduction in duration and severity of symptoms of the flu as well as a decrease in time off from work. More studies specifically looking at influenza, with clear diagnostic criteria for distinguishing flu from simple upper respiratory tract infection, are needed to confirm this finding. Caution is advised when taking andrographis, as adverse effects including drug interactions are possible. Andrographis should not be used if pregnant or breastfeeding unless otherwise directed by a doctor.

Astragalus: Astragalus (*Astragalus membranaceus*) is often used in Chinese medicine as a part of herbal mixtures to prevent or treat upper respiratory tract infections. Antiviral activity has been reported in laboratory and animal studies and in limited human reports. However, most studies have been small and poorly designed. Due to a lack of well-designed research, no firm conclusions can be drawn. Caution is advised when taking astragalus supplements, as adverse effects including drug interactions are possible. Astragalus should not be used if pregnant or breastfeeding unless otherwise directed by a doctor.

Boneset: Boneset (*Eupatorium perfoliatum*) is native to eastern North America and was used by Native Americans to treat fevers, including dengue fever and malaria. Boneset is used homeopathically, meaning in very dilute amounts. Homeopathic medicine is regulated by the FDA. Homeopathic boneset was found in one study to decrease the symptoms associated with colds and influenza. Homeopathic medicines do not have side effects due to the very small amount of substance, such as boneset, used in their preparation.

Cordyceps: Cordyceps (*Cordyceps sinensis*) is a fungus that naturally grows on the back of the larvae of a moth caterpillar (*Hepialus armoricanus*) found mainly in China, Nepal, and Tibet. Although traditional use of cordyceps includes lung conditions such as bronchitis, there is insufficient evidence from controlled clinical trials for the use of cordyceps for bronchitis. Most studies using cordyceps have found improved symptoms with cordyceps more than the prescription drugs. Caution is advised when taking cordyceps supplements, as adverse effects, including an increase in bleeding and drug interactions, are possible.

Echinacea: Echinacea (*Echinacea angustifolia, Echinacea purpurea, Echinacea pallida*) is one of the most widely used herbal supplements in the world. Echinacea seems to improve the body's natural immune system during colds and flu. However, preliminary studies have mixed results in using echinacea for preventing the common cold in adults. Although there are no human studies on using echinacea for influenza, animal studies support the antiviral effects of echinacea and echinacea does improve the response of the immune system to infection. Caution is advised when taking echinacea supplements, as adverse effects including drug interactions are possible. Echinacea supplements should not be used if pregnant or breastfeeding unless otherwise directed by a doctor.

Elderberry: Elderberry (*Sambucus nigra*) has been reported to have antiviral and antibacterial activity in laboratory studies. Laboratory studies suggest that elderberry may reduce mucus production and possess antiinflammatory and antiviral effects. One study reports that elderberry juice (Sambucol) may improve flulike symptoms, such as fever, fatigue, headache, sore throat, cough and ache, in less than half the time that it normally takes to get over the flu. However, this study was small with design flaws, and it should be noted that the berries must be cooked to prevent nausea or cyanide toxicity. It remains unclear whether there is any benefit from elderberry for the flu. Additional research is needed in this area before a firm conclusion can be reached. Elderberry should not be used in the place of other more proven therapies, and patients are advised to discuss influenza vaccination with their primary healthcare provider.

Guided Imagery: Therapeutic guided imagery may be used to help patients relax and focus on images associated with personal issues they are confronting. Experienced guided imagery practitioners may use an interactive, objective guiding style to encourage patients to find solutions to problems by exploring their existing inner resources. Biofeedback is sometimes used with imagery to enhance meditative relaxation. Interactive guided imagery groups, classes, workshops, and seminars are available as well as books and audiotapes. Preliminary research in children suggests that stress management and relaxation with guided imagery may reduce the duration of symptoms due to upper respiratory tract infections, including colds. Additional research is needed to confirm these results.

Kiwi: Kiwi (*Actinidia deliciosa, Actinidia chinensis*) may be beneficial in lung conditions such as upper respiratory infections (including colds). However, scientific data are lacking. One survey study suggests that kiwi and other fruits high in vitamin C may have a protective effect on lung conditions in children, especially wheezing. However, properly controlled studies are lacking at this time.

Mistletoe: Mistletoe (*Viscum album*) Iscador (preparation of *Viscum album* whole extract) has been reported to improve clinical symptoms and markers of immune function in children with recurrent respiratory disease exposed to the Chernobyl nuclear accident. There is insufficient evidence to recommend for or against mistletoe therapy for recurrent respiratory disease in general. Caution is advised when taking mistletoe supplements, as adverse effects including drug interactions are possible. Mistletoe supplements should not be used if pregnant or breastfeeding unless otherwise directed by a doctor. Mistletoe should not be used in seizure disorders, glaucoma (increased pressure in the eyes), diabetes, and hyperthyroidism (high thyroid hormone).

Moxibustion: Moxibustion is the application of heat to various points on the body. It is widely used traditionally in China for respiratory tract infections, including colds and flu, in children. However, at this time evidence is insufficient. Individuals not trained in moxibustion should not perform this procedure on themselves or others.

Nasal Irrigation: The three forms of nasal irrigation therapies used in clinical trials have been saline lavage, which uses a warm liquid solution of salt water; humidified warm air lavage (in hyperthermia or low body temperature); and large-particle nebulized aerosol therapy, which uses an aerosolized (droplets spread in the air) saline solution. Occasionally, antibiotics are added to the solution. Nasal saline irrigation is still the main treatment for acute rhinitis (runny nose) in infants since excessive usage of decongestant nose drops is contraindicated in early childhood. Studies support the usage of hypertonic saline for nasal irrigation. There is good evidence in support of nasal irrigation for allergic rhinitis and sinusitis. There is promising early evidence for using nasal irrigation in treating common colds, respiratory symptoms from occupational exposure, problems caused by influenza infection, and in postoperative care following sinus or nasal surgeries.

Vitamin E: Daily supplementation with oral vitamin E does not appear to affect the incidence, duration, or severity of pneumonia (lower respiratory tract infections) in elderly nursing home residents or alter patterns of antibiotic use, although there may be a protective effect against colds and influenza (upper respiratory tract infections). Additional research is warranted. Caution is advised when taking vitamin E supplements, as adverse effects, including an increase in bleeding and drug interactions, are possible. Vitamin E supplements should not be used if pregnant or breastfeeding unless otherwise directed by a doctor.

Zinc: Zinc lozenges are advertised as decreasing the symptoms, length, and severity of a cold. However, there are contradictory results regarding the efficacy of zinc formulations in treating duration and severity of common cold symptoms. Although zinc might be beneficial in the treatment of cold symptoms, more studies are needed to clarify which zinc formulations may be most effective, which rhinoviruses are affected by zinc, and if nasal sprays provide a useful alternative application route for zinc treatment. A recent study found no significant differences between zinc nasal spray and placebo. Negative results may be the cause of using doses of zinc that are too low or the presence of compounds like citric or tartaric acid, which may reduce efficacy of zinc.

Fair Negative Scientific Evidence

Echinacea: Initial research suggests that echinacea may not be helpful in children for treatment of upper respiratory tract infections. Additional research is needed in this area.

Traditional or Theoretical Uses Lacking Sufficient Evidence

Garlic: Garlic (*Allium sativum*) supplements may reduce the severity of upper respiratory tract infections, including colds and influenza. However, this has not been demonstrated in well-designed human studies. Garlic does help improve immune function in laboratory studies. Garlic may cause an increase in bleeding in sensitive individuals, including those taking medications for bleeding disorders, such as warfarin (Coumadin).

Goldenseal: Goldenseal (*Hydrastis canadensis*) has become a popular treatment for the common cold and upper respiratory tract infections and is often added to echinacea in commercial herbal cold remedies. Animal and laboratory research suggests that the goldenseal constituent, berberine, has effects against bacteria and inflammation. However, due to the very small amount of berberine in most goldenseal preparations, it is unclear whether goldenseal contains enough berberine to have the same effects or to be effective in influenza treatment. Caution is advised when taking goldenseal, as adverse effects including drug interactions are possible. Goldenseal should not be used if pregnant or breastfeeding unless otherwise directed by a doctor.

Hydrotherapy: Hydrotherapy is broadly defined as the external application of water in any form or temperature (hot, cold, steam, liquid, ice) for healing purposes. It may include immersion in a bath or body of water (such as the ocean or a pool), use of water jets, douches, application of wet towels to the skin, or water birth. These approaches have been used for the relief of various diseases and injuries or for general well being. There is preliminary evidence that daily showers with warm water followed by cold water, or cold water alone, may reduce the duration and frequency of common cold and influenza symptoms. Additional research is needed in this area before a clear conclusion can be drawn.

Peppermint: Peppermint (*Mentha piperita*) is a flowering plant that grows throughout Europe and North America. Peppermint is widely cultivated for its fragrant oil. Peppermint oil has been used historically for numerous health conditions, including common cold symptoms, viruses, cramps, headache, indigestion, joint pain, and nausea. Menthol, a constituent of peppermint oil, is sometimes included in inhaled preparations for nasal congestion, including "rubs" that are applied to the skin and inhaled. High-quality research is lacking in this area. Essential oils are not intended for internal use.

Slippery Elm: Slippery elm (*Ulmus fulva*) is commonly used to treat sore throats and is most typically taken as a lozenge. While anecdotally reported to be effective for sore throat and respiratory disorders such as bronchitis, supporting evidence is largely based on traditional evidence and the fact that the mucilages contained in the herb appear to possess soothing properties. Scientific evidence is necessary in this area before a clear conclusion can be drawn. Slipper elm throat lozenges are reported as safe in recommended dosages.

Vitamin C (Ascorbic Acid): Vitamin C, or ascorbic acid, is a water-soluble vitamin that is necessary for the body to form collagen in bones, cartilage, muscle, and blood vessels and additionally aids in the absorption of iron. Dietary sources of vitamin C include fruits and vegetables, particularly citrus fruits such as oranges. Scientific studies generally suggest that vitamin C does not prevent the onset of cold symptoms. However, in a subset of studies in people living in extreme circumstances (including soldiers, skiers, and marathon runners), significant reductions in the risk of developing colds by approximately 50% have been reported. This area merits additional study. Large doses of vitamin C may cause gastrointestinal upset, including diarrhea and vaginal yeast infections in sensitive women.

PREVENTION

Vaccination: One of the best ways to prevent the flu is to get a flu vaccination each year. There are two types of vaccines, including an injection (flu shot) and a nasal spray vaccine. The flu shot is an inactivated vaccine (containing killed virus) that is given with a needle. The flu shot is approved for use in people six months of age and older, including healthy people and people with chronic medical conditions such as diabetes, asthma, and heart disease. Target populations for the flu shot include children aged six month to five years; adults who are in close contact with children aged 6 months to five years, such as teachers and daycare workers; people 50 years of age and older; healthcare workers; all caregivers of high-risk people, such as those with HIV/AIDS or cancer; people with chronic health conditions such as asthma; and pregnant women. The best period to receive any of the influenza vaccines is soon after the vaccine becomes available in the fall of each year. Flu shots are given yearly to protect individuals against the strain of influenza prevalent for a particular year. The nasal spray flu vaccine is a vaccine made with live, weakened flu viruses that do not cause the flu (sometimes called live attenuated influenza vaccine or LAIV). The nasal flu vaccine is approved for use in healthy people five to 49 years of age who are not pregnant. Flu Mist is the first nasal spray vaccine for influenza and has been approved by the FDA for healthy people ages five to 49 years of age. The live virus is frozen and must remain that way until use. Healthcare professionals recommend thawing in a refrigerator. It should not be refrozen after thawing because of decreased vaccine potency. If the nasal vaccine is not available, the injection can be used where available. A prescription is needed for the influenza vaccine (both injection and nasal forms) and is available from a doctor or a "flu" clinic in the local area.

Healthcare professionals recommend that doctors, nurses, and other healthcare providers of high-risk persons should be immunized against the flu to protect themselves and high-risk patients. People who have close contact to infants and children, such as teachers and daycare workers, also should be immunized. Healthcare professionals recommend that some individuals should not be vaccinated. They include people who have a severe allergy to chicken eggs, people who have had a severe reaction to an influenza vaccination in the past, people who developed Guillain-Barré syndrome (a disorder where the immune system attacks the nervous system) within six weeks of getting an influenza vaccine previously, children less than six months of age (influenza vaccine is not approved for use in this age group), and people who have a moderate or severe illness with a fever should wait to get vaccinated until their symptoms lessen.

Cleanliness: Clean the hands thoroughly and often to prevent transmission of the influenza virus.

Carrying a bottle of alcohol-based hand rub containing at least 60% alcohol for times when soap and water are not available is a good idea. These gels kill most germs and are safe for older children to use themselves. Many healthcare professionals recommend not overusing antibacterial soaps and cleansers. The skin contains natural bacteria that can be harmed with repeated use of soaps. Keeping the kitchen and bathroom countertops clean, especially when someone in the family has the flu, is important. Wash children's toys before and after play when a cold is present in the house. Sneezing and coughing into tissues keeps the viruses from spreading. Used tissues should be discarded right away. A face mask can be worn to protect the individual from the influenza virus and to keep an infected person from transmitting the virus.

Avoiding Prolonged Contact: Healthcare professionals recommend to avoid close, prolonged contact with anyone who has the flu.

Careful Travel: Traveling to Southeast Asia or to any region with bird flu outbreaks puts an individual at risk. Healthcare professionals recommend to avoid domesticated birds such as pigeons, avoid open-air markets, wash the hands, watch children carefully, and stay clear of raw eggs.

IRRITABLE BOWEL SYNDROME (IBS)

BACKGROUND

Irritable bowel syndrome (IBS) may be referred to as spastic colon, mucous colitis, spastic colitis, nervous stomach, or irritable colon. IBS is a functional bowel disorder, a condition in which the bowel appears normal but does not function normally. IBS is fairly common and makes up 20-50% of visits to gastroenterologists (doctors who diagnose and treat digestive problems). Lower abdominal pain, bloating associated with alteration of bowel habits (constipation and/or diarrhea), and abdominal discomfort relieved with defecation are the most frequent symptoms. The colon, which is about five feet long, connects the small intestine to the rectum and anus. The major function of the colon is to absorb water, nutrients, and salts from the partially digested food that enters from the small intestine. Colon motility (the contraction of the colon muscles and the movement of its contents) is controlled by nerves, hormones, and the colon muscles. These contractions move the contents inside the colon toward the rectum. During this passage, water and nutrients are absorbed into the body, and what is left over is stool. A few times each day contractions push the stool down the colon, resulting in a bowel movement. However, if the muscles of the colon, sphincters, and pelvis do not contract in the right way (as in IBS), the contents inside the colon do not move correctly, resulting in abdominal pain, cramps, constipation, a sense of incomplete stool movement, or diarrhea.

Most people can control their symptoms with diet, stress management, lifestyle modification, and prescribed medications. For some people, however, IBS can be disabling. They may be unable to work, attend social events, or even travel short distances due to urgency to defecate (pass stool) and pain in the colon. IBS commonly starts between the ages of 20-30 and is twice as common in women as in men. The frequency of the condition in the general population is estimated to be somewhere between 10-20%. Up to 70% of people suffering from IBS are not receiving medical care for their symptoms. IBS tends to occur with other pain disorders, such as fibromyalgia (49% of patients also have IBS), chronic fatigue syndrome (51%), chronic pelvic pain (50%), and temporomandibular joint dysfunction (64%). IBS may also exist with psychiatric condi-

tions, such as depression, bipolar disorder (manic/depressive disorder), and anxiety.

The syndrome can be divided into four main types, depending on which symptom is reported. Symptoms include abdominal pain, diarrhea, constipation, or diarrhea alternating with constipation. The abdominal pain type is usually described in a patient as either diarrhea predominant (IBS-D), constipation predominant (IBS-C) or IBS with alternating stool pattern (IBS-A). In some individuals, IBS may have a sudden onset and develop after an infectious illness characterized by two or more of the following: fever, vomiting, acute diarrhea, or positive stool culture. This postinfective syndrome has consequently been termed postinfectious IBS (IBS-PI). Chronic functional abdominal pain is quite similar to, but less common than, IBS. Chronic functional abdominal pain can be diagnosed if there is no change in bowel habits (constipation, diarrhea). IBS is diagnosed by its signs and symptoms and by the absence of other diseases such as Crohn's disease, ulcerative colitis, and inflammatory bowel disease. These three diseases are inflammatory bowel conditions, whereas the colon is not inflamed in IBS. IBS does not seem to harm the intestines and does not lead to cancer.

RISK FACTORS AND CAUSES

Although the exact cause of IBS is unknown, contributors to IBS include poor dietary choices, neurotransmitter imbalances, and infection.

Neurotransmitter Imbalance: Up to 60% of individuals with the syndrome have psychological symptoms such as anxiety and depression. Research has reported that serotonin (a neurochemical for mood and intestinal movement) is linked with normal gastrointestinal functioning. Serotonin is a specialized type chemical called a neurotransmitter that delivers messages from one part of the body to another. Ninety-five percent of the serotonin in the body is located in the gastrointestinal tract, and the other 5% is found in the brain. Cells that line the inside of the bowel work as transporters and carry the serotonin out of the gastrointestinal tract. People with IBS, however, have fewer places for serotonin to bind, causing abnormal levels of serotonin to exist in the gastrointestinal tract. As a result, people with IBS experience problems with bowel movement, motility, and sensation. In addition, people with IBS frequently suffer from depression and anxiety, which can worsen symptoms. Similarly, the symptoms associated with IBS may cause a person to feel depressed and anxious.

Infection: IBS may develop after a gastrointestinal infection caused by bacteria (such as *Salmonella* or *Shigella*) or parasites (such as *Giardia*). Infection and treatment with antibiotics can disturb the digestive flora ("good" bacteria that live in the colon) that are necessary to help break down remaining nutrients (from foods) in the colon. These disturbances in normal flora may also decrease the immune response, which helps to keep the body healthy, and as a result a patient may be more prone to illness after the antibiotic is stopped.

Age and Gender: Gender plays a clear role, as more than 80% of IBS patients in the United States are women, according to the American College of Gastroenterology. Women with IBS appear to have more symptoms during their menstrual periods, suggesting that an imbalance of reproductive hormones such as estrogen and progesterone may increase symptoms of IBS. Age also seems to be a factor. IBS usually begins during the late teens or early 20s. Metabolism (the breaking down) of female hormones occurs in the intestines and is dependent upon the "good" bacteria for proper function. Disturbances in the "good" bacteria, such as with antibiotic use, may cause the hormones to not be broken down properly, leading to hormonal imbalances.

Diet: An increased sensitivity or intolerance to certain foods may trigger or worsen symptoms of IBS. The digestive system must work hard to break down large meals, meats, or meals eaten too quickly. Fatty foods, artificial sweeteners (sucralose [Splenda] and saccharine [Sweet'N Low]), chemical additives (dyes and preservatives), red meat, dairy products (milk, cheese, sour cream), chocolate, alcohol, and carbonated beverages (sodas) may trigger or aggravate episodes. Gluten contained in wheat and barley is also a common trigger for IBS. IBS may affect the absorption of nutrients, causing many individuals to have less of these nutrients available for use in the body.

Other Illnesses: Sometimes another illness, such as an acute episode of infectious diarrhea (gastroenteritis), may trigger IBS.

SIGNS AND SYMPTOMS

IBS symptoms include abdominal pain and occasional diarrhea, often alternating with constipation; rapid transit of food with frequent bowel movements; a sense of fullness (bloating); abdominal tenderness and swelling; a lack of awareness of the bowel action (the need to "go"); and often headache and anxiety. The pain is usually felt in one of the four corners of the abdomen, especially the lower left corner.

IBS may make bowel activity much more noisy than normal. Bowel noises, such as rumblings and squeaking caused by gases being propelled through the intestines by peristalsis (contraction of muscles in the intestines that move food through it) are called borborygmi. This may be embarrassing to people with the syndrome.

The stools are often ribbonlike or pelletlike and may contain mucus. They may also be large, dry stools which are hard to pass.

Other symptoms may include burping and bad breath.

Diarrhea-Predominant IBS (IBS-D): Symptoms associated with IBS-D include more than three bowel movements per day, loose watery stools, and urgency.

Pain-Predominant IBS: Symptoms associated with pain-predominant IBS include abdominal pain, cramping or aching that is relieved by a bowel movement or flatulence (gas), and cramping or aching that is relieved by a bowel movement or gas.

Bloating-Predominant IBS: Symptoms associated with bloating-predominant IBS include feeling full or bloated and excessive gas.

Predominant Rectal Dissatisfaction: Predominant rectal dissatisfaction is a feeling of incomplete evacuation of the colon contents.

Constipation-Predominant IBS (IBS-C): Symptoms associated with IBS-C include fewer than three bowel movements per week, lumpy hard stools, and straining during bowel movements.

IBS with Alternating Bowel Habit (IBS-A): Symptoms associated with IBS-A includes alternating episodes of diarrhea and constipation. Although the signs and symptoms for IBS may disappear for long periods of time, for most people IBS is a chronic (long-lasting) condition. Red flag symptoms that are not typical of IBS include pain that awakens/interferes with sleep, uncontrollable defecation, diarrhea that awakens/interferes with sleep, blood in the stool (visible or occult), weight loss, fever, and abnormal physical examination. People may experience symptoms from more than one of these categories, or their classification of IBS may change over time.

DIAGNOSIS

Medical History: To diagnosis IBS, a doctor must first rule out all other disease possibilities. Typically, the diagnosis begins with a medical history, including questions about the duration, severity, and characteristics of symptoms. The physician will ask about diet, stress, any medications currently being taken, and changes in bowel function. Most people with IBS have mild symptoms. Talking about bowel movements is not an easy subject for some to discuss, but it is very important to tell a doctor about symptoms.

Laboratory Tests: Laboratory tests, including complete blood count, food allergy tests, thyroid function, blood sugar levels, erythrocyte sedimentation rate, liver and kidney function tests, and fecal examination, may be performed to rule out other potential causes. The thyroid, adrenal glands, and pancreas are examined for disease. Depending on symptoms, additional testing may include a lactose tolerance test and a check for the presence of blood, bacteria, and parasites in feces. Celiac disease (nontropical sprue) is sensitivity to wheat protein that also may cause symptoms similar to those of IBS. Blood tests may help rule out that disorder.

Sigmoidoscopy or Colonoscopy: An examination of the rectum and lower (sigmoid) colon is called a sigmoidoscopy. An examination of the rectum and entire colon is called a colonoscopy. The individual will have a liquid dinner the night before a colonoscopy or sigmoidoscopy. A liquid diet means fat-free bouillon or broth, gelatin, strained fruit juice, water, plain coffee, plain tea, or diet soft drinks. Whole bowel irrigation with large quantities of fluid (usually one gallon) is performed using a solution of polyethylene glycol and electrolytes (GoLYTELY). Then, an enema (Fleet's Enema) is used early the next morning to ensure all contents are out of the colon. An enema an hour before the test may also be necessary. During a sigmoidoscopy, a long, flexible tube with a light on the end (called a sigmoidoscope) is used to view the rectum and lower colon. The patient may be lightly sedated before the exam (usually midazolam [Versed]) and can even watch the procedure on a screen. The procedure may cause abdominal pressure and a mild sensation of wanting to have a bowel movement. Air injected into the colon can cause cramping and gas.

During a colonoscopy, a flexible tube with a light on the end (called a colonoscope) is used to view the entire colon. This tube is longer than a sigmoidoscope. The patient lies on his or her side sedated, and a tube is inserted through the anus and rectum into the colon. If an abnormality is seen, the doctor can use the colonoscope to remove a small piece of tissue for examination (biopsy). Gas and bloating are common side effects with a colonoscopy. The individual would not be able to drive home alone after sedation.

Computed Tomography (CT) Scan: A CT scan uses x-rays to take many pictures of the body that are then combined by a computer to give a detailed picture. A CT scan can often show whether the cancer has spread to the liver, lungs, or other organs. CT scans can also be used to help guide a biopsy needle into a tumor. A new way to use a CT scan is to do a "virtual colonoscopy." After stool is cleaned from the colon and the colon is filled with air, a computer can put together a picture of the inside of the colon. This method requires the same preparation as for a colonoscopy, and there is some discomfort from the bowel being filled with air. If anything abnormal is seen, a follow-up colonoscopy will be needed.

Barium Enema: A barium enema, also called a lower gastrointestinal or gastrointestinal series, is an x-ray study in which liquid barium is inserted into the rectum and colon through the anus. Thorough cleaning of the large intestine is necessary for accurate pictures. Test preparations include a clear liquid diet, drinking a bottle of magnesium citrate (a laxative), and warm water enemas to clear out any stool particles. This test may be done in a hospital or clinic radiology department. The patient lies on the x-ray table and a preliminary x-ray is taken. The patient is then asked to lie on the side while a well-lubricated enema tube is inserted into the rectum. As the enema enters the body, the patient might have the sensation that their stomach is being filled. The barium, a radiopaque (shows up on x-ray) contrast medium, is then allowed to flow into the colon. A small balloon at the tip of the enema tube may be inflated to help keep the barium inside. The flow of the barium is monitored by the health care provider on an x-ray fluoroscope screen (like a TV monitor). Air may be puffed into the colon to distend it and provide better images (often called a "double-contrast" exam). If air is used, the enema tube will be reinserted (if it had been removed; whether it is depends on who does the exam) and a small amount of air will be introduced into the colon and more x-ray pictures are taken.

Lactose Intolerance Tests: Lactase is an enzyme needed to digest sugars found in dairy products. Individuals lacking this enzyme may have problems similar to those caused by IBS, including abdominal pain, gas, and diarrhea. Removing milk and dairy products from the diet for several weeks will rule out lactose intolerance. Also, a hydrogen breath test may be given. If the lactose cannot be digested, bacteria metabolize it and produce the gas hydrogen. This can be detected in the exhaled air. So a presence of hydrogen shows that lactose intolerance exists.

Rome II Criteria: Because there are usually no physical signs to definitively diagnose IBS, diagnosis is often a process of elimination. To help in this process, researchers have developed diagnostic criteria, known as Rome criteria for IBS and other functional gastrointestinal disorders (conditions in which the bowel appears normal but does not function normally). The most important symptoms to have for a diagnosis of IBS are abdominal pain and diarrhea or constipation lasting at least 12 weeks, though they do not have to occur consecutively. Other criteria include a change in the frequency or consistency of the stool, straining, urgency or a feeling that the bowels cannot be emptied completely, mucus in the stool, and bloating or abdominal distension.

The Manning Criteria: The Manning Criteria is another set of criteria established to distinguish organic causes for symptoms from those of IBS. Symptoms more likely to be found in IBS than in organic abdominal disease include pain eased after bowel movement, looser stools at onset of pain, more frequent bowel movements at onset of pain, abdominal distension, mucus per rectum, and a feeling of incomplete emptying.

COMPLICATIONS

Health complications arising from IBS include hemorrhoids (aggravated by diarrhea and/or constipation), depression, weight loss, vitamin and mineral deficiencies, and psychosocial problems such as interference with work, relationships, friends, and family.

TREATMENT

Diet: It is unclear from studies if diet has a great effect on the symptoms of IBS. Nevertheless, patients often associate their symptoms with specific foods (such as salads, fats, and spicy foods), and patients' symptoms improve when dietary changes are made. Dietary fiber is often recommended for patients with IBS. Fiber probably is of benefit to IBS patients with constipation, but it does not reduce abdominal pain and may even cause it. Eating foods high in pectin (such as apples) may help decrease diarrhea. A diet of bananas, rice, apple sauce, and dry toast may be helpful. Lactose (milk sugar) intolerance often is blamed for diarrhea-predominant IBS, but it does not cause IBS. Because they are both common, lactose intolerance and IBS may coexist. In this situation, restricting lactose will improve, but not eliminate, the symptoms. Lactose intolerance is easily determined by testing the effect of lactose (hydrogen breath testing) or following a strict lactose-free elimination diet. Intolerance to sugars other than lactose, specifically fructose, sucrose, and sorbitol, may cause symptoms that are similar to IBS or make IBS

worse. However, it has not been proven that these sugars cause IBS.

Constipation Treatments: Constipation is due to the slow transport of intestinal contents through the intestines, primarily the colon. This slow transit may be due to either abnormal function of the muscles of the entire colon or just the muscles of the anus and rectum. There are a number of prescription and over-the-counter (OTC) treatments for constipation available.

Enemas: Saline enemas cause water to be drawn into the colon. Phosphate enemas (Fleet Phospho-soda) stimulate the muscles of the colon. Mineral oil enemas lubricate and soften hard stool. Emollient enemas (Colace Microenema) contain agents that soften the stool. Enemas are particularly useful when there is impaction (hardening of stool in the rectum). Defecation (bowel movement) usually occurs between a few minutes and one hour after the enema is inserted. Enemas are meant for occasional rather than regular use. The frequent use of enemas may cause disturbances of the fluids and electrolytes in the body.

Suppositories: Different types of suppositories have different mechanisms of action. Bisacodyl (Dulcolax) is an example of a stimulant laxative suppository. Glycerin suppositories are believed to have their effect by irritating the rectum. They are commonly used in infants and children with constipation. The insertion of the finger into the rectum where the suppository is placed may itself stimulate a bowel movement.

Laxatives: If an individual with IBS needs a laxative, osmotic agents such as polyethylene glycol (Miralax), sorbitol, and lactulose (Cephulac) are good choices. Side effects may include diarrhea and abdominal discomfort (cramping, bloating).

Diarrhea Treatments: The most widely studied drug for the treatment of diarrhea in IBS is loperamide (Imodium). Loperamide appears to work by slowing down the contractions of the muscles of the small intestine and colon. Loperamide is approximately 30% more effective than a placebo in improving symptoms among patients who have diarrhea as the main symptom of their IBS. It is not clear if loperamide reduces abdominal pain. Dosages of loperamide include an initial dose of 4 mg (two capsules) followed by 2 mg (one capsule) after each unformed stool. The dose must be carefully adjusted and individualized for each patient. Another commonly used antidiarrheal drug is diphenoxylate/atropine (Lomotil). Lomotil is a controlled substance and may cause drug dependence. Other side effects may include dry mouth, headache, constipation, blurred vision, and drowsiness. Diarrhea may cause dehydration (loss of water and electrolytes such as sodium and potassium). The fluid and electrolytes lost during diarrhea need to be replaced quickly, as the body cannot function properly without them. Dehydration is particularly dangerous for infants and children, who may die from it within a matter of days. Although water is extremely important in preventing dehydration, it does not contain electrolytes. To maintain electrolyte levels, sports drinks (Gatorade, Powerade), broth or soups (which contain sodium), or fruit juices may be consumed. Consuming large amounts of water unbalanced by dietary electrolytes may result in a dangerous electrolytic imbalance, which in rare cases may prove fatal (water poisoning or water intoxication).

For children, doctors often recommend a special rehydration solution that contains the electrolytes and nutrients (vitamins and minerals) needed. Examples include Pedialyte, CeraLyte, and InfaLyte. A rehydration fluid sanctioned by the World Health Organization consists of sodium chloride, potassium chloride, glucose, and sodium bicarbonate.

Absorbents: Absorbents are compounds that absorb water. Absorbents that are taken orally bind water in the small intestine and colon and make loose stools less watery. They also may bind toxic chemicals produced by bacteria that cause the small intestine to secrete fluid. The OTC absorbents include attapulgite (clay) and calcium polycarbophil. Attapulgite (Kaopectate, Donnagel, Diasorb, Rhea-ban Maximum Strength) are considered by the U.S. Food and Drug Administration (FDA) as category 1 agents (safe and effective) for the treatment of acute diarrhea. Attapulgite is not absorbed systemically (into the body); therefore, side effects are minimal. Attapulgite may decrease the absorption of nutrients and other drugs. Because of this effect, individuals should not to take any other medications within two to three hours of taking attapulgite. Most experts agree not to use attapulgite preparations for more than two days unless doctor recommended, if blood or mucus is present in the stool, or in infants or children less than three years of age. Calcium polycarbophil (Mitrolan, Equalactin, FiberCon, Fiberall) is a bulk-forming laxative but can be used for diarrhea when the intestines are incapable of absorbing water at normal rates. Polycarbophil absorbs fecal water, forming a gel to aid in the production of formed stools. Like attapulgite, polycarbophil is not absorbed systemically. It can absorb up to 60 times its weight in water. Studies have demonstrated that polycarbophil decreases the frequency of bowel movements and improves stool consistency in patients with acute as well as chronic diarrhea. Side effects include epigastric (abdominal) pain and bloating.

Antimotility Drugs: Antimotility medications are drugs that relax the muscles of the small intestine and/or the colon. Relaxation results in slower flow of intestinal contents. Slower flow allows more time for water to be absorbed from the intestine and colon and reduces the water content of stool. Cramps, due to spasm of the intestinal muscles, also are relieved by the muscular relaxation. The two main antimotility medications are loperamide (Imodium), which is available without a prescription, and diphenoxylate/atropine (Lomotil), which requires a prescription. Loperamide, though related to opiates, does not cause addiction. Diphenoxylate is a man-made medication that at high doses can be addictive because of its opiatelike, euphoric (mood-elevating) effects. Diphenoxylate can cause drowsiness or dizziness, and caution should be used if driving or performing tasks that require alertness and coordination. Antimotility medications should not be used to treat diarrhea caused by inflammatory bowel diseases such as ulcerative colitis or Crohn's disease, *Clostridium difficile* colitis (inflammation of the colon caused by the bacterium *C. difficile*), and intestinal infections by bacteria that invade the intestine (*Escherichia coli, Salmonella, Shigella*). Their use can lead to more serious inflammation and prolong the infections. Antimotility medications are not to be used in children younger than two years of age.

Antispasmodics: The most widely studied drugs for the treatment of abdominal pain are a group of drugs called antispasmodics, which cause muscle relaxation. Muscle relaxation in the abdominal area helps decrease spasms and cramping. Commonly used smooth muscle relaxants are hyoscyamine (Levsin, Levsinex), dicyclomine (Bentyl), and methscopolamine (Pamine). Antispasmodic drugs are also available in combination with sedating or tranquilizing drugs, such as chlordiazepoxide and clidinium (Librax) and mixed salts of belladonna alkaloids and phenobarbital (Donnatal). Antispasmodics are generally taken 30-45 minutes before meals to relieve cramping that follows eating. Side effects may include drowsiness, dry mouth, blurred vision, and inability to urinate. For severe diarrhea, opiates (narcotics, normally used for pain control) may be used, including morphine or codeine. Opiates are habit forming and should be used with care. They may cause drowsiness.

Antidepressant Drugs: Patients with IBS are frequently found to be suffering from depression, but it is unclear if the depression is the cause of IBS, the result of IBS, or unrelated to IBS. Several trials have shown that antidepressants are effective in IBS in relieving abdominal pain and, perhaps, diarrhea. These drugs have been shown to alter the activity of nerves and to have analgesic (pain-relieving) effects as well, which may be why they work in some individuals with IBS. The most commonly used antidepressant drugs in IBS are the tricyclic antidepressants amitriptyline (Elavil) and desipramine (Norpramine). Side effects include constipation, dry mouth, blurred vision, dizziness, inability to urinate, and sedation. Although studies are encouraging, it is not yet clear whether the newer class of antidepressants, the selective serotonin-reuptake inhibitors, such as fluoxetine (Prozac), sertraline (Zoloft), and paroxetine (Paxil), are effective.

Alosetron (Lotronex) is used to treat diarrhea and abdominal discomfort that occurs in women with severe IBS that does not respond to other simpler treatments. Alosetron is a serotonin antagonist (blocks the effects of serotonin). It was approved by the FDA in February 2000 but was withdrawn from the market in November 2000 because of serious, life-threatening gastrointestinal side effects, including severe intestinal inflammation (in 10% of patients). In June 2002, it was approved again by the FDA for marketing but in a restricted manner as part of a drug company–sponsored program for managing the risks associated with treatment. Use of alosetron is allowed only among women with severe IBS-D who have failed to respond to conventional treatment. Cilansetron (Calmactin) is another serotonin antagonist for IBS-D in clinical trials. Recent studies have suggested that rifaximin (Xifaxan), a nonabsorbable antibiotic, may be used as an effective treatment for abdominal bloating and flatulence, giving more credibility to the potential role of bacterial overgrowth in some patients with IBS.

Psychotherapy: Psychotherapy includes cognitive-behavioral therapy (based on modifying everyday thoughts and behaviors, with the aim of positively influencing emotions), psychodynamic or inter-personal psychotherapy (working with an individual and their relationships with others), and relaxation/stress management. Psychotherapy has been used in patients with IBS who are psychologically distressed to the point that their quality of life is being impaired. A few studies have shown that psychological treatments may reduce anxiety and other psychological symptoms in addition to reducing IBS symptoms, particularly pain and diarrhea.

Other Treatments: Using a bench to elevate the feet increases the abdominal pressure on the colon and may help with constipation. Toilet paper may irritate the anus, so using baby wipes may be better. OTC creams or ointments containing hydrocortisone (Cortaid, Preparation H), applied sparingly to the affected area, may reduce inflammation and itching. A protective ointment that contains zinc oxide (Desitin, Balmex) also may help. If the symptoms are worse at night, an antihistamine (such as diphenhydramine [Benadryl]) may be prescribed to reduce itching until topical treatments take effect. With proper treatment, most individuals experience complete relief from anal itching in less than a month.

INTEGRATIVE THERAPIES
Good Scientific Evidence

Hypnotherapy: Hypnotherapy involves the power of suggestion during a deep state of relaxation. Early research suggests hypnotherapy may lower the sensory and motor component of the gastrocolonic (intestinal) responses in patients with IBS. Better studies are necessary to make a conclusion.

Peppermint: Peppermint (*Mentha piperita*) oil may improve IBS symptoms such as spasms (cramping) and bloating. Several clinical trials have used enteric-coated peppermint oil in IBS or recurrent abdominal pain in children. Significant improvements in symptoms of IBS were reported. Anti-spasmodics and serotonin agonists, both commonly used drugs for IBS, did not offer superior improvement rates over peppermint oil. However, more research is needed before a firm conclusion can be made. Caution is advised when taking peppermint supplements, as adverse effects, including heartburn, anal burning, and drug interactions, are possible. Peppermint oil by mouth may increase blood levels of the drugs felodipine (Plendil) and simvastatin (Zocor). Peppermint oil increases levels of cyclosporine in the blood. Peppermint oil used on the skin with 5-fluorouracil may increase the rate of absorption of 5-fluorouracil. Peppermint supplements should not be used if pregnant or breastfeeding unless otherwise directed by a doctor. Do not use peppermint oil in individuals with gallbladder problems.

Probiotics: Probiotics are beneficial bacteria (sometimes referred to as "friendly germs") that help to maintain the health of the intestinal tract and aid in digestion. They also help keep potentially harmful organisms in the gut (harmful bacteria and yeasts) under control. Most probiotics come from food sources, especially cultured milk products. Many varieties and combinations of probiotics have been studied in clinical trials for IBS. Findings frequently report reductions of symptoms, including pain, flatulence, bloating, and stool frequency. There is some evidence of reduced inflammation. The magnitude of benefit seen in most studies is modest. Not all studies, however, show beneficial effects. More studies are needed to determine the best protocols and the level of benefit that can be expected. Commonly used probiotics for IBS include *Lactobacillus acidophilus* and *Saccharomyces boulardii*. Probiotics are generally regarded as safe for human consumption. Probiotics may cause diarrhea in large doses.

Unclear or Conflicting Scientific Evidence

Acupressure, Shiatsu: The practice of applying finger pressure to specific acupoints throughout the body has been used in China for thousands of years, prior to the use of acupuncture. It is proposed that acupressure may reduce muscle pain and tension, improve blood circulation, release endorphins, and release/eliminate toxins. A small study suggests that acupressure may improve gastrointestinal motility. Additional research is necessary before a firm conclusion can be drawn.

Acupuncture: The practice of acupuncture originated in China 5,000 years ago. Acupuncture involves the use of needles to stimulate body function and bring the body into balance. Although limited evidence suggests benefit of acupuncture in IBS may be possible, more studies are needed.

Acustimulation: Acustimulation involves electrical stimulation at various points on the body (as an alternative to needles in acupuncture) and may be applied to reduce certain symptoms. One small study suggests that acustimulation to points on the wrist and below the knee may help patients with IBS to reduce symptoms and pain. However, the design was weak, and more studies are needed to determine benefits in IBS.

Agrimony: Anecdotally, agrimony (*Agrimonia eupatoria*) has been used for many gastrointestinal conditions such as appendicitis, mild diarrhea, stimulation of appetite, and ulcers. Human data are lacking for these uses. Caution is advised when taking agrimony supplements, as adverse effects, including increased bleeding, lowered blood pressure, and drug interactions, are possible. Agrimony supplements should not be used if pregnant or breastfeeding unless otherwise directed by a doctor.

Bacopa: Bacopa (*Bacopa monnieri*) is a commonly used herb in the Ayurvedic (Hindu or Indian) system of medicine. In one study, a combination of bacopa leaf and bael fruit (*Aegle marmelos correa*) was used to treat IBS. The effect of bacopa cannot be isolated in this study, and more high-quality studies using bacopa alone are needed. Caution is advised when taking bacopa supplements, as adverse effects including drug interactions are possible. Bacopa supplements should not be used if pregnant or breastfeeding unless otherwise directed by a doctor.

Chiropractic: Chiropractic is a health care discipline that focuses on the relationship between musculoskeletal structure (primarily the spine) and body function (as coordinated by the nervous system) and how this relationship affects the preservation and restoration of health. Although chiropractic is used anecdotally in colic therapy, there is not enough reliable scientific evidence on the effects of chiropractic techniques in the management of infantile colic.

Clay: There is not enough scientific evidence to recommend the medicinal use of clay by mouth in patients with gastrointestinal disorders. Some clay preparations have been found to be similar to Kaolin and Kaopectate, which are used to treat gastrointestinal disturbances including diarrhea. However, overall there are significant potential risks that accompany the use of clay, including intestinal blockage and injury as well as lead poisoning.

Globe Artichoke: Globe artichoke (*Cynara scolymus*) is a species of thistle that has been used for centuries for various gastrointestinal disorders. Several studies have found that globe artichoke supplements may decrease the symptoms associated with IBS, such as gas, bloating, and cramping. However, there is insufficient evidence from these controlled clinical trials to recommend for or against the use of artichoke in relieving the symptoms of IBS. Caution is advised when taking globe artichoke supplements, as adverse effects, including an increase in bleeding and drug interactions, are possible. Globe artichoke supplements should not be used if pregnant or breastfeeding unless otherwise directed by a doctor.

Reflexology: Reflexology involves the application of manual pressure to specific points or areas of the feet that are believed to correspond to other parts of the body. Preliminary study of reflexology in humans with IBS has not yielded definitive results. Better research is needed in this area.

Relaxation Therapy: There are many types of relaxation therapies, all with the goal of decreasing stress and relaxing the body and mind. Early research in humans suggests that relaxation may aid in the prevention and relief of IBS symptoms. Large, well-designed trials are needed to confirm these results.

Rhubarb: Rhubarb (*Rheum palmatum*) has been used by Chinese herbalists for thousands of years for various health conditions and has been used as a stimulant laxative.

Transcutaneous Electrical Nerve Stimulation (TENS): TENS is a noninvasive technique in which a low-voltage electrical current is delivered through wires from a small power unit to electrodes located on the skin. Wires may be connected to acupuncture needles and also inserted into the skin. There is conflicting evidence from clinical trials on the effectiveness of TENS in postoperative ileus (impairment of bowel movement). Well-designed, large studies are needed before a recommendation can be made.

White Horehound: White horehound (*Marrubium vulgare*) has been found to have antispasmodic properties and has been used traditionally to treat intestinal disorders. However, there are few well-designed studies in this area, and little information is available about the effectiveness of white horehound for this use. Caution is advised when taking white horehound supplements, as adverse effects including drug interactions are possible. White horehound supplements should not be used if pregnant or breastfeeding unless otherwise directed by a doctor.

Yoga: Yoga is an ancient system of relaxation, exercise, and healing with origins in Indian philosophy. Early evidence suggests that yoga may be beneficial in the management of IBS by helping to regulate colon function through exercise. Further research is needed in this area.

Fair Negative Scientific Evidence

Traditional Chinese Medicine (TCM): TCM has been studied for IBS-D, but herbal formulations used in available studies have not led to global symptom improvement. Further studies may be necessary to characterize the role of TCM in the management of IBS.

Turmeric: Preliminary clinical study investigated the effects of *Curcuma xanthorrhiza* on IBS and found that treatment did not show any therapeutic benefit over placebo. More studies are needed to verify these findings.

Strong Negative Scientific Evidence

Trigger Point Therapy: Clinical study demonstrated that trigger point therapy might be effective for treatment of abdominal pain. The results of this study warrant future investigations with more stringent study guidelines.

Traditional or Theoretical Uses Lacking Sufficient Evidence

Chamomile: Chamomile (*Matricaria recutita*) has been used medicinally for thousands of years and is widely used in Europe. Chamomile is used traditionally for numerous gastrointestinal conditions, including IBS, diverticulitis, intestinal cramps, stomach cramps, and intestinal spasms. However, reliable human research is currently unavailable in any of these areas. Additional study is needed. Caution is advised when taking chamomile supplements, as adverse effects, including drowsiness and drug interactions, are possible. Chamomile supplements should not be used if pregnant or breastfeeding unless otherwise directed by a doctor.

Fennel: For centuries, fennel (*Foeniculum vulgare*) has been used as traditional herbal medicine in Europe and China. An emulsion (oil and water mixture) of fennel seed oil and an herbal tea containing fennel has reduced colic in two randomized, double-blind, placebo-controlled trials. Additional studies are warranted in order to more conclusively confirm its benefits. Caution is advised when taking fennel supplements, as adverse effects, including an increase in bleeding and drug interactions, are possible. Fennel supplements should not be used if pregnant or breastfeeding unless otherwise directed by a doctor.

Slippery Elm: Slippery elm (*Ulmus fulva*) is traditionally used to treat inflammatory conditions of the digestive tract such as gastritis, peptic ulcer disease, or enteritis. It may be taken alone or in combination with other herbs. While anecdotally reported to be effective for IBS, supporting evidence is largely based upon traditional evidence and the fact that the mucilages (mucuslike components) contained in the herb appear to possess soothing properties. Scientific evidence is necessary in this area before a clear conclusion can be drawn. Caution is advised when taking slippery elm supplements, as adverse effects including drug interactions are possible. Slippery elm supplements should not be used if pregnant or breastfeeding unless otherwise directed by a doctor.

PREVENTION

Nutritional and lifestyle choices may help prevent or relieve symptoms of IBS.

Diet: Cutting out alcohol, caffeine, dairy products, refined sugars, and fatty foods may significantly reduce symptoms. Many individuals may have food sensitivities (allergies) that aggravate IBS or trigger episodes. Some common food triggers include dairy products, corn, peanuts, citrus, soy, eggs, fish, rye, barley, tomatoes, and wheat products (including gluten). Food allergy testing may be suggested by a doctor. A low-fat diet may also help relieve abdominal pain following meals.

Fiber: Eating sufficient amounts of fiber may alleviate constipation, improve diarrhea, and prevent muscle spasms. Soluble and insoluble fiber can be found in foods such as whole-grain cereals and breads, fruits, vegetables, and legumes (dried peas and beans). Fiber should be introduced gradually into the diet.

Exercise: Regular exercise (especially abdominal muscle exercises) and brisk walking are recommended according to the age and physical condition of the individual. Regular exercise may help reduce stress, decrease constipation, and improve physical performance.

Stress Reduction: Stress may be decreased through relaxation and meditation methods.

CONDITIONS: Kidney/Electrolyte Disorders, Fanconi Syndrome, Focal Segmental Glomerulosclerosis (FSGS), Glomerulonephritis, Kidney Cancer, Kidney Stones

BACKGROUND

Kidney disorders occur when the kidneys do not function normally. The kidneys, a pair of organs located on the left and right side of the abdomen, are an essential component of the urinary tract. The kidneys are responsible for removing toxins, chemicals, and waste products from the blood. These organs also regulate acid concentration and maintain water and electrolyte balance in the body by excreting urine. Nephropathy is a term that is used to describe kidney damage. Many diseases and disorders may lead to nephropathy or even kidney failure. Examples of kidney disorders include Fanconi syndrome, glomerulonephritis, focal segmental glomerulosclerosis, kidney cancer, kidney stones, and nephrotoxicity. These disorders may develop for a wide variety of reasons. Some disorders may be caused by exposure to toxic chemicals or medications, while others may be inherited. Treatment and prognosis vary depending on the type and severity of the kidney disorder. Most patients are able to recover completely if they are diagnosed and treated in the early stages of the disease. However, if left untreated, many disorders may lead to kidney failure, which is a fatal condition, unless the patient receives a kidney transplant.

COMMON TYPES AND CAUSES

Fanconi Syndrome: Fanconi syndrome occurs when the tubes in the kidneys do not work properly. Normally, the kidneys filter out waste products in the blood and regulate the amount of salt and other electrolytes in the body. They also reabsorb important molecules, including glucose, amino acids, small proteins, water, calcium, potassium, magnesium, bicarbonate, and phosphate. Patients with Fanconi syndrome are unable to reabsorb these molecules. As a result, the blood becomes overly acidic, and patients typically experience excessive thirst, increased urination, bone disease, and stunted growth.

Fanconi syndrome may be caused by inherited disorders. For instance, cystinosis galactosemia, glycogen storage disease, hereditary fructose intolerance, Lowe syndrome, Wilson disease, tyrosinemia, medullary cystic disease, and vitamin D dependency have been shown to cause Fanconi syndrome. In addition, some environmental factors may cause patients to develop Fanconi's syndrome later in life. For instance, exposure to heavy metals (e.g., cadmium, lead, mercury, platinum, or uranium), certain drugs (e.g., gentamicin), other substances (e.g., Lysol, paraquat, toluene, and lysine supplements), and kidney transplantation may cause Fanconi syndrome.

Glomerulonephritis: Glomerulonephritis is a kidney disease that occurs when the kidneys are unable to properly remove waste and excess fluids from the body. If the condition develops suddenly over a short amount of time it is considered acute. If glomerulonephritis develops gradually over a longer period of time, it is considered chronic. Sometimes glomerulonephritis occurs by itself. In some cases, the condition may be caused by other illnesses, such as an autoimmune disease called lupus, a lung and kidney disease called Goodpasture's syndrome, diabetes, or immunoglobulin A (IgA) nephropathy. IgA nephropathy occurs when the protein IgA builds up inside the kidneys. Glomerulonephritis may also develop with diseases that cause inflamed blood vessels (vasculitis). Examples of vasculitis disorders that may cause glomerulonephritis include polyarteritis and Wegener's granulomatosis. Glomerulonephritis may also develop after a bacterial or viral infection, such as streptococcus, human immunodeficiency virus, hepatitis B, or hepatitis C.

Focal Segmental Glomerulosclerosis (FSGS): FSGS is a type of glomerular disease (disease that affects the glomeruli) that can cause permanent kidney disease in children and adults. It affects kidney function by attacking the glomeruli, the tiny structures inside the kidneys where blood is filtered. The term glomerulosclerosis is used to describe the scarring or hardening of the tiny blood vessels inside the kidneys. Consequently, protein and sometimes red blood cells leak into the urine. The most common sign of FSGS is nephrotic syndrome, which is characterized by fluid in the body tissues that causes swelling (edema), excess protein in the urine (proteinuria), hypoalbuminemia (abnormally low levels of albumin, which is normally the most plentiful protein in the blood), and high cholesterol. The cause of FSGS is usually unknown. However, some cases may be inherited.

Kidney Cancer: The kidneys may develop cancer. The most common type of kidney cancer in adults is called renal cell carcinoma, which starts inside the cells that line tubes in the kidneys. The most common type of kidney cancer in children is called

Wilms' tumor. The exact cause of kidney cancer remains unknown. However, researchers believe that several factors, including smoking, obesity, high blood pressure, exposure to environmental toxins (e.g., asbestos), and exposure to radiation may increase a patient's risk of developing kidney cancer. In addition, patients who are undergoing dialysis or who have a history of von Hippel-Lindau disease or bladder cancer have an increased risk of developing kidney cancer. If diagnosed and treated quickly, most patients experience a full recovery. However, if left untreated, kidney cancer may spread to other parts of the body.

Kidney Stones (Renal Calculi): Kidney stones (also called renal calculi, urinary calculi, urolithiasis, or nephrolithiasis) usually develop when the urine becomes too concentrated. As a result, minerals and other substances in the urine form hard crystals on the inner surfaces of the kidneys. Over time, these crystals may combine to form a small, hard mass, or stone. There are four different types of kidney stones: calcium stones (also called calcium oxalate stones), struvite stones, uric acid stones, and cystine stones. Calcium stones are the most common type of kidney stones, accounting for 80% of cases. Calcium stones develop when there are high levels of calcium (hypercalcemia) and oxalate in the blood. Patients who consume excessive amounts of vitamin D or have overactive thyroids may have high levels of calcium in the blood. Vitamin D is found in many foods, including fish, eggs, fortified milk, and cod liver oil. The sun also helps the body produce vitamin D. Patients who consume large amounts of oxalic acid or undergo intestinal bypass surgery may have high levels of oxalate in the blood. Oxalic acid is found in some plants, such as spinach, alfalfa, angelica, black haw bark, and rhubarb. Struvite stones are usually caused by chronic urinary tract infections. The bacteria that cause these infections release enzymes that increase the amount of ammonia in the urine. This excess ammonia may form large, sharp stones that can potentially damage the kidneys. Uric acid stones form when there is excess uric acid in the urine. Uric acid is a waste product that is formed when the body breaks down proteins. These stones are usually caused by a cancer treatment called chemotherapy. It may also develop in patients who eat high-protein diets. Some patients are genetically predisposed to develop uric acid stones. Cystine stones develop in patients who have an inherited disorder called cystinuria. This disorder causes the kidneys to release too many amino acids, which then form stones.

Nephrotoxicity: Nephrotoxicity is a term used to describe toxic damage in the kidneys. When the kidneys become damaged, they are unable to remove excess fluid and waste from the blood. As a result, the electrolytes in the blood, including potassium and magnesium, will build up to toxic levels. When there are high levels of potassium in the blood, the condition is called hyperkalemia. Certain medications, such as cyclosporine (Neoral, Sandimmune), tenofovir (Viread), and gentamicin (Garamycin), may have a poisonous effect on the kidneys. This may occur if patients take doses that are too high. Patients with kidney disease have an increased risk of developing nephrotoxicity because their kidneys are already weakened.

Signs and Symptoms

Fanconi Syndrome: Symptoms of Fanconi syndrome typically include increased urination (diuresis), excessive thirst, dehydration, constipation, anorexia nervosa, and vomiting. Patients usually have high levels of sugar, phosphate (hypophosphatemia), calcium, uric acid, amino acids, and protein in the urine. High levels of chloride and low levels of phosphate and calcium in the blood are also common. As a result of these electrolyte imbalances, patients may develop bone disease.

FSGS: Common symptoms of FSGS include fatigue, nausea, headache, foamy urine, weight gain, and poor appetite. Patients with FSGS typically develop nephrotic syndrome, which is characterized by fluid retention that causes swelling (edema), foamy urine (caused by high levels of protein in the urine, also called proteinuria), abnormally low levels of albumin in the blood (hypoalbuminemia), and high cholesterol (hyperlipidemia). Edema generally develops over a few weeks, but initial symptoms may appear suddenly in some patients, with weight gain of 15 to 20 or more pounds. High blood pressure is common among most patients. It is especially common among African-American men with kidney insufficiency because this population is genetically predisposed to develop high blood pressure. Fluid in the lung cavity (pleural effusions) and fluid in the abdomen (ascites) may occur. In rare cases, fluid may build up in the sac that surrounds the heart, a condition called pericardial effusion.

Glomerulonephritis: In general, symptoms of glomerulonephritis may include dark-colored urine, foamy urine (from excess protein in the urine), high blood pressure, fluid retention that causes swelling (edema), fatigue, and less frequent urination.

Kidney Cancer: Most patients with kidney cancer do not experience any symptoms during the early stages of the disease. In the later stages, the most common symptom is blood in the urine (called hematuria). Other symptoms may include back pain (just below the ribs), weight loss, fatigue, and occasional fever.

Kidney Stones: If the kidney stone is small, patients do not experience any symptoms of the condition. The stone may pass in the urine without any pain. However, if the stone is large enough to block the tubes inside the kidney, patients may experience intense pains that come and go. Pain may last anywhere from five to 15 minutes at a time. The pain usually begins in the lower back. As the stone moves from the kidney toward the bladder, the patients may feel pain near the abdomen, groin, or genitals. Additional symptoms may include blood in the urine, cloudy or foul-smelling urine, nausea, vomiting, and constant urge to urinate. In some patients, the kidney stone may cause an infection. Symptoms of an infection include fever and chills.

Nephrotoxicity: Symptoms include increased urination, dark urine, blood in the urine, and frequent urge to urinate.

COMPLICATIONS

Bone Disease: Fanconi syndrome may lead to rickets in children and osteomalacia in adults. Both of these conditions cause the bones to become softer and less dense than normal. Rickets may lead to bone deformities, stunted growth, and difficulty walking in children. Osteomalacia (rickets in adults) may cause severe bone pain and spontaneous bone fractures. Unlike rickets, which is caused by poor nutrition, these conditions cannot be reversed with vitamin D supplementation.

High Blood Pressure: Some patients with kidney disorders, such as glomerulonephritis, may develop high blood pressure. If the kidneys do not filter the blood properly, the extra fluid and waste in the blood vessels may cause high blood pressure. Having high blood pressure may worsen symptoms of kidney disease. This is because high blood pressure damages the blood vessels throughout the body, including the kidneys.

Kidney Failure: Patients with kidney disease, including FSGS, glomerulonephritis, kidney cancer, and nephrotoxicity, may develop kidney failure. When this happens the kidneys are damaged beyond repair. Kidney failure is fatal unless treated with a kidney transplant. Symptoms may include altered mental status and advanced uremia (buildup of waste

in the blood due to severe kidney disease). Symptoms of uremia include nausea, vomiting, bleeding, and seizures.

DIAGNOSIS

Blood Urea Nitrogen Test: The blood urea nitrogen test measures the amount of nitrogenous waste in the patient's blood. If a patient has high levels of waste products in the blood, it indicates that the kidneys are not able to filter the blood. Healthy individuals usually have seven to 20 milligrams of waste per deciliter of blood. Elevated levels indicate kidney disease.

Creatine: A creatine test is used to measure the amount of creatine in a patient's blood or urine. This helps determine how well the kidneys are able to filter small molecules, such as creatine, out of the blood. Healthy individuals usually have about 0.8-1.4 milligrams of creatine per deciliter of blood. Elevated levels indicate kidney disease. A healthcare provider then uses the creatine test results, along with the patient's age, weight, and gender, to determine his/her estimated glomerular filtration rate. This rate represents how well the kidneys are able to filter the blood over a period of time. Healthy men typically have an estimated glomerular filtration rate of 97-137 milliliters per minute, while females have rates of about 88-128 milliliters per minute. Lower-than-normal results indicate kidney disease.

Imaging Studies: Imaging studies, such as a computerized tomography scan or magnetic resonance imaging scan, may be performed if cancer or kidney stones are suspected. These tests take pictures of the kidneys, allowing healthcare providers to detect tumors or kidney stones.

Kidney Biopsy: A kidney biopsy is the most definitive diagnostic test for most kidney disorders, including kidney cancer. During the procedure, which is performed at a hospital, a needle is inserted into the kidney and a small tissue sample is removed from either the kidney or a tumor on the kidney. Patients may be awake and receive medication to numb the area near the kidney, or patients may receive general anesthesia so that they are asleep during the procedure. The tissue is then analyzed in a laboratory. Kidney damage is indicated if scar tissue is revealed in the kidney tissue. If cancerous cells are present in the tumor tissue, cancer is diagnosed. Patients may have to stay overnight at the hospital. Most patients experience soreness near the biopsy site. Patients should tell their healthcare providers if there is blood in their urine more than 24 hours after the test, if they are unable to urinate, if they have a fever, if they experience increased pain at biopsy site, or if they feel dizzy. In rare cases, an infection may develop.

Urinalysis (Analysis of the Urine): A urinalysis, also called a urine sample test, is used to measure the levels of protein in the urine. Elevated levels of protein in the urine (with or without small amounts of blood) suggest kidney disease.

TREATMENT

Hemodialysis: In cases of severe kidney damage or kidney failure, hemodialysis may be administered. Dialysis is a method of removing toxic substances and waste from the blood because dysfunctional kidneys are unable to perform this function. During the procedure, a hollow tube, called a catheter, is inserted into a patient's vein at the hospital. The blood is then filtered through a dialysis machine to remove waste products from the blood. The filtered blood is then returned to the patient. This procedure typically lasts about three to four hours. In general, patients with kidney failure undergo dialysis about three times a week. Patients who develop nephrotoxicity may also require dialysis in order to remove toxic substances from the body.

Peritoneal Dialysis: Patients who have kidney failure may undergo peritoneal dialysis. This type of dialysis can be performed at home, but it must be done every day. During peritoneal dialysis, a catheter fills the abdomen with a dialysis solution, which removes toxins from the blood. The abdominal walls are lined with a membrane called the peritoneum. This membrane allows extra fluid to pass from the blood and into the dialysis solution. The dialysis solution collects the waste, and then the dialysis solution is drained from the body. The entire process takes about 30-40 minutes per day. Most patients have to repeat this process about four times a day. A type of peritoneal dialysis called continuous ambulatory peritoneal dialysis does not require a machine. Patients are able to go about their normal daily activities while the dialysis solution is in the abdomen. Another type of peritoneal dialysis, called continuous cycling peritoneal dialysis, involves a machine that fills and drains the abdomen, usually while the patient sleeps.

Diuretics: Diuretics, such as furosemide (Lasix) have been used to treat edema, which is associated with many types of kidney disorders, including FSGS and glomerulonephritis. These drugs signal the kidneys to increase urine output. This reduces the amount of fluid in the bloodstream, which subsequently reduces swelling and lowers blood pressure.

Antihypertensives (Angiotensin-Converting Enzyme Inhibitors): Antihypertensives (drugs that lower blood pressure) have been used to treat high blood pressure. When the kidneys do not filter the blood properly, the pressure in the blood vessels may increase, causing high blood pressure. One type of drug for high blood pressure, called an angiotensin-converting enzyme inhibitor, reduces the amount of protein in the urine by reducing the amount of pressure and resistance on blood as it circulates through the body.

Extracorporeal Shock Wave Lithotripsy: If patients with kidney stones are unable to pass their stones by drinking extra fluids, a procedure called extracorporeal shock wave lithotripsy may be performed. This is the most commonly used procedure to remove kidney stones. Sound waves (shock waves) are used to break the stone into smaller pieces. Patients will receive sedatives and/or anesthesia before the procedure. The patient will either be partially submerged in a tub of water or will lie on a soft cushion. Patients wear headphones because the shock waves are loud. High-energy sound waves then pass through the patient's body and break the stone into smaller pieces. The healthcare provider usually uses x-rays or an ultrasound to ensure that the stone breaks down. Treatment usually lasts for about one hour. Side effects of treatment include blood in the urine, bruising on the abdomen or back, bleeding around the kidney or nearby organs, and pain when the stone fragments are passed in the urine.

Transplant: Some patients with kidney disease may develop kidney failure. When this happens, the kidneys are no longer able to function properly. Kidney failure is fatal without a kidney transplant because these organs are vital for daily living. Since individuals can function with just one kidney, only one donated kidney must be transplanted into the patient. After the kidney transplant, patients will need to take drugs called immunosuppressants for the rest of their lives in order to prevent their bodies from attacking the transplanted organs. The most commonly prescribed oral immunosuppressants include tacrolimus (Prograf), mycophenolate mofetil (CellCept), sirolimus (Rapamune), prednisone (Prednisone Intensol), cyclosporine (Neoral, Sandimmune, Gengraf), and azathioprine (Imuran). In general, patients are typically prescribed two to three medications for long-term immunosuppression. Also, since kidney transplant recipients have only one functioning kidney after surgery, patients will need to alter their diets so the kidney is not overworked. For instance, alcohol and caffeine should be avoided because these products contain many toxins and wastes that are difficult for just one kidney to filter from the blood.

Not all kidney failure patients are suitable candidates for kidney transplantation. The transplant must come from a donor whose body tissues are a close biological match to the recipient. The donated kidney may come from a living relative who is a match or from a deceased donor. In order to receive an organ from a deceased donor, patients are added to a national waiting list. Members of the transplant center conduct medical tests and consider the patient's mental and physical health as well as his/her personal support system before adding him/her to the transplant list. There is no way to know how long a patient will wait. Some patients will wait weeks while others may wait years. Some patients die of kidney failure before they are able to receive an organ.

As with any major surgery, serious health risks are associated with the kidney transplantation. Individuals who have weakened immune systems are at risk of developing graft-versus-host disease after surgery. This condition occurs when the transplanted organ attacks the recipient's weakened immune system. Other recipients may experience transplant rejection, which occurs when the body's immune system attacks the donated organ.

Surgery: Patients with kidney cancer typically have their tumors surgically removed, if possible. If the tumor is very large, the kidney may also need to be removed. Individuals are able to live with just one kidney. However, if both kidneys are removed, the patient must receive a kidney transplant.

Radiation Therapy: Radiation therapy may be used along with surgery to treat patients with kidney cancer. During the procedure, the patient's kidney is exposed to high-energy beams, which kill cancerous cells. Patients typically receive treatment five days a week for several weeks. Side effects may include fatigue, skin rash, nausea, and vomiting.

Chemotherapy: Chemotherapy, which involves drugs that kill cancerous cells, is generally not used to treat kidney cancer. This is because chemotherapy has not been shown to be an effective treatment for patients with kidney cancer. Other therapies, such as surgery and immunotherapy, have been shown to be more effective treatments.

Arterial Embolization: Patients with kidney cancer may undergo a procedure called arterial embolization. A specialized healthcare professional, called a radiologist, injects a chemical into the main blood vessel that leads to the kidney. This substance clogs the blood vessel, which starves the tumor of nutrients. This procedure is typically used when the tumor cannot be surgically removed. Side effects may include temporary nausea, vomiting, or pain.

Cryoablation: A procedure called cryoablation may be performed if a kidney tumor cannot be removed. During the procedure, one or more specialized needles are inserted into the tumor. The needles contain a gas that causes the tumor to become so cold that it freezes. The needles are removed. Then, needles that contain a different kind of gas are inserted into the tumor. These needles warm the tumor. When the tumor is thawed, the process is repeated. The cycle of freezing and thawing the tumor eventually kills the tumor. Patients may experience pain after cryoablation. Rare side effects include infection, bleeding, and damage to the tissues surrounding the tumor.

Immunotherapy: Patients with kidney cancer may also receive immunotherapy, which helps the body's immune system fight against cancerous cells in the body. Patients receive injections with interferon and/or interleukin-2, which are normally produced by the body. Immunotherapy is usually administered in combination with surgery. The duration of treatment varies among patients. Medication may be given daily, weekly, or several times a week. Side effects may include nausea, vomiting, decreased appetite, fatigue, and fever. Some patients may bruise easily after treatment.

INTEGRATIVE THERAPIES

Strong Scientific Evidence

Phosphates, Phosphorus: Phosphorus is a mineral found in many foods, including milk, cheese, dried beans, peas, nuts, and peanut butter. Phosphorus plays an important role in the formation of bones and teeth. Phosphate is the most common form of phosphorus. Phosphate salts (except for calcium phosphate) have been shown to effectively reduce high levels of calcium in the blood, a condition called hypercalcemia. Hypercalcemia may occur as a result of kidney disorders such as Fanconi syndrome. High levels of calcium in the blood may also lead to kidney stones. However, intravenous phosphate may not be recommended as a treatment for hypercalcemia due to concerns about lowering blood pressure, excessively lowering calcium levels, heart attack, tetany, and kidney failure. Sudden low blood pressure, kidney failure, and death have been reported after phosphate infusion. The U.S. Food and Drug Administration has approved the use of phosphates for the treatment of hypophosphatemia in adults. Taking sodium phosphate or potassium phosphate has been shown to effectively prevent and treat most causes of hypophosphatemia. Patients should only take phosphate supplements under the guidance of their healthcare providers. The underlying cause of the hypophosphatemia should be identified and corrected whenever possible.

Avoid if allergic or hypersensitive to any ingredients in phosphorus/phosphate preparations. Use phosphorus/phosphate salts cautiously with kidney or liver disease, heart failure, chest pain (angina), recent heart surgery, hyperphosphatemia (high phosphate blood level), hypocalcemia (low calcium blood level), hypokalemia (low potassium blood level), hypernatremia (high sodium blood level), Addison's disease, intestinal obstruction or ileus, bowel perforation, severe chronic constipation, acute colitis, toxic megacolon, hypomotility syndrome, hypothyroidism, scleroderma, or gastric retention. Avoid sodium phosphate enemas with congenital (present at birth) abnormalities of the intestine. Too much phosphorus may cause serious or life-threatening toxicity.

Vitamin D: Vitamin D is found in many foods, including fish, eggs, fortified milk, and cod liver oil. The sun also helps the body produce vitamin D. Fanconi syndrome is a defect of the proximal tubules of the kidney that is associated with kidney tubular acidosis. Taking vitamin D by mouth has been shown to effectively treat hypophosphatemia associated with Fanconi syndrome.

Avoid if allergic or hypersensitive to vitamin D or any of its components. Vitamin D is generally well tolerated in recommended doses. Doses higher than recommended may cause toxic effects. Individuals with overactive thyroid glands, kidney disease, sarcoidosis, tuberculosis, or histoplasmosis have an increased risk of experiencing toxic effects. Vitamin D is generally considered safe for pregnant women. It may be necessary to give infants vitamin D supplements along with breast milk in order to prevent vitamin D deficiency.

Good Scientific Evidence

Chelation Therapy: During chelation therapy, ethylenediamine tetraacetic acid (EDTA), usually in combination with vitamins, trace elements, and iron supplements, is injected into the vein to treat a variety of diseases. Several studies support the use of EDTA chelation to reduce lead toxicity associated with chronic kidney insufficiency and to slow the progression of the disorder. More studies are needed to confirm these findings, but EDTA chelation can be considered a useful adjunctive therapy for the treatment of chronic kidney insufficiency. It is important to note that all reported trials were conducted by the same investigator.

Avoid with heart disease, liver disease, kidney disease, immune system disorders, bleeding disorders, or drugs that increase the risk of bleeding. Avoid if pregnant or breastfeeding due to potential toxic effects.

Rhubarb: In traditional Chinese medicine, rhubarb is used as an ulcer remedy, and it is considered a bitter, cold, dry herb used to "clear heat" from the liver, stomach, and blood. In laboratory studies, rhubarb has been shown to have positive effects on kidney failure. These studies show promise for human use. In some studies, rhubarb is more effective than captopril, and rhubarb combined with captopril is more effective than either substance alone. Higher quality studies are necessary to confirm this hypothesis.

Avoid if allergic or hypersensitive to rhubarb, its constituents, or related plants from the Polygonaceae family. Avoid using rhubarb for more than two weeks because it may induce tolerance in the colon, melanosis coli, laxative dependence, pathological alterations to the colonic smooth muscles, and substantial loss of electrolytes. Avoid with atony, colitis, Crohn's disease, dehydration with electrolyte depletion, diarrhea, hemorrhoids, insufficient liver function, intestinal obstruction or ileus, irritable bowel syndrome, menstruation, preeclampsia, kidney disorders, ulcerative colitis, or urinary problems. Avoid handling rhubarb leaves, as they may cause contact dermatitis. Avoid rhubarb in children younger than 12 years old. Use cautiously with bleeding disorders, cardiac conditions, or constipation. Use cautiously with a history of kidney stones or thin or brittle bones. Use cautiously if taking antipsychotic drugs, anticoagulants, or oral drugs, herbs, or supplements (including calcium, iron, and zinc) with similar effects. Avoid if pregnant or breastfeeding.

Unclear or Conflicting Scientific Evidence

Acupuncture: Acupuncture is commonly used throughout the world. According to Chinese medicine theory, the human body contains a network of energy pathways through which vital energy, called "chi," circulates. These pathways contain specific "points" that function like gates, allowing chi to flow through the body. Needles are inserted into these points to regulate the flow of chi. Illness and symptoms are thought to be caused by problems in the circulation of chi through the meridians. There has been limited research on acupuncture for the treatment of kidney disorders, such as gouty kidney damage. There is currently not adequate available evidence to recommend for or against acupuncture in these conditions.

Needles must be sterile in order to avoid disease transmission. Avoid with valvular heart disease, infections, bleeding disorders, medical conditions of unknown origin, and neurological disorders. Avoid on areas that have received radiation therapy and during pregnancy. Avoid if taking anticoagulants. Use cautiously with respiratory disease (e.g., asthma or emphysema). Use cautiously in elderly or medically compromised patients, diabetics, or with a history of seizures. Avoid electroacupuncture with arrhythmia (irregular heartbeat) or in patients with pacemakers.

Astragalus: In traditional Chinese medicine, astragalus is commonly found in mixtures with other herbs. Western herbalists began using astragalus in the 1800s as an ingredient in various tonics. Several animal and human studies report that kidney damage from toxins and kidney failure may be improved with the use of astragalus-containing herbal mixtures. Overall, this research has been poorly designed and reported. Astragalus alone has not been well evaluated. Better-quality research is necessary before a conclusion can be drawn.

Avoid if allergic to astragalus, peas, or any related plants. Avoid with a history of Quillaja bark–induced asthma. Avoid if taking aspirin, aspirin products, or herbs or supplements with similar effects. Avoid with inflammation, fever, stroke, transplant, or autoimmune diseases. Stop use two weeks before and immediately after surgery/dental/diagnostic procedures with bleeding risks. Use cautiously with bleeding disorders, diabetes, high blood pressure, lipid disorders, or kidney disorders. Use cautiously if taking blood thinners, blood sugar drugs, diuretics, or herbs and supplements with similar effects. Avoid if pregnant or breastfeeding.

Coenzyme Q10 (CoQ10): CoQ10, which is produced by the human body, is needed for the basic functioning of cells. Early research supports the use of CoQ10 supplements for the treatment of kidney failure. However, more research is needed before a firm conclusion can be made.

Reports on allergic reactions to CoQ10 supplements are lacking. However, there have been reports of rare cases of rash and itching after CoQ10 use. Stop use two weeks before and immediately after surgery/dental/diagnostic procedures that have bleeding risks. Use cautiously with a history of blood clots, diabetes, high blood pressure, heart attack, or stroke. Use cautiously if taking anticoagulants (blood thinners), antiplatelet drugs (e.g., aspirin, warfarin, or clopidogrel), blood pressure drugs, blood sugar drugs, cholesterol drugs, or thyroid drugs. Avoid if pregnant or breastfeeding.

Cordyceps: Cordyceps is a parasitic fungi that has been used as a tonic food in China and Tibet. In traditional Chinese medicine, cordyceps is used to strengthen kidney function. Two studies indicate that cordyceps may improve kidney function in patients with chronic kidney failure. More studies are needed to confirm these findings.

Avoid if allergic or hypersensitive to cordyceps, mold, or fungi. Use cautiously with diabetes, bleeding disorders, or prostate conditions. Use cautiously if taking immunosuppressants, anticoagulants, hormone replacement therapy, or birth control pills. Avoid with myelogenous-type cancers. Avoid if pregnant or breastfeeding.

Creatine: Creatine is an amino acid that is found in the muscles. One study suggests that creatine does not lower homocysteine levels in chronic hemodialysis patients. However, these patients were also taking vitamin B_{12} and folate. Therefore, a firm conclusion cannot be made until further research is performed.

Avoid if allergic or hypersensitive to creatine. Early research suggests that creatine may reduce muscle cramps that are often associated with hemodialysis. However, further studies are needed to confirm this claim. Avoid if taking diuretics (e.g., hydrochlorothiazide or furosemide). Use cautiously with asthma, diabetes, gout, kidney disease, liver disease, muscle problems, stroke, or with a history of these conditions. Avoid dehydration. Avoid if pregnant or breastfeeding.

Danshen: Danshen (*Salvia miltiorrhiza*) is widely used in traditional Chinese medicine, often in combination with other herbs. Although early evidence is promising, it is unknown whether danshen is a safe and effective treatment for kidney disease. Danshen injections may help patients recover kidney function after kidney transplants. Further research is needed to confirm these results.

Avoid if allergic or hypersensitive to danshen. Avoid if taking blood thinners (anticoagulants), digoxin, or hypotensive agents. Avoid with bleeding disorders and low blood pressure and following cerebral ischemia (inadequate blood flow to the brain). Use cautiously if taking sedatives, hypolipidemics (blood pressure–lowering medications), cardiac glycosides, agents metabolized by the liver, nitrate ester, steroidal agents, or some antiinflammatories (such as ibuprofen). Use cautiously with altered immune states, arrhythmia (irregular heartbeat), compromised liver function, or with a history of glaucoma, stroke, or ulcers. Stop use two weeks before and immediately after surgery/dental/diagnostic procedures that have bleeding risks. Use cautiously if driving or operating heavy machinery. Avoid if pregnant or breastfeeding.

Dong Quai: Dong quai (*Angelica sinensis*), also known as Chinese angelica, has been used for thousands of years in traditional Chinese, Korean, and Japanese medicine. It remains one of the most popular plants in Chinese medicine, and it is most commonly used for health conditions in women. There is insufficient evidence to support the use of dong quai as a treatment for kidney diseases, such as glomerulonephritis. Preliminary, poor-quality research of dong quai in combination with other herbs has reported unclear results.

Although dong quai is accepted as being safe as a food additive in the United States and Europe, it remains unknown if it is in larger doses as a medical treatment. There are no reliable long-term studies of side effects available. Avoid if allergic or hypersensitive to *Angelic radix* or members of the Apiaceae/Umbelliferae family (e.g., anise, caraway, carrot, celery, dill, or parsley). Avoid prolonged exposure to sunlight or ultraviolet light. Use cautiously with bleeding disorders, diabetes, glucose intolerance, or hormone-sensitive conditions (e.g., breast cancer, uterine cancer, or ovarian cancer). Use cautiously if taking blood thinners. Do not use immediately before or two weeks after dental or surgical procedures that have bleeding risks. Avoid if pregnant or breastfeeding.

Flaxseed: Flaxseed is a rich source of the essential fatty acid alpha-linolenic acid (omega-6). Alpha-linolenic acid is a building block in the body for omega-3 fatty acids. Flaxseed (not flaxseed oil) may help treat kidney diseases, such as lupus nephritis. However, further research is needed before a firm conclusion can be made.

Flaxseed has been well tolerated in studies for up to four months. Avoid if allergic to flaxseed, flaxseed oil, or other plants of the Linaceae family. Avoid with prostate cancer, breast cancer, uterine cancer, or endometriosis. Avoid ingestion of immature flaxseed pods. Avoid large amounts of flaxseed by mouth. Mix flaxseed with plenty of water or liquid before ingesting. Avoid flaxseed (not flaxseed oil) with a history of esophageal stricture, ileus, gastrointestinal stricture, or bowel obstruction. Avoid with a history of acute or chronic diarrhea, irritable bowel syndrome, diverticulitis, or inflammatory bowel disease. Avoid topical flaxseed in open wounds or abraded skin surfaces. Use cautiously with a history of bleeding disorders, high triglyceride levels, diabetes, mania, seizures, or asthma. Use cautiously if taking blood thinners or nonsteroidal antiinflammatory drugs. Avoid if pregnant or breastfeeding.

Hyssop: Hyssop is a blue-flowered plant of the mint family. It has dark-green, aromatic leaves that have a slightly bitter, minty flavor. A preliminary study using combination therapy with a decoction (a preparation made by boiling a plant in water) of qingre huoxue recipe, which contains less than 10% of giant hyssop herb, may improve kidney function in patients with mid-advanced crescentic nephritis (inflamed kidneys). Higher quality studies using hyssop alone are needed to further evaluate hyssop's effect on nephritis.

Avoid if allergic/hypersensitive to hyssop, any of its constituents, or any related plants in the Lamiaceae family. Use cautiously with diabetes or if taking antivirals or immunosuppressants. Avoid with seizure disorders, fever, high blood pressure, or medications that affect seizure threshold. Avoid in children. Avoid sustained use of hyssop oil (10 to 30 drops daily for adults). Avoid if pregnant or breastfeeding.

L-Carnitine: L-carnitine is an amino acid that is made in the liver and muscles. L-carnitine taken by mouth has been used in patients with hypertriglyceridemia who were receiving continuous ambulatory peritoneal dialysis. However, L-carnitine does not appear to effectively treat hypertriglyceridemia associated with continuous ambulatory peritoneal dialysis. Additional study is needed before a firm recommendation can be made.

Avoid with known allergy or hypersensitivity to carnitine. Use cautiously with peripheral vascular disease, high blood pressure, alcohol-induced liver cirrhosis, and diabetes. Use cautiously in low birth weight infants and individuals on hemodialysis. Use cautiously if taking anticoagulants (blood thinners), beta-blockers, or calcium channel blockers. Avoid if pregnant or breastfeeding.

Omega-3 Fatty Acids: Omega-3 fatty acids are found in fish oil and certain plant/nut oils. Fish oil contains both docosahexaenoic acid and eicosapentaenoic acid. Studies investigating the effect of omega-3 fatty acids on patients with IgA nephropathy have produced conflicting results. Further research is warranted in this area. Additional research is also needed to determine whether or not omega-3 fatty acids can effectively treat nephropathy in general.

Avoid if allergic or hypersensitive to products that contain omega-3 fatty acid, omega-6 fatty acid, or linolenic acid. This includes some fish and nuts.

Avoid during active bleeding. Use cautiously with bleeding disorders, diabetes, low blood pressure, or drugs, herbs, or supplements that treat any such conditions. Use cautiously before surgery. Omega-3 fatty acids are considered safe in pregnancy and breastfeeding when taken in the recommended doses.

Prayer: Prayer can be defined as a "reverent petition," the act of asking for something while aiming to connect with a higher power. Prayer on behalf of the ill or dying has played a prominent role throughout history and across cultures. Metaphysical explanations and beliefs often underlie the practice of prayer. Preliminary research shows positive trends associated with prayer and spirituality in patients with end-stage renal disease who are coping after kidney transplant. Further research is needed before conclusions can be drawn.

Prayer is not recommended as the sole treatment approach for potentially serious medical conditions and should not delay the time it takes to consult with a healthcare professional or receive established therapies. Sometimes religious beliefs come into conflict with standard medical approaches and require an open dialog between patients and caregivers.

Psychotherapy: Psychotherapy is an interactive process between a person and a qualified mental health professional. The patient explores thoughts, feelings, and behaviors to help with problem solving. Although individual and group psychotherapy may decrease depression associated with a kidney transplant, individual therapy may be more effective than group therapy. More research needs to be done in this area.

Psychotherapy cannot always fix mental or emotional conditions. Psychiatric drugs are sometimes needed. In some cases, symptoms may worsen if the proper medication is not taken. Not all therapists are qualified to work with all problems. Use cautiously with serious mental illness or some medical conditions because some forms of psychotherapy may stir up strong emotional feelings and expressions.

Reishi Mushroom: Reishi mushroom (*Ganoderma lucidum*), also known as ling zhi in China, grows wild on decaying logs and tree stumps. Reishi grows in six different colors. The red-colored mushroom is most commonly used and grown in East Asia and North America. One study investigated reishi mushroom for the treatment of proteinuria in patients with kidney disorders. Further research is needed in order to make a firm conclusion.

Avoid if allergic or hypersensitive to reishi mushroom, any of its constituents, or any members of its family. Use cautiously with diabetes, blood disorders (including hemophilia), low blood pressure, or ulcers. Avoid if pregnant or breastfeeding.

Rhubarb: In traditional Chinese medicine, rhubarb is used as an ulcer remedy, and it is considered a bitter, cold, dry herb used to "clear heat" from the liver, stomach, and blood. A preliminary study using a combination therapy with a decoction of qingre huoxue recipe, which contains less than 10% of rhubarb, may improve kidney function in patients with mid-advanced crescentic nephritis (inflamed kidneys). Higher quality studies using rhubarb as a monotherapy are needed to evaluate rhubarb's effect on nephritis.

Avoid if allergic or hypersensitive to rhubarb, its constituents, or related plants from the Polygonaceae family. Avoid using rhubarb for more than two weeks because it may induce tolerance in the colon, melanosis coli, laxative dependence, pathological alterations to the colonic smooth muscles, and substantial loss of electrolytes. Avoid with atony, colitis, Crohn's disease, dehydration with electrolyte depletion, diarrhea, hemorrhoids, insufficient liver function, intestinal obstruction or ileus, irritable bowel syndrome, menstruation, preeclampsia, kidney disorders, ulcerative colitis, and urinary problems. Avoid handling rhubarb leaves, as they may cause contact dermatitis. Avoid rhubarb in children younger than 12 years old. Use cautiously with bleeding disorders, cardiac conditions, constipation, or with a history of kidney stones or thin or brittle bones. Use cautiously if taking antipsychotic drugs, blood thinners, or oral drugs, herbs, or supplements (including calcium, iron, and zinc). Avoid if pregnant or breastfeeding.

Safflower: Safflower oil is ingested as a food or supplement, infused intravenously, or applied topically. There is currently insufficient available evidence to recommend for or against the use of safflower in the treatment of type II nephritic syndrome.

Avoid if allergic or hypersensitive to safflower (*Carthamus tinctorius*), safflower oil, daisies, ragweed, chrysanthemums, marigolds, or any related constituents. Use parenteral safflower oil emulsions cautiously in newborns. Use cautiously if taking anticoagulants (blood thinners) or antiplatelet drugs, immunosuppressants, or pentobarbital. Use cautiously with diabetes, low blood pressure, inadequate liver function, bleeding disorders, or skin pigmentation conditions. Use cautiously if pregnant or breastfeeding.

Selenium: Selenium is a mineral found in soil, water, and some foods. The benefits of selenium supplementation in dialysis patients remain unclear. Some methods of dialysis may lower plasma selenium levels.

Avoid if allergic or sensitive to products containing selenium. Avoid with a history of nonmelanoma skin cancer. Selenium is generally regarded as safe for pregnant or breastfeeding women. However, animal research reports that large doses of selenium may lead to birth defects.

Soy: Soy has been suggested for many conditions, including high cholesterol, cardiovascular health, menopausal symptoms, and diarrhea. Due to limited human study, there is not enough evidence to recommend for or against the use of soy in the treatment of kidney diseases, such as nephrotic syndrome. People with kidney disease should speak to their healthcare providers about recommended amounts of dietary protein, and they should bear in mind that soy is a high-protein food.

Avoid if allergic to soy. Breathing problems and rash may occur in sensitive people. Soy, as a part of the regular diet, is traditionally considered to be safe during pregnancy and breastfeeding, but there are limited scientific data. The effects of high doses of soy or soy isoflavones in humans are not clear, and therefore are not recommended. There has been a case report of vitamin D–deficiency rickets in an infant nursed with soybean milk (not specifically designed for infants). People who experience intestinal irritation (colitis) from cow's milk may experience intestinal damage or diarrhea from soy. It is unknown if soy or soy isoflavones share the same side effects as estrogens (e.g., increased risk of blood clots). The use of soy is often discouraged in patients with hormone-sensitive cancers, such as breast, ovarian, or prostate cancer. Other hormone-sensitive conditions, such as endometriosis, may also be worsened. Patients taking blood-thinning drugs (e.g., warfarin) should check with their doctors and/or pharmacists before taking soy supplementation.

Traditional Chinese Medicine (TCM): The idea of TCM is a recent development. In the 1940s and 1950s, the Chinese government blended many forms of Chinese medicine into a unified health system. TCM practitioners use a wide range of treatments, ranging from meditation and acupuncture to herbal therapy and martial arts. TCM herbs have been reported to improve the therapeutic effectiveness and counteract adverse reactions to hormone therapy in treating nephrotic syndrome and reduce the recurrence of symptoms. More studies are needed to confirm these findings.

Chinese herbs can be potent and may interact with other herbs, foods, or drugs. Consult a qualified healthcare professional before taking. There have been reports of manufactured or processed Chinese herbal products being tainted with toxins or heavy metals or not containing the listed ingredients. Herbal products should be purchased from reliable sources. Avoid ephedra (ma huang). Avoid ginseng if pregnant or breastfeeding.

Vitamin E: Vitamin E exists in eight different forms (called isomers): alpha, beta, gamma, and delta tocopherol and alpha, beta, gamma, and delta tocotrienol. Alpha-tocopherol is the most active form in humans. It has been suggested that proteinuria (protein in the urine) may be reduced with the use of vitamin E in patients with FSGS that is refractory to standard medical management. However, further research is necessary before a clear conclusion can be drawn.

Avoid if allergic or hypersensitive to vitamin E. For short periods of time, vitamin E supplementation is generally considered safe at doses up to 1,000 milligrams per day. Avoid doses higher than 1,000 milligrams a day. Avoid with retinitis pigmentosa (loss of peripheral vision). Use cautiously with bleeding disorders. The recommended dose of vitamin E for pregnant women of any age is 15 milligrams and for breastfeeding women of any age is 19 milligrams. Use beyond this level in pregnant women is not recommended.

Zinc: Zinc formulations have been used since ancient Egyptian times to enhance wound healing. Preliminary research suggests that zinc may improve uremia in patients with kidney disorders. Uremia is a condition that occurs with severe kidney disorders. This happens when the kidneys are unable to filter out a waste product, called urea, in the blood. As a result, urea builds up to toxic levels in the blood. Further research is needed to confirm these results. Zinc supplementation may be recommended only in the patients with proven zinc deficiency, but its use for all chronic renal failure patients is questionable.

Zinc is generally considered safe when taken at the recommended dosages. Avoid zinc chloride since studies have not been done on its safety or effectiveness. While zinc appears safe during pregnancy in amounts lower than the established upper intake level, caution should be used since studies cannot rule out the possibility of harm to the fetus.

Fair Negative Scientific Evidence

Arginine: L-arginine helps maintain the body's fluid balance (urea, creatinine) and aids in wound healing, hair growth, sperm production (spermatogenesis), and blood vessel relaxation (vasodilation).

It also helps fight infections. Animal studies report that arginine blocks the toxic effects of cyclosporine, a drug used to prevent organ transplant rejection. However, results from studies in humans have not found that arginine offers any protection from cyclosporine-induced toxicity. It has been suggested that arginine may be a useful supplement in people diagnosed with kidney failure. However, results from available studies do not support this claim. A small randomized, controlled clinical trial studied the ability of L-arginine to improve dilation of blood vessels in children with chronic renal (kidney) failure. Results showed that blood vessel dilation (endothelial function) was not improved with oral L-arginine, suggesting that dietary supplementation is not a beneficial or useful clinical approach in children with chronic renal failure. The contrast media or dye used during angiography to map a patient's arteries (or during some computerized tomographic scans) can be toxic to the kidneys, especially to people with preexisting kidney disease. A randomized, parallel, double-blind clinical trial studied the use of L-arginine to protect kidneys in patients with chronic renal failure undergoing angiography. The authors found no evidence that injections of L-arginine protect the kidney from damage due to contrast. Other therapies, such as *N*-acetylcysteine, have been found beneficial at protecting the kidneys from contrast-induced damage, particularly in patients at high risk (e.g., diabetics).

Avoid if allergic to arginine. Avoid with a history of stroke, liver disease, or kidney disease. Use cautiously if taking blood-thinning drugs (such as warfarin), blood pressure drugs, or herbs or supplements with similar effects. Check blood potassium levels. Avoid if pregnant or breastfeeding.

Iridology: Iridology is the study of the iris for diagnostic purposes. Iridology assumes that all bodily organs are represented on the surface of the iris via intricate neural connections. Preliminary study submitted photographs of irises of kidney disease patients to practicing iridologists and found no evidence of accurate detection of kidney disease. There is no evidence supporting iridology as a diagnostic tool in kidney disease.

Iridology should not be used alone to diagnose disease. Studies of iridology have reported incorrect diagnoses, and potentially severe medical problems may thus go undiagnosed. In addition, research suggests that iridology may lead to inappropriate treatment.

Trigger Point Therapy: Trigger point therapy is used by many healthcare practitioners, including medical doctors, osteopaths, chiropractors, and massage therapists, to relieve pain and dysfunction while re-educating the muscles into pain-free habits. Although many drugs have been used for the treatment of renal colic, none have been proven to relieve pain quickly and completely. The goal of trigger point therapy for renal colic is to eliminate the trigger points associated with renal colic and thus lessen the pain. One study demonstrated that trigger point therapy with lidocaine may effectively treat renal colic. The results of this study warrant future investigations with more stringent study guidelines.

Use cautiously with local or systemic infection, anticoagulation or bleeding disorders, or acute muscle trauma. Avoid aspirin ingestion within three days of injection. Avoid with extreme fear of needles, large bruises, phlebitis, varicose veins, undiagnosed lumps, or open wounds. Avoid if allergic to anesthetic agents (mainly caused by amino ester agents).

Zinc: Zinc formulations have been used since ancient Egyptian times to enhance wound healing. Based on one well-designed trial, zinc supplementation did not improve the nutritional status in patients undergoing continuous ambulatory peritoneal dialysis.

Zinc is generally considered safe when taken at the recommended dosages. Avoid zinc chloride since studies have not been done on its safety or effectiveness. While zinc appears safe during pregnancy in amounts lower than the established upper intake level, caution should be used since studies cannot rule out the possibility of harm to the fetus.

PREVENTION

Patients should use medications that are known to cyclosporine (Neoral, Sandimmune), the anti-HIV drug tenofovir (Viread), and the antibiotic gentamicin (Geramycin), cautiously.

Patients should avoid or minimize exposure to heavy metals and other toxins because they may lead to kidney disorders.

Patients should drink plenty of water to reduce the risk of developing kidney stones.

Patients who are diagnosed with kidney disease should visit their healthcare providers regularly and take their medications exactly as prescribed. This will help reduce the patients' risk of developing complications, including kidney failure.

CONDITION: Perimenopause, Postmenopause, Menopause

BACKGROUND

Menopause is when a woman's menstrual periods stop completely. It signals the end of the ovaries releasing eggs for fertilization. A woman is said to have gone through menopause when her menses have stopped for an entire year. Menopause generally occurs between the ages of 45-55, although it can occur as early as the 30s or as late as the 60s. It can also result from the surgical removal of both ovaries. A woman can still get pregnant during menopause until she has gone at least 12 months without menstruating (a period). Changes and symptoms include a change in menstruation (periods may be shorter or longer, lighter or heavier, with more or less time in between); hot flashes and/or night sweats; trouble sleeping; vaginal dryness; mood swings; trouble focusing; and, less commonly, hair loss on the head but increased hair on the face. About 85% of women experiencing menopause will have hot flashes.

All women will experience menopause. Menopause is not considered a disorder and most women do not need treatment for it. However, if symptoms are severe, medications may be used to help alleviate symptoms. Researchers have estimated that more than 1.3 million women in the United States and 25 million women worldwide experience menopause annually. There are about 470 million postmenopausal women worldwide, a number that is expected to increase to 1.2 billion by the year 2030. Some women take hormone replacement therapy (HRT) to relieve the symptoms associated with menopause. HRT is medication containing one or more female hormones, commonly estrogen plus progestin (synthetic progesterone). HRT may also protect against osteoporosis. However, HRT also has risks. It can increase the risk of breast cancer, heart disease, and stroke. Certain types of HRT have a higher risk, and each woman's own risks can vary depending upon her health history and lifestyle.

Perimenopause: During perimenopause, women may begin to experience menopausal physical and emotional signs and symptoms, such as hot flashes and depression, even though they still menstruate. The average length of perimenopause is four years, but for some women this stage may last only a few months or continue for 10 years. Perimenopause ends the first year after menopause, when a woman has gone 12 months without having her period. Periods (menstruation) tend to be irregular during this time and may be shorter or longer or even absent. Despite a decline in fertility during the perimenopause stage, individuals can still become pregnant. If the individual does not want to become pregnant, she should continue to use some form of birth control until menopause is reached.

Postmenopause: Postmenopause is a time when most of the distress of the menopausal changes have faded. Hot flashes may seem milder or less frequent and energy, emotional, and hormonal levels may seem to have stabilized. During postmenopause, women are at a higher risk for developing osteoporosis (bone loss) and heart disease due to the decrease in circulating estrogen. The postmenopausal phase begins when 12 full months have passed since the last menstrual period.

CAUSES AND RISK FACTORS

Menopause begins naturally when the ovaries start making less estrogen and progesterone, the hormones that regulate menstruation. The process usually begins in a woman's late 30s. By that time, fewer potential eggs for fertilization are found in the ovaries each month, and ovulation is less predictable. Progesterone (the hormone that prepares the body for pregnancy) levels drop and fertility declines. These changes are more pronounced in the 40s, as are changes in menstrual patterns. The woman's period may become longer or shorter, heavier or lighter, and more or less frequent. Eventually, the ovaries cease to function and there are no more periods. It is possible, but very unusual, to menstruate every month right up to the last egg is released; a gradual tapering off is more common.

Early menopause is associated with the following risk factors: smoking, nulliparity (never carrying a child to full term), medically treated depression, exposure to toxic chemicals (such as pesticides), and treatment of childhood cancer with pelvic radiation or chemotherapy.

Menopause is usually a natural process. But certain surgical or medical treatments or medical conditions can bring on menopause earlier than expected. An oophorectomy (also called ovariotomy) is the surgical removal of the ovaries. Oophorectomies are most often performed in women due to ovarian cysts or cancer, prophylactically to reduce the chances of developing ovarian cancer or breast cancer, or in conjunction with the removal of the uterus. A hysterectomy is a surgical procedure to remove the uterus but not the ovaries. A hysterectomy usually does not cause menopause. Although women no longer have periods, their ovaries still release eggs and produce estrogen and progesterone. However, surgery that removes the uterus and the ovaries (called a total hysterectomy and bilateral oophorectomy) does cause menopause without any perimenopausal phase. Instead, periods stop immediately and hot flashes and other menopausal signs and symptoms appear. Research suggests that women who have their ovaries removed are at a decreased chance of developing breast cancer, ovarian cancer, and endometriosis. Chemotherapy and radiation cancer therapies can induce menopause, causing symptoms such as hot flashes during the course of treatment or within three to six months.

SIGNS AND SYMPTOMS

Menstrual Changes: Many women experience irregular periods due to the changing hormone levels and the decreased frequency of ovulation (egg release). The changes may be subtle at first and then gradually become more noticeable. Common changes include short cycles (less than 28 days), bleeding for fewer days than usual, heavier than usual bleeding, lighter than usual bleeding, and missed periods. Although menstrual irregularities are expected during menopause, menstrual changes can also be caused by conditions such as fibroids or pregnancy. Women who experience heavy bleeding (usually with clots), periods that come more often than every three weeks, spotting between periods, or bleeding after intercourse should see their doctors or other healthcare providers. After menopause, women no longer menstruate. Any woman who experiences vaginal bleeding after menopause should see her doctor or other healthcare provider. Hormone treatments can sometimes cause vaginal bleeding to resume. Changes in the body during menopause are called climacteric symptoms. They include hot flashes, skin and hair changes, and vaginal changes.

Hot Flashes: As many as 85% of women experience hot flashes during menopause. Hot flashes are vasomotor symptoms that cause a warm or hot, flushed sensation that usually begins in the head and face and then radiates down the neck to other parts of the body. There may be red blotches on the skin. Each hot flash averages 2.7 minutes and is characterized by a sudden increase in heart rate, an increase in peripheral blood flow, which leads to a rise in skin temperature, and a sudden onset of sweating, particularly on the upper body. Hot flashes can occur before, during, or after menopause. Hot flashes can

begin when a woman's cycles are still regular or, more commonly, as menopause approaches and her cycles become irregular. They usually last for less than a year following the last menstrual period, although some women continue to experience hot flashes five to 10 years after menopause. Hot flashes can occur once a month, once a week, or several times an hour. They can happen any time of day or night. If they happen at night (such as night sweats), they can interrupt sleep and drench clothing and sheets. Loss of sleep can eventually lead to irritability and fatigue.

Skin and Hair Changes: The process of aging can cause many changes in the body that result in skin and hair changes. Estrogen helps keeps the skin smooth and moist. The loss of estrogen during menopause makes the skin dry, thin, lax, and transparent. The blood vessels are easier to see, and the skin bruises easily. The woman may experience growth of facial hair but thinning of hair in the temple region.

Vaginal Changes: Women may experience vaginal changes. In particular, the tissues of the vagina and vulva may become thin and dry (called vaginal atrophy), which can lead to itching and discomfort during sexual intercourse. In some women, vaginal dryness is the first sign of menopause.

Other Changes: Other changes that may occur during menopause include loss of bladder tone, resulting in stress incontinence (leaking urine when coughing, sneezing, laughing, or exercise); headaches; dizziness; loss of some muscle strength and tone; increasing bone loss, increasing the risk for osteoporosis; increasing risk for a heart attack when estrogen levels drop (however, the addition of estrogen as a prescribed medication after menopause can lead to an increase in heart attack and stroke); emotional changes associated with menopause such as irritability, mood changes, lack of concentration, difficulty with memory, tension, anxiety, and depression; and insomnia that may result from hot flashes that interrupt sleep.

COMPLICATIONS

Several chronic medical conditions tend to appear after menopause. By becoming aware of the following conditions, women can take steps to help reduce their risk.

Cardiovascular Disease: When estrogen levels decline, the risk of cardiovascular disease increases. Heart disease is the leading cause of death in women as well as in men. Risk-reduction steps for developing heart disease include stopping smoking, reducing high blood pressure, getting regular aerobic exercise, and eating a diet low in saturated fats and plentiful in whole grains, fruits, and vegetables.

Osteoporosis: During the first few years after menopause, women may lose bone density at a rapid rate, increasing their risk of osteoporosis. Osteoporosis is a condition that causes bones to become brittle and weak, leading to an increased risk of fractures. Postmenopausal women are especially susceptible to fractures of the hip, wrist, and spine. It is important for all women to get adequate calcium and vitamin D. It is recommended by healthcare professionals for postmenopausal women to have about 1,200-1,500 milligrams of elemental calcium and 800 IU (international units) of vitamin D daily. Healthcare professionals recommend regular exercise. Strength training and weight-bearing activities such as walking and jogging are especially beneficial in keeping the bones strong and healthy. It is important to check for the amount of elemental calcium on a supplement label.

Urinary Incontinence: Urinary incontinence is the loss of bladder control. As the tissues of the vagina and urethra lose their elasticity, postmenopausal women may experience a frequent, sudden, strong urge to urinate, followed by an involuntary loss of urine (urge incontinence), or the loss of urine with coughing, laughing, or lifting (stress incontinence).

Weight Gain: Many women gain weight during the menopausal transition. Individuals may need to eat less, perhaps as many as 200-400 fewer calories a day, and exercise more just to maintain their current weight.

DIAGNOSIS

A doctor will review the woman's medical history and perform a physical examination, including a pelvic exam. During the pelvic exam, a doctor will check for any abnormalities in the reproductive organs and look for indications of infection. There are no unique physical findings or laboratory tests to positively diagnose menopause.

The signs and symptoms of menopause, such as hot flashes and mood swings, are enough to tell most women they have begun going through the transition. Under certain circumstances, a doctor may check the level of follicle-stimulating hormone (FSH) and estrogen (estradiol) with a blood test. As menopause occurs, FSH levels increase and estradiol levels decrease. A doctor may also recommend a blood test to determine the level of thyroid-stimulating hormone, as hypothyroidism (low thyroid hormone levels) can cause symptoms similar to those of menopause, such as swelling, mood changes, and hot flashes.

The medical history and physical examination involve an evaluation of the symptoms and when they occur in relation to menstruation. Many healthcare providers advise women to keep a diary of menstrual cycles and the physical and psychological changes they experience over the course of several months. The menstrual diary provides clues to the physician and helps women understand and cope with the changes.

TREATMENT

Calcium Management: Adequate calcium intake is important to prevent osteoporosis and bone fractures. Daily elemental calcium intake for postmenopausal women should be around 1,200 milligrams. Women should eat foods rich in calcium (such as dairy products, leafy green vegetables, tofu, calcium-fortified foods) as well as foods that promote calcium absorption. A glass of milk provides about 300 milligrams of calcium. Intake of foods that rob the bones of calcium, such as animal protein and salt, should be limited. Vitamin D helps the body absorb calcium. Fifteen minutes of sun exposure every day provides sufficient vitamin D. Foods such as fortified milk, liver, and tuna contain vitamin D. Women should ask their healthcare providers or nutritionists if they should take a vitamin D supplement.

Calcium supplements are available in several forms: amino acid chelate, calcium carbonate, calcium chloride, calcium lactate, calcium gluconate, bone meal, dolomite, hydroxyapatite, and calcium citrate. To maximize absorption, supplements containing amino acid chelate, calcium citrate, gluconate, or hydroxyapatite should be taken. Make sure to look for elemental calcium amounts on the label.

Exercise: Exercise is an important part of preventative healthcare for postmenopausal women. By increasing cardiovascular fitness and strengthening the bones, exercise helps prevent heart disease and osteoporosis. Low-impact, weight-bearing exercises, such as walking, jogging, tennis, racquetball, and dancing, are helpful. Women diagnosed with osteoporosis or cardiovascular disease should consult with their healthcare providers before initiating an exercise program.

HRT: HRT uses estrogens and progestin (synthetic progesterone) to ease the symptoms of menopause. The hormones are available in a variety of forms: pills, vaginal creams, vaginal ring inserts, implants, injections, and patches worn on the skin.

HRT has many short-term and long-term side effects. It is important to weigh all of the potential benefits and risks, preferences, and needs before beginning HRT. The benefits and side effects vary considerably from woman to woman. Women who

M

take HRT should be closely monitored by a healthcare professional to ensure that they benefit as much as possible from the hormone therapy. Sometimes, changing the dosage or the way it is administered can help to control side effects. Minor side effects include bloating, breast tenderness, cramping, irritability, depression, and menstrual bleeding for months or years following menopause. More serious risks include: breast cancer; women who have not had a hysterectomy and use estrogen supplements are at increased risk for invasive breast cancer and cardiovascular disease. HRT causes an increased risk for stroke (neurological damage caused by a lack of oxygen to the brain), heart attack, and cardiovascular disease.

Endometrial cancer has been linked to high-dose estrogen supplements. Women who have not had their uterus removed are prescribed low doses of estrogen with progestin (progestin protects against endometrial cancer). Women who take HRT are at increased risk for deep vein thrombosis (blood clots). HRT may help to prevent or delay the development of many diseases, including osteoporosis, Alzheimer's disease, colon cancer, macular degeneration (the leading cause of visual impairment in persons over age 50), urinary incontinence, and skin aging.

Various types and dosages of estrogen and progestin are available, and the type of HRT often depends on particular symptoms. For example, women who experience vaginal dryness may opt for a vaginal cream or vaginal ring insert, both of which alleviate dryness. The vaginal ring insert can also help urinary tract problems. For women who suffer from hot flashes, pills or patches may be helpful.

Due to the potential health risks involved with taking HRT, doctors will prescribe the lowest possible dosage for the shortest period of time when treating symptoms of menopause. Topical application of progesterone is commonly used as an alternative to HRT, especially if vaginal dryness is present.

Hormonal Medications

Estrogen therapy remains, by far, the most effective treatment option for relieving menopausal hot flashes. Depending on the individual's personal and family medical history, a doctor may recommend estrogen in the lowest dose needed to provide symptom relief for the individual.

Conjugated Estrogens: Conjugated estrogens are a mixture of estrogens prescribed to treat menopausal symptoms. The conjugated estrogens in Premarin and Premarin Vaginal Cream are obtained from pregnant mare urine. The conjugated estrogens in Cenestin are synthetic.

Dienestrol: Dienestrol (Ortho-Dienestrol) is a synthetic, nonsteroidal, estrogen vaginal cream used to treat atrophic vaginitis. Side effects include vaginal discharge, increased vaginal discomfort, uterine bleeding, vaginal burning sensation, breast tenderness, and peripheral edema.

Esterified Estrogens: Esterified estrogens (Estratab, Menest) are estrogenic substances consisting of 75-85% natural estrogens and 15-25% equine (mare urine) estrogens. They are supplied in tablet form and are used to treat hot flashes and atrophic vaginitis and urethritis (infections due to thinning and drying of vaginal tissues).

Estradiol: Estradiol is one of the three major estrogens made by the human body and is the major estrogen secreted during the menstrual years. It is available as an oral pill (Estrace), transdermal skin patch (Climara, Estraderm, Vivelle), vaginal tablet (Vagifem), and vaginal cream (Estrace Vaginal Cream).

Estropipate (Estrone): Estropipate is an estrogenic substance derived from estrone, one of the three major estrogens produced by the body. Estrone is produced from estradiol and is a less potent estrogen. It is available in pill form (Ogen, Ortho-Est) and prescribed to treat hot flashes and vaginal atrophy and to help prevent osteoporosis.

Ethinyl Estradiol: Ethinyl estradiol (Estinyl) is a synthetic nonsteroidal estrogen available as a tablet that is prescribed to treat hot flashes (vasomotor symptom). It is administered on a cyclical basis (such as three weeks on and one week off) with attempts to discontinue or taper at three- to six-month intervals.

Testosterone: Testosterone is one of the androgens or male hormones and is also produced by women. Testosterone contributes to muscle strength, appetite, well-being, and sex drive (libido). The level of testosterone falls rapidly after menopause, and some women take testosterone supplements in addition to estrogen and progestin as part of HRT. However, supplemental testosterone can produce side effects and has potentially serious risks. Common side effects include weight gain, acne, facial hair, and liver disease. Testosterone can exacerbate estrogen's carcinogenic effect on breast and uterine tissue.

Other Medications

Low-Dose Antidepressants: Venlafaxine (Effexor) is an antidepressant in a group of drugs called selective serotonin and norepinephrine reuptake inhibitors. Effexor has been reported to decrease menopausal hot flashes. Selective serotonin reuptake inhibitors may be helpful, including fluoxetine (Prozac, Sarafem), paroxetine (Paxil), citalopram (Celexa), and sertraline (Zoloft). Side effects include drowsiness and fatigue.

Gabapentin (Neurontin): Gabapentin (Neurontin) is commonly used to treat seizures and for neuropathy (nerve pain), but it also has been reported to significantly reduce hot flashes. Side effects include drowsiness, sedation, blurred vision, nausea, vomiting, or tremor.

Clonidine (Catapres): Clonidine (Catapres) is typically used to treat high blood pressure. However, clonidine may significantly reduce the frequency of hot flashes. Side effects include slow heart rate, low blood pressure, fatigue, dizziness, headache, constipation, nausea, vomiting, diarrhea, insomnia, or a dry mouth.

Bisphosphonates: Alendronate (Fosamax), risedronate (Actonel), ibandronate (Boniva), and zoledronate (Zometa) are approved by the U.S. Food and Drug Administration for the prevention and treatment of osteoporosis in postmenopausal women. Alendronate is the only one currently approved for management of osteoporosis in men. Both alendronate and risedronate are approved for the prevention and treatment of steroid-induced osteoporosis in men and women. Bisphosphonates help slow down bone loss and have been shown to decrease the risk of fractures. All are taken on an empty stomach with water. Because bisphosphonates have the potential for irritating the esophagus, remaining upright for at least an hour after taking these medications is recommended by healthcare professionals. Alendronate and risedronate can be taken once a week, while ibandronate can be taken once a month. An intravenous form of ibandronate, given through the vein every three months, also has been approved for the management of osteoporosis. Another intravenous bisphosphonate being studied for osteoporosis is zoledronic acid or zoledronate (Zometa). This form is injected once yearly.

Side effects, which can be severe, include nausea, abdominal pain, and the risk of an inflamed esophagus or esophageal ulcers, especially if the individual has had acid reflux or ulcers in the past. If individuals cannot tolerate oral bisphosphonates, the doctor may recommend the periodic intravenous infusions of a bisphosphonate.

Use of bisphosphonates in women who are pregnant or breastfeeding is not well studied. Blood calcium levels in women who take bisphosphonates during pregnancy are usually monitored. Individuals using ibandronate injection will have blood levels of creatinine measured prior to each dose to determine kidney function. Creatinine is measured using blood tests.

Selective Estrogen Receptor Modulators: Selective estrogen receptor modulators mimic the positive effects of estrogen on bones without some of the serious side effects such as breast cancer and stroke. Raloxifene (Evista) decreases spine fractures in women and is approved for use only in women at this time. Hot flashes are a common side effect of raloxifene, and individuals with a history of blood clots should not use this drug.

Vaginal Estrogen: To relieve vaginal dryness, estrogen can be administered locally in the vagina using a vaginal tablet (Vagifem), ring (NuvaRing), or cream (Premarin vaginal cream). This treatment releases just a small amount of estrogen, which is absorbed by the vaginal tissue. It can help relieve vaginal dryness, discomfort with intercourse, and some urinary symptoms.

INTEGRATIVE THERAPIES

Good Scientific Evidence

Calcium: Calcium is the nutrient consistently found to be the most important for attaining peak bone mass and preventing osteoporosis. Adequate vitamin D intake is required for optimal calcium absorption. Adequate calcium and vitamin D are deemed essential for the prevention of osteoporosis in general, including postmenopausal osteoporosis. There is a link between lower dietary intake of calcium and symptoms of premenstrual syndrome (PMS). Calcium supplementation has been suggested in various clinical trials to decrease overall symptoms associated with PMS, such as depressed mood, water retention, and pain.

Sage: Sage (*Salvia officinalis*) may contain compounds with mild estrogenic activity. In theory, estrogenic compounds may decrease the symptoms of menopause. Sage has been tested against menopausal symptoms with promising results.

Soy: Soy (*Glycine max*) products containing isoflavones have been studied for the reduction of menopausal symptoms such as hot flashes. The scientific evidence is mixed in this area, with several human trials suggesting reduced number of hot flashes and other menopausal symptoms but more recent research reporting no benefits. Overall, the scientific evidence does suggest benefits, although better-quality studies are needed in this area in order to form a firm conclusion. It is currently unclear whether phytoestrogens from soy foods affect breast cancer risk. Studies looking directly at breast cancer risk and soy in the diet are not in agreement. Almost half of the studies have reported no effect of soy on breast cancer risk.

M

Unclear or Conflicting Scientific Evidence

Acupressure, Shiatsu: The practice of applying finger pressure to specific acupoints throughout the body has been used in China since 2000 BC, prior to the use of acupuncture. Acupressure techniques are widely practiced internationally for relaxation, wellness promotion, and the treatment of various health conditions. Based on initial research, acupressure may reduce menstrual pain severity, pain medication use, and anxiety associated with menstruation. Further research is needed.

Acupuncture: Acupuncture is a technique of inserting and manipulating needles into acupuncture points on the body with the aim of restoring health and well-being (e.g., treating pain and diseases). The practice of acupuncture originated in China 5,000 years ago. Today, it is widely used throughout the world and is one of the main pillars of Chinese medicine. Although some studies report beneficial results, currently there is not adequate available evidence to recommend for or against acupuncture in the treatment of dysmenorrhea related to PMS. Also, there has been limited research on acupuncture for menopausal symptoms such as hot flashes and menopause-related high blood pressure. There is insufficient evidence to make a firm conclusion.

Belladonna: Bellergal (a combination of phenobarbital, ergot, and belladonna) has been used to treat PMS symptoms. Bellergal also has been used historically to treat hot flashes. However, in human studies belladonna supplements have not shown effectiveness. More studies are needed.

Bilberry: Bilberry (*Vaccinium myrtillus*), a close relative of blueberry, has a long history of medicinal use. Preliminary evidence suggests that bilberry may be helpful for the relief of menstrual pain, although more research is necessary before a firm conclusion can be drawn. Bilberry supplements may lower blood sugar levels. Caution is advised in individuals taking bilberry and medications to lower blood sugar levels.

Black Cohosh: Black cohosh (*Actaea racemosa,* formerly known as *Cimicifuga racemosa*) is popular as an alternative to hormonal therapy in the treatment of menopausal (climacteric) symptoms such as hot flashes, mood disturbances, diaphoresis, palpitations, and vaginal dryness. Several studies have reported black cohosh to improve menopausal symptoms for up to six months, although the current evidence is mixed.

The mechanism of action of black cohosh remains unclear and the effects on estrogen receptors or hormonal levels (if any) are not definitively known. Recent publications suggest that there may be no direct effects on estrogen receptors, although this is an area of active controversy. Safety and efficacy beyond six months have not been proven, although recent reports suggest safety of short-term use, including in women experiencing menopausal symptoms for whom estrogen replacement therapy is contraindicated. Nonetheless, caution is advisable until better-quality safety data are available. Use of black cohosh in high-risk populations (such as in women with a history of breast cancer) should be under the supervision of a licensed healthcare professional.

Chasteberry: Chasteberry (*Vitex agnus-castus*) has been reported to inhibit prolactin secretion by competitively binding to dopamine receptors. Available evidence suggests that chasteberry may be an effective treatment option for hyperprolactinemic (elevated serum prolactin levels) conditions and PMS. Chasteberry does not appear to affect levels of luteinizing hormone or FSH. Most studies evaluating chasteberry in PMS have been of poor study design, although one recent trial demonstrating benefit is of high quality. Further evidence is necessary before a firm conclusion can be drawn. There is limited controlled trial evidence suggesting possible benefits of chasteberry in the alleviation of symptoms of premenstrual dysphoric disorder. Further evidence is necessary before a firm conclusion can be drawn.

Chasteberry supplements should be used with caution in individuals taking dopamine agonists, such as bromocriptine (Parlodel), or dopamine antagonists, including antipsychotic medications such as risperidone (Risperdal). Additionally, caution is advised in patients with Parkinson's disease and other illnesses of the central nervous system as medications used for these conditions often affect dopamine; taking them with chasteberry may increase effects and side effects.

Chiropractic: Chiropractic is a healthcare discipline that focuses on the relationship between musculoskeletal structure (primarily the spine) and body function (as coordinated by the nervous system) and how this relationship affects the preservation and restoration of health. The broad term "spinal manipulative therapy" incorporates all types of manual techniques, including chiropractic. Although used with positive results, there is not enough reliable scientific evidence to conclude the effects of chiropractic techniques in the management of dysmenorrhea and PMS.

Dehydroepiandrosterone (DHEA): DHEA is a hormone made in the human body and secreted by the adrenal gland. DHEA serves as precursor to male and female sex hormones (androgens and estrogens). Many different aspects of menopause have been studied using DHEA as a treatment, such as vaginal pain, osteoporosis, and hot flashes as well as emotional disturbances such as fatigue, irritability, anxiety, depression, insomnia, difficulties with concentration, memory, or decreased sex drive (which may occur near the time of menopause). Study results disagree and additional study is needed in this area.

Dong Quai: Dong quai (*Angelica sinensis*), also known as Chinese Angelica, has been used for thousands of years in traditional Chinese, Korean, and Japanese medicine. It remains one of the most popular plants in Chinese medicine and is used primarily for health conditions in women. Dong quai is used in traditional Chinese formulas for menopausal symptoms. It has been proposed that dong quai may contain phytoestrogens (chemicals with estrogenlike effects in the body). However, it remains unclear from laboratory studies if dong quai has the same effects on the body as estrogens, if it blocks the activity of estrogens, or if it has no significant effect on estrogens.

There is limited poor-quality study of dong quai as a part of herbal combinations given for amenorrhea. Additional research is necessary before a firm conclusion can be drawn. There are unclear results of preliminary, poor-quality human research of dong quai in combination with other herbs for dysmenorrhea. Reliable scientific evidence for dong quai alone in humans with dysmenorrhea is currently not available.

Dong quai supplements may increase the risk of bleeding in sensitive individuals, such as those taking medications to reduce blood clotting, including aspirin and warfarin (Coumadin).

Fennel: Fennel (*Foeniculum vulgare*) is native to the Mediterranean region. For centuries, fennel fruits have been used as traditional herbal medicine in Europe and China. Fennel has been used to treat dysmenorrhea. Although preliminary study is promising, there is currently insufficient evidence for the use of fennel in dysmenorrheal.

Flaxseed: Flaxseed (*Linum usitatissimum*) and its derivative flaxseed oil/linseed oil are rich sources of the essential fatty acid alpha-linolenic acid, which is a biological precursor to omega-3 fatty acids such as eicosapentaenoic acid. There is preliminary evidence from randomized, controlled trials that flaxseed oil may help decrease mild menopausal symptoms. Additional research is necessary before a clear conclusion can be drawn, and this remains an area of controversy. Patients should consult a doctor and pharmacist about treatment options before starting a new therapy. Overall, effects on bone mineral density and lipid profiles remain unclear. Also, early information from one study in women, the results of which have not been fully reported, suggests that flaxseed may reduce menstrual breast pain. However, further study is needed.

Gamma-Linolenic Acid (GLA): GLA is a dietary omega-6 fatty acid found in many plant oil extracts. One study has examined the effect of GLA (evening primrose oil) on menopausal flushing. No improvement in the number of flushes was noted as compared with placebo. More clinical trials are needed. A study using Efamol (a supplement containing GLA) suggests there may be benefit in terms of PMS symptoms. More studies are needed.

Gamma-Oryzanol: Gamma-oryzanol is a mixture of ferulic acid esters of sterol and triterpene alcohols, and it occurs in rice bran oil at a level of 1-2%, although it has been extracted from corn and barley oils as well. It is theorized that some of the health benefits from rice bran oil, namely its cholesterol-lowering effects, may be due to its gamma-oryzanol content. Gamma-oryzanol may reduce menopausal symptoms. However, these results must be viewed cautiously as a high placebo effect is associated with the treatment of menopause symptoms. Additional study is needed in this area to determine gamma-oryzanol's effect on menopausal symptoms.

Ginkgo: Ginkgo (*Ginkgo biloba*) has been used medicinally for thousands of years. Today, it is one of the top selling herbs in the United States. Initial study in women with PMS or breast discomfort suggests that ginkgo may relieve symptoms, including emotional upset. Further well-designed research is needed. Ginkgo supplements may increase the risk of bleeding in sensitive individuals, such as those taking medications to reduce blood clotting, including aspirin and warfarin (Coumadin).

Ginseng: Although ginseng (*Panax ginseng*) has been used for symptoms of menopause, evidence from a small amount of research is unclear in this area. Some studies report improvements in depression and sense of well-being, without changes in hormone levels.

Green Tea: Green tea supplements are made from the dried leaves of *Camellia sinensis,* a perennial evergreen shrub. Green tea has a long history of use, dating back to China approximately 5,000 years ago. Green tea, black tea, and oolong tea are all derived from the same plant. A study conducted in healthy

M

postmenopausal women showed that a morning/ evening menopausal formula containing green tea was effective in relieving menopausal symptoms, including hot flashes and sleep disturbance. Further studies are needed to confirm these results. Caffeine-free green tea supplements are available. Green tea supplements may increase the risk of bleeding in sensitive individuals, such as those taking medications to reduce blood clotting, including aspirin and warfarin (Coumadin).

Hypnosis: Early evidence shows that hypnotherapy may be beneficial in the treatment of hot flashes and may improve quality of life in women who are experiencing menopausal symptoms. Further research is needed.

Kudzu: Kudzu (*Pueraria lobata*) originated in China and was brought to the United States from Japan in the late 1800s. It is distributed throughout much of the eastern United States and is most common in the southern part of the continent. Kudzu contains chemicals called isoflavones, which are reported to have estrogenic activity. There is conflicting evidence regarding the effects of kudzu on menopausal symptoms. Additional study is needed to clarify these results.

Massage: Various forms of therapeutic superficial tissue manipulation have been practiced for thousands of years across cultures. Chinese use of massage dates to 1600 BC, and Hippocrates made reference to the importance of physicians being experienced with "rubbing" as early as 400 BC. Initial research of the effects of massage on mood in women with premenstrual dysphoric disorder is inconclusive. A recent study investigating abdominal meridian massage (Kyongrak) found positive effects for menstrual cramps and dysmenorrhea. Further study is needed.

Omega-3 Fatty Acids (Fish Oil): Dietary sources of omega-3 fatty acids include fish oil and certain plant/ nut oils. Fish oil contains both docosahexaenoic acid and eicosapentaenoic acid, while some nuts (English walnuts) and vegetable oils (canola, soybean, flaxseed/linseed, olive) contain alpha-linolenic acid. There is preliminary evidence suggesting possible benefits of fish oil/omega-3 fatty acids in patients with dysmenorrhea. Additional research is necessary before a firm conclusion can be reached. Omega-3 fatty acid supplements may increase the risk of bleeding in sensitive individuals, such as those taking medications to reduce blood clotting, including aspirin and warfarin (Coumadin).

Pycnogenol: Pycnogenol (Horphag Research, Berlin) is the patented trade name for a water extract of the bark of the French maritime pine (*Pinus pinaster* spp. *atlantica*), which is grown in coastal southwest France. Pycnogenol contains oligomeric proanthocyanidins as well as several other antioxidant bioflavonoids. Preliminary human data shows that Pycnogenol may have a potential analgesic (pain-relieving) effect on menstrual pain. Further research is needed to confirm these results. Pycnogenol may also effectively prevent cramps. Pycnogenol supplements may increase the risk of bleeding in sensitive individuals, such as those taking medications to reduce blood clotting, including aspirin and warfarin (Coumadin).

Red Clover: Red clover (*Trifolium pratense*) is a legume that, like soy, contains phytoestrogens (plant-based chemicals that are similar to estrogen and may act in the body like estrogen or may actually block the effects of estrogen). Laboratory research suggests that red clover isoflavones have estrogenlike activity. However, there is no clear evidence that isoflavones share the possible benefits of estrogens (such as effects on bone density). In addition, HRT itself is a controversial topic, with recent research reporting that the potential harm may outweigh any benefits. Red clover isoflavones are proposed to reduce symptoms of menopause (such as hot flashes), and are popular for this use. Blood pressure and triglyceride levels may be lowered. However, most of the available human studies are poorly designed and short in duration (less than 12 weeks of treatment). As results of published studies conflict with each other, more research is needed before a clear conclusion can be drawn. Red clover supplements may increase the risk of bleeding in sensitive individuals, such as those taking medications to reduce blood clotting, including aspirin and warfarin (Coumadin).

Reflexology: Reflexology involves the application of manual pressure to specific points or areas of the feet that are believed to correspond to other parts of the body. Preliminary human research reports that weekly reflexology sessions over a two-month period can reduce the severity of premenstrual symptoms in the short term. Further research is necessary before a firm conclusion can be reached in this area.

Relaxation Therapy: Relaxation techniques include behavioral therapeutic approaches that differ widely in philosophy, methodology, and practice. The primary goal is usually nondirected relaxation. Most techniques share the components of repetitive focus (on a word, sound, prayer phrase, body sensation, or muscular activity), adoption of a passive attitude towards intruding thoughts, and return to the focus. There is promising early evidence from human trials supporting the use of relaxation techniques to reduce menopausal symptoms, although effects appear to be short lived. Better-quality research is necessary before a firm conclusion can be drawn.

St. John's Wort: Extracts of St. John's wort (*Hypericum perforatum*) have been recommended traditionally for a wide range of medical conditions. The most common modern-day use of St. John's wort is the treatment of depression. Numerous studies report St. John's wort to be more effective than placebo and equally effective as tricyclic antidepressant drugs in the short-term treatment of mild-to-moderate major depression (one to three months). It is not clear if St. John's wort is as effective as selective serotonin reuptake inhibitor antidepressants such as sertraline (Zoloft). Although St. John's wort supplements have been used with effectiveness in treating depression associated with PMS and menopause, there is a lack of high-quality human studies supporting this therapy. More research is needed.

St. John's wort interferes with the way the body processes many drugs using the liver's cytochrome P450 enzyme system. As a result, the levels of these drugs may be increased in the blood in the short term (causing increased effects or potentially serious adverse reactions) and/or decreased in the blood in the long term (which can reduce the intended effects). Examples of medications that may be affected by St. John's wort in this manner include carbamazepine, cyclosporin, irinotecan, midazolam, nifedipine, birth control pills, simvastatin, theophylline, tricyclic antidepressants, warfarin, or HIV drugs such as non-nucleoside reverse transcriptase inhibitors or protease inhibitors. The U.S. Food & Drug Administration (FDA) suggests that patients with HIV/AIDS on protease inhibitors or nonnucleoside reverse transcriptase inhibitors avoid taking St. John's wort.

Transcutaneous Electrical Nerve Stimulation (TENS): TENS is a noninvasive technique in which a low-voltage electrical current is delivered through wires from a small power unit to electrodes located on the skin. Electrodes are temporarily attached with paste in various patterns, depending on the specific condition and treatment goals. TENS is often used to treat pain as an alternative or addition to pain medications. Therapy sessions may last from minutes to hours. TENS is usually a component of acupuncture treatment. TENS has been examined for the treatment of dysmenorrhea in several small studies. Research in this area suggests that the use of TENS may reduce short-term discomfort and need for pain medications. However, the available trials do not clearly describe study designs or results.

Vitamin E: Vitamin E is a fat-soluble vitamin with antioxidant properties. There is preliminary evidence of possible benefits of vitamin E supplementation to reduce chronic menstrual pain, although additional research is necessary in this area before a firm conclusion can be reached. Vitamin E supplements may increase the risk of bleeding in sensitive individuals, such as those taking medications to reduce blood clotting, including aspirin and warfarin (Coumadin).

Wild Yam: It has been hypothesized that wild yam (*Dioscorea villosa* and other *Dioscorea* species) possesses DHEA-like properties and acts as a precursor to human sex hormones such as estrogen and progesterone. Based on this proposed mechanism, extracts of the plant have been used to treat dysmenorrhea (painful menstruation), hot flashes, and headaches associated with menopause. However, these uses are based on a misconception that wild yam contains hormones or hormonal precursors—largely due to the historical fact that progesterone, androgens, and cortisone were chemically manufactured from Mexican wild yam in the 1960s. It is unlikely that this chemical conversion to progesterone occurs in the human body. The hormonal activity of some topical wild yam preparations has been attributed to adulteration with synthetic progesterone by manufacturers, although there is limited evidence in this area.

Fair Negative Scientific Evidence

Boron: Boron is a trace mineral found in soil, water, and some foods. It has been proposed that boron affects estrogen levels in postmenopausal women. However, preliminary studies have found no changes in menopausal symptoms.

Evening Primrose Oil: Available studies do not show evening primrose (*Oenothera biennis*) oil to be helpful with these potential complications of menopause. Small human studies do not report that evening primrose oil is helpful for the symptoms of PMS. A large, well-designed study is needed. Evening primrose oil supplements may increase the risk of bleeding in sensitive individuals, such as those taking medications to reduce blood clotting, including aspirin and warfarin (Coumadin).

Wild Yam: Despite popular belief, no natural progestins, estrogens, or other reproductive hormones are found in wild yam. Its active ingredient, diosgenin, is not converted to hormones in the human body. Artificial progesterone has been added to some wild yam products. The belief that there are hormones in wild yam may be due to the historical

M

fact that progesterone, androgens, and cortisone were chemically manufactured from Mexican wild yam in the 1960s.

Integrative therapies used in female conditions, such as menopause, that have historical or theoretical uses but lack sufficient clinical evidence include 55-hydroxytryptophan, homeopathic aconite (*Aconitum napellus*), African wild potato (*Hypoxis hemerocallidea*), alfalfa (*Medicago sativa*), anise (*Pimpinella anisum*), homeopathic arnica (*Arnica montana*), aromatherapy, ashwagandha (*Withania somnifera*), bay leaf (*Laurus nobilis*), bee pollen, black currant (*Ribes nigrum*), blue cohosh (*Caulophyllum thalictroides*), borage seed oil (*Borago officinalis*), boswellia (*Boswellia serrata*), bupleurum (*Bupleurum falcatum*), calendula (*Calendula officinalis*), cat's claw (*Uncaria tomentosa, Uncaria guianensis*), chamomile (*Matricaria recutita, Chamaemelum nobile*), chaparral (*Larrea tridentata*) and nordihydroguaiaretic acid, coleus (*Coleus forskohlii*), cramp bark (*Viburnum opulus*), dandelion (*Taraxacum officinale*), emu oil, fenugreek (*Trigonella foenum-graecum*), garcinia (*Garcinia cambogia*) and hydroxycitric acid, garlic (*Allium sativum*), ginger (*Zingiber officinale*), gotu kola (*Centella asiatica*), hops (*Humulus lupulus*), hydrotherapy, iron, kava (*Piper methysticum*), Kundalini yoga, licorice (*Glycyrrhiza glabra*) and deglycyrrhizinated licorice, magnet therapy, meditation, melatonin, methysulfonylmethane, muira puama (*Ptychopetalum olacoides*), oregano (*Origanum vulgare*), peppermint (*Mentha piperita*), physical therapy, polarity, pomegranate (*Punica granatum*), prayer, probiotics, raspberry (*Rubus idaeus*), resveratrol, S-adenosyl-L-methionine, selenium, tansy (*Tanacetum vulgare*), turmeric (*Curcuma longa*), uva ursi (*Arctostaphylos uva-ursi*), valerian (*Valeriana officinalis*), yarrow (*Achillea millefolium*), yoga, and zinc.

PREVENTION AND SELF-MANAGEMENT

Fortunately, many of the signs and symptoms associated with women's hormonal imbalances are temporary. Take these steps to help reduce or prevent the unwanted symptoms of menopause.

Decreasing Hot Flashes: Hot flashes are caused by rapid decreases in estrogen levels. Unfortunately, hot flashes cannot be prevented. However, they can be helped and made less uncomfortable. Techniques that can help individuals deal with hot flashes include wearing loose clothing and dressing in layers so the layers of clothing can be peeled off during a hot flash; wearing fabrics that absorb moisture and dry quickly; avoiding foods that may trigger hot flashes, such as hot drinks and spicy foods; splashing the face with cool water at the start of a flash; and avoiding stress.

Decreasing Vaginal Discomfort: Using over-the-counter water-based vaginal lubricants (Astroglide, K-Y) or moisturizers (Replens, Vagisil) can help relieve vaginal dryness associated with low estrogen levels such as in menopause. Staying sexually active also helps with dryness.

Optimizing Sleep: Healthcare professionals recommend avoiding caffeine, especially in the evening and at night. Exercise (during the day) can also help improve sleep. Relaxation techniques, such as deep breathing, guided imagery, and progressive muscle relaxation, can be very helpful.

Strengthening Pelvic Muscles: Pelvic floor muscle exercises, called Kegel exercises, can improve some forms of urinary incontinence. The exercises consist of the regular clenching and unclenching of the sex muscles that form part of the pelvic floor (sometimes called the Kegel muscles).

Eating Well: Eating a balanced diet that includes a variety of fruits, vegetables, and whole grains and that limits saturated fats, oils, and sugars is recommended by healthcare professionals. It is also recommended to consume 1,200-1,500 milligrams of elemental calcium and 800 IU (international units) of vitamin D a day. Eating smaller, more frequent meals each day may reduce bloating and the sensation of fullness. A high-protein diet or high coffee consumption increases calcium excretion and may increase the calcium needs for the body. Fiber, oxalates (in rhubarb, spinach, beets, celery, greens, berries, nuts, tea, cocoa), and high zinc foods (such as oysters and red meats) decrease absorption, requiring more calcium as a dietary supplement. The plant estrogens found in soy help maintain bone density and may reduce the risk of fractures, particularly in the first 10 years after menopause. It is recommended to limit salt and salty foods to reduce bloating and fluid retention; choose foods high in complex carbohydrates, such as fruits, vegetables, and whole grains; and choose foods rich in calcium. If the woman cannot tolerate dairy products or is not getting adequate calcium in the diet, a daily calcium supplement may be needed. Excessive alcohol has been associated with osteoporosis due to the degenerative metabolic effects of alcohol. Alcohol excess may inhibit calcium absorption and bone formation.

Weight Control: Being underweight is a risk factor for osteoporosis. Staying within a healthy weight is important for individuals experiencing menopause.

Smoking Cessation: Smoking increases the risk of heart disease, stroke, osteoporosis, cancer, and a range of other health problems. It may also increase hot flashes and bring on earlier menopause. It is never too late to benefit from stopping smoking. Smokers lose bone more rapidly than nonsmokers. Among 80-year-olds, smokers have up to 10% lower bone mineral density, which translates into twice the risk of spinal fractures and a 50% increase in risk of hip fracture. Fractures heal slower in smokers and are more apt to heal improperly.

Regular Exercise: It is recommended by healthcare professionals to get at least 30 minutes of moderate-intensity physical activity on most days to protect against cardiovascular disease, diabetes, osteoporosis, and other conditions associated with aging in women. More vigorous exercise for longer periods may provide further benefit and is particularly important if the individual is trying to lose weight. Exercise can also help reduce stress.

Regular Checkups: A doctor can advise the individual about mammograms, Pap tests, lipid level (cholesterol and triglyceride) testing, and other screening tests.

M

MIGRAINE

CONDITIONS: Migraine, Tension Headache, Cluster Headache

BACKGROUND

A migraine is not just headache pain. Migraine is thought to be a genetic neurological disease characterized by flare-ups often called "migraine attacks" or "migraine episodes." A headache can be one symptom of a migraine attack. Some individuals with migraine disease often have migraine attacks without having a headache. Migraine attacks, or episodes, occur in phases or parts. A typical migraine attack consists of four phases. Not every individual experiencing a migraine has all four phases. The four phases of a migraine attack are prodrome, aura, headache, and postdrome (see Signs and Symptoms). Individuals suffering from migraines tend to have recurring attacks triggered by a lack of food or sleep, certain food allergies, exposure to light, or hormonal changes in women, including puberty, menopause, and premenstrual syndrome (PMS). Anxiety, stress, or relaxation after stress can also be triggers. Exposure to a trigger does not always lead to a headache. Conversely, avoidance of triggers cannot completely prevent headaches. Different migraine sufferers respond to different triggers, and any one trigger will not induce a headache in every person who has migraine headaches. Attacks tend to become less severe as the migraine sufferer ages. The uncertainty of when attacks may occur leads to additional patient anxiety. Symptoms, incidence, and severity of migraine headaches vary by individual.

Migraine headaches are the second most common type of primary headache. An estimated 28 million people in the United States (about 12% of the population) will experience migraine headaches at one time in their lives. In the United States, migraine headaches often go undiagnosed or are misdiagnosed as tension or sinus headaches. As a result, many migraine sufferers do not receive effective treatment. Treatments for migraine attacks involve prevention of the attack and treatment of acute (immediate) symptoms such as the headache.

TYPES OF HEADACHES

A headache is pain in occurring in the head. There are two types of headaches: primary headaches and secondary headaches. Primary headaches are not associated with (caused by) other diseases. Examples of primary headaches are migraine headaches, tension headaches, and cluster headaches. Secondary headaches are caused by associated disease, such as brain tumors. The associated disease may be minor or serious and life threatening. Seven in 10 people have at least one type of headache a year.

Migraine Headaches

Migraine with Aura: Migraine with aura is a migraine headache characterized by a neurological (nervous system) experience originating in the brain called an aura. Most auras appear as bright shimmering lights around objects (halos) or at the edges of the field of vision (called scintillating scotomas), zigzag lines, wavy images, or other visual hallucinations. Other individuals may experience temporary vision loss. An aura is usually experienced 10-30 minutes before the headache. Nonvisual auras include muscle weakness, speech or language abnormalities, dizziness, and paresthesia (tingling or numbness) of the face, tongue, or extremities.

Migraine without Aura: Migraine without aura, or "silent" migraine, is the most prevalent type of migraine headache and may occur on one or both sides of the head. Tiredness or mood changes may be experienced the day before the headache. Nausea, vomiting, and sensitivity to light (also called photophobia) often accompany migraine without aura.

Basilar Migraine: Basilar migraine or basilar artery migraine, involves a disturbance of the basilar artery (blood vessel) in the brainstem. Symptoms include severe headache, vertigo (dizziness), double vision, slurred speech, and poor muscle coordination. Basilar migraines pain is usually bilateral, or on both sides of the head. This type occurs in any age, but mostly occurs in females.

Carotidynia: Carotidynia is also called lower-half headache or facial migraine. It produces deep, dull, aching, and sometimes piercing pain in the jaw or neck. There is usually tenderness and swelling over the carotid artery (blood vessel) in the neck. Episodes can occur several times weekly and last a few minutes to hours. This type occurs more commonly in older people.

Headache-Free Migraine: A headache-free migraine is characterized by the presence of aura without a headache. This occurs in patients with a history of migraine with aura.

Ophthalmoplegic Migraine: Ophthalmoplegic migraine begins with a headache felt in the eye and is accompanied by vomiting. As the headache progresses, the eyelid droops (ptosis), and the nerves

298

responsible for eye movement become paralyzed. Eyelid dropping may persist for days or weeks.

Status Migraine: Status migraine is a rare type involving intense pain that usually lasts longer than 72 hours. The patient may require hospitalization.

Other Primary Headaches

Tension Headaches: Tension headaches are the most common type of primary headache. As many as 90% of adults have had or will have tension headaches. Tension headaches are more common among women than men, possibly due to hormonal changes. Tension headaches often begin in the back of the head and upper neck as a band-like tightness or pressure. Tension headaches also are described as a band of pressure surrounding the head with the most intense pain over the eyebrows. The pain of tension headaches usually is mild (not disabling) and bilateral (affecting both sides of the head). Tension headaches are not associated with an aura or visual disturbances, and the patient normally has proper vision. Tension headaches are seldom associated with nausea, vomiting, or sensitivity to light and sound. Tension headaches usually occur sporadically (infrequently and without a pattern) but can occur frequently and even daily in some people. Most people are able to function despite their tension headaches. Tension headaches do not have a clear cause. Many healthcare professionals attribute tension headaches to excess stress during daily activities and anxiety.

Cluster Headaches: Cluster headaches are headaches that come in groups and last weeks or months, separated by pain-free periods of months or years. During the period in which the cluster headaches occur, pain typically occurs once or twice daily, but some patients may experience pain more than twice daily. Each episode of pain lasts from 30 minutes to one and one-half hours. Attacks tend to occur at about the same time every day and often awaken the patient at night from a sound sleep. The pain typically is excruciating and located unilaterally around or behind one eye. Some patients describe the pain as feeling like a hot poker in the eye. The affected eye may become red, inflamed, and watery. The nose on the affected side may become congested and runny. Unlike patients with migraine headaches, patients with cluster headaches tend to be restless. They often pace the floor, bang their heads against a wall, and can be driven to desperate measures. Cluster headaches are much more common in males than females. Cluster headaches do not have a clear cause, although alcohol and cigarettes can precipitate attacks. Many healthcare professionals believe that cluster and migraine headaches share a common cause that begins in the nerve that carries sensation from the head to the brain (trigeminal nerve) and ends with the blood vessels that surround the brain dilating (widening) and contracting (narrowing), which causes pain. Others believe that the pain arises in the deep vascular channels in the head and does not involve the trigeminal nerve. Cluster headaches are a rare type of primary headache, affecting 0.1% of the population. An estimated 85% of cluster headache sufferers are men. The average age of cluster headache sufferers is 28-30, although headaches may begin in childhood.

Secondary Headaches

Secondary headaches are headaches caused by conditions other than those related to primary headaches, such as migraine. Secondary headaches have diverse causes, ranging from serious and life-threatening conditions such as intracranial hemorrhage (bleeding within the skull), cerebral venous sinus thrombosis (blood clot within the membrane that covers the brain), cerebral stroke or infarct (lack of oxygen to the brain causing neurological damage), cerebral aneurysm (bulging blood vessel in the brain), Lyme disease (a bacterial disease from ticks), excess cerebrospinal fluid in the brain (hydrocephalus), meningitis (inflammation of the membranes of the brain or spinal cord), low level of cerebral spinal fluid, nasal sinus blockage, postictal headache (occurs after a stroke or seizure), temporomandibular joint dysfunction, and brain tumor. Secondary headache pain can vary in severity.

Less serious but common conditions may also cause headaches, such as withdrawal from caffeine and the discontinuation of pain medications. Overuse of pain relievers causes the pain relievers to become less effective. As the effect of the pain reliever wears off, headaches recur (rebound headache). These drugs include over-the-counter (OTC) or prescription pain relievers, such as acetaminophen (Tylenol), ibuprofen (Advil, Motrin), or opiates such as oxycodone (Percocet, OxyContin) and hydrocodone (Lortab, Vicodin). Medications such as estrogen, progestins, calcium channel blockers (commonly used for treating high blood pressure), and selective serotonin reuptake inhibitors (commonly used to treat depression) can cause secondary headaches. Individuals with a subarachnoid hemorrhage typically report having a sudden onset of severe headache. The pain of recurrent migraine headaches tends to build up gradually. Sometimes the headache of subarachnoid hemorrhage is triggered by exertion, such as exercise or sex. Musculoskeletal problems,

M

such as injuries or poor posture, can cause or contribute to headaches such as tension and migraine headaches. Headaches soon after trauma (injury) to the head may be caused by subdural (inner layer of the brain) or epidural (outer layer of the brain) hematomas (blood clots).

Headaches that persistently occur on the same side are often secondary headaches associated with conditions such as brain tumors or arteriovenous malformations (abnormal clusters of blood vessels in the brain).

Bacterial meningitis is a rapidly progressive and life-threatening disease with fever, headaches, stiff neck, and deterioration in mental function. Herpes simplex encephalitis (brain swelling caused by a herpes virus) is an infection of the brain that causes death of brain tissue. Symptoms include fever, headache, and deterioration in mental function. Early treatment with antibiotics and antiviral agents can decrease the extent of brain damage and improve survival.

Associated temporary weakness of the extremities or facial muscles can be symptoms of transient ischemic attacks (temporary lack of oxygen to the brain). Transient ischemic attacks are warning signals for future strokes that can cause permanent brain damage. Headache also can accompany strokes and intracerebral bleeding (bleeding into the brain).

RISK FACTORS AND CAUSES

Central Nervous System Disorder: The precise cause of a migraine attack is not completely understood. There appears to be general agreement, however, that a key element is change in the blood flow within the brain due to a variety of triggers. The most widely accepted theory suggests that a migraine attack is precipitated when pain-sensing nerve cells in the brain (called nociceptors) release chemicals called neuropeptides (nerve proteins) in response to stimulation of the trigeminal nerve system. At least one of the neurotransmitters (chemicals that transmit impulses to the brain), substance P, increases the pain sensitivity of other nearby nociceptors. Other neuropeptides act on the smooth muscle surrounding cranial (skull) blood vessels, causing inflammation. This smooth muscle regulates blood flow in the brain by causing vasodilation (relaxation of blood vessels) or vasoconstriction (contracting the blood vessel). At the onset of a migraine headache, neuropeptides are thought to cause muscle relaxation, allowing vessel dilation and increased blood flow. Other neuropeptides increase the permeability of cranial (skull) blood vessels, allowing fluid containing inflammatory chemicals to leak and promote inflammation and tissue

swelling. The pain of migraine is thought to result from this combination of increased pain sensitivity, tissue and vessel swelling, and inflammation.

Heredity: Susceptibility to migraine may be inherited. Children of migraine sufferers have as much as a 50% chance of developing a migraine attack in their lifetimes. If both parents are affected, the chance rises to 70%. However, the gene or genes responsible have not been identified. Genetics also increases the chances of having migraine attacks that are chronic (long term).

Neurotransmitters: Neurotransmitters are chemical messengers in the brain. Two important ones, serotonin and dopamine, appear to be critical in the processes leading to a migraine attack. Serotonin (also called 5-hydroxytryptamine) is involved in regulation of pain perception and mood, among other important functions. A number of studies have suggested that serotonin can stop the migraine process. To support this observation, higher-than-normal levels of a serotonin compound are excreted in urine and levels of serotonin in the blood drop during a migraine attack. Also, drugs that target receptors in the brain for serotonin are generally effective in stopping a migraine. The receptors for serotonin implicated in a migraine attack are found on the trigeminal nerve endings. Serotonin appears to block the peptides (including substance P) involved in overstimulating nerves and producing inflammation.

Dopamine, another important neurotransmitter, may act as a stimulant or accelerator of the migraine process. Some evidence suggests that certain genetic factors make people oversensitive to the effects of dopamine, which include nerve cell excitation. Such nerve cell overactivity could trigger the events in the brain leading to migraine. The prodromal symptoms (including mood changes, yawning, or drowsiness), for example, have been associated with increased dopamine activity. Dopamine receptors are also involved in regulation of blood flow in the brain, which may be of importance when dealing with vasoconstriction and vasodilation.

Calcium Channels: Some migraines may be due to abnormalities in the channels within cells that transport the electrical ions calcium, magnesium, sodium, and potassium. Calcium channels regulate the release of serotonin, an important neurotransmitter in the migraine process. Magnesium interacts with calcium channels, and magnesium deficiencies have been detected in the brains of migraine patients. Calcium channels also play a major role in cortical spreading depression, a brain event that includes a "wave" of nerve impulses (firing) that spreads across the surface of the brain, moving from the back (occipital region) of the cerebral cortex toward the front at about one-eighth to three-sixteenth inches (three to five millimeters) per minute. After the nerve excitation, a depression in nerve cell function occurs that can last for minutes. Cortical spreading depression is thought to be one of the causes of a migraine attack. Some individuals with migraine may inherit one or more factors that impair calcium channels, making them susceptible to headaches. For example, mutations in a gene that encodes calcium channels appears to be responsible for familial hemiplegic migraine.

Gender and Age: A migraine attack is three times more common in women than in men. Although the exact relationship between hormones and headaches is not clear, fluctuations in estrogen and progesterone seem to trigger headaches in many women with migraine headaches, including those with PMS and menopause. It seems to be hormonal fluctuations, or changes, that trigger migraine attacks, not the presence of the hormone. Prepubescent females, or females prior to reproductive maturity, can also suffer from migraines. Women with a history of migraines often have reported headaches immediately before or during their periods. Others report more migraines during pregnancy or menopause. Hormonal medications, such as oral contraceptives (birth control pills) and hormone replacement therapy (including estrogen and progesterone therapy), may also worsen migraines. In children younger than 10 years, boys appear to have migraines more often than girls. After puberty starts, migraine headaches are much more common in females (female-to-male ratio, 3:1), most likely due to hormonal changes.

In general, the rate of migraine occurrence in males drops to a low by age 28-29 years, with one case per 1,000 people in this age group. Migraine occurrence among females increases sharply up to age 40 years and then declines gradually. The age when migraine headache with aura begins appears to peak at or before age four to five years (6.6 cases per 1000 people in that age group), while the highest rate for migraine without aura occurs at age 10-11 years (10.1 cases per 1000 people in that age group). The severity and frequency of attacks tend to lessen with age. Data suggest that migraine attacks are a chronic (long-term) condition, although long remissions (illness-free periods) are common. One study showed that 62% of young adults were free of migraine headaches for more than two years, but only 40% continued to be free of them after 30 years.

Diet: Certain foods and beverages appear to trigger headaches in sensitive individuals. Common dietary triggers include alcohol (especially beer and red wine); aged cheeses, chocolate; fermented, pickled, or marinated foods (tofu, kim chee, miso); aspartame (an artificial sweetener); caffeine; monosodium glutamate (MSG, a key flavor enhancer in some Asian foods); and many canned and processed foods. Skipping meals or fasting also can trigger migraines. Eating proper food is very important in migraine prevention because a continuous supply of proper nutrients is essential to keeping chemical balance in the brain. Brain chemistry can be changed significantly by a single meal and, in turn, some changes in food composition can rapidly affect brain function. While all foods eaten modify brain function, some specifically alter mood or energy, such as caffeine or refined sugars. Eating unhealthy foods that do not supply adequate nutrients for proper brain function or foods that alter brain function can cause migraine attacks in susceptible individuals.

Magnesium Deficiency: Because levels of magnesium (a mineral involved in nerve cell function) also drop right before or during a migraine headache, it is possible that low amounts of magnesium may cause nerve cells in the brain to misfire. About 20% of the population consumes less than two-thirds of the recommended dietary allowance for magnesium.

Stress: A period of hard work followed by relaxation may lead to a weekend migraine headache. Acute (immediate) or chronic (long-term) stress at work or home also can set off a migraine.

Sensory Stimulus: Bright lights, sun glare, and unusual smells, including pleasant scents (such as perfume or flowers) and unpleasant odors (such as paint thinner and secondhand smoke), can trigger a migraine attack.

Physical Factors: Intense physical exertion, including sexual activity, may provoke migraines. Changes in sleep patterns, including too much or too little sleep, also can initiate a migraine headache. Sleep changes are usually seen in both adults and children with migraines. Healthcare professionals recommend eight hours of uninterrupted sleep nightly for adults. Sleep helps regulate certain neurochemicals (brain chemicals), including serotonin. Decreases in serotonin may cause a migraine attack.

Environmental Changes: A change of weather, season, altitude level, barometric pressure, or time zone can prompt a migraine headache. Environmental changes such as moving to a new area where the plants and pollens are different may also trigger a migraine attack.

Medications: Taking certain medications can aggravate migraines, including oral contraceptives (birth control pills), estrogen replacement therapy, nitrates (nitroglycerin), theophylline (Slo-Bid), reserpine (Serpasil), nifedipine (Procardia, Adalat), indomethacin (Indocin), cimetidine (Tagamet), decongestant overuse (such as pseudoephedrine or Sudafed), and antianxiety drug withdrawal, including alprazolam (Xanax) and diazepam (Valium). Caffeine withdrawal and the discontinuation of pain medications can trigger a migraine.

SIGNS AND SYMPTOMS

Prodrome: The prodrome (sometimes called preheadache) may be experienced hours or even days before a migraine attack. The prodrome is considered a warning sign for individuals suffering migraine attacks that an episode is imminent. For the 30-40% of individuals with migraines that experience prodrome, the warning signs can give the individuals opportunity to abort the migraine attack using conventional and integrative therapies. Symptoms typical of the prodrome include food cravings, constipation or diarrhea, mood changes (such as depression or irritability), muscle stiffness (especially in the neck), fatigue (excessive tiredness), and increased frequency of urination.

Aura: The aura is the most familiar of the phases. Auras are sensory phenomena that can follow the prodrome and usually last less than an hour. The symptoms and effects of the aura vary widely and include visual hallucinations (such as flashing lights, wavy lines, spots, partial loss of sight, blurry vision), olfactory hallucinations (smelling odors that are not there), tingling or numbness of the face or extremities on the side where the headache develops, difficult finding words and/or speaking, confusion, vertigo (dizziness), partial paralysis (loss of muscle coordination), auditory hallucinations (hearing noises that are not there), decrease in or loss of hearing, and reduced sensation or hypersensitivity to feel and touch. Approximately 20% of individuals with migraines experience aura. As with the prodrome, migraine aura can serve as a warning and sometimes allows the use of conventional or integrative therapies to abort the episode before the headache begins. Some individuals can experience aura without a headache, termed "silent" migraine.

Headache: The headache phase is generally the most unbearable part of a migraine episode. The effects of a headache are not limited to the head only, but affect the entire body. Migraine headaches usually are described as an intense, throbbing or pounding pain in the temple area, although the pain can be located in the forehead, around the eye, or the back of the head. The pain usually is on one side of the head (unilateral), although about a third of the time the pain is bilateral (both sides). Unilateral headaches typically change sides from one attack to the next. Although migraine headache pain can occur at any time of day, statistics have reported the most common time to be 6 a.m. It is not uncommon for individuals with a migraine headache to be awakened by the pain. The headache phase usually lasts from one to 72 hours. In less common cases where it lasts longer than 72 hours, it is termed status migrainosus, and medical attention should be sought. Symptoms of the headache phase of a migraine include pain worsened by physical activity, phonophobia (sensitivity to sound), photophobia (sensitivity to light), nausea and vomiting, diarrhea or constipation, nasal congestion and/or runny nose, depression or severe anxiety, hot flashes and chills, dizziness, confusion, and either dehydration or fluid retention, depending on the individual. The combination of disabling pain and symptoms such as nausea or vomiting often prevents sufferers from performing daily activities.

Postdrome: Once the headache is over, the migraine episode is still not over. The postdrome, or postheadache, follows immediately afterward. The majority of individuals with a migraine take hours to fully recover while others take days. Most individuals in a postdrome phase are fatigued (excessively tired) and have a "hangover" feeling. These feelings may often be attributed to medications taken to treat the migraine but may well be caused by the migraine itself. Postdromal symptoms have been shown to be accompanied and possibly caused by abnormal cerebral (brain) blood flow and altered electroencephalogram (a measure of brain electrical impulses) readings have been reported for up to 24 hours after the end of the headache stage. In cases where prodrome and/or aura are experienced without the headache phase, the postdrome may still occur. The symptoms of prodrome include decreased mood levels (especially depression) or feelings of well-being and euphoria, fatigue, poor concentration, and comprehension, and lowered intellect levels.

Migraine Headache Symptoms in Children: Migraines typically begin in childhood, adolescence, or early adulthood and, in general, may become less frequent and intense as the individual grows older. About half of all school-aged children in the United States have experienced some type of headache. During childhood, boys and girls suffer from migraine at about the same rate. However, during their adolescent years more girls are affected, most likely due to hormonal changes. Also, both aging men and women may suffer from secondary headaches, such as tension or cluster headaches, more often than children under 18 years of age.

Children's migraines tend to last for a shorter time, but the pain can be disabling and can be accompanied by nausea, vomiting, lightheadedness, and increased sensitivity to light. A migraine headache tends to occur on both sides of the head in children (bilateral), and visual auras are rare. Children often have premonition signs and symptoms, such as yawning, sleepiness or listlessness, and a craving for foods such as sugary foods and chocolate. Children may have all of the signs and symptoms of a migraine headache (nausea, vomiting, increased sensitivity to light and sound, aura) but no head pain. These migraines can be especially difficult to diagnose.

DIAGNOSIS

Diagnosis of a migraine headache is based on the history of symptoms, physical examination, and neurological (nerve) tests. The tests are performed to rule out other neurological and cerebrovascular (blood vessels in the brain) conditions, including bleeding within the skull (intracranial hemorrhage), blood clot within the membrane that covers the brain (cerebral venous sinus thrombosis), cerebral stroke or lack of oxygen to the brain (called an infarct), dilated blood vessel in the brain (cerebral aneurysm), excess cerebrospinal fluid in the brain (hydrocephalus), inflammation of the membranes of the brain or spinal cord (meningitis), low level of cerebral spinal fluid, nasal sinus blockage, postictal headache (occurs after a stroke or seizure), and brain tumor.

Computed Tomography (CT) Scan: A CT scan is an x-ray procedure that combines many x-ray images with the aid of a computer to generate cross-sectional views and, if needed, three-dimensional images of the internal organs and structures of the body. An intravenous (into the veins) dye is injected into the individual. Then the patient is placed under a large donut-shaped x-ray machine, which takes x-ray images at many different angles around the body. These images are processed by a computer to produce cross-sectional pictures of the body.

A CT scan is a very low-risk procedure. The most common problem is an adverse reaction to intravenous contrast material. Intravenous contrast is usually an iodine-based liquid given in the vein, which makes many organs and structures, such as the brain and blood vessels, much more visible on the CT scan. There may be resulting itching, a rash, hives, or a feeling of warmth throughout the body. These are usually self-limiting reactions and go away rather quickly. If needed, antihistamines

(such as diphenhydramine [Benadryl]) can be given by injection or orally to help relieve the symptoms. A more serious reaction to intravenous contrast is called an anaphylactic reaction. When this occurs, the patient may experience severe hives and/or extreme difficulty in breathing. This reaction is quite rare but is potentially life threatening if not treated. Medications taken to reverse this adverse reaction may include corticosteroids (steroids, such as prednisone [Deltasone]), antihistamines, and epinephrine. In migraine patients, a CT scan is performed to rule out an underlying brain abnormality, such as a tumor, when migraines are new or when there is a change in their character or frequency. CT scans may not be as reliable as newer diagnostic techniques, such as magnetic resonance imaging, but are less expensive.

Electroencephalogram (EEG): An EEG records electrical signals originating in the brain (called brain activity). This test is used to detect malfunctions in brain activity, such as seizures or migraines. EEGs are generally performed in a hospital or specialized laboratory. Sometimes the individual having the test will be told to stay up late the night before and to avoid caffeine drinks on the morning of the test. Some EEG tests are made with the patient sitting in a chair. Others are performed with the patient lying down on a couch. The EEG technologist applies small metal disks to several places on the scalp. The hair should be washed on the morning of the test with no additional chemicals, hair sprays, cleansers, cosmetics, or setting gels applied. A special glue, which is washed out afterwards, is used to attach the electrode disks to the scalp. A cap with the wires already attached may be used instead of the glue.

During the test, the technologist may ask the person to breathe deeply through the mouth for a short time. This may make the person feel slightly dizzy or produce a numb feeling in the hands or feet, but this goes away when normal breathing is started again. The technologist may shine a blinking light into the person's eyes, or ask him or her to open and close them rapidly a few times. The average EEG test may last 35-40 minutes. Children should be told what to expect during an EEG test and can be encouraged to "practice" on a doll or stuffed animal beforehand.

Lumbar Puncture: Lumbar puncture, or spinal tap, is performed to detect infection and determine levels of white blood cells (immune system cells), glucose, and protein in the cerebrospinal fluid. This test involves withdrawing a small amount of fluid from the spinal cord area and examining it under a microscope. The individual lies down on their side on an examination table. There are steps to make sure that the individual does not feel pain during the spinal tap. A topical anesthesia cream (such as EMLA) is applied on the skin of the back where the spinal tap will be performed (about 30 minutes to one hour before). After the skin is numbed, some doctors also inject liquid anesthesia such as lidocaine into the tissues right under the skin to prevent any further pain. Next, the doctor places a small needle through the skin and then forward through the space between the vertebrae (spine) in the lower back until it enters the space that contains the spinal fluid. When the needle goes into the skin, the individual will not feel sharp pain, only perhaps some pressure. The spinal fluid drips out through the needle into tubes, is collected, and sent to a lab for analysis. This procedure can be uncomfortable for the patient. Side effects can be headaches, pain, infection, or bleeding. Each of these complications is uncommon with the exception of headache, which can appear from hours to up to a day after LP. Headaches occur less frequently when the patient remains lying flat for one to three hours after the procedure. Patients may be given pain medications (such as morphine) or sedatives (such as alprazolam [Xanax]) before and after the procedure. These drugs can cause drowsiness or sedation and can lead to physical dependence.

Magnetic Resonance Imaging (MRI): An MRI can is a radiology technique that uses magnetism, radio waves, and a computer to produce images of body structures. The MRI scanner is a tube surrounded by a giant circular magnet. The patient is placed on a moveable bed that is inserted into the magnet. The patient may be given a sedative, such as alprazolam (Xanax), to decrease anxiety and stress associated with the procedure. The image and resolution produced by MRI is quite detailed and can detect tiny changes of structures within the body. An MRI in patient's with migraines may be performed for a more complete evaluation of the brain and can visualize blood vessels in the brain to detect aneurysms (tears in blood vessels) and other vascular abnormalities that can be causative agents in migraines.

TREATMENT

Many factors may contribute to the occurrence of migraine attacks, including diet, sleep, hormonal changes, changes in brain chemistry, and heredity. They are known as trigger factors. When identified, avoidance of trigger factors reduces the number of headaches a patient may experience. Trigger factors may be targets of drug therapy also.

Treatment for migraine attacks is divided into two categories, including acute (immediate) or prophylactic (preventative). Acute treatment is used during a migraine to stop or slow the progress of the attack, and preventative (or prophylactic) treatment tries to prevent migraine attacks from occurring.

Preventive (Prophylactic)

Preventative medication may be prescribed for patients who have frequent migraine attacks (three or more a month), those who do not respond consistently to acute treatment, and when specific medicines are contraindicated because of other medical conditions (such as stroke or bleeding in the brain). Studies have reported that as many as 40% of these patients may benefit from preventative treatment. The U.S. Food and Drug Administration (FDA) has approved four prescription drugs for migraine prevention. These include the beta-blockers propranolol (Inderal) and timolol (Blocadren), and the anticonvulsants topiramate (Topamax) and divalproex sodium (Depakote).

Anticonvulsants: Anticonvulsant medicines, normally used for seizures, have been used to prevent migraine headaches. Examples of anticonvulsants that have been used are valproic acid (Depakote, Depakote ER, Depakene), phenobarbital, gabapentin (Neurontin), and topiramate (Topamax). Control of the cortical spreading depression is thought to be the reason for anticonvulsant effectiveness in preventing migraine attacks. Side effects include fatigue (tiredness), nausea, vomiting, and trembling.

Beta-Blockers: Beta-blockers are a class of drugs that safely slow the heartbeat and decrease blood pressure. Beta-blockers have been used for many years to prevent migraine headaches. In migraine prevention, beta-blockers help dilate (open) blood vessels in the brain, which may prevent the vascular (blood vessel) symptoms associated with a migraine attack, including vasoconstriction (blood vessel narrowing) and vasodilation (blood vessel widening). Beta-blockers can also help reduce physical symptoms associated with migraine attacks, such as anxiety, heart palpitations, and shaking.

Beta-blockers used in migraine prevention include propranolol (Inderal), atenolol (Tenormin), metoprolol (Lopressor, Toprol XL), and nadolol (Corgard). Beta-blockers generally are well tolerated in most individuals. They can aggravate breathing difficulties in patients with asthma, chronic bronchitis (inflammation of the bronchial tubes), or emphysema (loss of lung function). In patients who already have slow heart rates (bradycardia) and heart block (defects in electrical conduction within the heart), beta-blockers can cause dangerously slow heartbeats. Beta-blockers can aggravate symptoms of heart failure. Other side effects include drowsiness, diarrhea, constipation, fatigue (tiredness), insomnia, nausea, depression, dreaming, memory loss, and impotence (loss of sexual performance).

Calcium Channel Blockers (CCBs): CCBs are a class of drugs normally used for high blood pressure, angina (chest pain), and arrhythmias (abnormal heart rhythms). CCBs also appear to alter serotonin (a brain chemical). Serotonin imbalances are a causative factor in developing a migraine. CCBs used in preventing migraine headaches are diltiazem (Cardizem, Dilacor, Tiazac), and verapamil (Calan, Verelan, Isoptin). The most common side effects of CCBs are constipation, nausea, headache, rash, edema (swelling of the legs with fluid), low blood pressure, drowsiness, and dizziness. Drinking grapefruit juice or eating grapefruit may cause levels of CCBs to rise, potentially leading to life-threatening arrhythmias (irregular heartbeats). Healthcare professionals recommend that individuals taking CCBs not consume grapefruit juice.

Hormone Replacement Therapy (HRT): For women with hormonal imbalances that may be causing the migraines, HRT may be used, including estrogen and progesterone. HRT, however, may cause side effects such as blood clots, an increased risk of developing some types of cancers, and heart disease. Menstruating women at risk for migraines may be placed on oral contraceptives for HRT. Prepubescent girls who are at risk for migraine attacks will not be treated with HRT but with other methods such as beta-blockers and anticonvulsants.

Lifestyle: Lifestyle changes, including decreasing stress levels, increasing exercise levels, and controlling the diet, have a major impact on migraine prevention and development. Lifestyle factors that are important in the prevention of migraines include regular sleep patterns, regular exercise (level depends upon the individual), limiting stress, limiting caffeine consumption to less than two caffeine-containing beverages a day, avoiding bright or flashing lights, and wearing sunglasses if sunlight is a trigger. Identifying and avoiding foods that trigger headaches is important. Healthcare professionals recommend keeping a food journal, where individuals write down everything they have for each meal of the day. Then review the diary with a healthcare professional. It is impractical to adopt a diet that avoids all known migraine triggers; however, it is reasonable to avoid foods that consistently trigger migraine headaches. Triggers vary from one individual to another.

Tricyclic Antidepressants (TCAs): TCAs are thought to prevent migraine headaches by altering the balance of serotonin, a neurotransmitter in the brain. Low levels of serotonin are thought to be a causative agent in migraine attacks. Chronic stress and depression can cause elevated levels of the stress hormone cortisol, which is produced in the adrenal glands. Cortisol can in turn cause imbalances in serotonin, leading to a migraine attack. The tricyclic antidepressants that have been used in preventing migraine headaches include amitriptyline (Elavil), nortriptyline (Pamelor, Aventyl), doxepin (Sinequan), and imipramine (Tofranil). Side effects include constipation, dry mouth, low blood pressure (hypotension), increased heart rate, (tachycardia), urinary retention, sexual dysfunction, and weight gain. TCAs may cause excessive sedation and fatigue (tiredness).

Others: Other drugs less commonly used for migraine prevention include antiserotonin medications, including methysergide (Sansert), which prevent migraine headaches by constricting (making smaller) blood vessels and reducing inflammation of the blood vessels. Cyproheptadine (Periactin) is an antihistamine that increases serotonin activity and is used occasionally in migraine prevention. Low levels of serotonin are a cause of migraine attacks.

Acute (Immediate)

OTC Treatments: The FDA has approved three OTC products to treat migraine attacks. Excedrin Migraine (a combination of aspirin, acetaminophen, and caffeine) is indicated for migraine and its associated symptoms such as head pain. Advil Migraine and Motrin Migraine Pain (both are ibuprofen) have antiinflammatory action and are approved to treat migraine headache and its pain.

Triptans: The triptans attach to serotonin receptors on the blood vessels and nerves and thereby reduce inflammation and constrict (narrow) the blood vessels. A reduction in inflammation decreases pressure on nerves in the trigeminal nerve system (nerves in the cranium or head), which decreases the pain signals to the brain and stops the headache. Traditionally, triptans, which are prescription medicines, were prescribed for moderate or severe migraines after OTC analgesics such as ibuprofen (Advil) and other simple measures failed. Newer studies suggest that triptans can be used as the first treatment for patients with migraines that are causing disability. Significant disability is defined as more than 10 days of at least 50% disability during a three-month period.

Triptans should be used early after the migraine begins, before the onset of pain or when the pain

M

is mild. Using a triptan early in an attack increases its effectiveness, reduces side effects, and decreases the chance of recurrence of another headache during the following 24 hours. Used early, triptans can be expected to abort more than 80% of migraine headaches within two hours. Triptans include sumatriptan (Imitrex), almotriptan (Axert), naratriptan (Amerge), rizatriptan (Maxalt), zolmitriptan (Zomig), frovatriptan (Frova), and eletriptan (Relpax).

The most common side effects of triptans are facial flushing, tingling of the skin, and a sense of tightness around the chest and throat. Other less common side effects include drowsiness, fatigue (tiredness), and dizziness. These side effects are short lived and are not considered serious. Triptans are not used in pregnant women and are not generally used in young children.

In patients with severe nausea, a combination of a triptan and an antinausea medication, such as prochlorperazine (Compazine), may be used.

Ergots: Ergots, like triptans, are medications that abort migraine headaches. Examples of ergots include ergotamine preparations (Cafergot) and dihydroergotamine preparations (Migranal, DHE-45). Ergots, like triptans, cause constriction (narrowing) of blood vessels, but ergots tend to cause more constriction of vessels in the heart and other parts of the body than the triptans, and they produce more negative effects on the heart than the triptans. Therefore, the ergots are not as safe as the triptans. Ergots are used to help stop the vasodilation (blood vessel widening) associated with a migraine attack. The ergots also are more prone to cause nausea and vomiting than the triptans. The ergots can cause prolonged contraction of the uterus and miscarriages in pregnant women.

Midrin: Midrin is used to abort migraine and tension headaches. It is a combination of isometheptene (a blood vessel constrictor), acetaminophen (a pain reliever), and dichloralphenazone (a mild sedative). The combination medication can help take care of three potential factors associated with a migraine attack: vasodilation, pain, and anxiety. Midrin is most effective if used early during a headache. However, because of its potent blood vessel constricting effect, it should not be used in patients with high blood pressure, kidney disease, glaucoma (increased pressure in the eyes), atherosclerosis (hardening of the arteries), or liver disease or in patients taking monoamine oxidase inhibitors, including phenelzine (Nardil), isocarboxazid (Marplan), and tranylcypromine sulfate (Parnate).

Other Prescription Medications: Some attacks may not be eliminated by acute therapy, and the individual requires pain-relieving measures. Due to the severity of the headaches, some patients may require a narcotic analgesic, including oxycodone (Percocet), codeine, or meperidine (Demerol). If the individual is experiencing frequent migraine attacks, the habitual use of opiate analgesics should be avoided. Opiates can cause addiction (both physical and mental) and may also cause rebound headaches, which are headaches that occur when the pain medicine no longer provides relief.

Butorphanol (Stadol NS) is an opiatelike drug available for injection and intranasal (in the nose) administration. The normal dosage of Stadol NS is one spray into the nostril, which usually relieves migraine symptoms in 15-30 minutes. This drug can be used every hour for relief. The use of Stadol NS may result in dependency if used regularly for pain relief. Side effects include nausea and vomiting, nasal irritation, and sedation.

Butalbital, a barbiturate medication, is also used for the immediate relief of migraine headache pain. It is used in various prescription combinations with aspirin, acetaminophen, caffeine, or codeine (an opiate pain medication). These medications are potentially addicting and are not used as initial treatment. They are sometimes used for patients whose headaches fail to respond to OTC medications but who are not candidates for triptans, either due to pregnancy or the risk of heart attack and stroke. Products include butalbital and acetaminophen (Axocet, Bupap, Cephadyn, Phrenilin or Sedapap); butalbital, acetaminophen, and caffeine (Fioricet, Esgic); butalbital and aspirin (Axotal); butalbital, aspirin, and caffeine (Fiorinal); butalbital, acetaminophen, caffeine, and codeine (Fioricet #3 with Codeine or Fioricet with Codeine); and butalbital, aspirin, caffeine, and codeine (Fiorinal #3 with Codeine or Fiorinal with Codeine).

INTEGRATIVE THERAPIES

Good Scientific Evidence

5-Hydroxytryptophan (5-HTP): Supplement use of 5-HTP may help balance serotonin in the body. Serotonin is the brain chemical associated with sleep, mood, movement, eating, and nervousness. There is evidence from several studies in both children and adults that 5-HTP may be effective in reducing the severity and frequency of headaches, including tension headaches and migraines. Fewer pain-relieving medications may be needed when taken with 5-HTP; however, many of the available studies show that more proven pharmaceutical drugs may work better than 5-HTP for headaches. Further research is needed. 5-HTP is generally safe when used in recommended dosages. Use with caution if taking antidepressant medications.

Butterbur: Butterbur (*Petasites hybridus*) is a perennial shrub found throughout Europe as well as parts of Asia and North America. Pain relief and headache prevention are traditional uses of butterbur. Recent preclinical studies suggest antiinflammatory and vasodilatory (blood vessel opening) properties of butterbur, thereby supporting a possible mechanism of action. A small number of human trials report efficacy of butterbur for migraine prevention when taken regularly for up to four months. This evidence is compelling enough to suggest benefits of butterbur for migraine prevention, although additional evidence from larger, well-designed studies is necessary. The use of butterbur during pregnancy and lactation should be avoided due to a lack of safety studies. Butterbur should not be used if there is an allergy to plants in the Aster family, including ragweed, marigolds, daisies, and chrysanthemums.

Chiropractic: Chiropractic is a healthcare discipline that focuses on the relationship between musculoskeletal structure (primarily the spine) and body function (as coordinated by the nervous system) and how this relationship affects the preservation and restoration of health. Manipulation is the skilled, gentle, passive movement of a joint (or spinal segment) either within or beyond its active range of motion. The use of spinal manipulative therapy for the relief of tension or migraine headache has been reported in several controlled human trials and systematic reviews. Overall, the quality of studies is not high, with incomplete reporting of design, inconsistent use of techniques between studies, and variable results. Despite these methodological problems, overall the evidence suggests some benefits in the prevention of episodic tension headache. Effects on migraine headache have not been demonstrated. Better-quality research is necessary in this area before a firm conclusion can be drawn.

Feverfew: Feverfew (*Tanacetum parthenium*) leaves have long been used orally for the treatment or prevention of headache, and there is a scientific basis for this use. Preclinical studies have reported antiinflammatory and blood vessel dilation (opening) effects. Several controlled human trials have been conducted in this area with mixed results. Overall, these studies suggest that feverfew taken daily as standardized capsules may reduce the incidence of attacks in patients who experience chronic migraine headaches. Feverfew may cause an increase in bleeding and drug interactions. Do not use feverfew if pregnant or nursing, or if allergic to plants in the aster family, including ragweed, marigolds, daisies, and chrysanthemums.

Guided Imagery: The term guided imagery may be used to refer to a number of techniques, including metaphor, story telling, fantasy, game playing, dream interpretation, drawing, visualization, active imagination, or direct suggestion using imagery. Therapeutic guided imagery may be used by therapists to help patients relax and focus on images associated with personal issues they are confronting. Initial research suggests that guided imagery may provide added benefits when used at the same time as standard medical care for migraine or tension headache.

Hypnotherapy: Hypnotherapy involves the power of suggestion while the individual is in a deep, relaxed state. Several studies report improvements in severity and frequency of tension headaches following several weekly hypnosis sessions. Early research suggests that hypnosis may be equivalent to other relaxation techniques, biofeedback, or autogenic training.

Unclear or Conflicting Scientific Evidence

Acupressure: Acupressure, or shiatsu, has been used in China and Japan for thousands of years for health and healing. Self-administered acupressure (in the temple region or others) is reported to help tension or migraine headaches in early studies.

Acupuncture: Acupuncture, or the use of needles to manipulate the "chi," or body energy, originated in China over 5,000 years ago. Although traditionally used to help patients with migraine headaches, there is inconclusive evidence in support of acupuncture for chronic migraine or tension headache. Although the majority of available studies have shown a trend in favor of acupuncture over placebo, most have been small and methodologically flawed. Blinding and follow-up have not been adequate in most studies, and approaches to placebo control are variable. Larger trials with clear blinding and controls are necessary before a recommendation can be made for or against acupuncture for this indication.

L-Arginine: L-arginine, or arginine, is a semi-essential amino acid needed by the body. Arginine is a precursor of nitric oxide, which causes blood vessel relaxation (vasodilation). Preliminary studies suggest that adding arginine to ibuprofen (Advil, Motrin) therapy may decrease migraine headache pain. Arginine is generally regarded as safe in recommended dosages.

Coenzyme Q10 (CoQ10): CoQ10 is produced by the human body and is necessary for the basic functioning of cells. There is promising good evidence from one randomized, controlled trial and one open-label trial to support the use of CoQ10 in migraine prevention or treatment. Properly designed, larger trials of longer treatment duration are needed to confirm these findings. CoQ10 is generally regarded as safe in recommended dosages.

Gamma-Linolenic Acid (GLA): GLA is a dietary omega-6 fatty acid found in many plant oil extracts. One open-label, uncontrolled study has examined the effect of fatty acids, including GLA, on severity, frequency and duration of migraine attacks. Better-designed clinical trials are required before recommendations can be made. Eighty-six percent of patients experienced a reduction in the severity, frequency, and duration of migraine attacks, while 90% of patients had reduced nausea and vomiting. GLA use may increase the chances of bleeding.

Melatonin: Melatonin is a natural hormone that is used for the improvement of sleep patterns. Several small studies have examined the possible role of melatonin in preventing various forms of headache, including migraine, cluster, and tension-type headache (in people who suffer from regular headaches). Limited initial research suggests possible benefits in all three types of headache, although well-designed controlled studies are needed before a firm conclusion can be drawn. Melatonin should not be used for extended periods of time. Caution is advised when taking melatonin supplements as numerous adverse effects including drug interactions are possible. Melatonin is not recommended during pregnancy or breastfeeding unless otherwise directed by a doctor.

Progressive Muscle Relaxation: Progressive muscle relaxation involves isolating one muscle group, creating tension for eight to 10 seconds, and then letting the muscle relax and the tension go. Individuals can sit (in a comfortable chair), lie on a bed, or lie on the floor (on a comfortable rug or carpet). Muscle groups (including the head, shoulders, arms, hands, stomach, legs, and feet), one at a time, are tensed, then relaxed. This technique has been reported effective in headache prevention, but more studies are needed.

Reflexology: Reflexology involves the application of manual pressure to specific points or areas of the feet that are believed to correspond to other parts of the body. Early research suggests that reflexology may relieve pain from migraine or tension headaches and that pain medication requirements may be reduced. However, study in this area has not been well designed or reported scientifically, and further evidence is necessary before a firm conclusion can be reached.

Relaxation Therapy: Relaxation techniques include behavioral therapeutic approaches that differ widely in philosophy, methodology, and practice. The primary goal is usually nondirected relaxation. Most techniques share the components of repetitive focus (on a word, sound, prayer phrase, body sensation, or muscular activity), adoption of a passive attitude towards intruding thoughts, and return to the focus. Preliminary evidence suggests that relaxation techniques may be helpful for the reduction of migraine headache symptoms in adults. Study of relaxation in children with headaches has yielded unclear results. Additional research is necessary before a firm conclusion can be drawn.

Riboflavin (vitamin B$_2$): Several studies suggest benefits of high-dose riboflavin in preventing migraine headaches. Further research is necessary before a firm conclusion can be drawn.

Soy: Soy (*Glycine max*) is a plant in the pea family (Fabaceae) and is native to southeastern Asia. Soy has been a dietary staple in Asian countries for at least 5,000 years. Soy supplements have been reported to help with symptoms associated with menopause, including headache. One study of a phytoestrogen (plant estrogen) combination showed a reduced number of migraine attacks suffered. Further research is needed. Use of soy supplements may cause drug interactions. Soy should not be used if the patient is pregnant or breastfeeding unless otherwise directed by a doctor. Until better research is available, it remains unclear if dietary soy or soy isoflavone supplements increase or decrease the risk of developing breast cancer.

Transcutaneous Electrical Nerve Stimulation (TENS): TENS is a noninvasive technique in which a low-voltage electrical current is delivered through wires from a small power unit to electrodes located on the skin. Acupuncturists can use TENS by sticking Japanese acupuncture needles into two sites and taping the needles down with surgical tape to prevent them from moving. Practitioners then hook the needles up to a TENS device and an electrical current is applied. The current now travels into the needles, which stimulates points on the body to get the "chi," or energy, to flow in a healthy manner. Preliminary controlled trials suggest that TENS may have some benefits in patients with migraine or chronic headache. Additional well-designed research is necessary before a firm conclusion can be reached in this area.

Therapeutic Touch: Therapeutic touch practitioners hold their hands a short distance from the patient without actually making physical contact. The purpose of this technique is to detect the patient's energy field, allowing the practitioner to correct any perceived imbalances. Therapeutic touch may reduce pain in patients with tension headache based on preliminary research.

Yoga: Yoga is an ancient system of relaxation, exercise, and healing with origins in Indian philosophy. Preliminary evidence suggests that yoga may effectively reduce the intensity and frequency of tension or migraine headaches and lessen the need for pain relief medications.

Prevention

Keeping a Diary: A diary can help an individual determine what triggers the migraine attack. Writing down when a migraine attack begins, how long each phase lasts, responses to medications, foods eaten in the 24 hours preceding an attack, any unusual stresses before the attack, and how the individual feels and what he or she was doing when a migraine attack begins is important.

Dietary Factors: Identifying and avoiding foods that consistently trigger headaches may be important in helping to reduce the occurrence of migraine headaches. Eat meals at regular times daily and do not skip meals.

Stress Reduction: Integrative therapies that reduce stress, such as yoga, therapeutic touch, and relaxation techniques, are important in reducing migraine attacks.

Regular Sleep Patterns: It is important for migraine sufferers to get adequate, consistent sleep every night. Healthcare professionals generally recommend eight hours of uninterrupted sleep nightly.

Regular Exercise: Regular aerobic exercise reduces tension and can help prevent migraines. If a doctor agrees, choosing an aerobic exercise, such as walking, swimming, or cycling, may help decrease migraine attacks. Warm up slowly, however, because sudden, intense exercise can cause headaches.

Caffeine Intake Reduction: Limiting caffeine consumption to less than two caffeine-containing beverages a day may be of benefit for reduction of migraine attacks.

Light Modification: Avoiding bright or flashing lights and wearing sunglasses, if sunlight is a trigger, may help reduce migraine attacks.

Smoking Cessation: Smoking cessation is important in decreasing migraine attacks, as smoke can be a potential allergen that triggers a migraine. Also, nicotine, one of the components of tobacco, stimulates vascular activity in the brain that may trigger a migraine attack.

M

CONDITIONS: Musculoskeletal Problems, Fibromyalgia, Muscular Dystrophy (MD), Temporomandibular Joint (TMJ) Disorder

BACKGROUND

The musculoskeletal system is a type of organ system that allows for movement and stability of the body and consists of bones, muscles, joints, tendons, cartilage, ligaments, bursae (fluid-filled sacs), and other connective tissue. Complications arising when individual parts of this bodily system are injured can range from minor discomfort to serious medical conditions. Symptoms of musculoskeletal disorders can be acute or chronic and may include inflammation, swelling, pain, fatigue, weakness, joint noises and stiffness, limited range of motion, and lack of coordination. The skeletal system serves many important functions, including providing structure, shape, form, support, and protection for the body. The skeletal system also allows for bodily movement, produces blood for the body, and stores minerals. The skeletal system consists of 206 bones that form a rigid framework as well as protect soft tissues and vital organs of the body. For example, the brain is protected by the skull, which surrounds it, and the heart and lungs are enclosed in the sternum and rib cage. Bodily movement is made possible by the interaction of the muscular and skeletal systems. For this reason, they are often grouped together as the musculoskeletal system. Muscles are connected to bones by tendons. Bones are connected to each other by ligaments. Where bones meet one another is called a joint. Muscles that cause movement of a joint are connected to two different bones. The muscles contract and relax to cause movement. An example would be the contraction of the biceps and a relaxation of the triceps. This produces a bend at the elbow. The contraction of the triceps and relaxation of the biceps produces the effect of straightening the arm.

Muscles are very specialized tissues that have the ability to contract and to conduct electrical impulses. Muscles are classified functionally as either voluntary or involuntary and structurally as either striated or smooth. From this organization, there are three types of muscles: smooth (involuntary) muscles, striated voluntary (skeletal) muscles, and striated involuntary (cardiac) muscles. Red blood cells are produced by the red marrow located in certain bones, including flat bones such as the hip bone, skull, and breastbone. An average of 2.6 million red blood cells is produced each second by the bone marrow

to replace those damaged and destroyed by the liver. Bones also serve as a storage area for minerals such as calcium and phosphorus. When an excess of these minerals is present in the blood, a buildup of the mineral will occur within the bones. When these minerals within the blood are low, they will be withdrawn from the bones to replenish the supply.

TYPES OF MUSCULOSKELETAL PROBLEMS

Arthritis: Arthritis is a disorder that involves joint inflammation or swelling. More than 100 different diseases fall under the general category of arthritis. Arthritis conditions affect the joints, the tissues surrounding the affected joints, and other connective tissues. Common forms of arthritis include rheumatoid arthritis, osteoarthritis, and periarthritis.

Muscular Dystrophy: Muscular dystrophy (MD) is a group of rare, inherited autoimmune muscle diseases in which muscle fibers are unusually susceptible to damage. Muscles, including primarily voluntary muscles, become progressively weaker due to muscle damage. In some types of MD, heart muscles, other involuntary muscles, and other organs are affected. The most common types of MD have been found to be due to a genetic deficiency of the muscle protein dystrophin. A cure for MD has not been found, but medications and therapy can slow the course of the disease.

Fibromyalgia: Fibromyalgia, also known as fibromyositis or fibrositis, is a chronic (long-term) condition characterized by widespread, long-term pain in the muscles, ligaments, and tendons as well as fatigue and multiple tender points (places on the body where slight pressure causes pain). In addition to muscular pain and fatigue, fibromyalgia can also cause sleep problems, depression, and an inability to think clearly. Although fibromyalgia affects about four million Americans, the vast majority of them are women in their mid-30s to late-50s. An estimate of the prevalence of fibromyalgia is as high as 3-5% of the population in the United States, or approximately six million people. Fibromyalgia symptoms may never completely resolve, and their intensity can vary. Although the symptoms of fibromyalgia may be hard to live with, the condition is not considered progressive or life threatening.

Joint Stiffness: Joint stiffness is the feeling that motion of a joint is limited or difficult. Some people with joint stiffness are capable of moving the joint through its full range of motion, but some individuals cannot move the joint due to the pain they are experiencing. Joint stiffness is common with arthritis and usually occurs immediately when rising after lying or sitting still.

Joint Noises: Joint noises, such as creaks and clicks, are common and harmless in many individuals, but they can also occur with specific problems of the joints. For example, the base of the knee cap may creak when it is damaged by osteoarthritis.

Temporomandibular Joint (TMJ) Disorder: TMJ disorder (TMJD, TMJ, or TMD), or TMJ syndrome, is an umbrella term covering acute or chronic inflammation of the TMJ, which connects the lower jaw to the skull. TMJ can result in significant pain and impairment. TMJ may require surgical repair.

Causes and Risk Factors

General

Individuals who are more susceptible to musculoskeletal problems tend to maintain fixed positions (such as sitting in a chair or standing), perform repetitive movements of the limbs (such as athletes or factory workers), overload particular muscle groups, apply pressure on body parts, and use forceful movements (such as in sports).

Musculoskeletal problems and pain can be caused by damage or injury to bones, joints, muscles, tendons, ligaments, bursae, or nerves. If no injury has occurred or if pain persists for more than a few days, then another cause is often responsible.

Bone pain is usually deep, penetrating, dull, or sharp. It commonly results from injury. Other less common causes of bone pain include bone infection (osteomyelitis), vitamin A toxicity, and tumors.

Muscle pain is often less intense than that of bone pain but can be very unpleasant. For example, a muscle spasm or cramp (a sustained painful muscle contraction) in the calf is an intense pain that is commonly called a charley horse. Pain can occur when a muscle is affected by an injury, an autoimmune reaction (for example, polymyositis or dermatomyositis), loss of blood flow to the muscle, dehydration and resulting electrolyte imbalances, infection, or invasion by a tumor.

Tendon and ligament pain is also often less intense than bone pain. This type of pain is often worse when the affected tendon or ligament is stretched or moved. Common causes of tendon pain include tendonitis, tenosynovitis, lateral and medial epicondylitis, and tendon injuries. Common causes of ligament pain include injuries (sprains).

Arthritis

The exact causes of osteoarthritis and rheumatoid arthritis remain unknown. Most researchers believe that several factors, including obesity, age, joint injury or stress, genetics, and muscle weakness, may contribute to the development of osteoarthritis. Some researchers believe that cartilage damage may occur when too many enzymes that allow for the natural breakdown and regeneration of cartilage are released.

Rheumatoid arthritis is considered an autoimmune disorder because the immune system does not function properly and attacks the body's own cells. Some researchers believe that this autoimmune process is triggered by an infection with a virus or bacterium. Heredity may also play a role in the development of rheumatoid arthritis.

Periarthritis typically occurs after a joint becomes injured, which causes scarring, thickening, and shrinkage of the joint. It may also occur after exposure to cold temperatures. Periarthritis typically affects the shoulder. Individuals who have other types of long-term arthritis that affect the shoulders have an increased risk of developing periarthritis of the shoulder.

Fibromyalgia

Gender: Although fibromyalgia may develop in men or women, statistics indicate that women are seven times more likely to develop the condition than men. Nine out of 10 fibromyalgia patients are women, and an estimated 3.4% of American women have the condition. Women's symptoms also tend to be more severe than men's. Women may be more prone to develop fibromyalgia during menopause.

Age: Individuals between the ages of 20-60 are at the highest risk of developing fibromyalgia, although it may occur at any age.

Genetic Factors: There is some indication that genetic factors may be involved in the development of fibromyalgia. Studies have shown that individuals with family members who have fibromyalgia are at a higher risk of developing it themselves.

Specific Lifestyle Factors: People who have recently experienced a traumatic physical or emotional event (such as a divorce, car accident, or death of a family member) may be at a higher risk of developing fibromyalgia.

Psychiatric Illness: While the majority of individuals with fibromyalgia report a history of psychiatric symptoms, such as depression or anxiety, many patients do not. There is no clear evidence that psychiatric illness causes fibromyalgia.

Aggravating Factors: Changes in weather, cold or drafty environments, infections, allergies, hormonal fluctuations (premenstrual and menopausal states), stress, depression, and anxiety may all contribute to fibromyalgia.

M

Muscular Dystrophy (MD)

MD refers to a number of diseases that are caused by genetic mutations that involve progressive weakness, degeneration, and wasting of muscles. The Duchenne and Becker types of MD (DBMD) have similar signs and symptoms, are caused by the same genetic mutation (dystrophin mutation) and occur more frequently in males than in females.

The particular gene that causes DBMD is found on the X chromosome, and so it is called X-linked. Females carry two X chromosomes. Males carry one X chromosome and one Y chromosome. Because males have only one X chromosome, a male carrying a copy with a DBMD mutation will have the condition. However, because females have two copies of the X chromosome, a female can have one copy with a DBMD mutation and one functional copy. Because the functional copy is usually enough to compensate, a female with a DBMD mutation usually has few or no symptoms. However, because she can pass the mutation on to her children, she is called a carrier. Each son born to a woman with the dystrophin mutation on one of her two X chromosomes has a 50% chance of inheriting the mutated gene and having DBMD. Each of her daughters has a 50% chance of inheriting the mutation and being a carrier. While most cases of DBMD occur by inheritance from the mother, in approximately one-third of boys with DBMD there is a new mutation that forms in the egg, and so the mother is actually not the carrier of the mutation.

TMJ Disorders

The cause of most TMJ disorders remains unknown. Some types of TMJ disorders appear to be caused by injury to the joint from a severe blow to the jaw or arthritis. Many behaviors, including frequently clenching the jaw or grinding the teeth (which may occur during sleep), poor posture that puts strain on the muscles and bones near the jaw, or other habits that overwork the jaw muscles (e.g., constantly chewing gum), may contribute to the development of TMJ disorders. However, further research is needed to definitively determine if these behaviors cause TMJ disorders.

SIGNS AND SYMPTOMS

General: Pain is the chief symptom of most musculoskeletal disorders. The pain may be dull, sharp, radiating, or local and may be mild or severe. Although pain may be acute (short lived), as is the case with most injuries, it may become chronic (ongoing) with illnesses such as rheumatoid arthritis. Muscle pain is known as myalgia.

Arthritis: Common symptoms of osteoarthritis include joint pain, swelling and/or stiffness in a joint (especially after use), joint discomfort before or during a change in the weather, bony lumps on the fingers, and loss of joint flexibility. The joints that are most often affected by osteoarthritis include the fingers, spine, and weight-bearing joints, such as the hips, ankles, feet, and knees.

Rheumatoid arthritis often affects many joints at the same time, and the severity of symptoms varies among patients. Symptoms, which may come and go, typically include pain and swelling in the joints (especially in the hands and feet), generalized aching or stiffness of the joints and muscles (especially after periods of rest), loss of motion of the affected joints, weakness in the muscles near the affected joints, low-grade fever, and general feeling of discomfort. Early in the disease, the joints in the hands, wrists, feet, and knees are most frequently affected. Over time, arthritis may develop in the shoulders, elbows, jaw, hips, and neck. In addition to the joints, rheumatoid arthritis may cause swelling in the tear ducts, salivary glands, the lining of the heart, the lungs, and occasionally, blood vessels.

Periarthritis causes swelling and pain in the joints. Most patients develop periarthritis of the shoulder. When the shoulder is affected, the joint's mobility is significantly or completely reduced and aggressive treatment is started.

MD: Signs and symptoms of MD vary according to the type of MD. In general, they may include muscle weakness, apparent lack of coordination, and progressive crippling, resulting in contractures of the muscles around the joints and loss of mobility.

Fibromyalgia: The primary symptoms of fibromyalgia include widespread musculoskeletal pain, severe fatigue (tiredness), and sleep disturbances. Fibromyalgia may cause pain in the muscles, tendons, or ligaments. The pain is usually in multiple locations and may be difficult to describe precisely. Most individuals with fibromyalgia complain of a total body ache. Their muscles may feel like they were pulled or overworked or feel as if they are burning. Other symptoms associated with fibromyalgia include irritable bowel syndrome (IBS). Symptoms of IBS include fluctuations between constipation and diarrhea, frequent abdominal pain, abdominal gas, and nausea. Symptoms of IBS are frequently found in roughly 40-70% of fibromyalgia patients.

Acid reflux, or gastroesophageal reflux disease, also occurs with the same high frequency. Recurrent migraine or tension-type headaches are seen in about 70% of fibromyalgia patients and can pose a major problem in coping for this patient group. TMJ disorder causes tremendous jaw-related face and head pain in one-quarter of fibromyalgia patients. Other common symptoms of fibromyalgia include premenstrual syndrome and painful periods, chest pain, morning stiffness, cognitive or memory impairment, numbness and tingling sensations, muscle twitching, irritable bladder, the feeling of swollen extremities (hands and feet), skin sensitivities, dry eyes and mouth, dizziness, and impaired coordination. Fibromyalgia patients are often sensitive to odors, loud noises, bright lights, and sometimes even the medications they are prescribed.

TMJ Disorder: Common symptoms of TMJ disorders include pain and soreness of the jaw (which may worsen when the individual chews food, talks, or yawns), pain in and around the ear, facial pain, an uneven bite or change in the way the lower and upper teeth fit together, jaw muscle stiffness, a clicking sound or grating sensation when the mouth is opened and closed (sometimes called jaw clicking), headache, tired facial muscles, and locking of the joint, which may temporarily limit the movement of the jaw. It is important to note that jaw clicking affects many individuals who do not have TMJ disorders. Individuals who do not experience pain or limited movement of the jaw when the jaw clicks most likely do not have TMJ disorders.

COMPLICATIONS

Depression: Some individuals with musculoskeletal problems may suffer from depression. This may happen if the musculoskeletal disorder interferes significantly with the patient's lifestyle, including causing pain. Individuals should consult their healthcare providers if they experience feelings of sadness, low self-esteem, loss of pleasure, apathy, and difficulty functioning for two weeks or longer with no known underlying cause. These may be signs of depression and suicidal thoughts.

Joint Damage: In some cases, musculoskeletal disorders can lead to severe joint damage. In such cases, surgery, such as a joint replacement, may be necessary. Individuals should regularly visit their healthcare providers to monitor their conditions.

Limited Mobility: Patients with musculoskeletal disorders may have limited mobility in their joints. Joint mobility decreases as the joint becomes more damaged.

DIAGNOSIS

A clinician can often diagnose a musculoskeletal disorder based on symptoms and the results of a physical examination. Laboratory tests, imaging tests, and other diagnostic procedures are sometimes necessary to help the clinician make or confirm a diagnosis.

Physical Examination: When a person complains of muscle weakness, the clinician checks muscles for bulk, texture, and tenderness. Muscles are also checked for twitches and involuntary movements, which may indicate a nerve disease rather than a muscle disease. Clinicians look for wasting away of muscle (atrophy), which can result from damage to the muscle or its nerves or from lack of use, as sometimes occurs with prolonged bed rest. Clinicians look for muscle enlargement (hypertrophy), which normally occurs with exercise such as weight lifting. However, when a person is ill, hypertrophy may result from one muscle working harder to compensate for the weakness of another. Muscles can also become enlarged when normal muscle tissue is replaced by abnormal tissue (increasing the size but not the strength of the muscle), which occurs in certain inherited muscle disorders, such as DBMD.

Clinicians try to establish which (if any) muscles are weak as well as the degree of weakness involved. The muscles can be tested systematically, usually beginning with the face and neck, then the arms, and finally the legs. Normally, a person should be able to hold the arms extended, palms up, for one minute without them sagging, turning, or shaking. Downward drift of the arm with palms turning inward is one sign of weakness. Strength is tested by pushing or pulling while the clinician pushes and pulls in the opposite direction. Strength is also tested by having the person perform certain maneuvers, such as walking on the heels and tiptoes, rising from a squatting position, or getting up and down from a chair rapidly 10 times. To assess eye muscle strength, the person is asked to look in all directions; if double vision develops, one or more eye muscles may be weak.

The clinician tests a joint's range of motion by moving the limb around a joint while the person is completely relaxed (passive movement). The clinician will check muscle tone by testing passive movement. Resistance to such movement (passive resistance) may be decreased when the nerve leading to the muscle is damaged. Resistance to such movement may be increased when the spinal cord or brain is damaged. If a person is weak, clinicians also tap the person's muscle tendon with a rubber hammer to assess reflexes. Reflexes may be slower than expected when the nerve leading to the muscle is damaged. Reflexes may be more rapid than expected when the spinal cord or brain is damaged.

M

Laboratory Tests: Laboratory tests are often helpful in making the diagnosis of a musculoskeletal disorder. A test called an erythrocyte sedimentation rate (ESR) test measures the rate at which red blood cells settle to the bottom of a test tube containing blood. The ESR is increased when inflammation is present. However, because inflammation occurs in so many conditions, the ESR alone does not establish a diagnosis. The level of creatine kinase (a normal muscle enzyme that leaks out and is released into the bloodstream when muscle is damaged) may also be tested. Levels of creatine kinase are increased when there is widespread and ongoing destruction of muscle. In rheumatoid arthritis, a blood test to identify rheumatoid factor or anticyclic citrullinated peptide antibody is helpful in making the diagnosis. In systemic lupus erythematosus (lupus), a blood test to identify autoimmune antibodies (antinuclear antibodies) is helpful in making the diagnosis.

Nerve Tests: Nerve conduction studies help determine whether the nerves supplying the muscles are functioning normally. Nerve conduction studies, together with electromyography, help indicate whether there is a problem primarily in the muscles (such as myositis or MD); in the nervous system, which supplies the muscles (such as a stroke, spinal cord problem, or polyneuropathy); or with the neuromuscular junction (such as myasthenia gravis). Electromyography, often performed at the same time as nerve conduction studies, is a test in which electrical impulses in the muscles are recorded to help determine how well the impulses from the nerves are reaching the connection between nerves and muscles (neuromuscular junction).

X-Rays: X-rays are most valuable for detecting abnormalities in bone and are taken to evaluate painful, deformed, or suspected abnormal areas of bone. Often, x-rays can help to diagnose fractures, tumors, injuries, infections, and deformities (such as congenital hip dysplasia). Also, x-rays may be helpful in showing changes that confirm a person has a certain kind of arthritis (for example, rheumatoid arthritis or osteoarthritis). X-rays do not show soft tissues such as muscles, bursae, ligaments, tendons, or nerves. To help determine whether the joint has been damaged by injury, a clinician may use an ordinary (non-stress) x-ray or one taken with the joint under stress (stress x-ray). Arthrography is an x-ray procedure in which a dye is injected into a joint space to outline the structures, such as ligaments inside a joint. Arthrography can be used to view torn ligaments and fragmented cartilage in the joint.

Dual-Energy X-Ray Absorptiometry (DEXA): The most accurate way to evaluate bone density, which is necessary when screening for or diagnosing osteoporosis, is with DEXA. In this test, low-dose x-rays are used to examine bone density at the lower spine, hip, wrist, or entire body. Measurements of bone density are very accurate at these sites. To help differentiate osteoporosis (the most common cause of an abnormal DEXA scan) from other bone disorders, doctors may need to consider the person's symptoms, medical conditions, medication use, and certain blood or urine test results as well as the DEXA results.

Computed Tomography (CT) and Magnetic Resonance Imaging (MRI): CT and MRI give much more detail than conventional x-rays. CT and MRI may be performed to determine the extent and exact location of musculoskeletal damage. These tests can also be used to detect fractures that are not visible on x-rays. MRI is especially valuable for imaging muscles, ligaments, and tendons. MRI can be used if the cause of pain is thought to be a severe soft-tissue problem (for example, rupture of a major ligament or tendon or damage to important structures inside the knee joint). The amount of time a person spends undergoing CT is much less than for MRI.

Bone Scanning: Bone scanning is an imaging procedure that is occasionally used to diagnose a fracture, particularly if other tests, such as plain x-rays and CT or MRI, do not reveal the fracture. Bone scanning involves the use of a radioactive substance (technetium-99 m–labeled pyrophosphate) that is absorbed by any healing bone. The technique can also be used when a bone infection or a metastasis (from a cancer elsewhere in the body) is suspected. The radioactive substance is given intravenously and is detected by a bone-scanning device, creating an image of the bone that can be viewed on a computer screen.

Joint Aspiration: Joint aspiration is used to diagnose certain joint problems. A needle is inserted into a joint space and fluid (synovial fluid) is drawn out (aspirated) and examined under a microscope. A doctor can often make a diagnosis after analyzing the fluid. For example, a sample of synovial fluid may contain bacteria, which confirms a diagnosis of infection. Joint aspiration is usually performed in a doctor's office and is generally quick, easy, and relatively painless. The risk of joint infection is minimal.

Arthroscopy: Arthroscopy is a procedure in which a small (diameter of a pencil) fiber optic scope is inserted into a joint space, allowing the doctor to look inside the joint and to project the image onto a television screen. The skin incision is very small. A person receives local, spinal, or general anesthesia. During arthroscopy, doctors can take a piece of tissue for analysis (biopsy) and, if necessary, perform surgery to correct the condition. Disorders commonly found during arthroscopy include inflammation of the synovium lining a joint (synovitis); ligament, tendon, or cartilage tears; and loose pieces of bone or cartilage. Such conditions affect people with arthritis or previous joint injuries as well as athletes. All of these conditions can be repaired or removed during arthroscopy. There is a very small risk of joint infection with this procedure.

TREATMENT

General: Musculoskeletal problems are generally managed with medications that reduce pain and inflammation. In severe cases, surgery may be necessary to repair damage. In order to properly manage pain and prevent joint damage, individuals should take their medications as prescribed by their healthcare providers. Individuals with musculoskeletal problems should also tell their healthcare providers if they are taking any other drugs (prescription, over-the-counter (OTC), or dietary supplements) because they may interfere with treatment.

Corticosteroids: Corticosteroids, such as prednisone (Deltasone) and methylprednisolone (Medrol), are occasionally used to reduce inflammation and pain and slow joint damage caused by musculoskeletal problems. These drugs are generally very effective when used short term. However, if used for many months to years, these drugs may become less effective and serious side effects may develop. Side effects may include easy bruising, thinning of bones, cataracts, weight gain, a "moon" face, and diabetes. Corticosteroids are usually prescribed for a certain amount of time, and then the individual is gradually tapered off the medication. Individuals should not stop taking corticosteroids suddenly or change their dosages without first consulting their healthcare providers.

Nonsteroidal Antiinflammatory Drugs (NSAIDs): NSAIDs have been used to relieve pain and inflammation caused by musculoskeletal problems. Commonly used OTC NSAIDs include ibuprofen (Advil, Motrin) and naproxen sodium (Aleve). Higher doses of these drugs are also available by prescription. Commonly prescribed NSAIDs include diclofenac (Cataflam, Voltaren), nabumetone (Relafen), and ketoprofen (Orudis). NSAIDs may be taken by mouth, injected into a vein, or applied to the skin. These medications are generally taken long term to manage symptoms. The frequency and severity of side effects vary among NSAIDs. The most common side effects include nausea, vomiting, diarrhea, constipation, decreased appetite, rash, dizziness, headache, and

drowsiness. The most serious side effects include kidney failure, liver failure, ulcers, heart-related problems, and prolonged bleeding after an injury or surgery. About 15% of patients who receive long-term NSAID treatment develop ulcers in the stomach or duodenum.

Pain Relievers: OTC pain relievers used in the treatment of musculoskeletal disorders include acetaminophen (Tylenol). Prescription pain relievers, including tramadol (Ultram), have been used to reduce pain caused by musculoskeletal problems. Although this drug, which is available by prescription, does not reduce swelling, it has fewer side effects than NSAIDs. Tramadol is generally taken as a short-term treatment to reduce symptoms of flare-ups. Narcotic pain relievers, such as acetaminophen/codeine (Tylenol with Codeine), hydrocodone/acetaminophen (Lorcet, Lortab, Vicodin), or oxycodone (OxyContin, Roxicodone), may be prescribed to treat severe musculoskeletal pain. However, they do not reduce swelling. These medications are only used short term to treat flare-ups. Common side effects include constipation, drowsiness, dry mouth, and difficulty urinating. Narcotic pain relievers should be used cautiously because individuals may become dependent upon them.

Selective Cyclooxygenase-2 (COX-2) Inhibitors: Celecoxib (Celebrex) has been taken by mouth to reduce pain and inflammation caused by musculoskeletal problems such as osteoarthritis. Celecoxib is currently the only COX-2 inhibitor that is approved by the U.S. Food and Drug Administration (FDA). Celecoxib is generally taken long term to manage symptoms. COX-2 inhibitors have been linked to an increased risk of serious heart-related side effects, including heart attack and stroke. Selective COX-2 inhibitors have also been shown to increase the risk of stomach bleeding, fluid retention, kidney problems, and liver damage. Less serious side effects may include headache, indigestion, upper respiratory tract infection, diarrhea, sinus inflammation, stomach pain, and nausea.

Topical Pain Relievers: Topical pain relievers are creams, ointments, gels, and sprays that are applied to the skin. Many OTC pain relievers may temporarily help reduce pain caused by osteoarthritis. Products such as Aspercreme, Sportscreme, Icy Hot, and Ben-Gay may help reduce arthritis pain. Capsaicin cream, which is made from the seeds of hot peppers, may reduce pain in joints that are close to the skin surface, such as the fingers, knees, and elbows. Lidocaine patches (Lidoderm) may also be used. Lidocaine is an anesthetic when applied topically and may decrease pain associated with musculoskeletal problems.

Antidepressants: Some individuals with musculo-skeletal problems may also suffer from depression. Commonly prescribed antidepressants for arthritis patients include amitriptyline, nortriptyline (Aventyl, Pamelor), and trazodone (Desyrel). These drugs may also help with nerve pain associated with musculo-skeletal disorders. Side effects of antidepressant medications include drowsiness, fatigue (excessive tiredness), constipation, dry mouth, and blurred vision.

Lifestyle Changes: Many lifestyle changes, includ-ing regular exercise, weight management, and consumption of a healthy diet may help reduce symptoms of musculoskeletal problems. A healthcare provider may recommend a physical therapist, nutritionist, or registered dietician to help determine the best treatment plan for the individual. Individuals with musculoskeletal problems such as osteoarthritis or rheumatoid arthritis should wear comfortable footwear that properly supports their weight. This may reduce the amount of strain put on the joints during walking. Individuals with musculoskeletal problems may require canes, walkers, or other devices to help them get around. If the hands are severely affected, braces may be beneficial. Individuals should talk to their healthcare providers about assistive devices that are available. Individuals with musculoskeletal problems should maintain good posture. This allows the body's weight to be evenly distributed among joints.

Cool Compress or Ice Pack: Applying a cool compress or ice pack to the affected joint during a flare-up may help reduce swelling and pain.

Heat: Applying a hot pack to affected joints may help reduce pain, relax muscles, and increase blood flow to the joint. It may also be an effective treatment before exercise. Alternatively, individuals may take a hot shower or bath before or after exercise to help reduce pain.

Fusing Bones: If there is serious joint damage, the bones of a joint, such as the ankle, may be surgically fused together in a procedure called arthrodesis. This surgery helps increase stability and reduces pain. However, the joint no longer has any flexibility and cannot bend or move.

Joint Replacement Surgery: In some cases, indivi-duals with osteoarthritis suffer from permanent joint damage. In such instances, joint replacement surgery may be necessary. During the procedure, the damaged joint is surgically removed, and it is replaced with a plastic or metal device called a prosthesis. The most commonly replaced joints are the hip and knee, but other joints, including the elbow, shoulder, finger, or ankle joints can be replaced as well. Joint replacement surgeries are generally most successful for large joints, such as the hip or knee. Researchers estimate that hip or knee replacements last at least 20 years in 80% of patients. After a successful surgery and several months of rehabilitation, individuals are able to use their new joints without pain. As with any major surgery, there are risks associated with joint replacements. Patients should discuss the potential health risks and benefits of surgery with their healthcare providers.

INTEGRATIVE THERAPIES

Strong Scientific Evidence

Chondroitin: Multiple clinical trials have examined the use of oral chondroitin in patients with osteo-arthritis of the knee and other locations (spine, hips, and finger joints). Most of these studies have reported significant benefits in terms of symptoms (such as pain), function (such as mobility), and reduced medi-cation requirements (such as antiinflammatories). The weight of scientific evidence points to a beneficial effect when chondroitin is used for six to 24 months. Longer-term effects are not clear. Preliminary studies of topical chondroitin have also been conducted. Chondroitin is frequently used with glucosamine. Glucosamine has independently been demonstrated to benefit patients with osteoarthritis (particularly of the knee). It remains unclear if there is added benefit of using these two agents together compared to using either alone. Chondroitin is currently manufactured from natural sources (shark/beef cartilage or bovine trachea) or by synthetic means.

Glucosamine: Glucosamine is a natural compound that is found in healthy cartilage. Based on human research, there is good evidence to support the use of glucosamine sulfate in the treatment of mild-to-moderate knee osteoarthritis. Most studies have used glucosamine sulfate supplied by one European manufacturer (Rotta Research Laboratorium), and it is not known if glucosamine preparations made by other manufacturers are equally effective. Although some studies of glucosamine have not found benefits, these have either included patients with severe osteoarthritis or have used products other than glucosamine sulfate. More well-designed clinical trials are needed to confirm safety and effectiveness and to test different formulations of glucosamine.

Avoid if allergic or hypersensitive to shellfish or iodine. Some reports suggest a link between glucosamine/chondroitin products and asthma. Use cautiously with diabetes or with a history of bleeding disorders. Avoid if pregnant or breastfeeding.

Willow Bark: Willow bark (*Salix alba*) contains salicin and has been used to treat many different kinds of pain. Willow bark is a traditional analgesic (pain relieving) therapy for osteoarthritis and musculoskeletal disorders. Several studies have confirmed this finding. Additional study comparing willow bark to conventional medicinal agents for safety and effectiveness is warranted.

Avoid if allergic/hypersensitive to aspirin, willow bark (*Salix* spp.), or any of its constituents, including salicylates. Use cautiously with gastrointestinal problems (e.g., ulcers), hepatic disorders, diabetes, gout, hypertension, or hyperlipidemia. Use cautiously with a history of allergy, asthma, or leukemia. Use cautiously if taking antihyperlipidemia agents, alcohol, leukemia medications, beta-blockers, diuretics, phenytoin (Dilantin), probenecid, spironolactone, sulfonylureas, valproic acid, or methotrexate. Use cautiously if taking tannin-containing herbs or supplements. Avoid use when operating heavy machinery. Avoid in children with chickenpox and any other viral infections. Avoid with blood disorders and renal disorders. Avoid if taking other NSAIDs, acetazolamide, or other carbonic anhydrase inhibitors. Avoid with elevated serum cadmium levels. Avoid if pregnant or breastfeeding.

Good Scientific Evidence

5-HTP: There is a small amount of research evaluating the use of 5-HTP for fibromyalgia, and early evidence suggests that 5-HTP may reduce the number of tender points, anxiety, and intensity of pain and may improve sleep, fatigue, and morning stiffness. Additional studies with larger numbers of people are needed to determine what dose may be safe and effective.

Acupuncture: Acupuncture is commonly used throughout the world. According to Chinese medicine theory, the human body contains a network of energy pathways through which vital energy, called chi, circulates. These pathways contain specific "points" that function like gates, allowing chi to flow through the body. Needles are inserted into these points to regulate the flow of chi. There has been substantial research into the efficacy of acupuncture in the treatment of osteoarthritis. Most studies focus on knee, cervical, and hip osteoarthritis symptoms. In recent years, the evidence has improved and is now considered strong enough to recommend trying acupuncture in osteoarthritis of the knee, which is one of the most common forms of this condition. There is also evidence from several studies suggesting that acupuncture may help with pain relief in fibromyalgia.

Avocado: A combination of avocado/soybean unsaponifiables has been found beneficial in osteoarthritis of the knee and hip. Additional study using avocado (*Persea Americana*) alone in OA is needed.

Borage Seed Oil: Borage (*Borago officinalis*) is an herb native to Syria that has spread throughout the Middle East and Mediterranean. Borage flowers and leaves may be eaten and borage seeds are often pressed to produce oil that is very high in gamma-linolenic acid (GLA). GLA has known antiinflammatory effects that may make it beneficial in treating rheumatoid arthritis. A few human studies have generally found positive results, and side effects were not reported. However, more research is needed to determine the optimal dose and administration.

Avoid if allergic or hypersensitive to borage, its constituents, or members of the Boraginaceae family. Avoid with a weakened immune system. Use cautiously with bleeding disorders, epilepsy, or drugs used to treat these disorders. Avoid if pregnant or breastfeeding.

Chlorella: Clinical evidence indicates that chlorella may reduce the tenderness associated with fibromyalgia. Although the results are promising, more high-quality studies are needed to confirm these findings.

Devil's Claw: Devil's claw (*Harpagophytum procumbens*) originates from the Kalahari and Savannah desert regions of South and Southeast Africa. There is increasing scientific evidence suggesting that devil's claw is safe and beneficial for the short-term treatment of pain related to degenerative joint disease or osteoarthritis (taken for eight to 12 weeks) and may be equally effective as drug therapies such as NSAIDs like ibuprofen (Advil, Motrin) or may allow for dose reductions or discontinuation of these drugs in some patients. However, most studies have been small, with flaws in their designs. Additional well-designed trials are necessary.

Glucosamine: Several human studies and animal experiments report benefits of glucosamine in treating osteoarthritis of various joints of the body, although the evidence is less plentiful than that for knee osteoarthritis. Some of these benefits include pain relief, possibly due to an antiinflammatory effect of glucosamine and improved joint function. Overall, these studies have not been well designed. Although there is some promising research, more study is needed in this area before a firm conclusion can be made.

Omega-3 Fatty Acids (Fish Oils): Multiple studies report improvements in morning stiffness and joint tenderness in patients with rheumatoid arthritis with the regular intake of fish oil supplements for up to three months. Benefits have been reported as additive with antiinflammatory medications, such as NSAIDs (such as ibuprofen). However, because of weaknesses in study designs and reporting, better research is necessary before a strong, favorable recommendation can be made. Effects beyond three months of treatment have not been well evaluated.

Avoid if allergic or hypersensitive to fish, omega-3 fatty acid products that come from fish, nuts, linolenic acid, or omega-3 fatty acid products that come from nuts. Avoid during active bleeding. Use cautiously with bleeding disorders, diabetes, low blood pressure, or drugs, herbs, or supplements that treat any such conditions. Use cautiously before surgery. Pregnant and breastfeeding women should not consume doses of omega-3 fatty acids that exceed the recommended dietary allowance.

Physical Therapy: The goal of physical therapy is to improve mobility, restore function, reduce pain, and prevent further injuries. Several techniques, including exercises, stretches, traction, electrical stimulation, and massage, are used. Physical therapy for osteoarthritis of the knee may provide short-term benefits, but long-term benefits do not appear better than standard treatments. Physical therapy, either as an individually delivered treatment or in a small group format, appears effective. Only one available study compared physical therapy to a sham group (subtherapeutic ultrasound) and found that a combination of manual physical therapy and supervised exercise was beneficial for patients with osteoarthritis of the knee. One method of physical therapy, infrared, short-wave diathermy-pulsed patterns and interferential therapy, showed more effectiveness than intraarticular hyaluronic drugs in two studies. More research using consistent treatment protocols and outcomes measures are needed.

Not all physical therapy programs are suited for everyone, and patients should discuss their medical history with their qualified healthcare professionals before beginning any treatments. Based on the available literature, physical therapy appears generally safe when practiced by a qualified physical therapist. Physical therapy may aggravate preexisting conditions. Persistent pain and fractures of unknown origin have been reported. Both morning stiffness and bone erosion in patients have been reported, although the cause is unclear. All therapies during pregnancy and breastfeeding should be discussed with a licensed obstetrician/gynecologist before initiation.

Psychotherapy: Psychotherapy is an interactive process between a person and a qualified mental health professional. The patient will explore thoughts, feelings, and behavior to help with problem solving. Although group therapy may somewhat decrease pain in people with rheumatoid arthritis and depression, individual therapy coupled with antidepressants may be more effective.

Rose Hips: Rose hips have traditionally been used by herbalists as an antiinflammatory and antiarthritic agent. A constituent isolated from dried and milled fruits of *Rosa canina* has demonstrated antiinflammatory properties, and Hyben Vital, a standardized rose hips extract, has been shown to have antioxidant properties. Rose hip extracts have been studied in patients with osteoarthritis, with some evidence of benefit. Additional high-quality clinical research is needed in this area to confirm these results.

S-Adenosylmethionine (SAMe): SAMe has been studied extensively in the treatment of osteoarthritis. SAMe reduces the pain associated with osteoarthritis and appears to be well tolerated in this patient population. Although an optimal dose has yet to be determined, SAMe appears as effective as NSAIDs. Additional study is warranted to confirm these findings.

Transcutaneous Electrical Nerve Stimulation (TENS): TENS is a noninvasive technique in which a low-voltage electrical current is delivered through wires from a small power unit to electrodes located on the skin. Electrodes are temporarily attached in various patterns depending on the specific condition and treatment goals. Preliminary studies of TENS in rheumatoid arthritis report improvements in joint function and pain. However, most research is not well designed or reported, and better studies are necessary before a clear conclusion can be reached.

Avoid with implantable devices, such as defibrillators, pacemakers, intravenous infusion pumps, or hepatic artery infusion pumps. Use cautiously with decreased sensation (such as neuropathy) or with seizure disorders. Avoid if pregnant or breastfeeding due to insufficient evidence of safety.

Unclear or Conflicting Scientific Evidence

Arnica: Arnica (*Arnica montana*) gel has been used on the skin for osteoarthritis pain and stiffness due to its antiinflammatory constituents. Although early study is promising, additional study is needed.

Ashwagandha: The use of ashwagandha in osteoarthritis has been suggested based on its reported antiinflammatory and antiarthritic properties. Well-designed human research is needed to confirm these results.

Astaxanthin: Astaxanthin is found in microalgae, yeast, salmon, trout, krill, shrimp, crayfish, crustaceans, and the feathers of some birds. Astaxanthin has been suggested as a possible treatment for rheumatoid arthritis. However, further research is warranted.

Avoid if allergic or hypersensitive to astaxanthin or related carotenoids, including canthaxanthin or an astaxanthin algal source. Use cautiously if taking 5-alpha-reductase inhibitors (used in prostate conditions), hypertensive agents, asthma medications, drugs that are broken down by the liver, menopausal agents, birth control pills, or medications that are used to treat *Helicobacter pylori* infections. Use cautiously with high blood pressure, parathyroid disorders, or osteoporosis. Avoid with hormone-sensitive conditions, immune disorders, or immuno-suppressive therapies. Avoid with previous experience of visual changes while taking astaxanthin and with low eosinophil levels. Avoid if pregnant or breastfeeding.

Beta-Carotene: Beta-carotene is a member of the carotenoid family, which contains highly pigmented (red, orange, yellow), fat-soluble compounds naturally present in many fruits, grains, oils, and vegetables (green plants, carrots, sweet potatoes, squash, spinach, apricots, and green peppers). Beta-carotene supplementation does not appear to prevent osteoarthritis, but it might slow progression of the disease. Well-designed clinical trials are needed before a conclusion can be drawn. Supplemental beta-carotene may increase the risk of lung cancer, prostate cancer, intracerebral hemorrhage, and cardiovascular and total mortality in people who smoke cigarettes or have a history of high-level exposure to asbestos. Beta-carotene from foods does not seem to have this effect.

Preliminary study has found that synthetic beta-carotene may increase cardiovascular mortality in people who smoke. In men who smoke and have had a prior myocardial infarction, the risk of fatal coronary heart disease increases by as much as 43% with low doses of beta-carotene. There is some evidence that beta-carotene in combination with selenium, vitamin C, and vitamin E might lower high-density lipoprotein-2 cholesterol levels. High-density lipoprotein levels are protective, so this is considered to be a negative effect. Dizziness and reversible yellowing of palms, hands, or soles of feet and, to a lesser extent, the face (called carotenoderma) can occur with high doses of beta-carotene. Loose stools, diarrhea, unusual bleeding or bruising, and joint pain have been reported.

Beta-Sitosterol: Beta-sitosterol is found in plant-based foods, such as fruits, vegetables, soybeans, breads, peanuts, and peanut products. It is also found in bourbon and oils, such as olive oil, flaxseed, and tuna. Beta-sitosterol has been shown to reduce inflammation, and it has therefore been suggested as a possible treatment for rheumatoid arthritis. Further research is needed to confirm these claims.

Avoid if allergic or hypersensitive to beta-sitosterol, beta-sitosterol glucoside, or pine. Use cautiously with asthma or breathing disorders, diabetes, primary biliary cirrhosis (destruction of the small bile duct in the liver), ileostomy, neurodegenerative disorders (such as Parkinson's disease or Alzheimer's disease), bulging of the colon, short-bowel syndrome, celiac disease, or sitosterolemia. Use cautiously with a history of gallstones. Avoid if pregnant or breastfeeding.

Black Cohosh: Although it has been suggested that black cohosh (*Actaea racemosa*) may help relieve joint pain associated with rheumatoid arthritis and osteoarthritis, further research is needed. High doses of black cohosh may cause frontal headache, dizziness, perspiration, or visual disturbances.

Use cautiously if allergic to members of the Ranunculaceae family, such as buttercup or crowfoot. Avoid with hormone conditions (e.g., breast cancer, ovarian cancer, uterine cancer, endometriosis). Avoid if allergic to aspirin products, NSAIDs (such as ibuprofen), or blood thinners (such as warfarin). Avoid with a history of blood clots, stroke, seizures, or liver disease. It is recommended to stop use of black cohosh two weeks before and immediately after surgery/dental/diagnostic procedures with bleeding risks.

Boron: Boron is a trace element that is found throughout the environment. Based on human population research, in a boron-rich environment people appear to have fewer joint disorders. It has also been proposed that boron deficiency may contribute to the development of osteoarthritis. However, there is no clear human evidence that supplementation with boron is beneficial as prevention against or as a treatment for osteoarthritis.

Boswellia: Resin extracts from the *Boswellia serrata* tree have been found to have antiinflammatory effects. Due to boswellia's potential antiinflammatory properties, boswellia has been suggested as a potential treatment for osteoarthritis. Further research is needed in this area. Boswellia may increase bleeding in sensitive individuals, such as those taking blood-thinning medications, including warfarin (Coumadin).

Bromelain: Bromelain is an herb that contains a digestive enzyme that comes from the stem and the fruit of the pineapple plant (*Ananas comosus*). When taken with meals, bromelain may aid in the digestion of proteins. When taken on an empty stomach, it acts as an antiinflammatory agent. In one study of the combination product ERC (enzyme-rutosid combination; rutosid, bromelain, trypsin), results showed that ERC may be considered as an effective and safe alternative to prescription NSAIDs such as diclofenac in the treatment of painful episodes of osteoarthritis of the knee. Further well-designed clinical trials of bromelain alone are needed to confirm these results.

Avoid if allergic to bromelain, pineapple, honeybee venom, latex, birch pollen, carrots, celery, fennel, cypress pollen, grass pollen, papain, rye flour, wheat flour, or other members of the Bromeliaceae family. Use cautiously with a history of bleeding disorders, stomach ulcers, heart disease, liver disease, or kidney disease. Use cautiously before dental or surgical procedures or while driving or operating machinery. Avoid if pregnant or breastfeeding.

Cat's Claw: Cat's claw is widely used in the United States and Europe, and it is one of the top herbal remedies sold despite a lack of high-quality human evidence. In Germany and Austria, cat's claw is only available by prescription. Several laboratory and animal studies suggest that cat's claw may reduce inflammation, and this has led to research of cat's claw for inflammatory conditions such as arthritis. Early research also suggests that cat's claw may reduce pain from knee osteoarthritis. Large, high-quality human studies are needed comparing the effects of cat's claw alone vs. placebo before a conclusion can be drawn.

Avoid if allergic to cat's claw, *Uncaria* plants, or plants in the Rubiaceae family (such as gardenia, coffee, or quinine). Avoid with a history of conditions affecting the immune system (such as AIDS, HIV, some types of cancer, multiple sclerosis, tuberculosis, or lupus). Use cautiously with bleeding disorders or with a history of stroke. Use cautiously if taking drugs that may increase the risk of bleeding. It is recommended to stop use of cat's claw two weeks before and immediately after surgery/dental/diagnostic procedures with a bleeding risk. Avoid if pregnant or breastfeeding. Cat's claw may be contaminated with other *Uncaria* species. Reports exist of a potentially toxic, Texan-grown plant, *Acacia greggii,* being substituted for cat's claw.

Chiropractic: Chiropractic is a healthcare discipline that focuses on the relationship between musculoskeletal structure (primarily the spine) and body function (as coordinated by the nervous system) and how this relationship affects the preservation and restoration of health. Promising results were obtained in the treatment of osteoarthritis using manual physical therapy and exercise. However, presently there is insufficient evidence to support the use of chiropractic manipulation for this condition.

Evening Primrose Oil: Evening primrose oil contains an omega-6 essential fatty acid called GLA, which is believed to be the active ingredient. Benefits of evening primrose oil in the treatment of arthritis have not been clearly shown. More information is needed before a recommendation can be made.

Avoid with seizure disorders. Use cautiously if taking mental illness drugs. It is recommended to stop use two weeks before surgery with anesthesia. Avoid if pregnant or breastfeeding.

Guggul: Guggul (gum guggul) is a resin produced by the mukul mirth tree. There is insufficient evidence to support the use of guggul or guggul derivatives for the management of rheumatoid arthritis. Avoid if allergic to guggul. Avoid with a history of thyroid disorders, anorexia, bulimia, or bleeding disorders. Signs of allergy to guggul may include itching and shortness of breath. Avoid if pregnant or breastfeeding.

Guided Imagery: Guided imagery refers to a number of techniques, including metaphor, storytelling, fantasy, game playing, dream interpretation, drawing, visualization, active imagination, and direct suggestion using imagery. Therapeutic guided imagery may be used to help patients relax and focus on images associated with personal issues they are confronting. Cognitive-behavioral interventions for pain may be an effective adjunct to standard pharmacological interventions for pain in patients with osteoarthritis. Further research is needed to confirm these results.

Guided imagery is usually intended to supplement medical care, not to replace it, and guided imagery should not be relied on as the sole therapy for a medical problem. Contact a qualified healthcare provider if mental or physical health is unstable or fragile. Never use guided imagery techniques while driving or doing any other activity that requires strict attention. Use cautiously with physical symptoms that can be brought about by stress, anxiety, or emotional upset because imagery may trigger these symptoms.

Magnet Therapy: Magnetic fields play an important role in Western medicine. For instance, they are used for MRI, pulsed electromagnetic fields, and experimental magnetic stimulatory techniques. Several studies have evaluated the use of magnetic field therapy applied to areas affected by osteoarthritis or degenerative joint disease. In particular, this research has focused on knee osteoarthritis. However, most studies have been small or poorly designed or reported. Efficacy remains unclear. Notably, one promising small study published in 2004 by Wolsko et al. reported some benefits. Larger and better-quality studies are needed before a recommendation can be made in this area. Initial evidence has failed to show improvements in knee pain with the use of magnet therapy. However, due to methodological weaknesses with this research, the conclusions cannot be considered definitive.

Avoid with implantable medical devices, such as heart pacemakers, defibrillators, insulin pumps, or hepatic artery infusion pumps. Avoid with myasthenia gravis or bleeding disorders. Avoid if pregnant or breastfeeding. Magnet therapy is not advised as the sole treatment for potentially serious medical conditions and should not delay the time to diagnosis a condition. It should not replace treatment with more proven methods. Patients are advised to discuss magnet therapy with their qualified healthcare providers before starting treatment.

Methysulfonylmethane (MSM): MSM is a form of organic sulfur that occurs naturally in a variety of fruits, vegetables, grains, and animals. MSM is a normal oxidation product of dimethyl sulfoxide. Preliminary study has used MSM, alone or in combination with glucosamine, in the treatment of osteoarthritis. The combination may provide pain relief and reduction in inflammation. Further studies on MSM and its effects on patients with osteoarthritis are warranted.

Niacin: Vitamin B_3 is made up of niacin (nicotinic acid) and its amide, niacinamide, and can be found in many foods, including yeast, meat, fish, milk, eggs, green vegetables, and cereal grains. Preliminary human studies suggest that niacinamide may be useful in the treatment of osteoarthritis. Further research is needed.

Pantothenic Acid (Vitamin B_5): Pantothenic acid is found in many foods, including meats, liver, kidney, fish/shellfish, chicken, vegetables, legumes, yeast, eggs, and milk. It has been reported that pantothenic acid levels are lower in the blood of patients with rheumatoid arthritis compared to healthy individuals. However, it is unclear if this is a cause, effect, or a beneficial adaptive reaction. There is currently insufficient scientific evidence in this area in order to form a clear conclusion. Pantothenic acid has also been suggested as a possible treatment for osteoarthritis. However, further research is needed to determine whether or not this treatment is effective.

Avoid if allergic or hypersensitive to pantothenic acid or dexpanthenol. Avoid with gastrointestinal blockage. Pantothenic acid is generally considered safe in pregnant and breastfeeding women when taken at recommended doses.

Probiotics: Probiotics are beneficial bacteria that are sometimes called friendly germs. They help maintain a healthy intestine and aid in digestion. They also help keep harmful bacteria and yeasts in the gut under control. Most probiotics come from food sources, especially cultured milk products. Probiotics can be taken as capsules, tablets, beverages, powders, yogurts, and other foods. In a small study, *Lactobacillus GG* was associated with improved subjective well-being and trends in reduced symptoms of rheumatoid arthritis. However, the results were not statistically significant. More studies on the effects of probiotics on rheumatoid arthritis are needed.

Probiotics are generally considered safe and well tolerated, but may cause diarrhea in sensitive individuals. Use cautiously if lactose intolerant.

Relaxation Therapy: Relaxation techniques include behavioral therapeutic approaches that differ widely in philosophy, methodology, and practice. The primary goal is usually nondirected relaxation. In a randomized study of patients with osteoarthritis pain, relaxation therapy was reported to lower the level of subjective pain over time. The study concluded that relaxation might be effective in reducing the amount of analgesic medication taken by participants. Further well-designed research is needed to confirm these results. Limited preliminary research reports that muscle relaxation training may improve function and well-being in patients with rheumatoid arthritis. Additional research is necessary before a conclusion can be reached.

Avoid with psychiatric disorders, such as schizophrenia or psychosis. Relaxation therapy, which involves flexing and relaxing specific muscles, should be used cautiously with illnesses, such as heart disease, high blood pressure, or musculoskeletal injury. Relaxation therapy is not recommended as the sole treatment approach for potentially serious medical conditions, and it should not delay the time to diagnosis or treatment with more proven techniques.

Tai Chi: Tai chi is a system of movements and positions believed to have developed in twelfth century China. Tai chi techniques aim to address the body and mind as an interconnected system and are traditionally believed to have mental and physical health benefits to improve posture, balance, flexibility and strength. A small trial in women with osteoarthritis reported that treatment with tai chi significantly decreased pain and stiffness compared

M

with a sedentary lifestyle. Women in the tai chi group also reported fewer perceptions of difficulties in physical functioning. Additional research is needed in this area.

Thymus Extract: Thymus extracts for nutritional supplements are usually derived from young calves (bovine). Thymus extract is commonly used to treat primary immunodeficiencies, bone marrow failure, autoimmune disorders, chronic skin diseases, recurrent viral and bacterial infections, hepatitis, allergies, chemotherapy side effects, and cancer. Further research is needed to determine whether or not thymus extract can effectively treat symptoms of rheumatoid arthritis.

Avoid if allergic or hypersensitive to thymus extracts. Use bovine thymus extract supplements cautiously due to potential for exposure to the virus that causes "mad cow disease." Avoid use with an organ transplant or other forms of allografts or xenografts. Avoid with thymic tumors, myasthenia gravis (neuromuscular disorder), or untreated hypothyroidism. Avoid if taking immunosuppressants or hormonal therapy. Avoid if pregnant or breastfeeding. Thymic extract increases human sperm motility and progression.

Turmeric: The rhizome (root) of turmeric (*Curcuma longa Linn.*) has long been used in traditional Asian medicine. Turmeric has been used historically to treat rheumatic conditions. Laboratory and animal studies show antiinflammatory activity of turmeric and its constituent curcumin, which may be beneficial in people with osteoarthritis. Reliable human research is lacking. Turmeric may increase bleeding in sensitive individuals, such as those taking blood thinning medications including warfarin (Coumadin).

Yoga: Yoga is an ancient system of relaxation, exercise, and healing, with origins in Indian philosophy. Yoga is often practiced by healthy individuals with the aim to achieve relaxation, fitness, and a healthy lifestyle. Based on a pilot study, yoga may help reduce pain and disability caused by knee osteoarthritis in some patients. Further research is needed.

Fair Negative Scientific Evidence

Arnica: Homeopaths believe that arnica may be effective in relieving pain due to delayed onset muscle soreness, which is defined by exercise to which subjects are unaccustomed. Currently, it is not recommended to give arnica for this indication, although it does not appear to be unsafe for use.

Chondroitin: Chondroitin sulfate is often used as an antiinflammatory and pain reliever for osteoarthritis, so chondroitin was thought to be beneficial for delayed onset muscle soreness. However, early

research does not support this use. More research is needed in this area to confirm these results.

Dehydroepiandrosterone (DHEA): DHEA does not seem to improve quality of life, pain, fatigue, cognitive function, mood, or functional impairment in postmenopausal patients with fibromyalgia.

Phenylalanine: In clinical study, D-phenylalanine has not been shown to affect symptoms in patients with chronic pain. Additional high-quality clinical research is needed to confirm these results.

Selenium: Selenium is a trace mineral found in soil, water, and some foods. It is an essential element in several metabolic pathways. Selenium-ACE, a formulation containing selenium with three vitamins, has been promoted for the treatment of arthritis. Research has failed to demonstrate significant benefits, with a possible excess of side effects compared to placebo.

Willow Bark: There is good evidence that willow bark may be effective in treating chronic pain from osteoarthritis; however, willow bark extract did not show efficacy in treating rheumatoid arthritis. Additional study is needed to confirm these results.

Traditional or Theoretical Uses Lacking Sufficient Evidence

Integrative therapies used in pain or related conditions causing pain and that have historical or theoretical uses but lack sufficient clinical evidence include homeopathic aconite (*Aconitum napellus*), acupressure (shiatsu), black currant (*Ribes nigrum*), black tea (*Camellia sinensis*), celery (*Apium graveolens*), chelation (ethylenediamine tetraacetic acid) therapy, Hellerwork (a form of body work), horse chestnut (*Aesculus hippocastanum*), Kundalini yoga, licorice (*Glycyrrhiza glabra*), mangosteen (*Garcinia mangostana*), massage, meadowsweet (*Filipendula ulmaria*), polarity therapy, rhubarb (*Rheum officinale, Rheum palmatum*), rutin, shark cartilage, and vitamin E.

PREVENTION

Preventing Sports Injury: Some musculoskeletal problems associated with injuries may be preventable. Care should be taken in sports and physical activities to prevent injuries, sprains, and the overuse of joints, such as in the ankle, wrist, knee, shoulder, and spine. Individuals participating in sports activities such as football, swimming, gymnastics, baseball, basketball, tennis, skiing, wrestling, and soccer may be at a greater risk of developing musculoskeletal problems.

Preventing Occupational Injury: Any job or activity that requires a fixed position over a long period of time can cause musculoskeletal discomfort. Poor job and workplace design appears to contribute to many reported discomforts. Important methods of preventing such discomfort include assuming a range of comfortable positions and having adjustable furniture, such as chairs, tables, and keyboard supports. However, the degree of adjustability for any furniture and visual display depends on how long and for what purpose they will be used. Prolonged work in the same position, whether seated or standing, can cause discomfort. Where possible, movement should be incorporated into the task to prevent discomfort and fatigue. It is best to avoid standing still in one place for long periods of time. The activity of the leg muscles acts as a pump and assists the veins in returning blood to the heart. Prolonged standing stops this pumping action and this may cause swelling of the lower extremities. Using a rubber or padded mat where prolonged standing cannot be avoided is recommended by healthcare providers. Mats help reduce fatigue and improve comfort. For those individuals who sit for long periods of time, a well-designed chair is very important.

Dietary Modification: Nutritional changes, along with the addition of supplements (vitamins, minerals and herbs), may be effective in reducing symptoms associated with musculoskeletal problems. It is best to limit caffeine and other stimulants, as well as alcohol, and to stop smoking. It may also be beneficial to eliminate potential food allergens, including dairy (milk, cheese, and sour cream), eggs, nuts, shellfish, wheat (gluten), corn, preservatives, and food additives (such as dyes and fillers). Additionally, it may be helpful to avoid refined foods such as white breads and pastas and foods with high levels of sugar or refined sugar, such as donuts, pastries, candy, and soft drinks.

Exercise: Maintaining physical fitness is important to those suffering from musculoskeletal problems. Those with musculoskeletal problems who exercise according to their healthcare professional's recommendations tend to do better, with less symptoms and a slower disease progression, than those who do not. A daily regimen of exercise can help the person feel better physically and mentally. Individuals should walk as much as possible, even if assistance is necessary. Regular exercise may also help individuals control their weight and decrease stress on the musculoskeletal system. There are many ways for people to exercise, including gardening, walking, sports activities, and dancing. Individuals who are beginning an exercise program should choose activities that fit their levels of strength and endurance. The type of exercise is not as important as a consistent exercise schedule. Most experts today agree that burning calories should not be the goal of exercise. Exercise that causes extreme pain or discomfort is considered by many experts as unhealthy and may even cause permanent damage to the body. Pilates is a body conditioning routine that seeks to build flexibility, strength, endurance, and coordination without adding muscle bulk. In addition, Pilates may increase circulation and may help to sculpt the body and strengthen the body's "core" (torso). People who engage in Pilates regularly report that they have better posture, are less prone to musculoskeletal injury, and experience better overall health. It is recommended for patients to consult with their healthcare providers before beginning any exercise program.

BACKGROUND

Obesity occurs when an individual has an increased amount of body fat. It is usually defined as being 20-30% above the normal body weight for someone of the same age, gender, and height. Morbid obesity is usually defined as being 50-100% above the normal body weight for someone of the same age, gender, and height. Many factors, including an individual's age, gender, and height, are considered to determine if he/she is overweight. People increase in weight until they are fully grown. On average, females tend to gain about 16 pounds of body weight from age 25-54. In contrast, males tend to gain about 10 pounds of body weight from age 25-45. By around age 55, both men and women start to decline in weight. Females naturally have more body fat and less muscles mass than men. It is also normal for taller individuals to weigh more than shorter individuals. Obesity is typically considered a long-term condition that often persists for many years. Researchers believe that many factors, including poor diet, overeating, pregnancy, medications, medical conditions, genetics, gender, and age, may contribute to a person becoming obese. Obesity can have serious long-term effects on health. Individuals who are overweight have an increased risk of developing many life-threatening illnesses, including heart disease, high blood pressure, stroke, obesity, diabetes, osteoporosis, and cancer. According to the American Heart Association, obesity was associated with nearly 112,000 deaths in 2005. In the United States, obesity is considered an epidemic. More than half of all Americans are considered overweight, and about 20% of children are overweight. In 2005, 140 million Americans were considered overweight or obese, according to the American Heart Association. Nearly 33% of Americans are considered obese, and these numbers continue to grow.

CAUSES

General: There are many potential causes of obesity. Some patients may be obese for multiple reasons.

Poor Diet: Individuals who regularly consume foods that are high in calories and saturated fats have an increased risk of becoming obese. Examples of foods and beverages that may lead to obesity include fast food, fried food, sodas, candy, and desserts. To

maintain a healthy weight, an individual's intake of calories should be about equal to the calories used or burned during the day. If an individual eats more calories than are burned, the body stores the extra calories as fat. That is why someone who leads a sedentary, or inactive, lifestyle would most likely gain weight if he/she ate the same amount of food as someone who goes running every day.

Overeating: Consistently eating too much food also increases the risk of becoming obese. Individuals who regularly eat extra-large portions of food, eat until they are full, or eat many times throughout the day are more likely to become obese.

Inactivity: Individuals who do not exercise regularly are more likely to become obese. Physical activity is needed to burn the calories that are consumed in the diet. If these calories are not burned, they will be stored as fat in the body. Most experts recommend at least 30 minutes of moderate exercise three or more times per week to help maintain a healthy weight.

Pregnancy: During pregnancy, the female's body weight increases, not only because she is carrying a baby, but also because the mother's body needs to support the growing fetus. The average weight gain during pregnancy is typically 25-35 pounds. Researchers believe that this weight gain may contribute to the development of obesity.

Medications: Some medications, including corticosteroids and tricyclic antidepressants, may cause weight gain as a side effect.

Medical Conditions: Although it is uncommon, sometimes obesity is caused by medical conditions. For instance, if the thyroid does not produce enough thyroid hormone, the metabolism slows down, leading to mild weight gain and difficulty losing extra weight. In addition, some long-term conditions, such as emphysema or arthritis, may limit an individual's ability to exercise. As a result, individuals may become overweight or obese.

Stress: Stress may also contribute to obesity. When an individual becomes stressed, it signals the adrenal glands to release a hormone called cortisol. Research suggests that increase in cortisol levels may lead to increased fat around the midsection. In addition, recent research suggests that there is a connection between high levels of stress and the desire to eat. It has been proposed that comfort foods, specifically those that are high in fats and sugars, may help reduce the body's response to stress and limit the amount of cortisol that is released. However, individuals who frequently indulge in these foods typically develop excess abdominal fat, which has been associated with an increased risk of heart disease and stroke.

Genetics: Genetics may also contribute to obesity. For instance, a patient's genetics may affect how much fat is stored and where it is distributed in the body. Genetics may also affect how quickly the body is able to convert food into energy and how efficiently the body is able to burn calories during physical activity. Although genetics can increase an individual's risk of becoming obese, it is not the only factor for the condition. In other words, individuals who are genetically predisposed to become obese will not always become obese, especially if they make the right lifestyle choices.

Gender: Women are more likely to become obese than men. This is because women naturally have more body fat and less muscle mass than men. In addition, women burn fewer calories at rest than men do. As a result, women are more likely to experience an increase in body fat than males.

Age: Age may also contribute to obesity. Muscle mass tends to decrease with age, which decreases the body's metabolism, or rate at which the body is able to process fats. In addition, most patients become less active as they age. All of these changes lead to a decrease in the amount of calories that body needs. If individuals do not decrease the amount of calories they consume, they will start to gain weight.

SIGNS AND SYMPTOMS

Patients who are obese have more fat than normal, healthy individuals of the same age, gender, and height. They may have difficulty walking, experience shortness of breath, and become tired after very little physical exertion.

COMPLICATIONS

Depression: Individuals who are obese often suffer from depression. This may occur if the patient's weight limits his/her ability to perform certain activities. Depression may also occur if the patient has poor self-esteem as a result of his/her weight.

Heart Disease: Obese individuals have an increased risk of developing high blood pressure. This is because the extra fat tissue, like other tissues in the body, requires oxygen from the blood. Therefore, the circulatory system is strained and the heart rate increases as it tries to supply a larger-than-normal body with enough oxygenated blood. In addition, obesity tends to increase the amount of insulin in the blood. High levels of insulin cause the body to retain sodium and water, which increases blood volume. Individuals who are overweight also have an increased risk of developing high cholesterol. High cholesterol can cause plaque deposits to form in the arteries. Plaque is composed of cholesterol, other fatty substances, fibrous tissue, and calcium. When plaque builds up in the arteries, it causes atherosclerosis (hardening of the arteries) or coronary artery disease. Atherosclerosis can lead to plaque ruptures and blockages in the arteries. If the blood supply to the heart is blocked, a heart attack may occur. If blood supply to the brain is blocked, a stroke may occur.

Sleep Apnea: Obese patients have an increased risk of developing sleep apnea, a serious condition that occurs when the individual stops breathing for short periods of time during sleep. In obese patients, sleep apnea typically occurs when excess fat in the upper airway obstructs breathing. Because sleep apnea causes individuals to wake up frequently throughout the night, patients are often drowsy during the day.

Diabetes: Obese patients are more likely to develop type 2 diabetes. This condition occurs when the body becomes resistant to a hormone called insulin. As a result, patients with type 2 diabetes have too much sugar in their bloodstream.

Cancer: Many types of cancer, including colon cancer, rectal cancer, esophageal cancer, kidney cancer, breast cancer, and prostate cancer, are associated with being overweight.

Physical Discomfort: Obese patients may suffer from chronic pain in various parts of the body. This is because fat eventually starts to crowd the space near the internal organs, impairs blood circulation, and puts extra strain and pressure on the body's joints. Sometimes the fat in the abdomen prevents patients from sitting comfortably. Pain is most likely to develop in the feet, joints, back, and muscles. It may be difficult for obese patients to breathe when they are sitting up.

Fertility Problems and Sexual Dysfunction: Men and women who are obese may suffer from fertility problems. In general, being obese decreases an individual's sex drive (libido). It may also make it difficult for males to achieve or maintain an erection. In addition, several studies have found that obesity may decrease an individual's sexual quality of life. Researchers have found that obesity is associated with a lack of enjoyment of sexual activity, lack of sexual desire, difficulties with sexual performance, and avoidance of sexual encounters. Many studies have also found that obese patients who lose weight experience an increase in their sexual quality of life.

Birth Defects: Obese females have an increased risk of having children with gestational diabetes or other complications during pregnancy that may lead to birth defects.

Osteoarthritis: Obese individuals are more likely to develop a degenerative joint disease called osteoarthritis. This is because being overweight increases the strain put on the weight-bearing joints, such as the knees and ankles.

Osteoporosis: Obese individuals have an increased risk of developing osteoporosis, which causes the bones to become weak and brittle. The bones become porous and less dense. As a result, individuals are more likely to fracture their bones if they slip, fall, or injure themselves. Some evidence suggests that osteoporosis may develop in obese patients because fat cells infiltrate the bone marrow. In addition, it has been shown that individuals who live sedentary lifestyles have an increased risk of developing osteoporosis.

DIAGNOSIS

A healthcare provider diagnoses obesity after measuring the patient's body mass index (BMI) and hip-to-waist ratio.

The BMI is a measurement of weight (in pounds) for height (in inches) in adults who are older than 20 years of age. BMI falls into one of these categories: below 18.5 units is underweight, 18.5-24.9 is normal, 25.0-29.9 is overweight, and 30.0 and above is obese. For adults, the accepted formula for BMI is: BMI = $703 \times$ [Weight in pounds/(Height in inches)^2].

Waist-to-hip ratio is the circumference of the waist divided by the circumference of the hips. For women, a healthy ratio is 0.8 or lower. For men, a healthy ratio is 1.0 or lower. A high ratio means that the patient is overweight or obese. A low ratio means that the patient is underweight.

TREATMENT

General: Most doctors believe that overweight individuals should try to lose weight gradually. This reduces the risk of nutritional deficiencies and increases the likelihood of long-term success. Individuals who are overweight should aim to lose about one-half to two pounds per week. The safest and most effective way to lose weight is to reduce the amount of calories in the diet and increase physical activity. Individuals should eat sensible portions of foods that are well balanced. In serious cases when obesity is causing life-threatening conditions or when all other options have failed, surgical weight-loss procedures (called bariatric surgeries) may be considered. However, individuals must meet specific criteria in order to qualify for weight-loss surgery.

In addition, bariatric surgeries, like all surgeries, have potential health risks. Patients should discuss the potential risks and benefits with their healthcare providers before making any decisions about medical treatments.

Exercise Programs: Patients who are overweight or obese are encouraged to exercise. Research shows that regular exercise can help individuals live longer, healthier lives. Exercise can help prevent illnesses, such as heart disease, stroke, diabetes, and cancer. In general, overweight patients should participate in 45-60 minutes of moderate exercise (e.g., brisk walking or jogging) each day in order to prevent becoming obese. Patients who were formerly obese are encouraged to participate in 60-90 minutes of moderate exercise each day along with a healthy, well-balanced diet in order to prevent gaining the weight back. Not everyone is able to perform intense types of exercise, such as tennis or running. The American Academy of Family Physicians recommends that individuals who are pregnant or have bone disease or nerve injuries participate in low-impact forms of exercise, such as walking or swimming. Individuals who are overweight or obese may have serious health conditions that limit the type or amount of exercise they can perform. Therefore, patients should talk to their healthcare providers before starting a new exercise plan, especially if they are pregnant, elderly, or have a critical illness or injury. A healthcare provider can work with a patient to design an individualized and safe exercise program.

Healthy Diet: In addition to regular exercise, a healthy diet is also important. Individuals should eat well-balanced meals in sensible portions. The U.S. government issued a revised Food Pyramid in 2005 to help Americans choose healthier eating habits. The new, updated MyPyramid provides 12 different models based on daily calorie needs, ranging from the 1,000-calorie diets for toddlers to 3,200-calorie diets for teenage boys. Overall, doctors suggest drinking six to eight glasses of water a day and eating lots of raw fruits and vegetables, especially green leafy vegetables. Some individuals may find it helpful to eat frequent small meals throughout the day to keep the body's energy and metabolism increased. Foods and drinks that contain a lot of sugar and little or no nutritional value should be consumed in moderation. This means individuals should limit their intakes of foods and drinks such as coffee, alcohol, soft drinks, fruits juices that are high in sugar, processed foods, white sugar, white flour, red meat, and animal fats.

A healthcare provider may recommend a nutritionist to help plan meals that are appropriate for the patient. A nutritionist can help teach the patient what foods are considered healthy and what are not. It is important for the patient to understand the negative impact that poor eating habits have on the body. Many experts recommend making gradual changes in the diet. This has been shown to help prevent or minimize food cravings. Individuals who slowly change their diets may be more likely to adopt these eating habits as part of their long-term lifestyle.

Appetite Suppressants: Appetite suppressants are medications, herbs, or supplements that decrease appetite or make the individual feel full. Some doctors prescribe appetite suppressant medications to help treat obese individuals. Most individuals who take these medications initially lose between five and 22 pounds. Weight loss is usually greatest during the first few weeks or months of treatment. After about six months, the patient's weight usually levels off. However, most people gain the weight back once they stop taking the medications. Appetite suppressants can be taken short term (few weeks to a few months) or long term (one year or more), depending on the specific medication prescribed. Diethylpropion (Tenuate, a short term medication. may increase blood pressure. Phentermine (Fastin), another short-term medication, has been taken off the market due to increased risk for heart valve disease. These medications may be taken for several months or years. Some individuals may need to take them their entire lives. There are also many appetite suppressants that are available over the counter. These products can be purchased at health food stores, local pharmacies, or nutrition stores. For instance, an herb called hoodia may cause individuals to feel full. As a result, patients may eat less food. However, no studies have been performed in humans to determine if hoodia is safe and effective in humans. Dietrine Carb Blocker with Phase 2 is also available over the counter. This product is made with an ingredient from white kidney beans that may prevent the body from storing sugar as fat in the body. While some side effects of U.S. Food and Drug Administration (FDA) approved medications are mild, and may usually go away as treatment is continued, some side effects may be severe and long-lasting. Symptoms may include sleeplessness and/or nervousness. There have also been reports of serious and deadly reactions to appetite suppressants, including primary pulmonary hypertension. Several previously approved drugs, such as phentermine (Fastin), have caused heart valve disease in patients, and are no longer available.

Other Medications: Orlistat (Xenical) is a lipase inhibitor, which reduces the amount of fat the body can absorb, and is used as long-term medication. About 30% of the fat from foods is excreted instead of being absorbed. Sibutramine (Meridia), also a long-term medication, aids in weight-loss by blocking the re-uptake of the neurotransmitters serotonin and norepinephrine. These long-term medications may be taken for several months or years. Some individuals may need to take them their entire lives.

Gastric Bypass Surgery: Gastric bypass surgery, which uses bands or staples to create food intake restriction, is the most common weight loss surgery. The bands or staples are surgically placed near the top of the stomach to section off a small portion that is often called a stomach pouch. A small outlet, about the size of a pencil eraser, is left at the bottom of the stomach pouch. Since the outlet is small, food stays in the pouch longer and the patient also feels full for a longer time. Next, a section of the small intestine is attached to the pouch. This allows food to bypass part of the intestine, resulting in fewer calories being absorbed. This surgery is often performed in those who have a BMI ≥40 (extremely obese) or in patients who have a BMI that is 35-39.9 along with weight-related health problems such as diabetes or high blood pressure.

Surgical candidates go through an extensive screening process. Not everyone who meets the criteria for the surgery is psychologically or medically ready for the surgical procedure. A team of professionals, including a physician, dietitian, psychologist, and surgeon, evaluate whether the surgery is appropriate. Following surgery, physical, nutritional, and metabolic counseling are given to prevent nutritional deficiencies. Lifelong use of nutritional supplements such as multivitamins, vitamin B_{12}, vitamin D, and calcium is recommended. Over two years, gastric bypass surgery patients have been shown to lose two-thirds of excess weight. The improvements observed in type 2 diabetes, high blood pressure, and high blood cholesterol may significantly decrease the risk of heart disease in individuals who have undergone gastric bypass surgery compared to those treated through other means. Gastric bypass surgery has also shown to improve mobility and quality of life for people who are severely overweight. However, individuals who continue to overeat after undergoing the surgery may stretch out the pouch. As a result, the stomach may become as large as it was prior to surgery, and the patient may gain back weight. There is a risk of death during gastric bypass surgery. The risk varies depending on age, general health, and other medical conditions. If the contents of the stomach leak out of one of the staple lines, the patient will receive antibiotics to prevent an infection. Most cases heal with time. Sometimes the leak can be serious enough to require emergency surgery. Excess weight places extra stress on the chest cavity and lungs. As a result, there is a higher risk of developing pneumonia during postoperative recovery when the patient is lying down. Narrowing of the opening between the stomach and small intestine has occurred. This rare complication may require either an outpatient procedure to pass a tube through the mouth to widen the narrowed opening or corrective surgery. Gastric bypass can also cause dumping syndrome, a condition where stomach contents move too quickly through the small intestine, causing nausea, vomiting, diarrhea, dizziness, and sweating. Other common complications include dehydration, gallstones, bleeding stomach ulcers, hernia at the incision site, and intolerance to certain foods.

Liposuction: Liposuction is the most frequent cosmetic operation in the United States in which fat tissue is removed. Relatively small amounts of total body fat can be removed safely. However, little weight is lost. Unless the patient makes lifestyle changes that include regular exercise and a healthy diet, the weight will return. Therefore, liposuction is categorized as a cosmetic surgery rather than a weight-loss surgery.

Adjustable Gastric Banding: A surgical procedure called gastric banding may also be performed. This surgery is designed to make the patient feel full quicker so he/she will eat less and lose weight. During the procedure, the surgeon uses an inflatable band to partition the stomach into two parts. The surgeon then wraps the band around the upper part of the stomach and pulls it tight, like a belt, creating a tiny channel between the two pouches. The band keeps the opening from expanding and is designed to stay in place indefinitely. However, it can be adjusted or surgically removed if necessary. Most surgeons perform this operation using a laparoscope.

Biliopancreatic Diversion: During a surgical procedure called biliopancreatic diversion, a portion of the stomach is removed. The remaining pouch is connected directly to the small intestine but completely bypasses the small intestine, where most nutrient absorption takes place. This weight-loss surgery offers sustained weight loss, but it presents a greater risk of malnutrition and vitamin deficiencies that requires close monitoring. Some patients may require vitamin

and/or nutritional supplements after the surgery. Other possible complications include infection, blood clot in the lung (called pulmonary embolism), as well as stomach contents leaking into the abdominal cavity.

Vertical Banded Gastroplasty: This operation divides the stomach into two parts, limiting space for food and forcing the patient to eat less. There is no bypass. Using a surgical stapler, the surgeon divides the stomach into upper and lower sections. The upper pouch is small and empties into the lower pouch. Surgeons use this procedure less frequently than gastric bypass partly because it does not lead to adequate long-term weight loss.

Jaw Wiring: Jaw wiring is another option, although it is used infrequently. This is a form of food intake restriction for temporary use in patients who do not have breathing problems. During the procedure, the patient's jaw is wired shut. While the jaw is wired, the patient is only able to consume liquid nutrition through a straw. The wires are typically removed every four to six weeks to allow the patient to exercise the jaw. Treatment may last anywhere from three to six months. Individuals regularly rinse their mouths with mouthwash and use antiseptic wipes on the front of their teeth. When the wires are removed, the patient can brush his/her teeth. It is recommended that individuals carry wire cutters with them at all times in case of an emergency such as the need to vomit. In general, breathing is not inhibited while the jaw is wired. However, activities that cause deep breathing, such as aerobic exercise, should be avoided. Although jaw wiring can be effective for short-term weight loss, weight regain occurs soon after the wires are removed. Therefore, it is not considered a conventional weight-loss procedure.

Antidepressants: Depression is commonly associated with obesity. Antidepressants may be prescribed to treat depression in some patients. Drugs called selective serotonin reuptake inhibitors (SSRIs) are the most common type of antidepressants used. Commonly prescribed SSRIs include fluoxetine (Prozac), fluvoxamine (Luvox), sertraline (Zoloft), and paroxetine (Paxil). Less commonly prescribed antidepressants include clomipramine (Anafranil), mirtazapine (Remeron), amitriptyline (Elavil), and bupropion (Wellbutrin). Side effects may include nausea, nervousness, insomnia, diarrhea, rash, agitation, or problems with sexual arousal or orgasm.

INTEGRATIVE THERAPIES

Although some integrative therapies have been shown to promote weight loss, not all treatments are safe. Most experts believe that overweight or obese individuals should aim to lose weight gradually with long-term lifestyle changes that include a healthy diet and regular exercise.

Strong Scientific Evidence

Ephedra: Ephedra contains the chemical ephedrine, which appears to cause weight loss when used in combination with caffeine, based on the available scientific evidence. The results of research on ephedrine alone (without caffeine) are unclear. The amounts of ephedrine in commercially available products have widely varied.

However, even though this herb has been shown to help reduce weight, it is unsafe for humans for this indication. Serious reactions, including heart attack, stroke, seizure, and death, have occurred with using ephedra. The U.S. Food and Drug Administration (FDA) has banned sales of ephedra dietary supplements in all states.

Good Scientific Evidence

5-Hydroxy-L-Tryptophan (5-HTP): 5-HTP is the precursor for serotonin. Serotonin is the brain chemical associated with sleep, mood, movement, feeding, and nervousness. 5-HTP may alter serotonin levels in the brain, which may then reduce eating behaviors and promote weight loss in obese individuals.

Avoid if allergic to 5-HTP. Use cautiously with a history of psychological disorders. Avoid if pregnant or breastfeeding.

The Atkins Diet: The Atkins diet is an eating style that radically departs from the FDA My-Pyramid. The Atkins diet advocates an increased consumption of fats as the primary source of energy while simultaneously restricting the intake of carbohydrates. This limitation is based on the premise that eating carbohydrates (e.g., bread, cereal, potatoes, or pasta) results in the excessive secretion of insulin, potentially resulting in increased fat stores. A carbohydrate-restricted diet has been shown to result in weight loss in obese and nonobese individuals. Effects at one year may be less and dropout rates are high. Overall the studies suggest that the Atkins diet does result in long-term weight loss. However, patients should consult with a qualified healthcare professional before beginning any new diet to discuss possible adverse effects and negative health consequences.

Avoid with severe kidney disease or kidney disorders. Avoid if taking growth hormone. Use cautiously with mood disorders (e.g., depression), schizophrenia, or bipolar disorders or if taking medications to treat these disorders. Use cautiously in athletes due to potential for muscle cramps, negative feelings towards exercise, fatigue, or hypoglycemia. Use cautiously with osteoporosis, gout, diabetes, menstrual disorders, gastrointestinal disorders, celiac disease, skin conditions, epilepsy, heart disease, anemia, thyroid disorders, or history of stroke or heart attack. Use cautiously in malnourished individuals, vegetarians, or in individuals with absorption concerns. Use cautiously if taking diuretics, medications that alter cholesterol, medications that alter blood sugar, medications for seizures, steroids, or nonsteroidal antiinflammatory drugs. Avoid if pregnant or breastfeeding.

Dehydroepiandrosterone (DHEA): DHEA is a hormone that is produced by the adrenal glands. Most human studies investigating the effects of DHEA on weight or fat loss support its use for this purpose.

Avoid if allergic to DHEA. Avoid with a history of seizures. Use cautiously with adrenal or thyroid disorders. Use cautiously if taking anticoagulants or drugs, herbs, or supplements that treat diabetes, heart disease, seizure, or stroke. Stop use two weeks before and immediately after surgery/dental/diagnostic procedures with bleeding risks. Avoid if pregnant or breastfeeding.

Psychotherapy: Psychotherapy is an interactive process between a person and a qualified mental health professional. The patient explores thoughts, feelings, and behaviors to help with problem solving. Several studies indicate that people who are overweight or obese may benefit from behavioral and cognitive-behavioral psychotherapy in combination with diet and exercise to lose weight.

Psychotherapy cannot always fix mental or emotional conditions. Psychiatric drugs are sometimes needed. In some cases, symptoms may worsen if the proper medication is not taken. Not all therapists are qualified to work with all problems. Use cautiously with serious mental illnesses or some medical conditions because some forms of psychotherapy may stir up strong emotional feelings and expression.

Unclear or Conflicting Scientific Evidence

Acupuncture: Acupuncture is commonly used throughout the world. According to Chinese medicine theory, the human body contains a network of energy pathways through which vital energy, called "chi," circulates. These pathways contain specific "points" that function like gates, allowing chi to flow through the body. Needles are inserted into these points to regulate the flow of chi. Studies have produced inconclusive evidence on whether acupuncture might contribute to weight loss. Some studies show modest benefit but others show none. Currently, there is insufficient available evidence to recommend either for or against acupuncture in weight loss.

Needles must be sterile in order to avoid disease transmission. Avoid with valvular heart disease, infections, bleeding disorders, medical conditions of unknown origin, or neurological disorders. Avoid on areas that have received radiation therapy and during pregnancy. Avoid if taking anticoagulants. Use cautiously with pulmonary disease (e.g., asthma or emphysema). Use cautiously in elderly or medically compromised patients, diabetics, and individuals with a history of seizures. Avoid electroacupuncture with arrhythmia (irregular heartbeat) or in patients with pacemakers.

Ayurveda: Ayurveda is a form of natural medicine that originated in ancient India more than 5,000 years ago. Evidence is inconclusive on whether the traditional herb guggul (Medohar) may contribute to weight loss in obese patients. More studies are needed to examine this treatment.

Ayurvedic herbs should be used cautiously because they are potent, and some constituents can be potentially toxic if taken in large amounts or for a long time. Some herbs imported from India have been reported to contain high levels of toxic metals. Ayurvedic herbs can interact with other herbs, foods, and drugs. A qualified healthcare professional should be consulted before taking. Use guggul cautiously with peptic ulcer disease. Avoid sour food, alcohol, and heavy exercise with guggul. Mahayograj guggul should not be taken for long periods of time. Avoid Ayurveda with traumatic injuries, acute pain, advanced disease stages, or medical conditions that require surgery.

Betaine Anhydrous: Betaine is found in most microorganisms, plants, and marine animals. There is currently insufficient available evidence supporting betaine for weight loss.

Avoid if allergic to betaine anhydrous or cocamidopropyl betaine, a form of betaine. Use cautiously with kidney disease, obesity, or psychiatric conditions. Avoid if pregnant or breastfeeding.

Bitter Orange: Bitter orange (*Citrus aurantium*) comes from a flowering, fruit-bearing evergreen tree native to tropical Asia. It is now widely grown in the Mediterranean region and elsewhere. Bitter orange is a common ingredient in dietary supplements as a weight loss aid and appetite suppressant. Since the ban on ephedra, some weight loss products previously containing ephedrine have been reformulated to include bitter orange. Although bitter orange is popularly used for weight loss, the effects of bitter orange are largely unknown, and more study is needed to make a strong recommendation.

Avoid if allergic or hypersensitive to bitter orange or any members of the Rutaceae family. Avoid with heart disease, narrow-angel glaucoma, intestinal colic, or long QT interval syndrome. Avoid if taking antiadrenergic agents, beta-blockers, QT-interval prolonging drugs, monoamine oxidase inhibitors, stimulants, or honey. Use cautiously with headache or overactive thyroid and in fair-skinned individuals. Avoid if pregnant or breastfeeding.

Calcium: Calcium is the most abundant mineral in the human body. Calcium is needed for muscle contraction, blood vessel contraction and expansion, the release of hormones and enzymes, and nervous system signaling. Diets with higher calcium density (high levels of calcium per total calories) have been associated with a reduced incidence of being overweight or obese in several studies. While more research is needed to understand the relationships between calcium intake and body fat, these findings emphasize the importance of maintaining an adequate calcium intake while attempting to diet or lose weight.

Avoid if allergic or hypersensitive to calcium or lactose. High doses taken by mouth may cause kidney stones. Avoid with high levels of calcium in the blood, high levels of calcium in urine, high levels of parathyroid hormone, bone tumors, digitalis toxicity, ventricular fibrillation (ventricles of the heart contract in unsynchronized rhythm), kidney stones, kidney disease, or sarcoidosis. Use cautiously with achlorhydria (absence of hydrochloric acid in gastric juices) or arrhythmia (irregular heartbeat). Calcium appears to be safe in pregnant or breastfeeding women. Talk to a healthcare provider to determine appropriate dosing during pregnancy and breastfeeding. Calcium supplements made from dolomite, oyster shells, or bone meal may contain unacceptable levels of lead.

Damiana: Damiana, which includes the aromatic species *Turnera diffusa* and *Turnera aphrodisiaca,* grows wild in the subtropical regions of the Americas and Africa. YGD, containing yerbe mate (leaves of *Ilex paraguayensis*), guarana (seeds of *Paullinia cupana*), and damiana (leaves of *Turnera diffusa* var. *aphrodisiaca*), is an herbal preparation frequently used for weight loss. More studies using damiana alone are needed before a recommendation can be made.

Avoid if allergic/hypersensitive to *Turnera diffusa, Turnera aphrodisiaca,* their constituents, or related plants in the Turneraceae family. Use cautiously with a history of breast cancer. Avoid with Alzheimer's disease or Parkinson's disease. Use cautiously with psychiatric disorders. Use cautiously if taking medications that alter blood sugar levels.

Evening Primrose: Evening primrose oil contains an omega-6 essential fatty acid called gamma-linolenic acid, believed to be the active ingredient. Initial human study suggests that evening primrose oil may have no effects on weight loss.

Avoid if allergic to plants in the Onagraceae family (e.g., willow's herb or enchanter's nightshade), or gamma-linolenic acid. Avoid with seizure disorders. Use cautiously if taking mental illness drugs. Stop use two weeks before surgery with anesthesia. Avoid if pregnant or breastfeeding.

Garcinia: *Garcinia cambogia* is an extremely small purple fruit that is naturally found in India and Southeast Asia. Evidence supporting hydroxycitric acid, the active ingredient in *Garcinia cambogia,* for weight loss is mixed. Additional study is warranted to clarify early findings.

Avoid if allergic or hypersensitive to *Garcinia cambogia*. Use cautiously with a history of diabetes, rhabdomyolysis (breakdown of skeletal muscle), or with 3-hydroxy-3-methylglutaryl coenzyme A reductase inhibitors (statins). Avoid with Alzheimer's disease. Avoid if pregnant or breastfeeding.

Green Tea: Green tea is made from the dried leaves of *Camellia sinensis,* an evergreen shrub. Green tea has a long history of use, dating back about 5,000 years ago in China. There are several small human studies addressing the use of green tea extract capsules for weight loss or weight maintenance in overweight or average-weight individuals. Study results are mixed. Better research is needed before a recommendation can be made in this area.

Avoid if allergic or hypersensitive to caffeine or tannin. Use cautiously with diabetes or liver disease.

Guarana: Guarana is a native species of South America and has stimulating properties when taken orally. Guarana has the same stimulatory effect as caffeine and is often used for energy, weight loss, and as an additive to soft drinks (e.g., Dark Dog Lemon, Guts, and Josta). Caffeine has been used as a weight loss agent due to its ability to burn calories by increasing heat output. In available studies, guarana has been studied with other herbs, making it difficult to draw a conclusion based on the effects of guarana alone. Additional study is needed in this area.

Avoid if allergic to guarana (*Paullinia cupana*), caffeine, tannins, or related species of the Sapindaceae family. Avoid with high blood pressure, psychological or psychiatric disorders, liver disorders, or irregular heartbeat. Avoid if taking other stimulatory agents, especially ephedra. Use cautiously with breast disease, impaired kidney function, diabetes, preexisting mitral valve prolapse, iron deficiency, gastric or duodenal ulcers, bleeding disorders, glaucoma, or risk for osteoporosis. Use cautiously if undergoing electroconvulsive therapy. Avoid if pregnant or breastfeeding.

Guggul: Guggul (gum guggul) is a resin produced by the mukul mirth tree. There is insufficient evidence to support the use of guggul or guggul derivatives for the management of obesity.

Avoid if allergic to guggul. Avoid with a history of thyroid disorders, anorexia, bulimia, or bleeding disorders. Avoid if pregnant or breastfeeding.

Hypnosis, Hypnotherapy: Hypnosis is a trancelike state in which a person becomes more aware and is more open to suggestion. Hypnotherapy has been used to treat health conditions or to change behaviors. Research suggests that hypnosis may be valuable as an adjunct to cognitive behavioral therapy for weight loss. However, it is unclear if hypnotherapy used alone is beneficial in this area.

Use cautiously with mental illnesses (e.g., psychosis/schizophrenia, bipolar disorder, multiple personality disorder, or dissociative disorders) or seizure disorders.

L-Carnitine: L-carnitine is an amino acid. Early evidence shows that L-carnitine may have no effect on weight loss in obese patients. Further studies are needed before a firm conclusion can be made.

Avoid if allergic or hypersensitivity to carnitine. Use cautiously with peripheral vascular disease, high blood pressure, alcohol-induced liver cirrhosis, or diabetes. Use cautiously in low birth weight infants and individuals on hemodialysis. Use cautiously if taking anticoagulants (blood thinners), beta-blockers, or calcium channel blockers. Avoid if pregnant or breastfeeding.

Licorice: Licorice is harvested from the root and dried rhizomes of the low-growing shrub *Glycyrrhiza glabra*. Preliminary data show that licorice may reduce body fat mass. Further research is needed to confirm these results.

Avoid if allergic to licorice, any component of licorice, or any member of the Fabaceae (Leguminosae) plant family. Avoid licorice with congestive heart failure, coronary heart disease, kidney disease, liver disease, fluid retention, high blood pressure, hormonal abnormalities, or diuretics. Licorice can cause abnormally low testosterone levels in men or high prolactin or estrogen levels in women. This may make it difficult to become pregnant and may cause menstrual abnormalities.

Lutein: Lutein and zeaxanthin are found in high levels in foods such as green vegetables, egg yolk, kiwifruit, grapes, orange juice, zucchini, squash, and corn. Currently, there is insufficient available evidence to recommend for or against the use of lutein for obesity.

Avoid if allergic or hypersensitive to lutein or zeaxanthin. Use cautiously if at risk for heart disease or cancer. Avoid if pregnant or breastfeeding.

Macrobiotic Diet: Macrobiotics is a popular approach to diet that stresses vegetarianism and consumption of whole, healthy foods. Proponents of macrobiotics advocate a flexible approach that allows supplementation with dairy, fish, or other supplements as needed on an individual basis. There is evidence that a macrobiotic diet may lead to reduced body size and obesity as well as increased leanness in preschool children compared to children on a normal diet. Studies are needed to determine whether or not these changes contribute to good health in children.

The macrobiotic diet poses a risk of nutrition deficiencies. However, this can be avoided with appropriate menu planning. Use cautiously with cancer or other medical conditions without expert planning or supplementation. Not recommended in children or adolescents without professional guidance or appropriate supplementation. Not recommended in pregnant or lactating women due to potential deficiencies unless properly supplemented.

Moxibustion: Moxibustion is a therapeutic method in traditional Chinese medicine, classical (five-element) acupuncture, and Japanese acupuncture. During moxibustion, an herb (usually mugwort) is burned above the skin or on the acupuncture points for the purpose of introducing heat into an acupuncture point to alleviate symptoms. It may be applied in the form of a cone, stick, or loose herb; or it may be placed on the head of an acupuncture needle to manipulate the temperature gradient of the needle. Evidence does not support use of moxibustion to aid in weight loss at this time, although it may contribute to increased psychological well-being and improved eating attitudes in obese patients. More studies are needed to determine whether or not moxibustion may play a role in weight loss.

Use cautiously over large blood vessels and on thin or weak skin. Avoid with aneurysms, any kind of "heat syndrome," heart disease, convulsions, cramps, diabetic neuropathy, extreme fatigue, anemia, fever, or inflammatory conditions. Avoid over allergic skin conditions, ulcerated sores, skin adhesions, areas of inflammation, or contraindicated acupuncture points. Avoid use on the face, genitals, head, nipples, or skin adhesions. Avoid in patients who have just finished exercising or taking a hot bath or shower. Use cautiously in elderly people with large vessels. It is not advisable to bathe or shower for up to 24 hours after a moxibustion treatment. Avoid if pregnant or breastfeeding.

Psyllium: Psyllium, also known as ispaghula, comes from the husks of the seeds of *Plantago ovata*. The reviewed evidence seems to show that psyllium may improve blood sugar and lipid levels, which have been associated with obesity in some children. However, further studies are needed to clarify its effects and the mechanisms involved. Body weight reduction has not been proven to be associated with psyllium use in adults.

Avoid if allergic or hypersensitive to psyllium, ispaghula, or English plantain (*Plantago lanceolata*). Prescription drugs should be taken one hour before or two hours after psyllium. Use cautiously if pregnant or breastfeeding because psyllium may lower blood sugar levels.

Rhubarb: In traditional Chinese medicine, rhubarb is used as an ulcer remedy, and it is considered a bitter, cold, dry herb used to "clear heat" from the liver, stomach, and blood. One three-stage study looked at the effects of rhubarb on simple obesity. Although the study indicates a positive effect compared to two other obesity treatments and a control group, more high-quality studies are needed to confirm rhubarb's role in weight gain and loss.

Avoid if allergic to rhubarb, its constituents, or related plants from the Polygonaceae family. Avoid using rhubarb for more than two weeks. Avoid with atony, colitis, Crohn's disease, dehydration, electrolyte depletion, diarrhea, hemorrhoids, insufficient liver function, intestinal obstruction, ileus, irritable bowel syndrome, menstruation, preeclampsia, kidney disorders, ulcerative colitis, or urinary problems. Avoid handling rhubarb leaves, as they may cause contact dermatitis. Avoid rhubarb in children younger than age 12 due to water depletion. Use cautiously with bleeding disorders, heart conditions, constipation, thin or brittle bones, or a history of kidney stones. Use cautiously if taking antipsychotic drugs or anticoagulants or oral drugs, herbs, or supplements (including calcium, iron, and zinc). Avoid if pregnant or breastfeeding.

Seaweed, Kelp, Bladderwrack: Bladderwrack (*Fucus vesiculosus*) is a brown seaweed found along the northern coasts of the Atlantic and Pacific oceans and North and Baltic seas. There is not enough scientific evidence to determine if bladderwrack can help obese patients lose weight. Further research is warranted in this area.

Avoid if allergic or hypersensitive to *Fucus vesiculosus* or iodine. Avoid with a history of thyroid disease, bleeding, acne, kidney disease, blood clots, nerve disorders, high blood pressure, stroke, or diabetes. Avoid if pregnant or breastfeeding.

Soy: Due to limited human study, there is not enough evidence to recommend for or against the use of soy for weight reduction. Further research is needed before a recommendation can be made.

In theory, soy supplements may interfere with the effects of some chemotherapy regimens or radiation therapy because of its antioxidant properties. Use cautiously if taking anticoagulants. The use of soy is often discouraged in patients with hormone-sensitive cancer (e.g., such as breast, ovarian, or uterine cancer) due to concerns about possible estrogenlike effects, which may theoretically stimulate tumor growth.

Spirulina: The term spirulina refers to a large number of cyanobacteria, or blue-green algae. Spirulina is a popular therapy for weight loss, and it is sometimes marketed as a "vitamin-enriched" appetite suppressant. However, little scientific information is available on the effects of spirulina on weight loss in humans.

Avoid if allergic or hypersensitive to spirulina or blue-green algae. Avoid with phenylketonuria. Avoid if pregnant or breastfeeding.

Taurine: Currently, there is insufficient available evidence to recommend for or against the use of taurine in the treatment of obesity.

Taurine is an amino acid, and it is unlikely that there are allergies related to this constituent. However, allergies may occur from multi-ingredient products that contain taurine. Use cautiously with high very-low-density lipoprotein cholesterol, hypertriglyceridemia, or with a history of low blood pressure, coagulation disorders, potential for mania, or epilepsy. Use cautiously if taking hypolipidemic medications or hypotensive, hypoglycemic, antiplatelet, or anticoagulant medications. Avoid consumption of energy drinks containing taurine, caffeine, glucuronolactone, B vitamins, and other ingredients before consuming alcohol or exercising. Use cautiously if pregnant or breastfeeding. Taurine is a natural component of breast milk.

Vitamin A (Retinol): Vitamin A is a fat-soluble vitamin that is derived from two sources: retinoids and carotenoids. Retinoids are found in animal sources (e.g., livers, kidneys, eggs, and dairy products). Carotenoids are found in plants (e.g., dark-colored or yellow vegetables). Daily vitamin A with calcium has been suggested for weight loss. In one study, an average loss of two pounds was reported after two years of supplementation in young women. However, further research is needed before a firm conclusion can be made in this area.

Avoid if allergic or hypersensitive to vitamin A. Vitamin A toxicity can occur if taken at high dosages. Use cautiously with liver disease or alcoholism. Smokers who consume alcohol and beta-carotene may be at an increased risk for lung cancer or heart disease. Vitamin A appears safe in pregnant women if taken at recommended doses. Use cautiously if breastfeeding because the benefits or dangers to nursing infants are not clearly established.

Yoga: Yoga is an ancient system of relaxation, exercise, and healing with origins in Indian philosophy. Yoga has been described as "the union of mind, body, and spirit," which addresses physical, mental, intellectual, emotional, and spiritual dimensions towards an overall harmonious state of being. Preliminary research does not provide clear answers. Yoga, in addition to healthy eating habits, may reduce weight. Better studies are necessary to form conclusions about the potential benefits of yoga alone.

Yoga is generally considered to be safe in healthy individuals when practiced appropriately. Avoid some inverted poses with disk disease of the spine, fragile or atherosclerotic neck arteries, extremely high or low blood pressure, glaucoma, detachment of the retina, ear problems, severe osteoporosis, cervical spondylitis, or risk for blood clots. Certain yoga breathing techniques should be avoided in people with heart or lung disease. Use cautiously with a history of psychotic disorders. Yoga techniques are believed to be safe during pregnancy and breastfeeding when practiced under the guidance of expert instruction. However, poses that put pressure on the uterus, such as abdominal twists, should be avoided in pregnancy.

Traditional or Theoretical Uses Lacking Sufficient Evidence

Gymnema: While preliminary research reports that gymnema may be beneficial in patients with type 1 or type 2 diabetes, there is currently no available clinical evidence with use of gymnema for obesity, a purported traditional or theoretical use. High-quality human research is needed in this area to further understand gymnema's potential use for obesity.

Hoodia: Hoodia (*Hoodia gordonii*) has purportedly been used and recently marketed as an appetite suppressant and weight reduction aid. Secondary sources note that the Bushmen of the Kalahari have eaten it to help ward off hunger and thirst during long trips in the desert. Unlike ephedra, hoodia does not appear to work as a stimulant, but rather it acts as an appetite suppressant. The pharmaceutical company Phytopharm (Godmanchester, UK) has found hoodia promising and is currently attempting to isolate the appetite-suppressing molecule, P57, to create a patented diet drug in the future. P57 was at one time licensed to Pfizer for development but was discontinued in 2003.

There are currently no available reliable human trials demonstrating efficacy and safety of hoodia for any indication. Additional research is needed in this area before a clinical recommendation can be made.

Fair Negative Scientific Evidence

Acupressure, Shiatsu: During acupressure, finger pressure is applied to specific acupoints on the body. Preliminary evidence suggests that acupressure may not be effective for weight loss.

With proper training, acupressure appears to be safe if self-administered or administered by an experienced therapist. No serious long-term complications have been reported, according to scientific data. Hand nerve injury and herpes zoster (shingles) cases have been reported after shiatsu massage. Forceful acupressure may cause bruising.

Beta-Glucan: Beta-glucan is a fiber derived that comes from the cell walls of algae, bacteria, fungi, yeast, and plants. Researchers suggest different types of fiber may have an effect on satiety and energy intake. Short-term use of fermentable fiber or nonfermentable fiber supplements does not appear to promote weight loss. More study is needed to confirm these findings.

Avoid if allergic or hypersensitive to beta-glucan. When taken by mouth, beta-glucans are generally considered safe. Use cautiously with acquired im-munodeficiency syndrome or related complex. Avoid using particulate insoluble beta-glucan, as preliminary evidence suggests intravenous beta-glucans in the microparticulate form may cause serious side effects, including hepatosplenomegaly (enlargement of both the liver and the spleen). Avoid if pregnant or breastfeeding.

PREVENTION

Awareness: Individuals should regularly visit their healthcare providers and know what their healthy weight should be. Individuals should also regularly weigh themselves so they can make lifestyle changes if they start to gain weight. Individuals who are overweight or obese should be aware of the health risks associated with these conditions, including high blood pressure, high cholesterol, diabetes, heart disease, stroke, and diabetes. In order to prevent these complications, overweight individuals should make lifestyle changes to promote weight loss.

Exercise: Regular exercise can help individuals maintain a healthy weight. It has also been shown to control diabetes, reduce stress, and reduce the risk of heart disease and stroke. Thirty minutes daily of exercise is normally recommended. Patients should talk to their healthcare providers before starting new exercise programs.

Diet: Eating a healthy and well-balanced diet is essential to maintaining a healthy weight. A healthy diet should include five or more daily servings of fruits and vegetables, foods rich in soluble fiber (such as oatmeal and beans), foods rich in calcium (such as dairy products, spinach), soy products (such as tempeh, miso, tofu, and soy milk), and foods rich in omega-3 fatty acids, including cold water fish (such as salmon, mackerel, and tuna).

Stress Management: Because stress may increase the risk of becoming obese, stress management is recommended.

OSTEOPOROSIS

CONDITION: Osteoporosis

BACKGROUND

Osteoporosis is a disease of the bones that makes them weak and prone to fracture. Osteoporosis is considered a silent disease because bone loss itself is gradual and painless. There are usually no symptoms to indicate that a person is developing osteoporosis early in the condition. Bone is living tissue that is in a constant state of formation and resorption. Bone resorption is the gradual loss of bone. As individuals age, formation lessens and after a peak bone mass is achieved, bone mass remains stable (resorption and formation are equal). Osteoclasts are the principal cells responsible for bone resorption. By their mid-30s, most individuals begin to gradually lose bone strength as the balance between bone resorption and bone formation shifts so that more bone is lost than can be replaced. As a result, bones become less dense and structurally weaker, called osteopenia. Osteopenia refers to mild bone loss that is not severe enough to be called osteoporosis but that increases the risk of developing osteoporosis. As this occurs, bones lose calcium, phosphorus, boron, and other minerals and become lighter, less dense, and more porous. This makes the bones weaker and increases the chance that they might break. If not prevented or if left untreated, osteopenia can progress painlessly into osteoporosis until a bone breaks or fractures.

Although any bone is susceptible to fracture, the most common fractures in osteoporosis occur at the spine, wrist, and hip. Spine and hip fractures in particular may lead to chronic pain, long-term disability, and even death. Osteoporosis is more common in older individuals and non-Hispanic white women but can occur at any age, in men as well as in women, and in all ethnic groups. In the United States, about eight million women and two million men have osteoporosis. Those over the age of 50 are at greatest risk of developing osteoporosis and suffering related fractures. In this age group, one in two women and one in six men will suffer an osteoporosis-related fracture at some point in their lives. Significant risk has been reported in people of all ethnic backgrounds. While osteoporosis is often thought of as a condition found in older individuals, it can strike at any age. Osteoporosis may also affect children, although it is rare. This is called juvenile osteoporosis. Juvenile osteoporosis is usually due to a medical condition, such as a thyroid condition or Cushing's disease (a rare condition involving insufficient adrenal hormone output), or medications, including corticosteroids. It's a significant problem because it occurs during the child's prime bone-building years. Conditions that may cause bone loss include osteomalacia, osteochondrosis, Kashin-Beck disease, and skeletal fluorosis. Osteomalacia is a softening of the bones resulting from defective bone mineralization. Osteomalacia may cause pain, weakness, and fragility of the bones. Osteomalacia is caused by insufficient nutritional quantities or faulty metabolism of vitamin D or calcium, following a parathyroidectomy (removal of the parathyroid gland), or in other conditions such as cystic fibrosis, renal osteodystrophy (failure of kidneys to maintain adequate blood nutrients for bone), and hepatic osteodystrophy (failure of the liver to produce adequate vitamin D). Kashin-Beck disease is a disorder of the bones and joints of the hands, fingers, elbows, knees, and ankles of children and adolescents who slowly develop stiff, deformed joints, shortened limb length, and short stature due to necrosis (death) of the growth plates of bones and of joint cartilage. Osteochondrosis is a disease that affects the progress of bone growth by killing bone tissue. Osteochondrosis is seen only in children and teens whose bones are still growing. Osteochondrosis is an inherited condition. Individuals with osteochondrosis nearly all have pain in the location of the bone damage. Some may involve considerable swelling, limping, bending, or kyphosis (exaggerated curve) of the upper spine. Skeletal fluorosis is the chronic intake of excessive fluoride. Skeletal fluorosis can lead to severe and permanent bone and joint deformations. This can lead to softening of the bone and increases in fractures. Skeletal fluorosis should not occur with fluorinated water or toothpaste use.

CAUSES AND RISK FACTORS

The strength of bones depends on their size and density. Bone density depends in part on the amount of calcium, phosphorus, boron, and other minerals that bones contain. When bones contain fewer minerals than normal, they are less strong and eventually lose their internal supporting structure. Genetic and environmental factors, such as diet and exercise, also affect bone strength. There are many reasons that bone becomes less dense than normal. Bone is continuously changing. New bone is made and old bone is broken down in a process called remodeling, or bone turnover.

O

A full cycle of bone remodeling takes about two to three months. When an individual is young, the body makes new bone faster than it breaks down old bone, and bone mass increases. Individuals reach their peak bone mass in the mid-30s. After that, bone remodeling continues, but slightly more bone is lost than is gained. In women at menopause, when estrogen levels drop, bone loss increases dramatically. Although many factors contribute to bone loss, the leading cause in women is decreased estrogen production during menopause. When women go through menopause, their estrogen levels drop to one-third of what these levels were during the childbearing years. Estrogen increases bone density by helping to block bone resorption.

The risk of developing osteoporosis depends on how much bone mass was attained between ages 25-35 (peak bone mass) and how rapidly the individual loses it later. The higher the peak bone mass, the more bone the individual has and less likely to develop osteoporosis as he/she ages and less likely to suffer major bone loss. Not getting enough vitamin D and calcium in the diet and enough exercise may lead to a lower peak bone mass and accelerated bone loss later in life.

Gender: Fractures from osteoporosis are about twice as common in women as they are in men. Although women are four times more likely than men to develop the disease, men also suffer from osteoporosis. Women develop osteoporosis more often because they start out with lower bone mass and tend to live longer. They also experience a sudden drop in estrogen at menopause that accelerates bone loss. Slender, small-framed women are particularly at risk. Men who have low levels of the male hormone testosterone also are at increased risk. From age 75 years on, osteoporosis is as common in men as it is in women.

It is estimated that around 40% of U.S. Caucasian women and 13% of U.S. Caucasian men aged 50 years and older will experience at least one fracture due to bone loss in their lifetimes. It is also estimated that in the United States, 54% of postmenopausal Caucasian women are osteopenic and 30% are osteoporotic, and by the age of 80, 27% of Caucasian women are osteopenic and 70% are osteoporotic.

Age: Bones weaken during normal aging in a process called resorption. As individuals age, whether male or female, there is an average loss of 0.5% bone mass every year after age 50.

Race: Caucasians and Southeast Asians are at the greatest risk of osteoporosis. African-American and Latino men and women have a lower but still significant risk of osteoporosis-related fractures.

Family History: Osteoporosis is, in part, hereditary. Having a parent or sibling (brother or sister) with osteoporosis puts the individual at greater risk, especially if the individual also has a family history of bone fractures. An individual with a family member who has osteoporosis has a 50-85% increased risk of developing osteoporosis.

Frame Size: Men and women who are exceptionally thin or have small body frames tend to have higher risk because they may have less bone mass to draw from as they age.

Smoking: The impact of cigarette smoking on bone health is not well understood. Smoking may cause a decrease in bone density due to smoking itself or to other risk factors, such as general health. Smokers are usually thinner than nonsmokers, tend to drink more alcohol, may be less physically active, and have poor diets. Women who smoke also tend to have an earlier menopause than nonsmokers. These factors place many smokers at an increased risk for osteoporosis apart from their tobacco use. In addition, most studies on the effects of smoking suggest that smoking increases the risk of having a fracture. Results have found that the longer an individual smokes and the more cigarettes consumed, the greater the risk of fracture in old age. Smokers who fracture may take longer to heal. Significant bone loss has been found in older women and men who smoke. Studies suggest secondhand smoke exposure during youth may increase the risk of developing low bone mass. Also, women who smoke often produce less estrogen and tend to experience menopause earlier than nonsmokers. Smoking cessations appears to reduce the risk of low bone mass and fractures.

Estrogen Levels: The longer a woman is exposed to estrogen, the lower her risk of osteoporosis. Women have a lower risk if they have a late menopause or they began menstruating at an earlier than average age. However, a history of abnormal menstrual periods, experiencing menopause earlier than the late 40s, or having the ovaries surgically removed before age 45 without receiving hormone therapy may also increase the risk of developing osteoporosis.

Health Conditions: Health conditions caused by hormone imbalances, such as hyperthyroidism (too much thyroid hormone), hyperparathyroidism (too much parathyroid hormone), and Cushing's syndrome (too much adrenal hormone) may increase the risk for osteoporosis because they interfere with the regulation of the hormones that regulate remodeling. Gastrointestinal disorders, such as celiac disease and Crohn's disease, which affect absorption of calcium and vitamin D, also increase the risk.

Early-onset menopause brought on by the removal of the uterus (hysterectomy) and the complete removal of the ovaries (oophorectomy) is associated with osteoporosis. For men, alcoholism is one of the leading risk factors for osteoporosis. Excess consumption of alcohol reduces bone formation and interferes with the body's ability to absorb calcium. Individuals who experience serious depression have increased rates of bone loss. Depression activates the sympathetic nervous system, which responds to impending danger or stress, causing the release of a chemical compound called noradrenaline that harms bone-building cells. Women and men with eating disorders, such as anorexia nervosa or bulimia, are at higher risk of lower bone density in their lower backs and hips. Eating disorders have significant physical consequences. Affected individuals can experience nutritional and hormonal problems that negatively impact bone density. Low body weight in females causes the body to stop producing estrogen, resulting in a condition known as amenorrhea, or absent menstrual periods. Low estrogen levels contribute to significant losses in bone density. In addition, individuals with anorexia often produce excessive amounts of the adrenal hormone cortisol, which is known to trigger bone loss. Other problems, such as a decrease in the production of growth hormone and other growth factors, low body weight, calcium deficiency, and malnutrition, all contribute to bone loss in individuals with eating disorders. Weight loss, restricted dietary intake, and testosterone deficiency may be responsible for the low bone density found in males with the disorder. Studies suggest that low bone mass (osteopenia) is common in people with anorexia and that it occurs early in the course of the disease. Girls with anorexia are less likely to reach their peak bone density and therefore may be at increased risk for osteoporosis and fracture throughout life.

Medications: Certain medications may decrease the body's ability to absorb calcium and may increase the risk of developing osteoporosis. Postmenopausal women who have had breast cancer are at increased risk of osteoporosis, especially if they were treated with medications such as anastrozole (Arimidex), letrozole (Femara), and exemestane (Aromasin), which suppress estrogen. Women treated with tamoxifen (Nolvadex) do not seem to develop an increase in bone loss. Diuretics, or medications that prevent buildup of fluids in the body can cause the kidneys to excrete more calcium, leading to thinning bones. Diuretics that cause calcium loss include furosemide (Lasix), bumetanide (Bumex), ethacrynic acid (Edecrin), and torsemide (Demadex). Long-term use of the blood-thinning medication heparin, the drug methotrexate (Rheumatrex), some antiseizure medications such as phenytoin (Dilantin), and aluminum-containing antacids such as Amphojel may also lead to bone loss. Cholestyramine (Cholestin), used to control blood cholesterol levels, may decrease calcium absorption, and increase the risk of osteoporosis. Gonadotropin-releasing hormones (such as Lupron) used for the treatment of endometriosis may also decrease calcium absorption and increase the risk of osteoporosis. Corticosteroids, such as prednisone (Deltasone), may lead to osteoporosis. Approximately 30-50% of individuals taking corticosteroids long term develop osteoporosis. Relatively short courses (two to three months) of more than 7.5 milligrams of prednisone (Deltasone) can cause significant bone loss. The common long-term use of corticosteroids in conditions such as rheumatoid arthritis results in a dramatic increase in vertebral and ultimately hip fracture rates.

Low Calcium Intake: A lifelong lack of calcium plays a major role in the development of osteoporosis. Low calcium intake contributes to poor bone density, early bone loss, and an increased risk of fractures.

Lack of Exercise: Exercise can increase bone density at any age. Children who are physically active and consume adequate amounts of calcium-containing foods have the greatest bone density.

Excess Soda Consumption: The link between osteoporosis and caffeinated sodas is not clear, but caffeine and phosphoric acid in the drinks may interfere with calcium absorption. Caffeine is also a diuretic, which may increase mineral loss.

SIGNS AND SYMPTOMS

In the early stages of bone loss, there usually is no pain or symptoms. Once bones have been weakened by osteoporosis, signs and symptoms may include back pain, which can be severe with a fractured or collapsed vertebra; loss of height over time, with an accompanying stooped posture; and fracture of the vertebrae, wrists, hips, or other bones.

While limb fractures (such as wrist or hip) are obvious, spine fractures can be more difficult to diagnose. Spinal fractures might either be painless, or if there is pain, a person may not know it is caused by a fracture because there are so many different causes of back pain. More obvious signs of spine fractures are loss of height and development of kyphosis or a curved upper back, sometimes called a dowager's hump.

COMPLICATIONS

Fractures: Fractures are the most frequent and serious complication of osteoporosis. Fractures often occur in the spine or hips, bones that directly support weight. Hip fractures, the second most common type of osteoporotic fracture, usually result from a fall. Although most individuals do relatively well in recovery with modern surgical treatment, hip fractures can result in disability and even death from postoperative complications, especially in older adults. Wrist fractures from falls are also common. Complications from osteoporotic fractures include chronic pain (neck, lower back), compressed or collapsed vertebrae, disability, depression, limited activity, dowager's hump, stooped posture, and loss of height.

DIAGNOSIS

Bone Mineral Density (BMD): BMD is a measurement of the amount of calcium in the bones. Various diagnostic tests exist to determine BMD in individuals susceptible to osteoporosis, such as dual-energy x-ray absorptiometry. The National Osteoporosis Foundation recommends a bone density test in women if they are not taking estrogen and any if the following conditions apply: they are taking medications such as corticosteroids (e.g., prednisone [Deltasone]) that can cause osteoporosis; they have type 1 diabetes, liver disease, kidney disease, or a family history of osteoporosis; they experience early menopause; they are postmenopausal (older than 50) and have at least one risk factor for osteoporosis; and if they are postmenopausal (older than 65) and have never had a bone density test. Doctors do not generally recommend osteoporosis screening for men because the disease is less common in men than it is in women.

Dual-Energy X-Ray Absorptiometry (DEXA): DEXA is the most accurate way to measure BMD. DEXA uses two different x-ray beams to estimate bone density in the spine and hip. Strong, dense bones allow less of the x-ray beam to pass through them. The amounts of each x-ray beam that are blocked by bone and soft tissue are compared to each other. DEXA can measure as little as 2% of bone loss per year. It is fast and uses very low doses of radiation but is more expensive than ultrasound testing. Single-energy x-ray absorptiometry (SXA) uses one x-ray beam and may be used to measure heel and forearm bone density. SXA is not used as often as DEXA due to less accuracy.

The results of the DEXA test are scored in comparison to the BMD of young, healthy individuals, resulting in a measurement called a T-score. If the T-score is −2.5 or lower, the individual is considered to have osteoporosis and therefore at high risk for a fracture. T-scores between −1.0 and −2.5 are generally considered to show osteopenia. The risk of fractures generally is lower in individuals with osteopenia when compared with those with osteoporosis but, if bone loss continues, the risk for fracture increases.

Peripheral DEXA (P-DEXA): P-DEXA is a type of DEXA test. P-DEXA measures the density of bones in the arms or legs, such as the wrist. P-DEXA cannot measure the density of the bones most likely to break, such as the hip and spine. P-DEXA machines are portable units that can be used in a doctor's office. P-DEXA also uses very low doses of radiation, and the results are ready faster than standard DEXA measurements. P-DEXA is not as useful as DEXA for finding out how well medicine used to treat osteoporosis is working. P-DEXA may be used in less serious cases of osteoporosis.

Dual-Photon Absorptiometry (DPA): DPA uses a radioactive substance to measure bone density. The radioactivity passes through the body similar to an x-ray. DPA can measure BMD in the hip and spine. DPA also uses very low doses of radiation but has a slower scan time than the other methods.

Quantitative Ultrasound: Ultrasound uses sound waves to measure BMD, usually in the heel. If results from an ultrasound test find low bone density, DEXA is recommended to confirm the results. Machines pass the sound waves through air and some pass them through water. Ultrasound is quick, painless, and does not use potentially harmful radiation like x-rays. One disadvantage of ultrasound is it cannot measure the density of the bones most likely to fracture (the hip and spine) from osteoporosis.

Quantitative Computed Tomography (QCT): QCT is a type of computed tomography scan that measures the density of a bone in the spine (vertebra). A form of QCT called peripheral QCT measures the density of bones in the arms or legs, usually the wrist. QCT is not usually used because it is expensive, uses higher radiation doses, and is less accurate than DEXA, P-DEXA, or DPA.

X-Rays: X-rays are low doses of radiation that are used to create an image of a body part, organ, or bodily system on film paper or fluorescent screens. X-rays show the alignment of the spine and may reveal degenerative joint disease, fracture, or tumor. X-rays cannot determine BMD but can determine if a fracture has occurred.

TREATMENT

Nutrition and Lifestyle

Dietary Factors: It is important to that there is enough calcium in the diet for proper bone health.

Healthcare professionals recommend calcium intakes of at least 1,000 mg daily for everyone over eight years of age. Higher calcium intakes of 1,200 mg daily are recommended for adults over 50 years and 1,300 mg daily for teens nine to 18 years. Adequate vitamin D intake is also important for calcium absorption and to maintain muscle strength. Healthcare professionals recommend 400 international units of vitamin D daily until age 60, then 600-800 international units per day after age 60. Doses can be adjusted by a doctor according to blood levels of vitamin D. Milk and milk products are calcium-dense foods providing about 300 milligrams calcium per serving. These foods also contain other nutrients important to bone health such as vitamin D (if fortified), phosphorus, and magnesium. Approximately 73% of calcium in the food supply comes from dairy products, 9% from fruits and vegetables, 5% from grain products, and 12% from all other sources, such as dietary supplements.

Weight-Bearing Exercises: Exercise is an important treatment for osteoporosis to maintain healthy bones. Weight-bearing aerobic activities involving the bones supporting body weight have been shown to have a positive effect in maintaining and increasing bone mass and preventing osteoporosis. These activities include weightlifting, jogging, hiking, stair climbing, step aerobics, dancing, racquet sports, and other activities that require muscles to work against gravity. Swimming and simply walking, although good for cardiovascular fitness, are not the best exercises for building bone. Individuals who live a sedentary lifestyle have weaker bones and are subjected to a higher risk of sustaining fractures.

Medications

Bisphosphonates: Alendronate (Fosamax), risedronate (Actonel), ibandronate (Boniva), and zoledronate (Zometa) are approved by the U.S. Food and Drug Administration for the prevention and treatment of osteoporosis in postmenopausal women. Alendronate is a drug currently approved for management of osteoporosis in men. Both alendronate and risedronate are approved for the prevention and treatment of steroid-induced osteoporosis in men and women. Bisphosphonates help slow down bone loss and have been shown to decrease the risk of fractures. All are taken on an empty stomach with water. Because bisphosphonates have the potential for irritating the esophagus, remaining upright for at least an hour after taking these medications is recommended by healthcare professionals. Alendronate and risedronate can be taken once a week, while ibandronate can be taken once a month. An intravenous form of ibandronate, given through the vein every three months, also has been FDA approved for the management of osteoporosis. Another intravenous bisphosphonate being studied for osteoporosis is zoledronic acid or zoledronate (Zometa). This form is injected once yearly. Side effects, which can be severe, include nausea, abdominal pain, and the risk of an inflamed esophagus or esophageal ulcers, especially if the individual has had acid reflux or ulcers in the past. If individuals cannot tolerate oral bisphosphonates, the doctor may recommend the periodic intravenous infusions of a bisphosphonate.

Use of bisphosphonates in women who are pregnant or breastfeeding is not well studied. Blood calcium levels in women who take bisphosphonates during pregnancy are usually monitored. Individuals using Boniva injection will have blood levels of creatinine measured prior to each dose to determine kidney function. Creatinine is measured using blood tests.

Calcitonin (Miacalcin): Calcitonin is a naturally occurring hormone produced by the thyroid gland that can be given as an injection or taken as a nasal spray. Calcitonin also inhibits the function of the cells that break down bone, the osteoclasts. Calcitonin has long been known to be beneficial in individuals with osteoporosis, but the injections were difficult to administer and had unpleasant side effects. The nasal spray has greatly improved the use of calcitonin, and it is much more commonly used today. Calcitonin has been reported to slow bone loss and also decrease pain associated with osteoporosis fractures.

Hormone Replacement Therapy (HRT): Estrogen therapy alone or in combination with another hormone, progestin, has been reported to decrease the risk of osteoporosis and osteoporotic fractures in women. However, the combination of estrogen with a progestin has been shown to increase the risk for breast and ovarian cancer, strokes, heart attacks, and blood clots. Estrogens alone may increase the risk of strokes. Healthcare professionals recommend weighing all options before choosing HRT as part of osteoporosis prevention.

Selective Estrogen Receptor Modulators (SERMs): SERMs mimic the positive effects of estrogen on bones without some of the serious side effects such as breast cancer and stroke. Raloxifene (Evista) decreases spine fractures in women and is approved for use only in women at this time. Hot flashes are a common side effect of raloxifene, and individuals with a history of blood clots should not use this drug.

Teriparatide (Forteo): Teriparatide is a form of parathyroid hormone that helps stimulate bone formation. Teriparatide is approved for use in post-menopausal women and men at high risk for osteo-porotic fracture. It is given as a daily injection under the skin and can be used for up to two years. Individuals who have ever had radiation treatment or have parathyroid hormone levels that are already too high may not be able to take this medication.

Tamoxifen (Nolvadex): Tamoxifen (Nolvadex) is a synthetic hormone used to treat breast cancer and is given to certain high-risk women to help reduce their chances of developing breast cancer. Although tamoxifen blocks estrogen's effect on breast tissue, it has an estrogenlike effect on other cells in the body, including bone cells. As a result, tamoxifen appears to reduce the risk of fractures, especially in women over age 50. Possible side effects of tamoxifen include hot flashes, stomach upset, and vaginal dryness or discharge.

Surgery

Vertebroplasty: Vertebroplasty is a minimally in-vasive procedure used to reinforce vertebrae with compression fractures. Compression fractures are common in individuals with osteoporosis. Vertebro-plasty involves injecting an acrylic compound into the collapsed vertebrae to stabilize the weakened bone. The procedure is performed in an operating room or radiology suite, and treatment of each affected vertebra takes approximately one hour.

Local anesthesia, usually lidocaine (Xylocaine), is injected into the vertebra. Then, a small incision is made, and a bone biopsy needle is inserted. Several small syringes of the acrylic cementing material are then injected through the needle into the vertebra. The cement hardens almost immediately.

Approximately 70-90% of individuals experience pain relief after vertebroplasty, and most are released from the hospital the same day. Antiinflammatory medications such as ibuprofen (Motrin, Advil) may be used to relieve pain after the procedure. Complications from a vertebroplasty are rare. Bone cement may enter the lung, spinal cord, or epidural space surrounding the vertebrae. Other possible complications associated with vertebroplasty include nerve irritation, punctured lung (pneumothorax), and spinal cord injury.

Kyphoplasty: Multiple spinal compression fractures caused by osteoporosis may lead to height loss, kyphosis (extreme curvature of the spine), and pain. Kyphoplasty is a minimally invasive procedure that is used to restore the height of the vertebrae

and stabilize weakened bone. Kyphoplasty cannot correct established spine deformities and is used in individuals who have experienced recent fractures, usually within two to four months. The procedure is usually performed in the hospital under local or general anesthesia and takes approximately one hour for each affected vertebra. A small incision is made and a fluoroscope (device that consists of a screen and an x-ray tube) is used to guide the insertion of a balloon catheter into the vertebra. The balloon is inflated slowly to raise the compressed vertebra and is deflated. An acrylic compound (cementing material) is then injected into the vertebra through a bone biopsy needle. The material hardens almost immediately. Pain relief usually occurs within two days.

Most individuals are released from the hospital the day after kyphoplasty and can resume daily activities upon discharge. Strenuous activity, such as heavy lifting, should be avoided for at least six weeks.

INTEGRATIVE THERAPIES
Strong Scientific Evidence

Calcium: Calcium is the nutrient consistently found to be the most important nutrient for attaining peak bone mass and preventing osteoporosis. Adequate vitamin D intake is required for optimal calcium absorption. Adequate calcium and vitamin D are deemed essential for the prevention of osteoporosis in general, including postmenopausal osteoporosis. Although calcium and vitamin D alone are not recommended as the sole treatment of osteoporosis, they are necessary additions to pharmaceutical treatments. The vast majority of clinical trials investigating the efficacy of pharmaceutical treatments for osteoporosis have investigated these agents in combination with calcium and vitamin D. So, although calcium alone is unlikely to have an effect on the rate of bone loss following menopause, osteoporosis cannot be treated in the absence of calcium. Treatment of postmenopausal osteoporosis should only be done under the supervision of a qualified healthcare professional. Multiple studies of calcium supplementation in the elderly and postmenopausal women have found that high calcium intakes can help reduce the loss of bone density. Studies indicated that bone loss could be prevented in many areas, including ankles, hips, and spine.

Vitamin D: Vitamin D is found in numerous dietary sources such as fish, eggs, fortified milk, and cod liver oil. The sun is also a significant contributor to our daily production of vitamin D, and as little as 10 minutes of exposure is thought to be enough to prevent deficiencies. In adults with severe vitamin D deficiency, bone mineral is lost (hypomineralization) and results in bone pain and osteomalacia (soft bones). Osteomalacia may result from deficiency of vitamin D in elderly patients, decreased absorption of vitamin D, patients with chronic malabsorption syndrome secondary to jejunoileal bypass, patients with partial gastrectomy, aluminum-induced bone disease, chronic liver disease, or kidney disease with renal osteodystrophy. Treatment for osteomalacia depends on the underlying cause of the disease and often includes pain control and orthopedic surgical intervention as well as vitamin D and phosphate binding agents.

Good Scientific Evidence

Vitamin D: Without sufficient vitamin D, calcium absorption cannot be maximized, and the resulting elevation in parathyroid secretion by the parathyroid glands results in increased bone resorption, which may weaken bones and increase the risk of fracture. Vitamin D supplementation has been demonstrated to slow bone loss and reduce fracture, particularly when taken with calcium. Oral calcifediol or ergocalciferol may help manage hypocalcemia and prevent renal osteodystrophy in people with chronic renal failure undergoing dialysis. Renal osteodystrophy is a term that refers to all of the bone problems that occur in patients with chronic kidney failure.

Unclear or Conflicting Scientific Evidence

Black Tea: Black tea (*Camellia sinensis*) is from the same shrub as green tea and oolong tea. Each is processed differently. Preliminary research suggests that chronic use of black tea may improve BMD in older women. Better research is needed in this area before a conclusion can be drawn. Caffeine is a stimulant of the central nervous system and may cause insomnia in adults, children, and infants (including nursing infants of mothers taking caffeine). Caffeine acts on the kidneys as a diuretic (increasing urine and urine sodium/potassium levels, and potentially decreasing blood sodium/potassium levels), and may worsen incontinence. Caffeine-containing beverages may increase the production of stomach acid and may worsen ulcer symptoms. Tannin in tea can cause constipation. Caffeine in certain doses can increase heart rate and blood pressure, although people who consume caffeine regularly do not seem to experience these effects in the long term. There are many drug interactions possible when using caffeinated beverages.

Boron: Boron is a trace mineral found in the global environment. Animal and preliminary human studies report that boron may play a role in mineral metabolism, with effects on calcium, phosphorus, and vitamin D. However, research of BMD in women taking boron supplements does not clearly demonstrate benefits in osteoporosis. Additional study is needed before a firm conclusion can be drawn.

Calcium: Calcium is the nutrient consistently found to be the most important for attaining peak bone mass and preventing osteoporosis. Adequate vitamin D intake is required for optimal calcium absorption. Adequate calcium and vitamin D are deemed essential for the prevention of osteoporosis in general, including postmenopausal osteoporosis. Calcium supplementation in patients on long-term, high-dose inhaled steroids for asthma may reduce bone loss due to steroid intake. Treatment using the prescription drug pamidronate with calcium has been shown to be superior to calcium alone in the prevention of corticosteroid-induced osteoporosis. Inhaled steroids have been reported to disturb normal bone metabolism, and they are associated with a decrease in BMD. Results suggest that long-term administration of high-dose inhaled steroid induces bone loss that is preventable with calcium supplementation with or without the prescription drug etidronate. Long-term studies involving more patients should follow to confirm these preliminary findings.

Rickets and osteomalacia (bone softening) are commonly thought of as diseases due to vitamin D deficiency; however, calcium deficiency may also be another risk factor in sunny areas of the world where vitamin D deficiency would not be expected. Calcium gluconate is used as an adjuvant in the treatment of rickets and osteomalacia as well as a single therapeutic agent in non-vitamin D–deficient rickets. Research continues into the importance of calcium alone in the treatment and prevention of rickets and osteomalacia. Treatment of rickets and osteomalacia should only be done under supervision of a qualified healthcare professional.

Copper: Copper is a mineral that occurs naturally in many foods, including vegetables, legumes, nuts, grains, and fruits, as well as shellfish, avocado, and beef (organs such as liver). Osteopenia and other abnormalities of bone development related to copper deficiency may occur in copper-deficient low birth weight infants and young children. Supplementation with copper may be helpful in the treatment and/or prevention of osteoporosis, although early human evidence is conflicting. The effects of copper deficiency or copper supplementation on bone metabolism and age-related osteoporosis require further research before clear conclusions can be drawn.

Dehydroepiandrosterone (DHEA): Laboratory studies have found that DHEA may improve BMD. The ability of DHEA to increase bone density in humans is under investigation. Effects are not clear at this time.

Gamma-Linolenic Acid (GLA): Some evidence from a clinical trial along with observations of clinicians and dieticians have suggested that GLA and eicosapentaenoic acid enhance the effects of calcium supplementation in elderly patients with osteoporosis. More clinical studies are required to produce results to determine effectiveness in diverse elderly and middle-age populations.

Horsetail: Silicon may be beneficial for bone strengthening. Because horsetail (*Equisetum arvense*) contains silicon, it has been suggested as a possible natural treatment for osteoporosis. Preliminary human study reports benefits, but more detailed research is needed before a firm recommendation can be made. People with osteoporosis should speak with a qualified healthcare provider about possible treatment with more proven therapies.

Physical Therapy: Supervised or home-based physical therapy has been used in combination with resistance and endurance training in physically frail elderly women taking HRT to improve bone density. Long-term, high-intensity, weight-bearing exercise programs have also been used in rheumatoid arthritis patients with some success. Although early study is promising, more studies are needed in this area.

Red Clover: It is not clear if red clover (*Trifolium pratense*) isoflavones have beneficial effects on bone density. Most studies of isoflavones in this area have looked at soy, which contains different amounts of isoflavones, as well as other nonisoflavone ingredients. More research is needed. Red clover extract may increase bleeding in sensitive individuals, including those taking blood-thinning medications such as warfarin (Coumadin).

Soy: It has been theorized that soy (*Glycine max*) phytoestrogens (plant-based compounds with weak estrogen like properties), such as isoflavones, may increase BMD in postmenopausal women and reduce the risk of fractures. However, most studies have not been well designed or reported. Until better research is available, a firm conclusion cannot be drawn. Individuals at risk for osteoporosis should speak with a qualified healthcare provider about the therapeutic options for increasing BMD.

Tai Chi: Preliminary research suggests that tai chi may be beneficial in delaying early bone loss in postmenopausal women. Additional evidence and long-term follow-up are needed to confirm these results.

Tamarind: Preliminary study has examined the use of tamarind (*Tamarindus indica*) for fluorosis prevention. Although beneficial outcomes have been reported, these results are not conclusive. Additional study is needed in this area.

Vitamin D: Some evidence implies that steroids may impair vitamin D metabolism, further contributing to the loss of bone and development of osteoporosis associated with steroid medications. There is limited evidence that vitamin D may be beneficial to bone strength in individuals taking long-term steroids. Osteoporosis is common in patients with cystic fibrosis due to fat malabsorption, which leads to a deficiency of fat-soluble vitamins such as vitamin D. Oral calcitriol administration appears to increase absorption of calcium and lower parathyroid concentrations.

Vitamin K: Vitamin K appears to prevent bone resorption, and adequate dietary intake is likely necessary to prevent excess bone loss. Elderly or institutionalized patients may be at particular risk, and adequate intake of vitamin K–rich foods should be maintained. Unless patients have demonstrated vitamin K deficiency, there is no evidence that additional vitamin K supplementation is helpful. However, vitamin K may play a role in the prevention and treatment of glucocorticoid-induced bone loss. Further research is needed to confirm these results. Over-the-counter vitamin K_1–containing multivitamin supplements may disrupt warfarin anticoagulation in vitamin K_1–depleted patients. Vitamin K–depleted patients are sensitive to even small changes in vitamin K_1 intake.

Fair Negative Scientific Evidence

Selenium: Selenium is a trace mineral found in soil, water, and some foods. It is an essential element in several metabolic pathways. Kashin-Beck disease is an osteoarthropathy endemic in selenium- and iodine-deficient areas. Preliminary evidence suggests that selenium supplementation does not significantly improve this disease.

Traditional or Theoretical Uses Lacking Sufficient Evidence

Integrative therapies used in pain, or related complications of osteoporosis causing pain, that have historical or theoretical uses but lack sufficient clinical evidence include the Alexander technique, anise (*Pimpinella anisum*), applied kinesiology, arginine

(L-arginine), black cohosh (*Actaea racemosa*), bovine colostrum, chelation (ethylenediamine tetraacetic acid) therapy, dong quai (*Angelica sinensis*), folate (folic acid), glucosamine, green tea (*Camellia sinensis*), hops (*Humulus lupulus*), kudzu (*Pueraria lobata*), Kundalini yoga, maca (*Lepidium meyenii*), magnet therapy, melatonin, mistletoe (*Viscum album*), octacosanol, omega-3 fatty acids (fish oil, alpha-linolenic acid), probiotics, resveratrol, rosemary (*Rosmarinus officinalis*), shiitake (*Lentinula edodes*), vitamin B_{12} (cyanocobalamin), vitamin C (ascorbic acid), and yoga.

PREVENTION

Smoking Cessation: Smokers lose bone more rapidly than nonsmokers. Among 80-year-olds, smokers have up to 10% lower BMD, which translates into twice the risk of spinal fractures and a 50% increase in risk of hip fracture. Fractures heal slower in smokers and are more apt to heal improperly.

Alcohol in Moderation: Excessive alcohol has been associated with osteoporosis due to the degenerative metabolic effects of alcohol. Alcohol excess may inhibit calcium absorption and bone formation.

Healthy Body Weight: Being underweight is a risk factor for osteoporosis. Staying within a healthy weight for an individual is important. Extreme thinness is a risk factor for osteoporosis. The onset of anorexia nervosa frequently occurs during puberty, the time of life when maximal bone mass accrual occurs, thereby putting adolescent girls with anorexia nervosa at high risk for reduced peak bone mass.

Sunlight: Healthcare professionals recommend sun exposure of 15 minutes a day to hands and face to help the body make vitamin D. Vitamin D helps calcium be absorbed and used by the body. Avoid overexposure to the sun.

Diet: A high-protein diet or high coffee consumption increases calcium loss and may increase the calcium needs for the body. Fiber, oxalates (in rhubarb, spinach, beets, celery, greens, berries, nuts, tea, cocoa), and high-zinc foods (such as oysters and red meats) decrease absorption, requiring taking more calcium in dietary supplement form. The plant estrogens found in soy help maintain bone density and may reduce the risk of fractures, particularly in the first 10 years after menopause.

Exercise: The amount and type of exercise will vary depending on age and bone health. An exercise program should be individually tailored to the individual's needs and capabilities. Overall, most individuals should aim to exercise for 30-40 minutes three to four times each week, with some weight-bearing and resistance exercises in the program. Although exercise is important in the prevention of osteoporosis, women and teenage girls who exercise to an extreme degree can develop amenorrhea (cessation of menstruation) due to estrogen deficiency. Estrogen deficiency in younger women contributes to bone loss in much the same way that estrogen deficiency after menopause does. Both male and female athletes who practice excessive exercise without adequate caloric intake are at heightened risk of osteoporosis. Athletes who train hard while trying to keep their weight below a certain level for competitive reasons are at particularly high risk.

Eliminating Fall Hazards: If an individual has osteoporosis, it is important not only to help prevent further bone loss, but also to prevent a fracture. Eliminating hazards in the house that can increase the risk of falling is important. Removing loose wires or throw rugs, installing grab bars in the bathroom and nonskid mats near sinks and in the tub, and not walking in slick shoes or socks are recommended by healthcare professionals. Healthcare professionals also recommend caution when carrying or lifting items, as this could cause a spinal fracture. Wearing sturdy shoes is important. Using a cane or walker is recommended by healthcare professionals if the individual has balance problems or other difficulties walking.

O

PARKINSON'S DISEASE

BACKGROUND

Parkinson's disease (PD) is a movement disorder that is chronic and progressive, meaning that symptoms continue and worsen over time. PD affects nerve cells in a part of the brain that controls muscle movement.

PD occurs when a group of cells in an area of the brain called the substantia nigra begins to malfunction and die. The cells in the substantia nigra produce a chemical called dopamine. Dopamine is a neurotransmitter, or chemical messenger, that sends information to the parts of the brain that control movement and coordination. When an individual has PD, their dopamine-producing cells begin to die and the amount of dopamine produced in the brain decreases. Messages from the brain telling the body how and when to move are therefore delivered more slowly, leaving a person incapable of initiating and controlling movements in a normal way.

PD is the most common form of parkinsonism. Parkinsonism is a group of movement disorders that have similar features and symptoms. When the cause of PD is unknown, it is called idiopathic PD.

The four primary symptoms of PD are tremor, or trembling in hands, arms, legs, jaw, and face; rigidity, or stiffness of the limbs and trunk; bradykinesia, or slowness of movement; and postural instability, or impaired balance and coordination (parkinsonian gait). As these symptoms become more severe, patients may have difficulty walking, talking, or completing other simple tasks. Early symptoms of PD are subtle and occur gradually. In some people, the disease progresses more quickly than in others. As the disease progresses, the shaking, or tremor, which affects the majority of PD patients may begin to interfere with daily activities. Other symptoms may include depression and other emotional changes; difficulty in swallowing, chewing, and speaking; urinary problems or constipation; skin problems; and sleep disruptions.

PD usually affects people over the age of 50. There are one to one and one-half million people in the United States living with PD. The disorder occurs in all races but is somewhat more prevalent among Caucasians. Men are affected slightly more often than women.

Symptoms of PD may appear at any age, but the average age of onset is 60. It is rare in people younger than 30 and risk increases with age. It is estimated that 5-10% of patients experience symptoms before the age of 40.

There are currently no blood or laboratory tests that have been proven to help in diagnosing PD. Therefore, the diagnosis is based on medical history and a neurological examination. The disease can be difficult to diagnose accurately. Doctors may sometimes request brain scans or laboratory tests in order to rule out other diseases.

RISK FACTORS AND CAUSES

Age: Age is one of the main risk factors for PD. Although the disease can rarely affect adults in their 20s, it ordinarily starts in middle or late life. The risk of developing PD continues to increase with age.

Heredity: Having one or more close relatives with PD increases the chances that the individual will also develop the disease. The risk of developing PD is still less than 5% if a relative has the condition.

Sex: Men are more likely to develop PD than women, possibly due in part to decreased levels of estrogen in men.

Exposure to Pesticides and Herbicides: Ongoing exposure to herbicides and pesticides puts an individual at slightly increased risk of developing PD. There is also an increased risk if the individual is involved in farming, lives in a rural area, or drinks well water. Local health departments can test well water for contaminants such as pesticides.

Reduced Estrogen Levels: Reduced estrogen levels may increase the risk of PD. Menopausal women who receive little or no hormone therapy (such as estrogen and progesterone) and those who have had a hysterectomy may be at an increased risk for developing PD. Menopausal women using hormonal therapy appear to have a decreased risk, as do women taking birth control pills. However, taking hormonal therapy as a combination therapy (estrogen plus progestin) can increase the risk of serious side effects such as heart disease and cancer.

Medications: A number of drugs taken for long periods of time or in excessive dosages can cause symptoms of PD. These include medications such as haloperidol (Haldol) and chlorpromazine (Thorazine), which are prescribed for certain psychiatric disorders. Other medications used to treat nausea, such as prochlorperazine (Compazine) and metoclopramide (Reglan), may also cause symptoms of PD. The antiseizure drug valproic acid (Depakene, Depakote) may cause some of the features of parkinsonism, especially severe tremor. These medications do not cause PD, and the symptoms of PD disappear when the drugs are stopped.

SIGNS AND SYMPTOMS

Individuals with idiopathic (unknown cause) PD may develop several symptoms over time, but they typically develop the primary symptoms: brady-kinesia, tremor, rigidity, and parkinsonian gait, or manner of walking. Most individuals with PD do not develop all of the symptoms associated with the disease.

Primary Symptoms

Not every person with PD develops all signs or symptoms of the disease. Some individuals experience tremor as the primary symptom, while others may not have tremor but do have balance problems. The disease may progress quickly or gradually over years. Many people become profoundly disabled and others function relatively well.

Symptoms may vary from day to day or even moment to moment. There is no clear reason for the fluctuation of symptoms. Variance may be attributable to the disease process or to anti-parkinsonian medications.

Tremor: In the early stages of the disease, about 70% of individuals experience a slight tremor in the hand or foot on one side of the body, or less commonly in the jaw or face. It appears as a slight beating or pulsing movement in the cheek, face, or jaw. Because the Parkinson's tremor usually appears when an individual's muscles are relaxed, it is called resting tremor. The affected body part trembles when it is not doing work, and it usually subsides when a person begins an action. The tremor often spreads to the other side of the body as the disease progresses but remains most apparent on the original side of occurrence. Hand tremors are often referred to as a "pill rolling" motion, as if the individual is rolling a pill between the thumb and fingers.

Rigidity: Rigidity, also called increased muscle tone, means stiffness or inflexibility of the muscles. Muscles normally stretch when they move and then relax when they are at rest. In rigidity, the muscle tone of an affected limb is always stiff and does not relax, sometimes resulting in a decreased range of motion. An individual with rigidity may not be able to swing the arms when walking because the muscles are too tight. Rigidity can cause pain and cramping.

Bradykinesia: Bradykinesia is the phenomenon of an individual experiencing slow movement. In addition to slow movements, an individual with bradykinesia will probably also have incomplete movement, difficulty initiating movements, and sudden stopping of ongoing movement. Individuals who have bradykinesia may walk with short, shuf-fling steps (called festination). Bradykinesia and rigidity can occur in the facial muscles, reducing an individual's range of facial expressions.

Impaired Balance and Coordination: Individuals with PD often experience instability when standing or impaired balance and coordination. These symptoms, combined with other symptoms such as bradykinesia, increase the probability of falling. Individuals with balance problems may have difficulty making turns or abrupt movements. They may go through periods of freezing, which is when the individual feels stuck to the ground and finds it difficult to start walking. The slowness and incompleteness of movement can also affect speaking and swallowing.

Secondary Symptoms

Secondary symptoms of PD can be, for many, as troublesome as the primary movement symptoms of the disease. Secondary symptoms include speech changes; loss of facial expression, or masking; micrographia or small, cramped handwriting; difficulty swallowing; drooling; pain; dementia or confusion; sleep disturbances; constipation; skin conditions such as boils or eczema; depression and anxiety; sexual dysfunction; urinary problems; a soft, whispery voice, termed hypophonia; fatigue or excessive tiredness; compulsive behavior; and cramping.

DIAGNOSIS

Because no definitive tests exist for PD, the condition can be difficult to diagnose, especially in the early stages. Signs and symptoms of PD, including gait changes, trembling, and trouble speaking or writing, may be generally thought of as the effects of aging, particularly in older adults with the disease. PD in younger adults may also be misdiagnosed by doctors due to the misconception that only older adults get the condition.

Medical History and Physical Examination: A diagnosis of PD is based on the individual's medical history, observations of signs and symptoms, and a neurological examination. As part of the medical history, a doctor will discuss past and present medical conditions, surgeries, and medications. The doctor will also discuss the family history of the individual to determine if heredity may play a role in developing PD.

The neurological examination includes an evaluation of walking, coordination, and simple tests for dexterity. A doctor may also notice subtle signs of parkinsonism, such as reduced facial expressions, a lack of gestures, or a subtle tremor when taking the medical history.

Diagnosis is based on symptoms and ruling out other disorders that produce similar symptoms.

An individual must have two or more of the primary symptoms, including tremor, rigidity, bradykinesia (resting tremor), and impaired balance and coordination. In many cases, this diagnosis is made after observing that symptoms have developed and become established over a period of time.

Imaging Techniques: After a thorough medical history, physical, and neurological exam, the doctor may order a computerized tomography or magnetic resonance imaging scan to determine if other criteria for a diagnosis of PD exists, such as ruling out a brain tumor or stroke (a lack of oxygen to the brain causing neurological damage) that produces parkinsonian symptoms.

Blood Tests: Blood tests may include a complete blood count, a creatine kinase test, and a DNA analysis (to determine if the disorder is genetic). In some cases, a cerebrospinal fluid analysis also is performed.

Spinal Tap: Cerebrospinal fluid (surrounds the brain and spinal cord) analysis involves performing a spinal tap or lumbar puncture. In this procedure, about two tablespoons of cerebrospinal fluid are drawn into a needle, which is inserted between two lumbar vertebrae. The fluid is then examined under a microscope. This procedure is usually performed in a hospital or clinic under local anesthesia, although general anesthesia can be used. Side effects include pain and tenderness in the area of puncture.

COMPLICATIONS

Depression and Emotional Disturbances: As many as half of the individuals with PD develop depression. In some cases, depression may occur months or even years before PD is diagnosed. Although physical limitations resulting from PD can be frustrating and stressful, depression in someone with PD isn't usually a reaction to physical disability. Instead, it more likely arises from underlying brain changes associated with the disease itself.

Dementia: In addition, some people with PD eventually develop dementia, a condition that can include memory loss, impaired judgment, and personality changes.

Other Complications: Other complications of PD may include difficulty chewing and swallowing. In the later stages of the condition, the muscles used to swallow may be affected, making eating more difficult.

PD may also cause either urinary incontinence (difficulty controlling the urine flow) or urine retention (difficulty to urinate). Certain medications used to treat the disease, especially anticholinergic drugs (such as tolterodine [Detrol]), may also cause difficulty in urinating.

Many individuals with PD develop constipation because the digestive tract works more slowly. Constipation may also be a side effect of medications used to treat the disease. Studies have found that chronic (long-term) constipation may be a risk factor associated with the development of PD, but further research needs to be performed in this area.

Individuals with PD often have trouble falling asleep and may wake up frequently throughout the night.

Some individuals with PD may notice a decrease in libido or sexual desire. This may be caused by a combination of psychological and physical factors, or it may be the result of physical factors alone. Medications may also cause a decrease in libido, including antidepressant medications such as fluoxetine (Prozac) or amitriptyline (Elavil).

TREATMENT

There is no cure for PD. Treatment for PD is built around medications to relieve the symptoms. The U.S. Food and Drug Administration (FDA) also has approved a surgically implanted device that lessens tremors. In some severe cases, brain surgery may offer the greatest benefit.

Medications

Medication selection and dosage are tailored to the individual. The doctor considers factors such as severity of symptoms, age, and presence of other medical conditions. No two individuals will respond identically to a particular drug or dosage level, so this process involves experimentation, persistence, and patience. As the disease progresses, drug dosages may have to be modified and medication regimens changed.

Levodopa/Carbidopa: Sometimes a combination of drugs is given. Combination levodopa and carbidopa (Sinemet, Sinemet CR) is the main drug treatment for PD. Levodopa is rapidly converted into dopamine by enzymes in the body. Because PD is caused by too little dopamine, this increase helps balance the levels of dopamine, decrease symptoms such as bradykinesia (slow trembling) and rigidity and, less effectively, reduce tremor. Levodopa is often ineffective in relieving problems with balance. Carbidopa helps decrease the metabolism of levodopa, thereby increasing the amount available for the brain. Side effects include nausea and vomiting (especially early in treatment), hypotension (low blood pressure), and dyskinesias (abnormal movements). Slow dosage adjustment and taking medication with food can reduce these effects. Using the lowest effective dose may prevent or delay the appearance of motor dysfunction. Levodopa may become ineffective over time. Depression, confusion, and visual hallucinations also may occur when using levodopa, especially in the elderly.

Dopamine Agonists: Dopamine agonists mimic dopamine's function in the brain. They are used primarily as adjuncts to levodopa/carbidopa therapy. They can be used as monotherapy but are generally less effective in controlling symptoms. Side effects are similar to those produced by levodopa and include nausea, sleepiness, dizziness, and headache. Dopamine agonists include bromocriptine (Parlodel), pramipexole (Mirapex), ropinirole (Requip), and rotigotine (Neupro). The FDA approved rotigotine transdermal system (Neupro) for the treatment of early PD in May 2007. Neupro, which is a medicated patch that is applied to the skin once a day, provides the dopamine agonist rotigotine continuously over a 24-hour period. Redness and tenderness are common at the site of application on the body.

Amantadine: Amantadine (Symmetrel) is an antiviral drug with dopamine agonist properties. It increases the release of dopamine. It is often used to treat early-stage PD, either alone, with an anticholinergic drug, or with levodopa. Generally, it loses its effectiveness within three to four months. Doctors may cycle individuals on and off amantadine. Side effects include spotting of the skin, edema, confusion, blurred vision, insomnia, and anxiety.

Monoamine Oxidase B (MAO-B) Inhibitors: Dopamine is oxidized by MAO-B. Selegiline (Carbex) inhibits MAO-B, increasing the amount of available dopamine in the brain. MAO-B inhibitors boost the effects of levodopa. Side effects may include nausea, dizziness, abdominal pain, confusion, hallucinations, and dry mouth.

Anticholinergics: Anticholinergics reduce the overactivity of the neurotransmitter acetylcholine to balance the reduced dopamine levels. This class of drugs is most effective in the control of tremors, and they are used in combination with levodopa. Anticholinergic drugs include benztropine mesylate (Cogentin), diphenhydramine (Benadryl), and trihexyphenidyl (Artane). Side effects associated with anticholinergic drugs include dry mouth, blurred vision, constipation, and urinary retention.

Catechol-*O*-Methyl Transferase (COMT) Inhibitors: COMT inhibitors help increase levodopa therapy by inhibiting the COMT enzyme, which metabolizes levodopa before it reaches the brain. Inhibiting COMT increases the amount of levodopa that enters the brain. These drugs are only effective when used with levodopa. COMT inhibitors include entacapone (Comtan) and tolcapone (Tasmar). But because tolcapone has been linked to liver damage and liver failure, the drug is normally used only in people who are not responding to other therapies. Entacapone is a COMT inhibitor that shares some of the properties of tolcapone but does not seem to cause liver problems. Entacapone is now combined with carbidopa and levodopa in a medication called Stalevo. Side effects include vivid dreams, visual hallucinations, nausea, sleep disturbances, daytime drowsiness, headache, and dyskinesias (difficulty in performing movements).

Surgery

Surgery is another method of controlling symptoms and improving quality of life when medication ceases to be effective or when medication side effects, such as jerking and dyskinesias (difficulty in performing movements), become intolerable.

Not every individual suffering from PD is a good candidate for surgery. Surgery has not been found to be effective in those who respond poorly to levodopa/carbidopa. Only about 10% of Parkinson's patients are estimated to be suitable candidates. There are three surgical procedures for treating PD: ablative surgery, stimulation surgery or deep brain stimulation, and transplantation or restorative surgery.

Doctors will help individuals with PD to determine if surgery is appropriate for them. Seeking more than one opinion may be helpful.

Deep Brain Stimulation (DBS): DBS involves a surgically implanted, battery-operated medical device (called a neurostimulator) used to deliver electrical stimulation to areas of the brain that control movement. The electrical charge blocks nerve signals that trigger abnormal movement. In DBS, an electrode (lead) is inserted through a small incision in the skull and is implanted in the targeted area of the brain. An insulated wire (extension) is then passed under the skin in the head, neck, and shoulder, connecting the lead to the neurostimulator, which is surgically implanted in the chest or upper abdomen. Side effects of DBS include bleeding at the implantation site, depression, impaired muscle tone, infection, loss of balance, paresis (slight paralysis), dysarthria (slurred speech), and paresthesia (tingling) in the head or the hands.

Ablative Surgery: Ablative surgery locates, targets, and then ablates (destroys) the clearly defined area of the brain that produces chemical or electrical impulses that cause abnormal movements. In this surgery, a heated probe or electrode is inserted into the targeted area. The individual remains awake during the procedure to determine if the problem has been eliminated. A local anesthetic is used to dull the outer part of the brain and skull. The brain is insensitive to pain, so the individual does not feel the actual procedure. In some cases, it may be difficult to estimate how much tissue to destroy and the amount of heat to use.

This type of surgery involves either ablation in the part of the brain called the globus pallidus (called pallidotomy) or ablation of brain tissue in the thalamus (called thalamotomy). A related procedure, cryothalamotomy, uses a supercooled probe that is inserted into the thalamus to freeze and destroy areas that produce tremors.

Pallidotomy may be used to eliminate uncontrolled dyskinesia (difficulty in movement) and thalamotomy may be performed to eliminate tremor. These procedures are successful in approximately 75% of cases.

Cryothalamotomy uses a super-cooled probe that is inserted into the thalamus to freeze and destroy areas that produce tremors. Ablative surgery is safe and rarely causes complications such as affecting other areas of the brain.

Transplantation or Restorative Surgery: In transplantation (or restorative) surgery, dopamine-producing cells are implanted into the striatum. The cells used for transplantation may come from one of several sources, including the individual's own body, human embryos, and pig embryos.

Using cells from the individual's body has been unsuccessful so far because of an insufficient supply of dopamine cells and the inability of the implanted cells to survive.

To use fetal cells, between three and eight embryos are needed per procedure, and even under the most favorable conditions 90% of transplanted cells do not survive. This procedure is only moderately effective in some patients and usually in those younger than age 60. Preliminary studies have shown that pig embryo cells do survive transplantation and have an effect on symptoms. Stem cells, primitive cells that can grow into nerve cells, are able to survive and reproduce. Once they grow as nerve cells, they can be transformed into dopamine-producing cells. Stem cells are obtained from discarded blood in a newborn's umbilical cord, the bone marrow of an adult, unused embryos from fertility clinics, or an aborted embryo. There is much controversy surrounding the use of stem cells.

Nutrition and Lifestyle Changes

Proper diet and exercise are very important for individuals with movement disorders, including PD. In helping individuals to eat, caregivers should allow plenty of time for meals. Food can be cut into small pieces, softened, or pureed to ease swallowing and prevent choking. While some foods may require the addition of thickeners, other foods may need to be thinned. Dairy products, in particular, tend to increase the secretion of mucus, which in turn increases the risk of choking.

Some individuals may benefit from swallowing therapy, which is especially helpful if started before serious problems arise. Suction cups for plates, special tableware designed for people with disabilities, and plastic cups with tops can help prevent spilling. The individual's doctor can offer additional advice about diet and about how to handle swallowing difficulties or gastrointestinal problems that might arise, such as incontinence or constipation.

Maximizing physical activity is a goal in all movement disorders. Patients should perform daily activities to the extent possible. If they cannot, a regular exercise program or physical therapy may help condition them physically and teach them adaptive strategies. Because the disease, medications, and inactivity can lead to constipation, patients should consume a high-fiber diet, such as bran cereals, whole wheat bread, fresh vegetables, and brown rice. Dietary supplements, including psyllium and stimulant laxatives (such as bisacodyl [Dulcolax]), may be needed for constipation.

Although their coordination may be poor, individuals should continue walking, with assistance if necessary. Those who want to walk independently should be allowed to do so as long as possible. Careful attention should be given to keeping their environment free of hard, sharp objects to help ensure maximal independence while minimizing the risk of injury from a fall. Individuals can also wear special padding during walks to help protect against injury from falls. Some individuals have found that small weights around the ankles can help stability. Wearing sturdy shoes that fit well can help as well, especially shoes without laces that can be slipped on or off easily. Velcro shoes may help provide extra stability.

Speech Therapy: Some movement disorders, such as PD, can impair speech, affecting the ability of the individual to express complex thoughts. Speech therapy may improve the individual's ability to communicate and swallow. It is important for caregivers to understand that individuals with these movement disorders may not be communicating due to the disease and not due to a lack of sociability.

Social Activity: Unless and until the disease's progression prohibits it, people with movement disorders should participate in outside activities, socialize, and pursue hobbies and interests. These activities also give family members and caregivers valuable time for themselves.

Caregiver Support: Movement disorders confront individuals and their caregivers with many complex problems that must be dealt with for the life of the patient. While it may be emotionally difficult, it is important for patients and caregivers to make informed, carefully considered decisions regarding the future while the patient is capable of making his or her contribution to a planned course of action.

Physical Therapy: According to the American Physical Therapy Association, the goal of physical therapy or physiotherapy is to improve mobility, restore function, reduce pain, and prevent further injury by using a variety of methods, including exercises, stretches, traction, electrical stimulation, and massage. Physical therapy has been reported useful in neurological disorders.

INTEGRATIVE THERAPIES

Although there are a few clinical studies using integrative therapies for the treatment of PD, there have been studies in other neurological disorders that may present with similar symptoms as PD. Listed below are integrative therapies that have been studies clinically in various movement disorders, including PD.

Good Scientific Evidence

5-Hydroxy-L-Tryptophan (5-HTP): Cerebral ataxia results from the failure of part of the brain to regulate body posture and limb movements. 5-HTP has been observed to have benefits in some people who have difficulty standing or walking because of cerebral ataxia. Some research shows that 5-HTP may allow individuals with unsteady movements to stand alone without assistance, walk without aid, or improve coordination. Other research shows no benefit. Further research is needed before a conclusion can be drawn. 5-HTP may interact with other mood-altering medications such as antidepressants and antianxiety drugs.

Music Therapy: Music therapy has been reported to improve symptoms in people with PD. Modest

improvement in symptoms, including motor coordination, speech intelligibility and vocal intensity, bradykinesia (slow movement), emotional functions, activities of daily living, and quality of life, were seen.

Unclear or Conflicting Scientific Evidence

Acupressure, Shiatsu: The practice of applying finger pressure to specific acupoints (energy points) throughout the body has been used in China since 2000 B.C. Shiatsu technique involves finger pressure at acupoints and along body meridians (energy lines). It can incorporate palm pressure, stretching, massaging, and other manual techniques. Shiatsu practitioners commonly treat musculoskeletal and psychological conditions, including neck/shoulder and lower back problems, arthritis, depression, and anxiety. Preliminary clinical evidence from one small study with individuals with facial spasm report improvement when using Shiatsu acupressure. Further research is needed.

Acupuncture: Acupuncture has been reported to help relieve symptoms of some neurological disorders, including cerebral palsy, hemiplegia (full or partial paralysis of one side of the body due to disease, trauma, or stroke), PD (characterized by fine muscle coordination and tremors), spinal cord injury, Tourette's syndrome (characterized by tics), and trigeminal neuralgia. One study found that parents were impressed with acupuncture therapy on functional well-being in Huntington's disease in children. There is insufficient evidence available from well-designed studies for using acupuncture in neurological disorders such as Tourette's syndrome. More trials need to be performed.

Alexander Technique: The Alexander technique is an educational program that teaches movement patterns and postures with an aim to improve coordination and balance, reduce tension, relieve pain, alleviate fatigue, improve various medical conditions, and promote well-being. Preliminary research suggests that Alexander technique instruction may improve fine and gross movements and reduce depression in patients with PD. Well-designed human trials are necessary.

Chiropractic: Chiropractic is a healthcare discipline that focuses on the relationship between musculoskeletal structure (primarily the spine) and body function (as coordinated by the nervous system) and how this relationship affects the preservation and restoration of health. Although there is not enough reliable scientific evidence to conclude the effects of chiropractic techniques in the management of

PD, anecdotal reports suggest a positive impact on fine muscle coordination in some individuals. More clinical research is necessary.

Coenzyme Q10 (CoQ10): CoQ10 is produced by the human body and is necessary for the basic functioning of cells. There is promising evidence from one case-control study and two case series to support the use of CoQ10 in the treatment of symptoms associated with PD. These studies are lacking in sample sizes. A future randomized, controlled trial with a substantial number of participants is necessary for proper evaluation of efficacy of CoQ10 in PD. Further research using CoQ10 for neurological conditions is necessary.

Cowhage: Traditional Ayurvedic medicine and preliminary evidence suggests that cowhage (*Mucuna pruriens*) contains 3.6-4.2% levodopa, the same chemical used in several PD drugs. Cowhage treatments have yielded positive results in early studies. However, additional high-quality clinical research is needed to confirm these results.

Avoid if allergic or hypersensitive to cowhage, its constituents, or members of the Fabaceae family. Use cautiously with PD and/or when taking levodopa, dopamine, dopamine agonists, dopamine antagonists, or dopamine reuptake inhibitors, as cowhage seeds contain the dopamine precursor levodopa. Use cautiously if taking MAO inhibitors or other antidepressants. Use cautiously if taking anticoagulants (blood thinners) or with diabetes. Avoid with psychosis or schizophrenia. Avoid if pregnant or breastfeeding, as cowhage may inhibit prolactin secretion.

Ginseng: A clinical study found that patients with neurological disorders may improve when taking Asian ginseng (*Panax ginseng*). This supports research findings that report *Panax ginseng* improving cognitive function. More research is needed in this area.

Melatonin: Melatonin is a naturally occurring hormone that helps regulate sleep/wake cycles (circadian rhythm). Melatonin has been reported useful in neurological conditions including PD, periodic limb movement disorder, and tardive dyskinesia. The use of melatonin in these conditions, however, is not supported by rigorous scientific testing. Better-designed research is needed to determine if melatonin is beneficial in individuals with neurological disorders.

Reiki: Reiki is a system of lying on of the hands that originated as a Buddhist practice approximately 2,500 years ago. One randomized trial suggests that Reiki may have an effect on autonomic nervous system functions such as heart rate, blood pressure, or breathing activity, important in neurological disorders

that may damage autonomic function, including neurological conditions. Large, well-designed studies are needed before conclusions can be drawn.

Taurine: Taurine may affect cellular hyperexcitability by increasing membrane conductance to potassium and chloride ions, possibly by altering intracellular (within the cell) availability of calcium. Results from a single, nonrandomized trial suggest that taurine supplementation may result in improvements in myotonic (slow relaxation after contraction of muscles) complaints. Well-designed clinical trials are needed.

Vitamin B_6: Vitamin B_6 (pyridoxine) is required for the synthesis of the neurotransmitters serotonin and norepinephrine and for myelin formation. Pyridoxine deficiency in adults principally affects the peripheral nerves, skin, mucous membranes, and the blood cell system. In children, the central nervous system is also affected. Major sources of vitamin B_6 include cereal grains, legumes, vegetables (carrots, spinach, peas), potatoes, milk, cheese, eggs, fish, liver, meat, and flour. Some prescription drugs called neuroleptics, which are used in psychiatric conditions, may cause movement disorders as an unwanted side effect. Vitamin B_6 has been studied for treatment of acute neuroleptic-induced akathisia (a neuromuscular disorder characterized by a feeling of "inner restlessness" or a constant urge to be moving) in schizophrenic and schizoaffective disorder patients. Preliminary results indicate that high doses of vitamin B_6 may be useful additions to the available treatments for neuroleptic-induced akathisia, perhaps due to its combined effects on various neurotransmitter systems. Further research is needed to confirm these results.

Vitamin E: Vitamin E has been studied in the management of tardive dyskinesia and has been reported to significantly improve abnormal involuntary movements, although the results of exiting studies are not conclusive enough to form a clear recommendation. Vitamin E may be more effective in higher doses and in people who have had tardive dyskinesia for less than five years.

Other supplements that have unclear or conflicting scientific evidence include ashwagandha root (*Withania somniferum*), dehydroepiandrosterone, dong quai root (*Angelica sinensis*), homeopathic dilutions of belladonna (*Atropa belladonna*), choline, psychotherapy, selenium, and yohimbe bark (*Pausinystalia yohimbe*).

Historical or Theoretical Uses Lacking Sufficient Evidence

Integrative therapies used in neurological disorders such as PD that have historical or theoretical uses but lack sufficient clinical evidence include aloe (*Aloe vera*), arabinoxylan, aromatherapy, art therapy, asparagus (*Asparagus officinalis*), arnica (*Arnica montana*), bacopa (*Bacopa monnieri*), bitter orange (*Citrus aurantium*), black cohosh (*Actaea racemosa*), cat's claw (*Uncaria tomentosa*), chelation therapy (ethylenediamine tetraacetic acid), chondroitin sulfate, cordyceps (*Cordyceps sinensis*), devil's claw (*Harpagophytum procumbens*), horse chestnut (*Aesculus hippocastanum*), hypnosis, kava kava (*Piper methysticum*), kudzu (*Pueraria lobota*), lycopene, magnet therapy, massage, muira puama (*Ptychopetalum olacoides*), omega-3 fatty acids, prayer, qi gong, relaxation, St. John's wort (*Hypericum perforatum*), and valerian (*Valeriana* spp.).

PREVENTION

Proper Diet: It is best to avoid stimulants, alcohol, and smoking.

It may be best to eliminate potential food allergens, including dairy (e.g., milk, cheese, and sour cream), eggs, nuts, shellfish, wheat (gluten), corn, preservatives, and food additives (such as dyes and fillers). A clinical study found a higher risk of PD among dairy product consumers in both men and women, suggesting that dairy consumption may increase the risk of PD, particularly in men. Dairy may increase mucus production. More studies are needed.

Studies suggest that moderate consumption of coffee may actually help reduce the chances of developing PD. Research suggests it is the caffeine content that offers protection, so decaffeinated coffee may offer no benefits in PD prevention.

Preventing complications of PD, such as inability to swallow foods, is important. Food can be cut into small pieces, softened, or pureed to ease swallowing and prevent choking. While some foods may require the addition of thickeners, other foods may need to be thinned. Dairy products, in particular, tend to increase the secretion of mucus, which in turn increases the risk of choking.

Weight Control: Body mass index is associated with a risk of PD. Losing weight may reduce the chances of developing PD.

Exercise: Maintaining physical fitness is important to those suffering from movement disorders such as PD. Those with movement disorders who exercise and keep active tend to do better, with fewer symptoms and a slower disease progression, than those who do not. A daily regimen of exercise can help the person feel better physically and mentally. Individuals should walk as much as possible, even if assistance is necessary. Talking with a healthcare provider about an exercise program is important.

Mobility: PD can cause the sense of balance to be off, making it difficult to walk with a normal gait or stride. If shuffling of the feet is noticed, slow down and check the posture. It is best to stand up straight with the head over the hips and the feet eight to 10 inches apart. It can also help to purchase a good pair of walking shoes. If the individual becomes frozen in place, rocking gently from side to side may help decrease the time of inability to move.

In the later stages of the disease, the individual may fall more easily. PD may affect the balance and coordination centers in the brain. In fact, a person may be thrown off balance by just a small push or bump. The following suggestions may help:

Wearing rubber-soled shoes is recommended by healthcare professionals. This type of shoe is less likely to slip than are shoes with leather soles. Rugs should be removed from the home to avoid tripping and falling. Carpeting should be secured firmly to the floor. It is recommended that handrails be installed, especially along stairways and in the bathroom, and that electrical and telephone cords be kept out of the way.

Daily Activities: Dressing can be the most frustrating of all activities for someone with PD. The loss of fine motor control makes it hard to button and zip clothes and even to step into a pair of pants. A physical therapist can point out techniques that make daily activities easier. It is best to allow plenty of time so as not to feel rushed when dressing. Clothing may be laid nearby for ease of putting it on. Clothes that can be slipped on easily, such as sweat pants and t-shirts, simple dresses, or pants with elastic waistbands, are recommended.

Even in the early stages of PD, the voice may become very soft or hoarse. To communicate more easily, healthcare professionals recommend facing the individual and deliberately speak louder than necessary. Practicing reading or reciting out loud, focusing on breathing, and a using a strong voice may be beneficial. A speech pathologist may be consulted to improve verbal communication skills in individuals with PD.

PNEUMONIA

BACKGROUND

Pneumonia is an infection of one or both lungs that is usually caused by bacteria, viruses, or fungi. Pneumonia can also be caused by the inhalation of food, liquid, gases, or dust. Approximately 50% of pneumonia cases are believed to be caused by viruses and tend to result in less-severe illness than bacteria-caused pneumonia. Most pneumonia in the very young is caused by viral infection, including respiratory syncytial virus (RSV). The symptoms of viral pneumonia are similar to influenza symptoms and include fever, dry cough, headache, muscle pain, weakness, and increasing breathlessness. More than a million people in the United States are hospitalized each year for pneumonia, making it the third most frequent reason for hospitalizations (after births and heart disease). Although the majority of pneumonias respond well to treatment, the infection can still be a very serious problem. Pneumonia kills between 40,000-70,000 individuals in the United States each year. Pneumonia is spread by close person-to-person contact, usually when an infected person coughs or sneezes on another person.

Individuals considered at high risk for pneumonia include the elderly, infants, and those with underlying health problems, such as chronic obstructive pulmonary disease, diabetes mellitus, congestive heart failure, and sickle cell anemia. Other conditions that may increase an individual's chance of developing pneumonia include impairment of the immune system, such as in acquired immunodeficiency syndrome (AIDS), or those undergoing cancer therapy or organ transplantation. Currently, over three million people develop pneumonia each year in the United States. Over a half a million of these people are admitted to a hospital for treatment. Although most of these people recover, approximately 5% will die from pneumonia. Pneumonia is the sixth leading cause of death in the United States. Pneumonia is often a complication of a preexisting condition or infection. Pneumonia is triggered when an individual's defense system is weakened, most often by a simple viral upper respiratory tract infection or a case of influenza. Pneumonia can be caused by bacteria, viruses, mycoplasma, and fungi. The onset of bacterial pneumonia can vary from gradual to sudden. In most severe cases, the patient may experience shaking/chills, chattering teeth, severe chest pains, sweats, cough that produces rust colored or greenish mucus, increased breathing and pulse rate, and bluish colored lips or nails due to a lack of oxygen.

TYPES AND CAUSES

The lungs are two spongy organs surrounded by a moist membrane, called the pleura. When an individual inhales, air is carried through the windpipe (trachea) to the lungs. Inside the lungs, there are major airways called bronchi. The bronchi repeatedly subdivide into many smaller airways, called bronchioles, which finally end in clusters of tiny air sacs called alveoli.

The body has mechanisms to protect the lungs from infection. Individuals are frequently exposed to bacteria and viruses that can cause pneumonia, but a body normally prevents most of these organisms from invading and overwhelming the airways.

Bacterial Pneumonia: The bacteria *Streptococcus pneumoniae,* also called pneumococcal pneumonia, is the most common cause of bacterial pneumonia acquired outside of hospitals (also called community-acquired pneumonia). Pneumonia bacteria are present in some healthy throats. The bacteria can multiply and cause serious damage to a healthy individual's lungs, bloodstream, and brain as well as other parts of the body. If the immune system is weakened, individuals are especially susceptible to pneumonia. Pneumococcal pneumonia accounts for 25-35% of all community-acquired pneumonia. With an estimated 40,000 deaths yearly, this can be a serious form of pneumonia. Another bacteria, *Haemophilus influenzae* or *H. influenza,* can also cause pneumonia.

Bacterial pneumonia can also be considered hospital-acquired pneumonia. Hospital-acquired pneumonia develops at least 48 hours after hospitalization. The most common causes are bacteria such as *Staphylococcus aureus.*

Viral Pneumonia: Half of all pneumonias are believed to be caused by viruses. More and more viruses are being identified as the cause of respiratory infection, and though most attack the upper respiratory tract, some produce pneumonia, especially in children. Most of these pneumonias are not serious and last a short time. Infection with the influenza virus may be severe, but the likelihood of death is rare. The virus invades the lungs and multiplies, but there are almost no physical signs of lung tissue becoming filled with fluid. It finds many of its victims among those who have preexisting heart or lung disease or are pregnant.

Viral conditions that may lead to pneumonia include influenza virus, RSV, severe acute respiratory distress syndrome, human parainfluenza virus, adenoviruses, and herpes viruses.

Walking Pneumonia: Walking pneumonia is caused by *Mycoplasma pneumoniae*. Mycoplasmas are the smallest free-living agents of disease in man. Mycoplasma infections generally cause a mild and widespread pneumonia. Mycoplasmas are responsible for approximately 3% of all cases of pneumonia. The most prominent symptom of walking pneumonia is a cough that tends to come in violent attacks but produces only sparse whitish mucus.

Other Types of Pneumonia: Certain types of fungus, including *Histoplasma capsulatum, Coccidioides immitis, Blastomyces dermatitidis,* and *Paracoccidioides brasiliensis,* also can cause pneumonia. Pneumonia caused by fungi is much less common than pneumonia caused by bacteria or viruses. Another type of fungal pneumonia is caused by *Pneumocystis carinii. Pneumocystis carinii* pneumonia (PCP) primarily affects AIDS patients. Certain diseases, such as tuberculosis, can also predispose someone to pneumonia. PCP may be the first sign of illness in many persons with AIDS. PCP can be successfully treated in many cases. It may recur a few months later, but treatment can help to prevent or delay its recurrence.

Other less-common pneumonias may be quite serious and are occurring more often. Various special pneumonias are caused by the inhalation of food, liquid, gases, or dust and by fungi. Obstruction of the lungs, such as a tumor, may promote the occurrence of pneumonia, although obstructions are not causes of pneumonia.

Rickettsia (an organism somewhere between a virus and bacteria) causes Rocky Mountain spotted fever, Q fever, typhus, and psittacosis, all diseases that may have mild or severe effects on the lungs.

Chemical exposure, such as to chlorine gas, can cause inflammation and pneumonia. Workers exposed to cattle are at a risk for pneumonia caused by anthrax from the bacterium *Bacillus anthracis.*

Aspiration Pneumonia: Aspiration pneumonia occurs when foreign matter is inhaled into the lungs, most often when the contents of the stomach enter the lungs after vomiting. This commonly happens when a brain injury or other condition affects the normal gag reflex.

Another common cause of aspiration pneumonia is consuming too much alcohol. This happens when the inebriated person passes out and then vomits due to the effects of alcohol on the stomach. If someone is unconscious, it's possible to aspirate the liquid contents and possibly solid food from the stomach into the lungs, causing aspiration pneumonia.

SIGNS AND SYMPTOMS

The symptoms of pneumonia can vary and generally overlap with other symptoms of the common cold or flu. This variability makes it sometimes difficult to recognize pneumonia. Many people attribute the symptoms to a cold that just won't go away. However, pneumonia can be life-threatening if it is not properly treated.

Some symptoms of pneumonia include shaking and chills; fever; a cough that produces mucus or phlegm, which usually appears rust colored or burnt orange; shortness of breath; chest pain worsened by deep breathing or coughing; and night sweats. When pneumonia is caused by bacteria, an infected individual usually becomes sick relatively quickly and experiences the sudden onset of high fever and unusually rapid breathing. When pneumonia is caused by viruses, symptoms tend to appear more gradually and are often less severe than in bacterial pneumonia. Wheezing may be more common in viral pneumonia. In extreme cases, the individual has a desperate need for air and extreme breathlessness. Viral pneumonias may be complicated by an invasion of bacteria, with all the typical symptoms of bacterial pneumonia.

Mycoplasma, or walking pneumonia, causes signs and symptoms similar to those of other bacterial and viral infections, although symptoms appear more gradually and are often mild and flulike. Individuals may not be sick enough to stay in bed or to seek medical care and may never even know they have had pneumonia.

The incubation period for pneumonia varies depending on the type of virus or bacteria causing the infection. Some common incubation periods are four to six days for RSV and 18-72 hours for influenza. With treatment, most types of bacterial pneumonia can be cured within one to two weeks. Viral pneumonia may last longer. Mycoplasma pneumonia may take four to six weeks to resolve completely.

COMPLICATIONS

The seriousness of pneumonia depends on the individual's overall health and the type and severity of the pneumonia. If the person is young and healthy, pneumonia can usually be treated successfully. In those with other health conditions, especially from smoking, or if older, pneumonia may be harder to cure. These individuals are also more likely to develop lung complications, some of which can be life threatening.

Sepsis: Sepsis, or bacteremia, is bacteria in the bloodstream. Pneumonia can be deadly when inflammation fills the air sacs in the lungs and interferes with the individual's ability to breathe. In some cases the infection may invade the bloodstream. It can then spread quickly to other organs.

Fluid Accumulation: Pleural effusion is when fluid accumulates between the thin, transparent membrane covering the lungs and the membrane that lines the inner surface of the chest wall. Normally, the pleurae are silky smooth, allowing the lungs to slide easily along the chest wall when the individual breathes in and out. But when the pleurae around the lungs become inflamed (called pleurisy), often as a result of pneumonia, fluid can accumulate and may become infected (called empyema).

Lung Abscess: A lung abscess, or a cavity containing pus that forms within the area affected by pneumonia, is another potential complication. Abscesses usually are treated with antibiotics, but in rare cases they may need to be removed surgically.

Mechanical Breathing: Some individuals with pneumonia who cannot breathe on their own may require the assistance of a mechanical ventilator. Ventilator-associated pneumonia has a high mortality rate (up to 40%) and has serious complications, such as acute respiratory distress syndrome (ARDS).

DIAGNOSIS

A doctor may first suspect pneumonia based on a medical history and a physical exam. During the exam, the doctor will listen to the lungs with a stethoscope to check for abnormal bubbling or crackling sounds and for rumblings that signal the presence of thick liquid. Both these sounds may indicate inflammation caused by infection. A chest x-ray is usually used to confirm the presence of pneumonia and to determine the extent and location of the infection. Blood tests are usually performed to check white blood cell count or to look for the presence of viruses, bacteria, or other organisms. A doctor may examine a sample of phlegm (mucus) or blood to help identify the microorganism that is causing the pneumonia.

TREATMENT

Bacterial Pneumonia

Antibiotics: Doctors use antibiotics to treat pneumonia caused by bacteria, the most common cause of the condition. The individual usually will continue to take antibiotics for five to 14 days, although the person may take them longer if the immune system is impaired. The doctor will choose an antibiotic based on a number of factors, including age, symptoms, how severe the symptoms are, what the cause of the pneumonia is, whether the pneumonia is hospital acquired or community acquired, and whether

the individual needs to be hospitalized. Although individuals may start to feel better shortly after beginning the medication, healthcare professionals recommend completing the entire course of antibiotics. Stopping medication too soon may cause the pneumonia to return. It also helps create strains of bacteria that are resistant to antibiotics, an increasingly serious problem in the United States.

Antibiotics used for bacterial pneumonia include macrolides, such as erythromycin (Ery-Tab), clarithromycin (Biaxin, Biaxin XL), and azithromycin (Zithromax); tetracyclines, such as doxycycline (Vibramycin, Doryx); and fluoroquinolones, such as levofloxacin (Levaquin) and moxifloxacin (Avelox). Others include cephalosporins, such as cefaclor (Ceclor), cefadroxil (Duricef), and cefuroxime (Ceftin); penicillins, such as amoxicillin (Amoxil), amoxicillin/clavulanic acid (Augmentin), and ticarcillin/clavulanate (Timentin); and vancomycin (Vancocin). Side effects of antibiotics include nausea, vomiting, stomach discomfort, cramping, and diarrhea. A serious but less common side effect of vancomycin (Vancocin) can be loss of hearing.

Antibiotics usually work well with younger, otherwise healthy people with strong immune systems. Individuals usually see some improvement in symptoms within two to three days. Unless the individual gets worse during this time, a doctor usually will not change the treatment for at least three days. If there is no improvement or if symptoms get worse, the individual may need further testing. These tests help identify the organism that is causing symptoms and determine whether the bacteria may be resistant to the antibiotic.

Individuals are usually hospitalized with pneumonia if they are older than 65; have other health problems, such as chronic obstructive pulmonary disease, heart failure, asthma, diabetes, long-term (chronic) kidney failure, or chronic liver disease; cannot care for themselves, or would not be able to tell anyone if the symptoms got worse, such as in dementia; have severe illness with less oxygen getting to the tissues (hypoxia); have chest pain caused by inflammation of the lining of the lung (pleurisy) and therefore not able to cough up mucus effectively and clear the lungs; are being treated outside a hospital and are not getting better (such as shortness of breath not improving); or are not able to eat or keep food down so that the individual needs to take fluids through a vein (intravenous).

Viral Pneumonia

Pneumonia also can be caused by viruses, such as those that cause influenza (flu), herpes, and chickenpox (varicella). At this time, there is no proven medication to treat pneumonia caused by the influenza virus. Home treatment, such as rest and taking care of the cough, is the only treatment. Expectorants, such as guaifenesin (Robitussin), can be used to loosen phlegm. Patients should drink plenty of fluids.

Varicella pneumonia, which is rare, can be treated with the antiviral medication acyclovir (Zovirax).

Walking Pneumonia

Walking pneumonia, also known as *Mycoplasma pneumonia,* is treated with antibiotics, such as those for bacterial pneumonias. Even so, recovery may not be immediate. In some cases, fatigue may continue long after the infection itself has cleared.

Fungal Pneumonia

If the pneumonia is caused by a fungus, the individual will likely be treated with an antifungal medication such as fluconazole (Diflucan) or itraconazole (Sporanox). Side effects of antifungal medications include nausea, vomiting, diarrhea, and headache.

In addition to these treatments, a doctor may recommend over-the-counter (OTC) medications to reduce fever and treat aches and pains, such as aspirin or acetaminophen (Tylenol), and soothe the cough associated with pneumonia, such as guaifenesin (Robitussin). Coughs should not be suppressed completely, as coughing helps clear the lungs of phlegm (mucus). Dextromethorphan (Robitussin DM) is a commonly used OTC cough suppressant.

INTEGRATIVE THERAPIES

Unclear or Conflicting Scientific Evidence

Chiropractic: Chiropractic is a healthcare discipline that focuses on the relationship between musculoskeletal structure (primarily the spine) and body function (as coordinated by the nervous system) and how this relationship affects the preservation and restoration of health. The broad term "spinal manipulative therapy" incorporates all types of manual techniques, including chiropractic. Although used with limited success, there is not enough reliable scientific evidence to draw a conclusion on the effects of chiropractic techniques in the management of pneumonia in the elderly.

Chlorophyll: Chlorophyll is a chemoprotein commonly known for its contribution to the green pigmentation in plants and is related to protoheme, the red pigment of blood. It can be obtained from green leafy vegetables (broccoli, Brussels sprouts, cabbage, lettuce, and spinach), algae (Chlorella and Spirulina), wheat grass, and numerous herbs (alfalfa, damiana, nettle, and parsley). Chlorophyll may help to regulate immunity in patients with active destructive pneumonia. Further studies are required to further elaborate on the immune-modifying effects of chlorophyll.

Iodine: Based on one prospective, randomized study, regular oropharyngeal application of povidone-iodine may decrease the prevalence of ventilator-associated pneumonia in patients with severe head trauma. Evidence in this area is not conclusive.

Physical Therapy: Early evidence suggests that chest physiotherapy techniques such as postural drainage, external help with breathing, percussion, and vibration are not better that receiving advice of deep breathing instructions in the treatment of serious pneumonia. Additional evidence is needed in this area.

Probiotics: Probiotics are beneficial bacteria (sometimes referred to as "friendly germs") that help to maintain the health of the intestinal tract and aid in digestion. They also help keep potentially harmful organisms in the gut (harmful bacteria and yeasts) under control. Most probiotics come from food sources, especially cultured milk products. Probiotics can be consumed as capsules, tablets, beverages, powders, yogurts, and other foods. Although some clinical studies support the use of probiotics for pneumonia, there is insufficient evidence to draw any firm conclusions. Probiotics may also be helpful in relieving gastrointestinal side effects, such as nausea and vomiting, caused by antibiotics used to treat pneumonia. More research is necessary.

Sea Buckthorn: Sea buckthorn (*Hippophae rhamnoides*) is found throughout Europe and Asia, particularly eastern Europe and central Asia. The plant's orange fruit and the oil from its pulp and seeds have been used traditionally for lung conditions, including coughing and phlegm reduction. One clinical study supports the use of sea buckthorn in pneumonia, although more clinical research is necessary.

Vitamin A: One study found no effect of a moderate dose of vitamin A supplementation on the duration of uncomplicated pneumonia in underweight or normal-weight children aged younger than five years. However, a beneficial effect was seen in children with high basal serum retinol concentrations.

Vitamin A toxicity, or hypervitaminosis A, is rare in the general population. Vitamin A toxicity can occur with excessive amounts of vitamin A taken over short or long periods of time. Consequently, toxicity can be acute or chronic. An infant with acute toxicity can develop a bulging fontanelle (the soft spot on the head) and symptoms similar to a brain tumor. Adults experience less-specific symptoms such as headache, dizziness, fatigue, malaise, blurry vision, bone pain and swelling, nausea, and/or vomiting. Severe toxicity can lead to eye damage, high levels of calcium, and liver damage. Persons with liver disease and high alcohol intake may be at risk for hepatotoxicity (liver damage) from vitamin A supplementation. Smokers who consume alcohol and beta-carotene may be at an increased risk for lung cancer or cardiovascular disease.

Yerba Santa: Chumash Native Americans and other California tribes have used yerba santa (*Eriodictyon californicum*) and other related species (*Eriodictyon crassifolium, Eriodictyon trichocalyx*) for many centuries in the treatment of pulmonary (lung) conditions and saliva production as well as to stop bleeding of minor cuts and scrapes. There is an extensive clinical history of the use of *Eriodictyon* extracts in pulmonary conditions such as influenza, bacterial pneumonia, asthma, bronchitis, and tuberculosis. However, additional study is needed.

Yoga: Yoga is an ancient system of relaxation, exercise, and healing with origins in Indian philosophy. Limited adult human study exists for the treatment of lung conditions such as bronchitis, fluid around the lungs (pleural effusion), or airway obstruction. Better-designed research is necessary.

Zinc: Results from large clinical trials suggest that supplementation with zinc may reduce the incidence of lower respiratory infections. Some studies suggest these effects to be only apparent in boys and not girls. A trend toward increased respiratory infections in children has been noted in one study. A recent study does not support the use of zinc supplementation in the management of acute lower respiratory infections requiring hospitalization in indigenous children living in remote areas. Due to conflicting results, further research is needed before a conclusion can be drawn. Future studies could examine whether these adult populations have a similar response.

Fair Negative Scientific Evidence

Zinc: One study found that zinc supplementation does not seem to lessen the duration of tachypnea, hypoxia, chest indrawing, inability to feed, lethargy, severe illness, or hospitalization in children with pneumonia.

Traditional or Theoretical Uses Lacking Sufficient Evidence

Integrative therapies used in pneumonia that have historical or theoretical uses but lack sufficient clinical evidence include homeopathic aconite (*Aconitum napellus*), beta-carotene, blue flag (*Iris versicolor*), coenzyme Q10, garlic (*Allium sativum*), ginseng (*Panax ginseng*), goldenseal (*Hydrastis canadensis*), ozone therapy, selenium, spirulina, vitamin C, and white horehound (*Marrubium vulgare*).

PREVENTION

Because pneumonia is a common complication of the flu, getting a flu shot every fall may help prevent pneumonia.

A vaccine is also available to help fight pneumococcal pneumonia, a type of bacterial pneumonia. A doctor can help individuals decide if they, or a member of their family, need the vaccine against pneumococcal pneumonia. The vaccine is usually given only to people at high risk of getting the disease, such as those with lung conditions, the elderly, smokers, or those with AIDS. The vaccine is not recommended for pregnant women or children under age two. Unlike vaccination with the "flu shot," the pneumococcal vaccine does not need to be given each year. One dosage of the vaccine is usually sufficient, but sometimes doctors recommend a second dose of the vaccine.

A vaccine known as pneumococcal conjugate vaccine can help protect young children against pneumonia. The vaccine is recommended by healthcare professionals for all children younger than age two and for children two years and older who are at particular risk of pneumococcal disease, such as those with an immune system deficiency, cancer, cardiovascular disease, or sickle cell anemia. Side effects of the pneumococcal vaccine are generally minor and include mild soreness or swelling at the injection site.

Since pneumonia often follows ordinary respiratory infections, the most important preventive measure is to be alert to any symptoms of respiratory trouble that linger more than a few days. Good lifestyle habits, such as proper diet and hygiene, rest, and regular exercise, increase resistance to all respiratory illnesses. They also help promote fast recovery when illness does occur.

Individuals with pneumonia should try to stay away from anyone with a compromised immune system, such as those with AIDS. If that is not possible, protecting others by wearing a face mask and always coughing into a tissue is important.

PROSTATE CONDITIONS

BACKGROUND

The prostate is part of a man's reproductive (genitourinary) system and is located in front of the rectum and under the bladder. It surrounds the urethra, the tube through which urine flows. A healthy prostate is about the size of a walnut. Male hormones (androgens, particularly testosterone) normally produced by the body stimulate the growth of the prostate. The testicles are the main source of male hormones, including testosterone. The prostate changes size very little from birth until puberty, but at puberty it increases in weight and doubles in size. In general, the size of the prostate remains constant after puberty for the next 30 or more years. In some men, in fact, the prostate never again increases in size. Unfortunately, however, this is not the case for most men, who will develop some form of noncancerous enlargement of the prostate, medically known as benign prostatic hyperplasia (BPH). Half of all men in their 50s and 80% of men in their 80s have some symptoms of BPH. The prostate makes part of the seminal fluid. During ejaculation, seminal fluid helps carry sperm out of the man's body as part of semen. In the adult male, the glandular tissue of the prostate secretes a fluid that contributes 20-30% of the total volume of the seminal fluid released when a man ejaculates. This prostate fluid is continuously generated by the prostate but increases during sexual excitement. The combination of spermatozoa, seminal vesicle fluid, and prostatic fluid, in addition to a tiny amount of fluid from some minor glands, constitutes semen. The prostate gland fluid is a thin, milky substance that gives semen its characteristic color and odor. Some common prostate problems include prostatitis (inflammation of the prostate, usually caused by bacterial infection), BPH (an enlarged prostate, which may cause dribbling after urination or a need to urinate often, especially at night), and prostate cancer (a common cancer that responds best to treatment when detected early).

TYPES AND CAUSES

Prostatitis: Prostatitis is inflammation of the prostate gland usually caused by an infection that often affects younger men. With treatment, prostatitis should generally be alleviated within several days to two weeks. Treatment of chronic (long-term) bacterial prostatitis usually involves antimicrobial medication for four to 12 weeks. This type of prostatitis is difficult to treat and recurrence is possible. Prostatitis usually results from blockage or irritation of some of the ducts within the prostate gland, and the cause may be mechanical (such as narrowing of the urethra) or infectious. The infectious causes may be viral or bacterial, including *Escherichia coli* or sexually transmitted infections such as *Chlamydia*.

There are four types of prostatitis: acute bacterial prostatitis (the least common of the four types, but the most common in men under 35), chronic bacterial (not very common, but affects mostly men between 40-70 years), asymptomatic inflammatory prostatitis (produces no outward symptoms and occurs mainly in men aged 60 and over), and chronic nonbacterial/prostadynia (most common type). Prostadynia, also known as chronic pelvic pain syndrome, is a condition associated with similar symptoms as chronic nonbacterial prostatitis but that has no evidence of prostate inflammation.

BPH: BPH is a normal, gradual enlargement of the prostate caused by hormonal fluctuations, such as decreases in testosterone and increases in dihydrotestosterone (DHT) and estrogen in prostate tissue. BPH usually beings in middle age. BPH does not lead to cancer. BPH does not generally cause pain, but discomfort (a feeling of pressure) in the groin area is generally found. As the prostate enlarges, it presses against the urethra and interferes with urination. At the same time, the bladder wall becomes thicker and irritated and begins to contract, even when it contains small amounts of urine, which causes more frequent urination. And, as the bladder continues to weaken, it may not empty completely, leaving some urine behind. Blocking or narrowing of the urethra by the prostate and partial emptying of the bladder cause many of the problems associated with BPH.

BPH affects about half of men aged over 60 and 80% of men aged 80 or older; it is considered to be a condition related to aging. Almost every man over 45 has some prostate enlargement, but symptoms are rarely felt before the age of 60. BPH affects all men differently and therefore treatment varies.

Prostate Cancer: As men get older (after age 50), their risk of prostate cancer increases. Men above 50 years of age should be checked for prostate cancer routinely by their doctors, and men with risk factors for developing prostate cancer (including family history of prostate cancer, multiple family members with prostate cancer, and/or African heritage),

P

should talk to their doctors about starting this screening at a younger age, such as 40.

Prostate cancer exhibits tremendous differences in incidence among populations worldwide. Asian men typically have a very low incidence of prostate cancer, with age-adjusted incidence rates ranging from two to 10 per 100,000 men. Higher incidence rates are generally observed in northern European countries. African men, however, have the highest incidence of prostate cancer in the world. In the United States, African-American men have a 60% higher incidence rate compared with Caucasian men.

Prostate cancer is the most common non-skin cancer in America, affecting one in six men. More than 218,000 men in the United States will be diagnosed with prostate cancer in 2007. Healthcare professionals recommend men 50 years of age and older get screened for prostate cancer. If an immediate family member such as a father or brother has prostate cancer, the risk of developing the disease is greater than that of the average American man. Between 5-10% of prostate cancer cases are believed to be due primarily to high-risk inherited genetic factors or prostate cancer susceptibility genes. The survival rate indicates the percentage of patients who live a specific number of years after the cancer is diagnosed. For prostate cancer, the 10-year survival rate is 93% and the 15-year survival rate is 77%.

A high-fat diet and obesity may increase the risk of prostate cancer. Researchers theorize that fat increases production of the hormone testosterone, which may promote the development of prostate cancer cells. Obese men who are diagnosed with prostate cancer have more than two-and-a-half times the risk of dying from the disease as compared to men of normal weight at the time of diagnosis. Scientists believe that obesity increases the risk of prostate cancer by increasing inflammation and steroid hormones, such as testosterone.

Because testosterone naturally stimulates the growth of the prostate gland, men who have high levels of testosterone and men who use testosterone (steroid) therapy are more likely to develop prostate cancer than are men who have lower levels of testosterone. Long-term testosterone treatment could cause prostate gland enlargement (BPH). Also, doctors are concerned that testosterone therapy might fuel the growth of prostate cancer that is already present.

SIGNS AND SYMPTOMS
Prostatitis
Symptoms of prostatitis may include painful, burning, or frequent urination; weak urine flow or incomplete emptying; fever and chills; lower abdominal pain or pressure; painful ejaculation; impotence; and low back pain.

Acute Bacterial Prostatitis: Although the least common of all types of prostatitis, acute bacterial prostatitis occurs in men at any age and often with sudden onset and severe symptoms. Men may find urination difficult and extremely painful. Other symptoms of acute bacterial prostatitis include fever, chills, lower back pain, pain in the genital (between the legs) area, urinary frequency, burning during urination, and/or urinary urgency at night, coupled with aches and pains throughout the body.

Chronic Bacterial Prostatitis: Although fairly uncommon, chronic bacterial prostatitis is a recurrent infection of the prostate gland that is difficult to treat. Symptoms of the infection are often similar to but less intense than acute bacterial prostatitis. However, symptoms of chronic bacterial prostatitis generally last longer and often fever is absent, unlike during an acute infection.

Chronic Prostatitis/Chronic Pelvic Pain Syndrome: Chronic prostatitis/chronic pelvic pain syndrome is likely the least understood form of prostatitis, but the most common form of the disease. Symptoms may resolve and then reappear without warning. The infection may be considered inflammatory, in which urine, semen, and other secretions are absent of a known infecting organism but do contain infection-fighting cells, or the infection may be considered noninflammatory, in which inflammation and infection-fighting cells are both absent.

Asymptomatic Inflammatory Prostatitis: Asymptomatic inflammatory prostatitis may be diagnosed when infection-fighting cells are present, but common symptoms of prostatitis, such as difficulty with urination, fever, and lower back and pelvic pain, are absent. A diagnosis of asymptomatic inflammatory prostatitis is made most often during an examination for other conditions, such as infertility or prostate cancer.

BPH: Common symptoms of BPH include having to wait for the urine stream to start, poor urinary flow and a variable flow rate, frequent urination, difficulty postponing urination (urgency), dribbling of urine at the end of urination, and having to wake at night to urinate multiple times (nocturia).

Prostate Cancer
Cancer of the prostate often grows slowly, especially in older men. Symptoms may be mild and occur over many years. Early symptoms of prostate cancer can mimic other prostate conditions, such as BPH and prostatitis. In later stages, prostate cancer cells may

spread to the bones, causing pain in the back, hips, pelvis, and other bony areas.

DIAGNOSIS

Digital Rectal Exam (DRE): The DRE is a procedure commonly performed during routine physical examinations. During a DRE, a doctor feels the prostate gland by passing a gloved finger into the individual's rectum to find hard or lumpy areas of the gland, which may represent an abnormality. If there is suspicion of an abnormal prostate, the doctor may analyze urine and prostate fluid after massaging the prostate gland. The doctor may also assess the degree of pain or discomfort the individual experiences as he presses the muscles and ligaments of the pelvic floor and perineum. If a man has prostatitis, this examination may produce momentary pain or discomfort but it causes neither damage nor significant prolonged pain.

Prostate-Specific Antigen (PSA) Test: PSA is an enzyme normally made by cells in the prostate gland that helps break down proteins in seminal fluid to aid with fertility. PSA levels can be measured by drawing blood from a vein, which is then sent for a PSA laboratory test. It is normal for the bloodstream to contain some PSA. However, if the PSA level is found to be elevated, it may be an indication of prostate infection, inflammation, enlargement (BPH), or cancer. However, in the United States, a generally accepted standard PSA level is considered to be 4.0 nanograms per milliliter (ng/mL). If the PSA level is above 4.0, further evaluation will often be recommended, for example with an ultrasound and prostate biopsy by an urologist. Even if the PSA is less than 4.0, if the PSA has risen a concerning amount since a prior measurement, further evaluation may be recommended. PSA values tend to be lower in younger men, and it has been suggested that the PSA level at which to consider a biopsy should be lower for younger men than for older men. Even if the PSA is elevated, it does not necessarily mean that cancer is present since there are other causes of PSA elevations. This is why further evaluation with a biopsy is often recommended.

Using the PSA test to screen men for prostate cancer is controversial because it has not clearly been proven that this test actually saves lives. Moreover, it is not clear if the benefits of PSA screening outweigh the risks of follow-up diagnostic tests and cancer treatments. For example, the PSA test may detect small cancers that would never become life threatening. This situation, called overdiagnosis, might put men at risk for complications from unnecessary treatments such as surgery or radiation, although this is unproven. Regardless of these concerns, at this time PSA screening is recommended by most professional organizations and is considered the standard of care.

Prostate Biopsy Procedure: If the DRE and/or PSA blood test results are suspicious for a possible prostate cancer, a doctor may recommend a prostate biopsy. The patient will be prescribed antibiotics, usually a three-day course, before the procedure. Most individuals receive local anesthesia, such as lidocaine (Xylocaine). To do a biopsy, a doctor inserts a small, lubricated probe about the size and shape of a cigar into the rectum (called transrectal ultrasound). The probe uses sound waves that are converted to visual data in order to see a picture of the prostate gland, which is then analyzed for changes. If an abnormal area is seen on the transrectal ultrasound, the doctor will likely biopsy that area. Then a fine, hollow needle is aimed at these areas of the prostate. A spring propels the needle into the prostate gland and retrieves a very thin section of tissue. Biopsies are generally obtained from multiple areas of the prostate, and it is important that all relevant areas be included (this should be discussed with the urologist). Biopsies are often done with the guidance of a transrectal ultrasound. Biopsies in general take 15-45 minutes to complete depending upon the procedure. The procedure may cause side effects, including bleeding and infection. Approximately 55% of men report discomfort during the biopsy. Some men also experience pain in the rectal area or penis following biopsy, which should be reported to a doctor if it does not resolve. Biopsies can also be performed through the perineum area (between the anus and the scrotum, called transperineal biopsy) or through the urethra (canal that the urine travels through for elimination, called transurethral biopsy).

Prostate Biopsy Analysis: Prostate biopsy specimens are examined by pathologists using a microscope and chemical staining in order to make a diagnosis. The pathologist may determine that the prostate looks normal, or that there are precancerous areas called high-grade prostatic intraepithelial neoplasia, or that there is prostate cancer present. If there is high-grade prostatic intraepithelial neoplasia, a repeat biopsy or close follow-up will usually be recommended. If there is prostate cancer present, the pathologist will assign Gleason grades to evaluate the aggressiveness of the cancer. For each biopsy core, two numbers will be assigned that are then added together for the total Gleason grade for that core. The first number represents the most common level of aggressiveness of cancer cells for that core,

P

and the second number represents the second most common level of aggressiveness for that core. These individual numbers can range between 3 and 5, and therefore the total Gleason sums range between 6 and 10. For example, if there is a core with the most common cancer cell type being 3 and the second most common being 4, then the total Gleason grade for that core is $3 + 4 = 7$. Each core gets its own grade. Sometimes the pathologist will note the third most common level of aggressiveness for a core; this is called the tertiary Gleason grade.

Transrectal Ultrasound (TRUS): If the doctor requires a closer look at the prostate gland or decides that a biopsy is necessary, he may order a TRUS, which allows visualization of the prostate gland. A TRUS is a five- to 15-minute outpatient procedure that uses sound waves to create a video image of the prostate gland. A small, lubricated probe placed into the rectum releases sound waves, which create echoes as they enter the prostate. Prostate tumors sometimes create echoes that are different from normal prostate tissue. The echoes that bounce back are sent to a computer that translates the pattern of echoes into a picture of the prostate. While the probe may be temporarily uncomfortable, TRUS is usually a painless procedure.

Imaging: If prostate cancer is diagnosed with a biopsy, depending on the Gleason grade and PSA values, a physician may recommend a bone scan and computerized tomography scan of the abdomen and pelvis. The bone scan is to evaluate for potential spread of cancer to the bones. The CT scan should be done using intravenous contrast for eligible patients and can evaluate the lymph nodes, liver and, to a limited extent, the prostate area. Even if there is a very low chance of spreading, these scans can be helpful to get baseline images for later comparisons if necessary. Increasingly, magnetic resonance imaging of the prostate is being used to obtain views of the prostate to plan treatment, with good supporting evidence. This is usually done with a thin probe that is placed into the rectum to get the best picture possible.

COMPLICATIONS

Biopsy Complications: Biopsy complications can include pain (which can persist after the biopsy), bleeding (which can appear in the stool or semen), and infection. Ongoing discomfort or bleeding should be evaluated by a clinician.

Prostate Cancer Complications: Prostate cancer can metastasize (spread to areas of the body other than the prostate, such as lymph nodes, bone, lung, or liver) and can be life threatening. Metastasis can take months to years to occur depending on the individual. Although early-stage prostate cancer typically is not painful, once it has spread to bones it may produce pain, which can be intense. Local growth of prostate cancer or treatment of prostate cancer can lead to urinary incontinence (leakage), erectile dysfunction (impotence), and other serious complications.

TREATMENT
Prostatitis
Pain relievers and several weeks of treatment with antibiotics are typically needed for category 1 and 2 prostatitis, which are bacterial infections. A variety of treatments as well as self-care measures also can provide relief. Treatment for category 3 prostatitis (nonbacterial) is less clear and mainly involves relieving symptoms. Category 4 prostatitis is usually found during examination for another reason and often does not require treatment.

Acute bacterial prostatitis (infectious prostatitis) is treated with oral antibiotics for one to two weeks. The commonly used antibiotics include quinolones, such as norfloxacin (Noroxin), ciprofloxacin (Cipro), or levofloxacin (Levaquin). In severe cases, treatment with intravenous antibiotics may be necessary. Chronic bacterial prostatitis is also treated with oral antibiotics for four to 12 weeks. Other medications used to treat infectious prostatitis include stool softeners, such as docusate sodium (Colace); antiinflammatory medications, such as ibuprofen (Motrin); analgesics or pain medications, such as hydrocodone (Vicodin, Lortab); alpha-blockers such as tamsulosin (Flomax); and 5-alpha reductase inhibitors, such as finasteride (Proscar) or dutasteride (Avodart).

If the individual has noninfectious prostatitis, he will not need antimicrobial medication. Treatment depends upon the symptoms that are present. If the condition responds to muscle relaxation, the individual may be given an alpha-blocker, a drug that can relax the muscle tissue in the prostate and reduce the difficulty in urination.

Asymptomatic inflammatory prostatitis and chronic prostatitis may respond to multidisciplinary approaches incorporating exercise, progressive relaxation, and counseling.

BPH
Drug Therapy: The U.S. Food and Drug Administration (FDA) has approved multiple drugs to relieve common symptoms associated with an enlarged prostate. Finasteride (Proscar), FDA approved in

1992, and dutasteride (Avodart), FDA approved in 2001, inhibit the production of the hormone DHT, which is involved with prostate enlargement. The use of either of these drugs can either prevent the progression of growth of the prostate or actually shrink the prostate in some men.

The FDA also approved the drugs terazosin (Hytrin) in 1993, doxazosin (Cardura) in 1995, tamsulosin (Flomax) in 1997, and alfuzosin (Uroxatral) in 2003 for the treatment of BPH. All four drugs act by relaxing the smooth muscle of the prostate and bladder neck to improve urine flow and to reduce bladder outlet obstruction. The four drugs belong to the class known as alpha-blockers. Terazosin and doxazosin were developed first to treat high blood pressure. Tamsulosin and alfuzosin were developed specifically to treat BPH. Because drug treatment is not effective in all cases, researchers in recent years have developed a number of procedures that relieve BPH symptoms but are less invasive than surgery.

Transurethral Resection of the Prostate (TURP): This is a surgical procedure to remove tissue from the prostate that may be blocking urine flow using a resectoscope (a thin, lighted tube with a cutting tool) inserted through the urethra. This surgery is sometimes performed to relieve symptoms caused by benign (noncancerous) tumors. TURP may also be done in men who cannot have a radical prostatectomy because of age or illness.

Transurethral Microwave Procedures: In May 1996, the FDA approved the Prostatron (EDAP TMS, Lyon, France), a device that uses microwave-generated heat to destroy excess prostate tissue. In the procedure, called transurethral microwave thermotherapy, the Prostatron sends computer-regulated microwaves through a catheter to heat selected portions of the prostate to at least 111° F. The temperature becomes high enough inside the prostate to kill some of the tissue. As this part of the prostate heals, it shrinks, reducing the blockage of urine flow. A cooling system protects the urinary tract during the procedure.

A similar microwave device, the Targis System (Urologix Inc., Minneapolis, MN), received FDA approval in September 1997. Like the Prostatron, the Targis System delivers microwaves to destroy selected portions of the prostate and uses a cooling system to protect the urethra. A heat-sensing device inserted in the rectum helps monitor the therapy.

Both procedures take about one hour and can be performed on an outpatient basis without general anesthesia. Neither procedure has been reported to lead to impotence or incontinence.

While microwave therapy does not cure BPH, it reduces urinary frequency, urgency, straining, and intermittent flow. It does not correct the problem of incomplete emptying of the bladder. Ongoing research will determine any long-term effects of microwave therapy and who might benefit most from this therapy.

Transurethral Needle Ablation: In October 1996, FDA approved the minimally invasive transurethral needle ablation (TUNA) system for the treatment of BPH. The TUNA system delivers low-level radiofrequency energy through twin needles to burn away a well-defined region of the enlarged prostate. Shields protect the urethra from heat damage. The TUNA system improves urine flow and relieves symptoms with fewer side effects compared with TURP. No incontinence or impotence has been observed.

Prostate Cancer

Overview of Management Options: When prostate cancer is localized (not spread beyond the prostate), most practitioners will discuss options with patients that include surgical removal of the prostate (prostatectomy), radiation treatment, or active surveillance (also called watchful waiting or observation). The goal of prostatectomy or radiation treatment is to cure the patient by eradicating the cancer. There are other, less well-established approaches, including cryotherapy and high-intensity focused ultrasound, for which there is less scientific evidence available compared to prostatectomy or radiation therapy.

Prostatectomy: Radical prostatectomy is a surgical procedure to remove the prostate, surrounding tissue, seminal vesicles, and pelvic lymph nodes. Prostatectomy is performed by a urologist. The traditional open surgery is also called radical retropubic prostatectomy, during which a three- to four-inch incision is made below the belly button, through which the prostate and nearby lymph nodes are removed. Less common is the perineal prostatectomy, which is an open surgical procedure to remove the prostate and nearby lymph nodes through an incision made in the perineum (area between the scrotum and anus). More recently, laparoscopic prostatectomy and robotic laparoscopic prostatectomy approaches have become more common. For these procedures, several small incisions are made in the abdomen, through which instruments are inserted to perform the surgery. For nonrobotic prostatectomy, the surgeon operates these instruments by hand, while in robotic prostatectomy the surgeon operates controls that move a robotic arm to perform the surgery. Most likely, these approaches are all equivalent in terms of effectiveness and side effects, although the least scientific evidence is available on robotic prostatectomy as it is a recently developed technique. Most scientific evidence suggests that the most important factor when selecting a surgical approach is the experience of the surgeon, not the specific surgical technique. Several studies show that the more prostatectomies a surgeon does each year, the better the outcomes for patients. Therefore, patients are advised to undergo surgery with a physician with a lot of experience removing prostates.

Surgery Complications: Surgery for prostate cancer can cause problems such as erectile dysfunction (impotence) and leakage of urine from the bladder (incontinence). Levels of severity are highly variable. In many cases, doctors may use a technique known as nerve-sparing surgery to save the nerves that control erection. These surgeries are performed under general anesthesia, which may also cause complications. The risk of complications should be discussed with the surgeon during initial meetings. Preoperative clearance by an internal medicine physician or cardiologist should be considered and discussed with the surgeon.

Radiation Therapy: Radiation therapy is a cancer treatment that uses high-energy radiation to kill cancer cells and shrink tumors. It is performed by a radiation oncologist. There are two main types of radiation therapy. External beam radiation therapy (EBRT) uses a machine outside the body to send radiation toward the cancer. Most commonly, EBRT is performed using "conformal" approaches that customize the radiation to the shape of each patient's prostate and location of tumor, and particularly intensity-modulated radiation therapy. Internal radiation therapy (or brachytherapy) involves surgically implanting tiny, radioactive capsules (called "seeds") into the cancerous prostate gland. The seeds emit radiation that kills the malignant tumor. The type of radiation therapy used depends on the type and stage of the cancer being treated. For some prostate tumors, a combination of EBRT and seeds may be considered by the radiation oncologist. For cancers that are higher risk (higher Gleason grades, higher PSA scores, and/or greater amounts of cancer in the prostate or surrounding area), hormone therapy may be recommended by the radiation oncologist to be given during treatment and for a period of time after the radiation is completed. Recently, proton beam therapy has been suggested for localized prostate cancer, but evidence is limited

and this approach is generally reserved for other types of cancers, such as small tumors in children.

Radiation Complications: Side effects during radiation treatment can include diarrhea, skin burns, sexual dysfunction, and urinary discomfort or urgency. Normal tissue can be damaged by radiation. Like prostatectomy, possible long-term complications include urinary incontinence (leakage) and erectile dysfunction (impotence). There is also a very small chance of long-term blood in the stool due to radiation damage to the lining of the rectum (radiation proctitis). New developments in radiation delivery have decreased the chances of these complications. The risks of these complications should be discussed with the radiation oncologist during an initial meeting.

Active Surveillance, Watchful Waiting, Observation: For selected patients with low-grade cancers (Gleason 3 + 3 = 6 in few cores with low PSA), active surveillance may be appropriate. Surveillance is usually under the supervision of a urologist and involves regular follow-up of the PSA, DRE, periodic rebiopsy, and consideration of periodic imaging with magnetic resonance or computed tomography scans. If concerning changes occur suggesting that the cancer is progressing, then proceeding with prostatectomy or radiation treatment will be considered. For older patients with limited life expectancy (less than five to 10 years) and low-grade cancers, observation may be considered if the potential risks of treatment are felt to outweigh potential benefits.

Cryosurgery: Cryosurgery is a treatment that uses an instrument to freeze and destroy prostate cancer cells. This type of treatment is also called cryotherapy. There is less scientific evidence available to support this therapy than there is for prostatectomy or radiation. It is sometimes used for cancer that has recurred after radiation or surgery, but it is associated with high levels of incontinence.

High-Intensity Focused Ultrasound: High-intensity focused ultrasound is a new treatment that uses ultrasound (high-energy sound waves) to destroy cancer cells. To treat prostate cancer, an endorectal (inside the rectum) probe is used to make the sound waves. Scientific evidence supporting this approach is limited.

Choosing a Management Approach: Selecting between the available options for localized prostate cancer can be very difficult, especially because for many men there may be no clear advantage of one approach over another. The choice of treatment should be made after discussion with physicians and reading about the different options. Regardless of the approach selected, it should be under the care of a physician with experience treating prostate cancer.

Metastatic Prostate Cancer

Overview of Management Options: When prostate cancer has spread beyond the prostate, it is said to be metastatic or to have metastasized. The most common areas of metastasis are the bones (especially ribs, spine, skull, and pelvis), lymph nodes and, less commonly, the lungs and liver. Once the cancer spreads to the bones, liver, or lungs, it cannot be cured, and treatments are aimed at controlling the growth of the cancer for as long as possible. The standard initial treatment for metastatic prostate cancer is hormonal therapy. Chemotherapy is generally not given unless the cancer becomes resistant to the effects of hormonal therapy. Generally, the prostate area itself is not treated if the cancer has metastasized, although in some cases if there is a lot of cancer in the prostate area, radiation may be given for local control to avoid complications from the cancer growing too large in the pelvis area.

Hormonal Therapy: Hormone therapy is a potentially confusing term, as the goal of this treatment approach is actually to block the effects of the normal male hormone, testosterone, on prostate cancers. This is because testosterone stimulates the growth of prostate cancer cells. There are several stages of hormone therapy that can be used as the cancer becomes resistant to each prior stage.

Castration (Surgical or with Medications): The initial stage of hormonal therapy involves blocking most of the body's production of testosterone (castration). This can either be done by surgical castration (surgical removal of the testicles) or with injected medications (pharmacological or chemical castration). The medications are called luteinizing hormone–releasing hormone agonists or gonadotropin-releasing hormone antagonists and include leuprolide (Eligard, Lupron, Lupron Depot, Viadur), goserelin (Zoladex), and buserelin (Suprefact). Side effects most commonly include hot flashes, erectile dysfunction (impotence), loss of sexual desire, weight gain, and fatigue. Less commonly men may experience diminished concentration and skin changes. Bone loss occurs and therefore a baseline bone mineral density test should be conducted, treatment with calcium and vitamin D should be started, and a bone-strengthening medicine such as a bisphosphonate should be considered. Recently, hormonal therapy has been linked to a possible increased risk of diabetes or heart disease, although further studies are necessary to determine if a link truly exists. Therefore, people with increased risk of these conditions should discuss the risks vs. potential benefits of this therapy with a doctor. Patients who begin hormone therapy may experience an increase in prostate cancer symptoms for approximately two weeks after starting this treatment due to a temporary increase in testosterone levels, and therefore two to four weeks of a different medication (antiandrogen) may be given initially to mute this effect.

Antiandrogens: Antiandrogens are pills that block the action of testosterone on prostate cells. Examples are bicalutamide (Casodex), nilutamide (Nilandron, Anadron), and flutamide (Eulexin). They are often added when a prostate cancer becomes resistant to castration treatment alone. Breast enlargement and tenderness can occur, and to prevent breast enlargement, some patients undergo a single radiation treatment to the breast area (which should be given before starting the antiandrogen). Patients taking antiandrogens should undergo periodic liver function tests and should report symptoms such as nausea, vomiting, stomach pain, fatigue, appetite loss, dark urine, or yellowing of the eyes to a physician immediately. Diabetic patients should follow blood sugars closely when beginning therapy. If a cancer progresses during treatment with an antiandrogen, withdrawal of the antiandrogen should be done to see if the action of taking away the antiandrogen shrinks the cancer. If the cancer grows again, then a different antiandrogen may be considered.

Adrenal Agents: Drugs that can prevent the adrenal glands from making androgens (male sex hormones) include ketoconazole. An adrenal agent can be considered if a cancer progresses despite treatment with castration plus an antiandrogen. The adrenal agent should be started at a low dose and gradually increased by the treating physician as appropriate. At higher doses, a steroid pill such as hydrocortisone should be given with the adrenal therapy. Side effects can include drowsiness, dizziness, headache, weakness, nausea, or loss of appetite, especially during the first few weeks of treatment. If these symptoms are severe, a physician should be contacted immediately. Liver function tests should be monitored during this treatment.

Estrogens: Estrogens (hormones that promote female sex characteristics) were previously used to treat prostate cancer but are seldom used today because of the risk of serious side effects, including blood clots.

Chemotherapy: Chemotherapy is a cancer treatment that uses drugs to stop the growth of cancer cells, either by killing the cells or by stopping them from dividing. Chemotherapy is often used to treat advanced prostate cancers that are resistant to hormonal treatments. A medical oncologist (cancer specialist) will usually recommend a single drug or a combination of drugs.

P

As of 2008, the only FDA-approved chemotherapy for prostate cancer shown to lengthen life and improve quality of life is docetaxel (Taxotere). Mitoxantrone (Novantrone) has also been approved by the FDA for prostate cancer but has not been shown to lengthen life and is only beneficial in a small percent of patients. Other chemotherapy medications sometimes used to treat prostate cancer include paclitaxel (Taxol), carboplatin and, less commonly, doxorubicin (Adriamycin) or oral etoposide. For rare cases of small-cell or neuroendocrine prostate cancer, intravenous etoposide and a platinum agent may be used. Side effects of chemotherapy depend on the type of drug used, dosage, and length of treatment. The most common side effects are fatigue, nausea and vomiting, diarrhea, hair loss, anemia, and increased susceptibility to infection due to lowered white blood cell counts. Radiopharmaceuticals such as samarium (Quadramet) may be used as a palliative measure to treat bone pain.

Clinical Trials: Many new drugs, including "targeted" agents, vaccine-type therapies, and new chemotherapies, are in development. A treating oncologist may offer enrollment in a trial to patients with prostate cancer. An informed consent document will be given to a patient that explains the potential risks and benefits of the trial. Information from clinical trials is used to improve therapies for future patients and is an opportunity to receive a new treatment approach that is not otherwise available.

Hospice and End-of-Life Care: When a patient has not responded to treatment methods, is too frail to receive further therapy, or the prognosis is not good, palliative care can be started with a goal of comfort and to provide symptomatic relief and dignity. Hospice services are available as inpatient facilities or in the home with hospice nurses visiting as necessary. Hospice options can be discussed with an oncologist's office.

INTEGRATIVE THERAPIES

Strong Scientific Evidence

Saw Palmetto: Numerous human trials report that saw palmetto (*Serenoa repens*) improves symptoms of BPH such as nighttime urination, urinary flow, and overall quality of life, although it may not greatly reduce the size of the prostate. Although the quality of these studies has been variable, overall they suggest effectiveness. There is no evidence that saw palmetto is beneficial in the treatment of prostate cancer, and theoretically it may lower PSA values, making it more difficult to determine when a cancer is growing.

Good Scientific Evidence

Beta-Sitosterol: Beta-sitosterol and beta-sitosterol glucoside have been used to treat symptoms of BPH. Additional clinical study is needed before a firm recommendation can be made.

Lycopene: Lycopene is a carotenoid (in the vitamin A family) antioxidant found in processed tomato products, such as canned tomato sauces. Laboratory studies have reported that lycopene inhibits the growth of prostate cancer cells. There is evidence from studies observing large populations that lycopene may prevent the development of prostate cancer. There is ongoing research in this area. Scientific evidence suggests that the best source of lycopene is in processed tomato products rather than fresh tomatoes. However, caution is urged because many of these products are high in salt.

Pygeum: Pygeum (*Pygeum africanum*) has been observed to moderately improve urinary symptoms associated with enlargement of the prostate gland or prostate inflammation. Numerous human studies report pygeum to significantly reduce the number of nighttime urinary episodes, urinary hesitancy, urinary frequency, and pain with urination in men who experience mild-to-moderate symptoms. However, pygeum does not appear to reduce the size of the prostate gland. It is unclear how pygeum compares to the effectiveness or safety of other medical therapies, such as prescription drugs (e.g., alpha-adrenergic blockers or 5-alpha reductase inhibitors), surgical approaches, or other herbs/supplements such as saw palmetto. Caution is advised when taking pygeum, as adverse effects including drug interactions are possible. Pygeum has not been shown to have effects on prostate cancer.

Selenium: There is evidence that low selenium levels are associated with an increased risk of prostate cancer. In human studies, initial evidence has suggested that selenium supplementation reduces the risk of developing prostate cancer in men with normal baseline PSA levels and low selenium blood levels. Selenium deficiency may be diagnosed by measuring the selenium in the blood where the normal level is 70 nanograms per milliliter (ng/mL) in blood plasma (liquid component) or 90 ng/mL in red blood cells, where the normal values are indicated. Laboratory studies have reported several potential mechanisms for selenium's beneficial effects in prostate cancer, including a decrease in androgen receptors and PSA production, angiogenesis (growth of new blood vessels in tumors) inhibition, and increased antioxidant effects, including cancer cell apoptosis (cell death). There is ongoing research in this area.

Unclear or Conflicting Scientific Evidence

Green Tea: Green tea (*Camellia sinensis*) is reported to have antioxidant and immune-stimulating properties. It has been proposed that drinking green tea may decrease cancer and cardiovascular disease risks, although further evidence is needed in these areas. One clinical trial reported minimal benefit using green tea extract capsules for the treatment of hormone-refractory prostate cancer. Further research is needed before a clear conclusion can be reached. Caution is advised when drinking green tea, as adverse effects, including an increased risk of bleeding and drug interactions, are possible. Caffeine-free products are available.

Modified Citrus Pectin: Pectins are gel-forming polysaccharides from plant cell walls, especially apple and citrus fruits. Modified citrus pectin has been suggested to reduce the metastasis (spread to other areas of the body) of certain types of cancers, including lung, prostate, and breast, although further scientific evidence is necessary before a clear conclusion can be drawn.

Pomegranate Juice: Pomegranate juice has received publicity for being possibly helpful for prostate cancer. In laboratory study, flavonoid compounds from pomegranate fruit have been shown to have anticancer activity against prostate cancer cells. The scientific evidence is limited in this area, and further research is necessary before a clear conclusion can be drawn.

Stinging Nettle: Stinging nettle is used rather frequently in Europe in the treatment of symptoms associated with BPH (enlarged prostate). Early evidence suggests an improvement in symptoms, such as the alleviation of lower urinary tract symptoms associated with stage I or II BPH, as a result of nettle therapy. Additional study is warranted in this area.

Vitamin E: The role of vitamin E supplementation in the prevention of prostate cancer is controversial. There are numerous laboratory studies that suggest possible anticancer properties. However, the results of population research and human research have been mixed, with some studies reporting benefits and others finding no effects. Vitamin E succinate (one specific form of vitamin E) has been reported in laboratory studies to inhibit the growth of human prostate cancer cells.

Traditional or Theoretical Uses Lacking Sufficient Evidence

Maitake Mushroom: Maitake mushroom has been suggested to help the body fight infections and cancer. Further evidence is necessary before a

clear conclusion can be drawn about its effects in preventing or treating conditions of the prostate.

Milk Thistle: Milk thistle (*Silybum marianum*) has been used traditionally to "detoxify" the liver and as an antioxidant. Recent laboratory studies have reported that milk thistle may be effective against prostate cancer cells, but further evidence is necessary before clear conclusions can be drawn. Caution is advised when taking milk thistle, as adverse effects including drug interactions are possible.

Panax Ginseng: Compounds found in *Panax ginseng* have been reported in laboratory studies to enhance immunity cell function and to cause cancer cell apoptosis (cell death). This research is very preliminary and additional study is necessary before a clear conclusion can be reached. Caution is advised when taking *Panax ginseng,* as adverse effects including drug interactions are possible.

Prayer: Initial studies in patients with cancer (such as prostate cancer) report variable effects on disease progression and death rates when intercessory prayer is used. Better-quality research is necessary before a firm conclusion can be drawn.

Quercetin: There is some evidence that quercetin, a bioflavonoid and antioxidant, may be useful for the treatment of chronic prostatitis (inflammation of the prostate). Further research is needed to confirm these results. Quercetin is reported safe in recommended dosages.

Shiitake Mushroom: Shiitake mushroom (*Lentinus edodes*) has been suggested to help the body fight infections and cancer. Further evidence is necessary before a clear conclusion can be drawn about its effects in preventing or treating conditions of the prostate. Caution is advised when taking shiitake, as adverse effects, including an increase in bleeding and drug interactions, are possible.

Fair Negative Scientific Evidence

Vitamin D: Although there was preliminary evidence based on laboratory and limited human studies that high-dose vitamin D was possibly beneficial in the treatment of metastatic prostate cancer, a large study reported that patients taking high-dose calcitriol along with chemotherapy did worse than patients taking chemotherapy alone. Therefore, this treatment should be discouraged.

PREVENTION

Generally, BPH and prostatitis cannot be prevented. Proper nutrition is important, such as eating plenty of fresh vegetables and decreasing the amounts of refined carbohydrates, such as sugars and white breads.

Prostate Screening: The American Urological Association encourages men who are in good health to have annual PSA testing starting at age 50, or at age 40 if they are in high-risk groups, such as African-American men or those with a father, brother, or son with BPH.

Vaccine: The FDA has begun the process of approving a new vaccine aimed at extending survival for patients with deadly metastatic prostate cancer. The vaccine, called Provenge, on average increases the survival of prostate cancer victims by 18% compared to those on a placebo. That equals 4.5 months of extra survival time or 25.9 months for those receiving Provenge vs. 22 months for those not taking the vaccine. The vaccine is targeted at individuals with prostate cancer who have ceased responding to hormone therapy and have cancer that has spread to other organs and tissues. Side effects include fever, chills, and fatigue (tiredness).

Lifestyle Changes: Diets should include less high-fat dairy products, such as cheese, sour cream, and ice cream. High-fat dairy products and the calcium contained in dairy may increase the risks of developing prostate cancer.

Cruciferous vegetables (such as broccoli, cabbage, and cauliflower) have been reported to contain cancer-fighting phytochemicals that may decrease the chances of developing prostate cancer. Antioxidant-containing foods, including fruits (such as berries, grapes, and tomatoes) and vegetables (such as peppers and carrots) may help prevent the development of prostate cancer.

Dietary consumption of red meat and/or processed meats may increase the risks of developing cancer of the colon, rectum, stomach, pancreas, bladder, ovaries, prostate, breasts, and lungs and other diseases such as heart disease, rheumatoid arthritis, type 2 diabetes, and Alzheimer's disease.

Exercise (at least 30 minutes daily for five days a week), smoking cessation, and relaxation all may contribute to decreasing the risk of developing prostate cancer.

SEXUALLY TRANSMITTED DISEASES (STDs)

CONDITIONS: Sexually Transmitted Diseases (STDs), Chlamydia, Gonorrhea, Human Papilloma Virus (HPV), Pelvic Inflammatory Disease (PID), Syphilis, Trichomoniasis

BACKGROUND

Sexually transmitted diseases (STDs) are infections that can be transmitted through oral, anal, and vaginal sex. These diseases may be transmitted from person to person through blood, semen, vaginal secretions, and breast milk. STDs are sometimes called sexually transmitted infections because they involve passing a disease-causing microorganism (e.g., bacteria or virus) to another person during sex. STDs are among the most common infectious disease in the United States. Researchers estimate that 13 million Americans become infected with STDs each year.

There are more than 20 different STDs. Examples of common STDs include chlamydia, genital herpes, gonorrhea, human immunodeficiency virus (HIV), human papilloma virus (HPV), pelvic inflammatory disease (PID), syphilis, and trichomoniasis. HIV is the most dangerous STD because it progresses to acquired immune deficiency syndrome (AIDS), which is an incurable and fatal disease. However, many other STDs, such as syphilis, may also be life threatening if left untreated. Certain patients have an increased risk of developing STDs. This includes patients who have multiple sexual partners, engage in unprotected sex (oral, anal, or vaginal), or who have sexual partners who have or have previously had an STD. In addition, men who have sex with men are more likely to develop many STDs because they are more likely to engage in risky or unsafe sexual behavior. It is important that patients, especially those at high risk, are regularly tested for STDs. This is because patients do not always experience symptoms of diseases or infections. If a patient has an STD and is not tested, he/she may unknowingly pass the disease to his/her sexual partner(s). Treatment and prognosis depend on the specific type of STD. Not all STDs can be cured. Some STDs, such as HIV, HPV, and genital herpes, require lifelong medication and treatment to manage symptoms and prevent complications. Patients should always take medications exactly as prescribed. This is especially important for patients who are taking antibiotics to treat bacterial infections, such as gonorrhea or syphilis. Even if symptoms go away, medications should not be stopped early because the bacteria may still be present in the body. If the medication is stopped too early, the remaining bacteria in the body may mutate and become resistant to treatment. Once the bacteria are resistant to a medication, the antibiotic is no longer effective. There are many ways to reduce the risk of developing STDs. Individuals should practice safe sex, avoid risky behaviors (e.g., sharing needles or having multiple sex partners), and undergo routine screenings for STDs. Patients should also follow the recommended safety precautions to avoid exposure to blood or other bodily fluids. For instance, individuals should wear rubber gloves when applying first aid to someone who is bleeding.

CHLAMYDIA

Overview: Chlamydia is a curable sexually transmitted infection of the genital tract. If left untreated, chlamydia may damage the genital tract and lead to serious illnesses, including PID in females and inflammation of the tubes that carry semen (epididymitis) in males. According to the U.S. Centers for Disease Control and Prevention (CDC), nearly three million Americans become infected with chlamydia each year. Although chlamydia can affect people of all ages; in the United States it is most common among teenagers.

A bacterium called *Chlamydia trachomatis* causes chlamydia. Most cases of chlamydia are transmitted from person to person through oral, anal, or vaginal sex. Pregnant women may also pass the infection to their babies during vaginal childbirth. This is because the newborn is exposed to the mother's blood and other bodily fluids during birth.

Symptoms: During the early stages of chlamydia, most patients experience few or no symptoms of an infection. In general, symptoms usually develop one to three weeks after the bacteria have entered the body.

If patients develop the infection after vaginal sex, common symptoms include painful urination, vaginal or penile discharge, lower abdominal pain, painful sexual intercourse in women, and testicular pain in men.

If patients develop the infection after anal sex, rectal inflammation usually occurs. This inflammation typically causes pain and mucus discharge.

If patients touch their eyes after touching bodily secretions (e.g., semen or vaginal discharge) that are infected with chlamydia, they may develop an eye infection called pinkeye (conjunctivitis). Left untreated, pinkeye may lead to permanent blindness.

S

Newborns who contract chlamydia during childbirth usually develop pneumonia and/or severe eye infections, which may lead to blindness.

Complications: Patients infected with chlamydia are more vulnerable to other STDs, including HIV, gonorrhea, and syphilis, if they are exposed to them. Therefore, patients who test positive for chlamydia are often tested for other STDs.

Females with untreated chlamydia may develop PID. This is an infection of the fallopian tubes, uterus, and cervix. If left untreated, PID may cause permanent damage to the reproductive tract, which may lead to infertility. It may also lead to long-term pelvic pain.

Males with untreated chlamydia may develop a condition called epididymitis. This condition is characterized by inflammation of the tubes near the testicles that carry semen. Symptoms may include fever, scrotal pain, and swelling. The infection may also spread to the prostate gland in males, causing inflammation (prostatitis). Symptoms of prostatitis may include pain during or after sex, fever, painful urination, and lower back pain.

Diagnosis: Patients should talk to their healthcare providers to determine how often they should be tested for chlamydia. Patients who have symptoms of chlamydia or suspect that they may have been exposed to chlamydia should be tested. The CDC recommends that all pregnant women be screened for chlamydia during the first prenatal examination and possibly later on in the pregnancy.

The standard diagnostic test for chlamydia is a culture swab. For females, the healthcare provider may swab the discharge from the cervix. For males, the healthcare provider inserts a thin swab into the tip of the penis to retrieve a sample of fluid from the urethra. In some cases, the healthcare provider may swab the anus. The sample is then rubbed on a Petri dish. If the patient has chlamydia, *Chlamydia trachomatis* will grow on the Petri dish. A urine analysis may also be performed. A sample of the patient's urine is analyzed in a laboratory for the presence of the disease-causing bacteria.

Treatment: Chlamydia is curable. Patients take prescription antibiotics, such as azithromycin (Zithromax), doxycycline, or erythromycin (ERYC, Ery-Tab), by mouth. Treatment may last up to 10 days. Patients should take their medications exactly as prescribed. Even if symptoms go away, medications should not be stopped early because the bacteria may still be present in the body.

The patient's sexual partner(s) will also require treatment, even if they do not have symptoms of the infection. Otherwise, the patient may become reinfected with chlamydia.

Genital Herpes

Overview: Genital herpes, also called herpes simplex type 2, is an incurable viral infection that is characterized by painful sores on the genitals. Genital herpes can only be contracted through direct sexual contact, including genital-to-genital, mouth-to-genital, or hand-to-genital contact with an infected partner. Individuals cannot contract the virus through kissing. Occasionally, oral-genital contact can spread oral herpes to the genitals (and vice versa). Individuals with active herpes lesions on or around their mouths or on their genitals should only engage in oral sex if they use a condom or place a small piece of latex, called a dental dam, over the vagina or anus.

The chance of a pregnant woman passing herpes to her baby is highest if the first infection occurs near the time of delivery. The virus can be transmitted to the fetus through the placenta during pregnancy or during vaginal childbirth. First-time infection during pregnancy leads to an increased risk of miscarriage, decreased fetal growth, and preterm labor. About 30-50% of infants who are born vaginally to a mother with first-time infection become infected with the herpes virus. Of babies born to women experiencing recurrent outbreaks at the time of birth, 1-4% become infected with the herpes simplex virus.

After an initial or primary infection, herpes viruses establish a period called latency, during which the virus is present in the cell bodies of nerves that attach to the area of the original viral outbreak (e.g., genitals, mouth, and lips). At some point, this latency ends and the virus becomes active again. While active, the virus begins to multiply (called shedding) and becomes transmittable again. This shedding may or may not be accompanied by symptoms. During reactivation, the virus multiplies in the nerve cell and is transported outwardly via the nerve to the skin. The ability of herpes virus to become latent and reactive explains the long-term, recurring nature of a herpes infection.

Recurrence of the viral symptoms is usually milder than the original infection. Recurrence may be triggered by menstruation, sun exposure, illnesses that cause fevers, stress, immune system imbalances, and other unknown causes. However, not all patients experience a second outbreak.

Symptoms: Genital herpes typically causes painful, watery blisters to develop on the skin, mucous membranes (e.g., the mouth or lips), or genitals. The location of these blisters depends on where contact was made during transmission. Lesions heal with a crust-forming scab, the hallmark of herpes. Many individuals with recurrent disease develop pain in the area of the infection even before any blisters or ulcers can be seen. This pain is due to irritation and inflammation of the nerves leading to the infected area of skin. These are signs that an outbreak is about to start. An individual is particularly contagious during this period even though the skin still appears normal.

Diagnosis: A viral culture uses specimens taken from the blister, fluid in the blister, or sometimes spinal fluid. The samples are sent to a laboratory where they are analyzed. It takes between one and 14 days to detect the virus in the preparation made from the specimen. This test is useful, but it is sometimes difficult to detect the virus in the sample.

An immunofluorescence assay is a diagnostic technique used to identify antibodies to herpes simplex type 2. These antibodies are proteins that help the body fight against the infection. If the specific antibodies are present, a positive diagnosis is made. This test is less expensive, more accurate, and faster than a viral culture. However, it may take up to 30 days for antibodies to build up to detectable levels. Therefore, if herpes is highly suspected and results are negative soon after possible exposure to the virus, a repeat test may be recommended.

A polymerase chain reaction test may also be performed to determine whether the virus itself is present in the patient's blood. A sample of the patient's blood is taken and sent to a laboratory. If the virus's genetic makeup (DNA) is present, a positive diagnosis is made. The virus can even be detected during the latent stages of the infection.

Treatment: Although there is no cure for genital herpes, medications are available to minimize the number of outbreaks, reduce the likelihood of viral shedding, and decrease the likelihood of transmission.

There are three antiviral medications that the U.S. Food and Drug Administration (FDA) has approved for the treatment of genital herpes. Approved antiviral drugs include acyclovir (Zovirax), valacyclovir (Valtrex), and famciclovir (Famvir). Antiviral medication is commonly prescribed for patients having a first episode of genital herpes, but it can be used for recurrent episodes as well. There are two kinds of treatment regimens: episodic therapy and suppressive therapy.

With episodic therapy, the patient begins taking the medication at the first sign of an outbreak. The medication is then taken for several days to hasten the recovery or healing or to prevent a full outbreak from fully occurring. All three of the approved medications help shorten the amount of time that a person may experience symptoms of herpes. However, results may vary from person to person.

Suppressive therapy is used in individuals with recurrent genital herpes who want to prevent outbreaks. Patients who have six or more outbreaks per year may take antiviral medications on a regular basis, before symptoms appear. For these individuals, studies have reported that suppressive therapy may reduce the number of outbreaks by at least 75% while the medication is being taken. Suppressive therapy may completely prevent outbreaks in some patients. Suppressive therapy may need to be taken for the rest of the patient's life. Side effects of antiviral medicines include stomach upset, loss of appetite, nausea, vomiting, diarrhea, headache, dizziness, and/or weakness.

Gonorrhea

Overview: Gonorrhea, sometimes called the clap, is a curable bacterial infection that affects the sex organs. If left untreated, gonorrhea may lead to infertility.

Gonorrhea is caused by a bacterium called *Neisseria gonorrhoeae*. Gonorrhea is transmitted through contact with the penis, vagina, mouth, or anus. Ejaculation does not have to occur for gonorrhea to be transmitted or acquired.

Pregnant females with untreated gonorrhea may pass the infection onto their babies during vaginal childbirth (not cesarean section).

The bacterium can only live outside of the body for a few seconds. Therefore, the infection cannot be transmitted through toilet seats or other objects such as towels or clothing.

Symptoms: Most patients develop symptoms of gonorrhea one to 10 days after the bacteria enter the body. Some patients may be infected for months before symptoms develop. More than 50% of females with gonorrhea do not experience any symptoms.

Common symptoms of gonorrhea include thick or bloody discharge from the penis or vagina, pain or burning sensation during urination, frequent urination, and pain during sexual intercourse.

Anorectal gonorrhea may develop in males or females after anal intercourse with an infected person. In some cases, the infection may spread from the genitals to the anus. Anorectal gonorrhea may cause some discomfort in and discharge from the anal area, but many patients do not experience any symptoms.

Oral sex can cause pharyngeal gonorrhea. Symptoms of pharyngeal gonorrhea commonly include pain when swallowing and redness of the throat and tonsils.

If a patient touches an eye after touching bodily fluids that contain the bacteria, it may cause pinkeye (conjunctivitis). Symptoms may include reddening and inflammation of the eye(s).

Newborns with gonorrhea may develop permanent blindness and infection of the joints and blood.

Complications: In females, untreated gonorrhea may lead to PID. This is an infection of the fallopian tubes, uterus, and cervix. If left untreated, PID may cause permanent damage to the reproductive tract, which may lead to infertility. It may also lead to long-term pelvic pain.

Males with untreated gonorrhea may develop a condition called epididymitis. This condition is characterized by inflammation of the tubes near the testicles that carry semen. Symptoms may include fever, scrotal pain, and swelling.

In rare cases, *Neisseria gonorrhoeae* may enter the bloodstream and infect other parts of the body, such as the skin, joints, or internal organs. Symptoms may include fever, swelling, joint pain and stiffness, rash, and skin sores.

Diagnosis: Patients should talk to their healthcare providers to determine how often they should be tested for gonorrhea. Patients who have symptoms of gonorrhea or suspect they may have been exposed to gonorrhea should be tested.

The standard diagnostic test for gonorrhea is a culture swab. For females, the healthcare provider may swab the discharge from the cervix. For males, the healthcare provider inserts a thin swab into the tip of the penis to retrieve a sample of fluid from the urethra. In some cases, the healthcare provider may swab the anus. The sample is then rubbed on a Petri dish. If the patient has gonorrhea, *Neisseria gonorrhoeae* will grow on the Petri dish. A urine analysis may also be performed. A sample of the patient's urine is analyzed in a laboratory for the presence of the disease-causing bacteria.

Treatment: Gonorrhea is curable. Patients typically take antibiotics, such as ciprofloxacin (Cipro, Cipro XR), ofloxacin (Floxin), and levofloxacin (Levaquin).

Babies with gonorrhea also receive antibiotics. In addition, medication, such as silver nitrate, is usually applied to the baby's eyes immediately after birth. This has been shown to help prevent the infection from spreading into the eyes.

Even if symptoms go away, medications should not be stopped early because the bacteria may still be present in the body. If the medication is stopped too early, the remaining bacteria in the body may mutate and become resistant to treatment. Once the bacteria are resistant to a medication, the antibiotic is no longer effective.

HIV/AIDS

Overview: HIV is a virus that progresses to AIDS. HIV primarily attacks the immune defense system, making the patient extremely vulnerable to opportunistic infections. Opportunistic infections are illnesses that occur in individuals who have weakened immune systems.

HIV primarily infects and destroys immune cells called CD4 T-cells. Healthy individuals have a CD4 cell count between 600 and 1,200 cells per microliter of blood. HIV patients who are not receiving treatment have less than 600 CD4 cells per microliter of blood. AIDS patients who have CD4 cell counts that are lower than 200 have the greatest risk of developing opportunistic infections that may be fatal.

HIV is transmitted from person to person via bodily fluids, including blood, semen, vaginal secretions, and breast milk. Therefore, it can be transmitted through sexual contact with an infected person, by sharing needles/syringes with someone who is infected, through breastfeeding, during vaginal birth or, less commonly (and rare in countries where blood is screened for HIV antibodies), through transfusions with infected blood.

Symptoms: Many patients experience no symptoms when they first become infected with HIV. After one or two months, an estimated 80-90% of HIV patients develop flulike symptoms, including headache, fever, fatigue, and enlarged lymph nodes. These symptoms usually disappear after one week to one month and are often mistaken for another viral infection, such as the flu. Despite having minimal or no symptoms during this stage, individuals are very infectious because the virus is present in large quantities in bodily fluids.

After the initial infection with HIV, the next stage is called clinical latency. Although patients experience few or no symptoms during the clinical latency stage, the infection may still be passed to others. Once infected with HIV, the clinical latency stage may last 10 or more years in adults or up to two years in children who are born with HIV infection. The length of this asymptomatic period varies in individuals. Some people may start to experience more serious symptoms within a few months, while others may be symptom free for several years. The virus can also hide inside infected cells and lay dormant. Patients can still transmit the virus to others when the virus is dormant.

As the immune system continues to weaken, many symptoms appear, including inflamed lymph nodes (swollen glands) that may be enlarged for longer than three months. Other symptoms often experienced months to years before the onset of AIDS include fatigue, weight loss, frequent fevers and sweats, persistent or frequent yeast infections (oral or vaginal), persistent skin rashes, flaky skin, PID in women that does not respond well to treatment, and short-term memory loss.

In addition, some individuals develop a painful nerve disease called shingles or frequent and severe herpes infections that cause sores to develop on the mouth, genitals, or anus. Infected children may be sick often, grow or gain weight slowly, or take longer to develop important mental and motor skills.

Although treatment can slow the progression of HIV, nearly all patients eventually develop AIDS. Once the patient's CD4 T-cell count is less than 200 cells per microliter of blood, their condition has progressed to AIDS, the final stage of the disease. Some patients are diagnosed with AIDS after they develop an AIDS-defining illness, such as *Pneumocystis jiroveci* pneumonia (formerly called *Pneumocystis carinii*). The first symptoms of AIDS often include moderate and unexplained weight loss, recurring respiratory tract infections, and oral ulcerations.

Patients with AIDS have the greatest risk of developing opportunistic infections and tumors. Opportunistic infections and tumors may include tuberculosis, thrush, herpes viruses, shingles, Epstein-Barr virus, pneumonia, and a type of cancer called Kaposi's sarcoma. In the last stages of AIDS, it is common for individuals to develop respiratory infections, including cytomegalovirus or *Mycobacterium avium* complex infections.

Diagnosis: HIV is diagnosed after HIV antibodies or HIV itself is detected in the patient's body. As soon as the virus enters the body, the immune system produces antibodies, which are proteins that detect and bind to HIV. The presence of these antibodies, which may take months to build up to detectable levels in the blood, oral fluid, and urine, can be used to determine whether HIV is in the body.

It may take some time for the immune system to produce enough antibodies for the antibody test to detect them. This time period, known as the window period, varies among patients. Most people will develop detectable antibodies two to eight weeks after exposure, with the average being 25 days. However, some individuals might take longer to develop detectable antibodies. Ninety-seven percent of patients develop antibodies within the first three months following the time of their infection. In very rare cases, it can take up to six months to develop antibodies to HIV. Therefore, if a patient tests negative for HIV in the first three months after possible exposure, repeat testing should be considered longer than three months after the exposure. In the United States, the test results must remain confidential. Individuals who are younger than 18 years old can consent to or refuse to be tested for HIV without the involvement of their legal guardians. Test results may not be released to the patient's legal guardian(s) without his/her consent.

Treatment: Currently, there is no cure for HIV/AIDS. Patients may receive a combination of anti-HIV drugs called antiretrovirals. These drugs interfere with the virus's ability to multiply, which subsequently boosts the immune system. HIV patients typically receive a combination of antiretroviral drugs, called highly active antiretroviral therapy (HAART), because a single patient may have several different strains (types) of the virus circulating in the blood. The combination of drugs also helps prevent mutations from occurring. The different strains of the virus may respond differently to specific types of drugs. HAART is a combination of at least three drugs from at least two different classes. There are four major classes of antiretrovirals: fusion inhibitors, protease inhibitors, nucleoside reverse transcriptase inhibitors, and nonnucleoside reverse transcriptase inhibitors. Each drug class disrupts different stages of HIV's life cycle.

Although HAART may help patients live longer lives, these drugs do not reduce the risk of transmitting the disease to someone else.

Many new HIV drugs are under investigation. The FDA approved a CCR5 receptor antagonist called maraviroc (Celsentri) and an integrase inhibitor called raltegravir (Isentress) in late 2007.

HUMAN PAPILLOMA VIRUS (HPV)

Overview: HPV is a viral infection that sometimes causes genital warts (also called venereal warts). There are more than 100 different types of HPV, but only a few cause genital warts. HPV is highly contagious. The infection may be transmitted through direct contact with the virus during oral, anal, or vaginal sex. It may also be transmitted after touching objects (e.g., towels, bed linens, or clothing) that have come into contact with an infected person.

There is currently no cure for HPV. Although treatment can help manage symptoms, females with HPV have a much greater risk of developing cervical cancer than females who are not infected with HPV. It has also been associated with other types of genital cancers, including cancer of the penis, anus, vulva, and vagina.

In June 2006, the FDA approved the first HPV vaccine, called Gardasil. The vaccine is expected to prevent most cases of cervical cancer due to HPV types included in the vaccine. However, patients will not be protected if they have been infected with the HPV type(s) prior to vaccination, and the drug does not protect against less-common types of HPV.

Symptoms: Most patients develop symptoms within three months of exposure to HPV. However, some patients may not develop symptoms for several years, and others may not experience any symptoms at all.

Common symptoms include small swellings in the genital area, multiple warts that form cauliflower-shaped clusters, itching or discomfort in the genital area, and bleeding during intercourse. Warts may spread to other areas of the body. Symptoms may worsen during pregnancy.

Complications: HPV has been shown to cause cervical cancer in females. In addition, certain types of HPV have also been associated with cancer of the anus, vagina, vulva, and penis. Regular pelvic exams and Pap tests are recommended to diagnose and treat infections quickly.

Genital warts may also lead to complications during pregnancy. In some patients, the warts may enlarge, making it difficult to urinate. Also, warts on the vaginal wall may reduce flexibility of the vaginal tissues during childbirth. In rare cases, a baby born to a mother with genital warts may develop warts in the throat. In such cases, surgery may be required to remove the warts and prevent airway obstruction.

Diagnosis: An acetic acid solution may be applied to the patient's genitals. This solution helps the healthcare provider detect warts because it turns warts a white color. Then, a specialized microscope, called a colposcope, is used to view the warts. If they are characteristic of HPV, a positive diagnosis is made. It is especially important for women to undergo routine pelvic exams and Pap tests because HPV increases a female's risk of developing cervical cancer. Patients diagnosed with HPV may need to have a Pap test every three to six months. Patients should talk to their healthcare providers to determine how often they should be screened.

Treatment: There is currently no cure for HPV. However, many treatments are available to manage symptoms. Even if genital warts are no longer present, the virus is never eliminated from the body. This means warts may come back in the future.

Patients should not use over-the-counter wart removers for genital warts. These products are not designed for genital warts and they may cause serious side effects. Patients should consult their healthcare providers to determine the safest and most effective way to remove warts.

Many creams and ointments, such as imiquimod (Aldara) and podofilox (Condylox), may be applied directly to the skin to remove warts. Healthcare providers may also apply a chemical called trichloroacetic acid to the skin to burn off warts. These medications may damage condoms, making them less effective.

Many surgical procedures, including cryotherapy, electrocautery, surgical incision, and laser removal, are available to remove warts. During cryotherapy, a healthcare provider applies liquid nitrogen to freeze off the wart. During electrocautery, an electrical current is used to burn off warts. Surgical incisions, which involve using a scalpel and other surgical instruments to remove the wart, may also be used. During laser treatments, the warts are removed with an intense beam of light. These procedures are usually only performed for severe warts that do not respond to other types of treatment.

Patients should not have sex while they are receiving treatment. Sexual partners of patients who have been diagnosed with HPV should be tested and treated for STDs.

PELVIC INFLAMMATORY DISEASE (PID)

Overview: PID is an infection of the female reproductive organs that causes pain and swelling. If left untreated, PID may cause scarring and permanently damage the reproductive organs. Without treatment, some patients may become infertile or experience complications during pregnancy. PID usually develops when a sexually transmitted bacteria enters the uterus and reproduces in the upper genital tract. The most common bacteria that causes PID also cause the STDs gonorrhea and chlamydia.

Symptoms: Common symptoms of PID include pain in the lower abdomen and pelvis, irregular menstrual bleeding, foul-smelling vaginal discharge, lower back pain, fever, fatigue, diarrhea, vomiting, pain during intercourse, and difficulty or pain during urination. Up to 50% of females with PID develop chronic pelvic pain that may last for months or years.

PID may cause scarring in the fallopian tubes and other organs that may cause pain during exercise, ovulation, and sexual intercourse.

Diagnosis: PID is diagnosed after a pelvic examination, cervical cultures, and/or analysis of the vaginal discharge. The reproductive organs, including the uterus, will appear inflamed during a pelvic exam. Cervical cultures and/or analyses of vaginal discharge are performed to detect the presence of bacteria known to cause PID. If bacteria are present, a positive diagnosis is made.

Treatment: Antibiotics are the standard treatment for PID. These medications, which are usually taken by mouth, kill the disease-causing microorganism. Severe infections that have spread to the kidneys may require hospitalization and intravenous antibiotics. Commonly prescribed antibiotics include amoxicillin (Amoxil, Trimox), nitrofurantoin (Furadantin, Macrodantin), trimethoprim (Proloprim), and trimethoprim/sulfamethoxazole (Bactrim, Septra). Symptoms usually start to improve after a few days of treatment.

Patients should take medications exactly as prescribed. Even if symptoms appear to go away, patients should take all of their medication because there may still be bacteria in the body. Stopping medication early may allow the infection to return. Also, stopping medication early may lead to antibiotic resistance. The few remaining bacteria in the body that survive most of the antibiotic therapy are the most difficult to kill. If the bacteria become resistant to treatment, the medications will no longer be effective if taken in the future.

Treating STDs, such as gonorrhea, promptly reduces the risk of developing PID.

Sexual partners of patients who have been diagnosed with PID should be tested and treated for STDs.

SYPHILIS

Overview: Syphilis is a bacterial infection that initially causes skin sores and rashes to form on the genitals, skin, and mucous membranes. Although this infection is curable, it can be fatal if it is not treated quickly. If left untreated, syphilis may cause permanent damage to other organs, such as the brain and heart. Syphilis is caused by a bacterium called *Treponema pallidum*. There are four different stages of syphilis: primary, secondary, latent, and tertiary. The disease is contagious during the primary and secondary stages and sometimes the latent period. Most cases of syphilis are transmitted during oral, anal, or vaginal sex. A patient may also acquire the infection if his/her blood comes into contact with an infected patient's blood. It may also be transmitted through direct contact with an infected person's skin sore. An infected pregnant woman may also transmit the infection to her fetus during pregnancy. This is because the mother's infected blood passes through the placenta and to the baby. *Treponema pallidum* is not able to survive outside of the body. Therefore, the disease cannot be transmitted by sharing clothing, toilet seats, or other objects with an infected person.

Symptoms: Symptoms of syphilis vary with each stage. Initial symptoms during the primary stage typically develop 10 days to three months after exposure. Symptoms commonly include enlarged lymph nodes near the groin and a small painless chancre sore on the part of the body where the bacterium was transmitted. Chancre sores are most common on the tongue, lips, genitals, or rectum. Some patients may develop several sores. If patients do not receive treatment, the symptoms will go away on their own within three to six weeks. However, this does not mean that the infection is gone. In fact, it means that the infection is progressing to the secondary stage.

Symptoms of secondary syphilis develop two to 10 weeks after the first chancre sore appears. Symptoms may include a skin rash that causes small reddish-brown sores, fever, fatigue, general feeling of discomfort, soreness, and aching. If the patient does not receive treatment during this stage, symptoms may go away within a few weeks or repeatedly go away and come back for as long as one year. Even if symptoms are not present, the infection will continue to worsen without treatment.

Some patients experience a period called latent syphilis before tertiary symptoms develop. During the clinical latency stage, no symptoms are present. This stage may last one to two years.

The tertiary stage may develop immediately after the secondary stage or one to two years after the latent stage. This is the final and most severe stage of the infection. During the tertiary stage, syphilis may cause permanent organ damage and death. It often causes brain (neurological) problems, which may include stroke, infection and inflammation of the membranes that surround the brain and spinal cord (meningitis), numbness, poor muscle coordination, deafness, visual problems or blindness, changes in personality, and dementia. Syphilis may also affect the heart, causing bulging (aneurysm) and inflammation of blood vessels, including the aorta, which is the body's main artery. It may also cause

S

valvular heart disease, such as aortic valve stenosis (when the valve becomes narrowed). All of these symptoms are potentially life threatening.

Babies born with syphilis may develop symptoms that are apparent at birth or several weeks after birth. Syphilis progresses much quicker and is more likely to cause complications in infants than adults. If the baby does not receive prompt treatment, serious and life-threatening complications may develop. Symptoms may include bone abnormalities, depressed nose bridge (saddle nose), vision and hearing problems (that may lead to deafness or blindness), swollen joints, screwdriver-shaped teeth (Hutchinson's teeth), and scarring where chancre sores developed.

Complications: In general, patients with syphilis have an increased risk of contracting HIV. This is because a syphilis chancre sore provides an easy way for HIV to enter the body.

Diagnosis: In order to prevent life-threatening complications of syphilis, patients should be tested if they have symptoms of syphilis or suspect that they were exposed to syphilis. Doctors recommend annual STD screenings for patients who have increased risks of developing STDs. This includes patients who have multiple sexual partners, engage in unprotected sex, or who have sexual partners who have or previously had an STD. Routine testing is especially important for detecting syphilis because symptoms may come and go.

If the patient has sores that are characteristic of syphilis, a healthcare provider may scrape a small sample of cells from affected skin. The cells are then analyzed under a microscope for the presence of *Treponema pallidum*. If the bacteria are present, a positive diagnosis is made. If patients do not have sores, a blood test may be used to diagnose syphilis. A sample of blood is taken from the patient and analyzed for antibodies to the bacterium that causes syphilis. These antibodies are proteins that are specialized to detect and help destroy the bacterium. If the antibodies are present, a positive diagnosis is made.

If it is suspected that the infection has spread to the brain, a healthcare provider may recommend a test called a lumbar puncture. During the procedure, a long, thin needle is inserted into the lower back. A small sample of fluid from the spine (cerebrospinal fluid) is removed and analyzed under a microscope for the disease-causing bacteria.

Treatment: If treated early, patients with syphilis can expect a full recovery. Patients receive one to three injections of an antibiotic called penicillin. This medication kills the bacterium and cures syphilis. Even if a pregnant mother receives treatment for syphilis, the newborn should also receive antibiotics as a precautionary measure. Patients should avoid sexual contact with their partners during treatment in order to prevent transmitting the infection.

During the first day of antibiotic treatment, many patients experience the Jarisch-Herxheimer reaction. Researchers believe that this reaction occurs because so many bacteria are dying at once. Symptoms, which usually only last one day, may include fever, nausea, aching pain, and headache.

Sexual partners of patients who have been diagnosed with syphilis should be tested and treated for STDs.

TRICHOMONIASIS

Overview: Trichomoniasis is a sexually transmitted infection that usually causes pain, inflammation, and irritation in the vagina, penis, and urethral tissues. Although trichomoniasis may affect males or females, symptoms are more common among females. Trichomoniasis is caused by *Trichomonas vaginalis,* a microscopic parasite called a protozoan.

Symptoms: Females typically develop foul-smelling vaginal discharge that may appear foamy and yellow or green in color. Vaginal itching and pain during urination may also occur. Males typically experience penile discharge, pain during urination, and pain and swelling of the scrotum (caused by epididymis).

Diagnosis: For females, the healthcare provider may swab the discharge from the cervix. For males, the healthcare provider inserts a thin swab into the tip of the penis to retrieve a sample of fluid from the urethra. The sample is then analyzed under a microscope. If the parasite is present, a positive diagnosis is made.

Treatment: Patients take the antibiotic metronidazole (Flagyl) by mouth to kill the parasite and cure the infection. This drug is not safe during pregnancy. Pregnant females who are infected typically apply an antibiotic cream called clotrimazole (Gyne-Lotrimin, Mycelex-7) to the genitals. Patients should abstain from sex while they are receiving treatment. Sexual partners of patients who have been diagnosed with trichomoniasis should be tested and treated for STDs.

INTEGRATIVE THERAPIES

Unclear or Conflicting Scientific Evidence

Hydrotherapy: Hydrotherapy is broadly defined as the external application of water in any form or temperature (hot, cold, steam, liquid, or ice) for healing purposes. It may include immersion in a bath or body of water (such as the ocean or a pool), use of water jets, douches, application of wet towels to the skin, or water birth. Studies have evaluated hydrotherapy as a possible treatment for PID. However, further research is needed before a firm conclusion can be made.

Avoid sudden or prolonged exposure to extreme temperatures in baths, wraps, or saunas, especially with heart disease, lung disease, or if pregnant. Avoid with implanted medical devices, such as pacemakers, defibrillators, or liver infusion pumps. Vigorous use of water jets should be avoided with fractures, known blood clots, bleeding disorders, severe osteoporosis, open wounds, or pregnancy. Use cautiously with Raynaud's disease, chilblains, acrocyanosis, erythrocyanosis, or impaired temperature sensitivity, such as neuropathy. Use cautiously if pregnant or breastfeeding. Hydrotherapy should not delay the time to diagnosis or treatment with more proven techniques or therapies, and it should not be used as the sole approach to illnesses. Patients with known illnesses should consult their physicians before starting hydrotherapy.

Traditional or Theoretical Uses Lacking Sufficient Evidence

Barberry: Barberry has been used in Indian folk medicine for centuries, and the Chinese have used berberine, a constituent of barberry, since ancient times. Barberry has been suggested as a possible treatment for STDs, including chlamydia. However, human studies are lacking.

Because of the lack of available evidence investigating barberry, no firm recommendations can be made regarding barberry's safety. Avoid if allergic or hypersensitive to barberry, any of its constituents (including berberine), or any member of the Berberidaceae family. Use cautiously with heart disease, gastrointestinal disorders, or kidney disease. Use cautiously in children due to a lack of sufficient available evidence. Barberry has exhibited uterine stimulant properties, and berberine has been shown to have antifertility activity. Avoid if pregnant or breastfeeding.

Boswellia: Historically, boswellia has been used to treat STDs, including genital warts and syphilis. However, further research in humans is needed to determine if it is a safe and effective treatment.

Avoid if allergic to boswellia. Avoid with a history of stomach ulcers or gastroesophageal reflux disease. Avoid if pregnant or breastfeeding.

Kava: Kava is a member of the pepper family and is native to many Pacific Ocean islands.

Traditionally, kava has been used to treat syphilis. However, human studies have not tested the safety and effectiveness of this treatment. Further research is warranted.

Avoid if allergic to kava or kava pyrones. Avoid with a history of liver disease, Parkinson's disease, heart disease, lung disease, eye disease, depression, bipolar disease, or blood cell disorders. Avoid while driving or operating heavy machinery because kava may cause drowsiness. Avoid if pregnant or breastfeeding.

Neem: Neem is thought to have originated in Assam (a state in northeast India) and Myanmar. Neem has been used to treat infections, skin conditions, and reduce inflammation. Although neem has been traditionally used to treat STDs, studies have not been performed to determine if it is effective.

Avoid if allergic or hypersensitive to neem (*Azadirachta indica*) or members of the Meliaceae family. Use cautiously with liver disease. Avoid in children and infants. Avoid if pregnant or breastfeeding.

Reiki: Reiki is a Buddhist practice that is about 2,500 years old. Treatments involve the systematic placing of hands in varying positions either directly on a clothed patient or held above the skin. Sessions may last 30-90 minutes. Reiki has been suggested as a possible treatment for venereal diseases, but human evidence is currently lacking. Further research is warranted in this area.

Reiki is not recommended as the sole treatment approach for potentially serious medical conditions, and it should not delay the time it takes to consult with a healthcare professional or receive established therapies. Use cautiously with psychiatric illnesses.

PREVENTION

Routine Testing: According to the CDC guidelines, patients who are either at risk for acquiring HIV or are between the ages of 13-64 should be tested for HIV annually. Patients should talk to their doctors to determine how often they should be tested for other STDs.

If a patient has symptoms of an STD or suspects he/she was exposed to an STD, the patient should be tested.

Patients who test positive for STDs should tell their partners. Their partners should be tested and treated to prevent reinfection.

Females should undergo annual Pap smears.

Safe Sex: Avoid unprotected sexual contact, including vaginal, anal, and oral sex, with an infected person or with someone who has not been tested for STDs.

Wear gloves when in contact with blood or other body fluids that could possibly contain blood, such as urine, feces, or vomit.

Patients should limit the number of sexual partners they have. Having multiple sexual partners increases a patient's risk of developing STDs.

Know your partner and his/her STD status and health.

Avoid Risky Behavior: Do not share needles or syringes.

Avoid excessive use of alcohol or other drugs, which can cloud judgment and lead to unsafe sexual practices.

Practices that increase the likelihood of blood contact, such as the sharing of razors, toothbrushes, and nail clippers, should be avoided.

Safety Precautions: Cuts, scrapes, sores, or breaks on the exposed skin of both the caregiver and patient should be covered with bandages.

Wash any part of the body that comes into contact with blood or other body fluids. Surfaces that have been tainted with blood should be disinfected with antibacterial soap.

Females should not douche because it decreases the number of good bacteria in the vagina. As a result, douching may increase the risk of infection.

Needles and other sharp instruments should be used only when medically necessary and handled appropriately.

In 1985, the CDC issued a list of routine precautions for all personal service workers, such as hairdressers, barbers, cosmetologists, and massage therapists. Instruments that penetrate the skin, such as tattoo and acupuncture needles or ear-piercing guns, should either be used once and disposed of or thoroughly sterilized. Instruments that are not meant to penetrate the skin but may come in contact with blood (such as razors) should not be shared unless thoroughly sterilized.

Preventing Transmission During Pregnancy: Antiviral therapy during pregnancy can significantly lower the chance that the HIV will be passed to the infant before, during, or after birth. The treatment is most effective if it is started as early as possible during pregnancy. However, there are still health benefits if treatment is begun during labor or shortly after the baby is born. This treatment has been shown to be safe and effective for the mother and her baby.

Delivering the baby by cesarean section has been shown to reduce the risk of transmission of HIV to the newborn. However, this is not the standard preventative care for HIV-infected pregnant women. It should only be considered in certain clinical circumstances, such as for patients who have a very high viral overload or for patients who do not take their medications exactly as prescribed.

Mothers with STDs should not breastfeed their newborn(s) because infections, such as HIV, may be transmitted to their babies. In addition, many medications used to treat STDs may be excreted in the breast milk and cause harm to the baby.

HPV: In June 2006, the FDA approved the first HPV vaccine, called Gardasil. The drug, developed by Merck & Co. Inc., is a recombinant vaccine. This means that the vaccine does not contain the live virus, so there is no chance that patients who receive the vaccine can become infected with HPV.

The vaccine is expected to prevent most cases of cervical cancer due to HPV types included in the vaccine. However, patients will not be protected if they have been infected with the HPV type(s) prior to vaccination, and the drug does not protect against less-common types of HPV.

The vaccine is given as three injections over the course of six months. The National Advisory Committee on Immunization Practices recommends routine vaccination for females who are 11 and 12 years old, as well as females ages 13-26 if they have not already received the vaccine. According to researchers, the vaccine is most effective if it is given to females before they are sexually active.

Possible side effects may include pain or swelling at the injection site, mild fever, nausea, vomiting, dizziness, stuffy nose, sore throat, cough, or muscle pain.

Skin Rash

BACKGROUND

Rash is a general term that describes a change in color and texture in the skin. A rash generally causes temporary red patches or bumps in the skin and may be itchy and/or tender. The affected skin is often swollen.

A rash is a symptom of an underlying medical condition. There are hundreds of conditions that are known to cause rashes. Among the most common causes are allergies, autoimmune disorders (like lupus), infections, irritants (like sun exposure), poisonous plants (like poison ivy), and skin disorders (like eczema).

There are many forms of rashes, which differ depending on the cause. Rashes vary in appearance, location, severity, and duration. Some rashes may contain blisters, flat or raised bumps, pimples, or dry or flaky skin. The amount of skin affected may be limited to an isolated area or it may affect multiple areas of the body.

While the duration of a skin rash varies depending on the cause, most rashes resolve either on their own or with treatment within one to 14 days. Some rashes, including those caused by conditions like lupus and rosacea, are long term but they can be managed with medications. Once the underlying cause is treated, symptoms will begin to subside.

CAUSES

There are hundreds of conditions that have been shown to causes rashes. Some of the most common causes include allergies, autoimmune disorders, infections, irritants, poisonous plants, and skin disorders.

Allergies: An allergic reaction, which occurs when the body's immune system overreacts to a harmless substance (like pollen or dust mites), may cause a skin rash. Common triggers of allergic reactions include insect stings (bees, wasps, etc.), medications (like antibiotics and seizure medications), foods (especially peanuts, seafood, and eggs), and latex (like rubber gloves and condoms).

Autoimmune Disorders: Autoimmune disorders, which occur when the immune system mistakenly identifies the body's own cells as foreign invaders (like bacteria), may also cause skin rashes. Rashes are a common feature of autoimmune disorders such as rheumatoid arthritis and lupus.

Infections: Many infections caused by bacteria, fungi, or viruses may cause skin rashes. Infections such as chickenpox, Lyme disease (bacterial infection), ringworm (parasitic infection), shingles (chickenpox in adults), measles, fifth disease (flulike illness that causes reddening of the cheeks), and herpes (viral infection) are among the most common causes of rashes.

Irritants: Rashes may develop if the skin becomes irritated. For instance, some patients develop rashes after exposure to heat or sun. Some babies develop diaper rash if the diaper rubs against the skin or is not changed frequently enough.

Poisonous Plants: Exposure to poison ivy, poison oak, and poison sumac plants may lead to an itchy skin rash. These plants produce oil called urushiol, which may trigger an allergic reaction. Patients who are allergic to these plants may experience a rash that consists of swollen, itchy, red bumps and blisters that appear wherever the oil has touched the skin.

Skin Disorders: Other potential causes include skin disorders like acne (pimples), psoriasis, rosacea, and atopic dermatitis (eczema).

SYMPTOMS

General: While the duration of a skin rash varies depending on the cause, most rashes resolve either on their own or with treatment within one to 14 days. Some rashes, including those caused by conditions like lupus and rosacea, are long term but they can be managed with medications. There are many different forms of rashes that vary in their appearance, location, severity, and duration. The skin may be red and/or itchy. If the skin itches, it is called pruritus. If a butterfly-shaped, red rash develops on the cheek and nose, it is called a malar rash.

Dermatologists classify rashes based on their physical appearance. The main types of rashes include discoid rashes, macular rash, maculopapular rash, papular rash, papulosquamous rash, and vesicular rash.

Discoid Rash: A discoid rash is characterized by red and scaly patches of skin on the face and scalp that can lead to scarring and temporary hair loss.

Macular Rash: When the skin has areas of flat, red spots, it is called a macular rash.

Maculopapular Rash: A maculopapular rash occurs when a patient has areas of flat, red spots combined with areas of small, raised, solid bumps on the skin.

Papular Rash: A papular rash causes small, raised, solid bumps on the skin.

Papulosquamous Rash: A papulosquamous rash occurs when the patient has a combination of pimples and dry, flaky skin.

Vesicular Rash: A vesicular rash occurs when a patient has small, raised, fluid-filled blisters.

Other Symptoms: A rash is usually just one symptom of an underlying medical condition. Some of the most common symptoms associated with rashes include fever and enlarged lymph nodes.

COMPLICATIONS

Anaphylaxis: A skin rash may be a symptom of a severe and potentially life-threatening reaction called anaphylaxis. The most serious symptoms of anaphylaxis include low blood pressure, breathing difficulties, shock, and loss of consciousness, all of which can be fatal. Patients should seek immediate medical treatment if these symptoms develop.

Psychological Symptoms: Some patients who have long-term skin conditions like lupus, chronic acne, or rosacea may suffer from low self-esteem.

Secondary Infections: Secondary infections may develop if the patient's rash has open sores or blisters. Patients should not scratch irritated skin because it may cause the skin to break. If bacteria or viruses enter the body through the open skin, an infection may develop. Antibiotics are used to treat bacterial infection, antifungals are used to treat fungal infections, and antivirals are used to treat viral infections. Specific treatment and duration depend on the type and severity of infection and overall health of the patient.

Stevens-Johnson Syndrome: A severe skin rash called Stevens-Johnson syndrome (SJS) may develop as an allergic reaction to medication. SJS is potentially life threatening because in severe cases the lesions can cause significant scarring of the involved organs, which often leads to loss of function of the organ systems. SJS typically starts with a nonspecific upper respiratory tract infection. The patient may experience flulike symptoms, including fever, sore throat, chills, headache, and general feeling of discomfort for one to 14 days. Some individuals will also experience diarrhea and vomiting. As the disease progresses, skin lesions quickly develop. Patients may experience extensive shedding of the skin. Skin lesions may occur anywhere, but they are most common on the palms, soles of the feet, back of the hands, and extremities. Mucosal involvement may include reddening of the skin, edema (fluid in body tissues), blistering, open sores on the skin, and dead skin.

DIAGNOSIS

General: A rash is easily identified during a physical examination. However, because it is a symptom of an underlying medical condition, the cause must be identified in order to treat it. During a physical examination, a healthcare provider will take a careful medical history to determine the underlying cause. Medical tests may be necessary.

Medical History: The healthcare provider will ask whether the patient has a history of allergies, infections, or skin diseases or has been exposed to chemicals or irritants. A healthcare provider will also ask about the patient's daily activities. For instance, individuals who spend time in wooded areas have an increased risk of developing rashes from exposure to poisonous plants.

Physical Examination: The healthcare provider will ask when the rash first developed. It is important to know if it started after the patient ate a new food, tried a new skin product, or took a new drug, herb, or supplement.

The location and pattern of the rash are also important. For instance, a heat rash will only be present on areas of the skin that were exposed to the sun. Certain patterns are associated with specific diseases. For instance, patients who have lupus often develop a butterfly-shaped rash on their cheeks and nose. Reactions to poisonous plants often have a streaky pattern where the plant brushed against the skin.

Depending on the underlying cause, certain rashes typically last longer than others. For instance, a rash caused by a viral infection called roseola usually only lasts a couple of days, whereas fifth disease (flulike illness) may cause a rash for a week. Patients with lupus will have symptoms that persist until they receive treatment.

The healthcare provider will also take into account other symptoms (if any) that accompany the rash. For instance, if patients also have a fever and enlarged lymph nodes, an infection may be suspected.

Allergen-Specific Immunoglobulin E (IgE) Test: An IgE test, commonly referred to as radioallergosorbent test, may also be used to determine whether the patient is allergic to particular substances. This test is less accurate than a skin test. It is usually performed in patients who have coexisting severe skin diseases (like eczema or psoriasis) that make it difficult to interpret a skin test. During the procedure, a sample of the patient's blood is sent to a laboratory for testing. The allergen is combined with the blood to determine whether the patient has IgE antibodies to the allergen. Antibodies are substances that identify and bind to foreign invaders in the body. If the patient has IgE antibodies, an allergy is diagnosed.

Blood Test: A blood tests may be performed to determine whether the patient has a bacterial or viral infection. A blood test may also be performed if an autoimmune disorder (like lupus) is suspected. A sample of the patient's blood is analyzed for the presence of autoantibodies. These autoantibodies in the blood mistakenly destroy the patient's own body cells if they have the disorder.

Potassium and Hydroxide (KOH) Preparation: A KOH preparation test is used to determine whether a fungal infection is causing the rash. During this test, a healthcare provider will gently scrape the skin with a blunt edge (like the edge of a microscope slide). The sample of scraped skin is then combined with KOH. This solution allows the healthcare provider to see the fungus (if it is present) under a microscope. This procedure is not painful because only a tiny amount of skin is needed. Patients may feel a slight pressure sensation when the skin is scraped.

Skin Biopsy: A skin biopsy may also be performed. During the procedure, a healthcare provider will inject an anesthetic into the skin, which numbs the area. Then a small sample of skin is removed and analyzed under a microscope to determine whether the patient has a skin disorder, such as psoriasis.

Skin Test: A skin test may be used to determine whether the rash is caused by an allergic reaction. During the test, the skin is exposed to the suspected allergens (substances that may be triggering an allergic reaction) and observed for an allergic reaction. If the allergen triggers an allergic reaction, the patient will develop reddening, swelling, or a raised, itchy red wheal (bump) that looks similar to a mosquito bite. The healthcare provider will measure the size of the wheal and record the results. The larger the wheal, the more severe the allergy.

Tzanck Test: A Tzanck test is used to determine whether a viral infection called herpes is causing a rash. The virus may be suspected if the patient has a rash that contains blisters. During the procedure, a small area of the skin is numbed and a blister is opened. The healthcare provider will scrape a small sample of the fluid and skin from the blister, and it will be analyzed under a microscope for the virus. If the virus is present, a positive diagnosis for herpes is made.

Wood Lamp: A wood lamp test may be performed if a healthcare provider suspects the patient has a bacterial or fungal infection of the skin. The procedure is performed in a dark room, at a doctor's office. The healthcare provider shines an ultraviolet light onto the patient's rash. The rash is then observed for color changes when it comes into contact with the light. If a bacterial or fungal infection is present, the skin will appear to glow under the light.

Before undergoing this test, patients should not wash their skin because it may alter test results. Skin products, such as soap, deodorant, makeup, or lotion, should not be applied to the skin prior to testing. These products may glow under the light and cause false-positive results. Also, if the room is not dark enough, a patient may receive false-negative results. This means the patient has the infection even though he/she tests negative.

TREATMENT

General: Treatment depends on the cause of the rash. If an allergic reaction causes a rash, oral antihistamines may be taken or hydrocortisone may be applied to the skin. Anaphylaxis, the most severe allergic reaction, must be treated with an injection of epinephrine as soon as possible. Antimicrobials are used to treat infections that cause rashes. Autoimmune disorders are treated with corticosteroids and other medications. Rashes caused by poisonous plants may be treated with antihistamines, calamine lotion, hydrocortisone, and/or baking soda solutions. Diaper rash may be treated with zinc oxide ointments. Skin disorders like atopic dermatitis may be treated with topical corticosteroids. If a patient develops SJS in response to medication, the patient should stop taking the offending drug immediately. No specific drug treatment exists for SJS. Recovery may take two to six weeks. Severe cases may require hospitalization in an intensive care unit or burn unit where the patient will receive intravenous fluids and nutritional supplements.

Antihistamines: Oral antihistamines like diphenhydramine (Benadryl) have been used to treat skin rashes caused by an allergic reaction. Antihistamines decrease redness and itchiness associated with the rash.

Antimicrobials: Medications called antimicrobials are used to treat skin rashes caused by infection. Antibiotics are used for bacterial infections (like Lyme disease), antifungals are used to treat fungal infections (like yeast infections), and antivirals are used to treat viral infections (like herpes). Depending on the type and severity of the condition, these agents may be administered in topical, oral, or injectable forms. Treatment duration and doses also depend on the type and severity of the infection. Many viral infections will resolve on their own and do not require medications.

Aloe Vera Gel: Aloe vera gel has been applied to affected areas of the skin to relieve itching and help rashes heal. Aloe vera is used most often to treat rashes from sunburn, heat rash, or poisonous plants. Aloe vera gel should not be applied to open cuts, blisters, or sores on the skin.

S

Baking Soda: A solution of baking soda and water may help treat allergic skin reactions caused by poisonous plants. Three teaspoons of baking soda have been mixed with one teaspoon of water and applied to affected areas of the skin.

Calamine Lotion: Calamine lotion (Calamox) can be applied to the skin to reduce itching and blistering caused by poisonous plant exposure.

Cool Compress: Applying a cool compress to affected areas of the skin may help relieve itching and swelling associated with rashes.

Epinephrine: A medication called epinephrine is used to treat anaphylaxis. Epinephrine is injected into the skin at a hospital. Patients with a history of anaphylaxis should carry an autoinjectable epinephrine (EpiPen) with them at all times. If symptoms of anaphylaxis appear after exposure to an allergen, the patient uses the device to inject the epinephrine into his/her thigh. Epinephrine acts as a bronchodilator because it opens the patient's airway. It also constricts the blood vessels, which increases blood pressure. Patients who experience anaphylaxis may also be admitted to the hospital to have their blood pressure monitored and possibly to receive breathing support.

Hydrocortisone: Hydrocortisone cream has been applied to the affected area to temporarily relieve itching associated with allergic reactions and exposure to poisonous plants. Hydrocortisone 1% cream, which is available over the counter, has antiinflammatory effects and relieves swelling and redness in addition to itching. Prescription hydrocortisone has been used to relieve itching, redness, dryness, crusting, scaling, inflammation, and discomfort associated with the reaction.

Sunscreen: Patients who are sensitive to sun exposure should wear ultraviolet-blocking sunscreens to prevent or reduce the development of a skin rash.

Oral Corticosteroids: Autoimmune disorders are often treated with oral corticosteroids like methyl-prednisolone (Adlone, Medrol, Solu-Medrol, Depopred) and prednisone (Deltasone, Orasone, Meticorten) to suppress the body's immune system and decrease skin inflammation. These medications may also be used short term to treat severe rashes caused by poisonous plants. Patients should slowly taper off medication to avoid serious side effects.

Topical Anesthetics: Topical anesthetics like lidocaine (Lidoderm) have been applied to the skin to relieve pain associated with SJS lesions.

Topical Corticosteroids: Topical (applied to the skin) corticosteroids (like hydrocortisone, betamethasone, or fluticasone propionate) are the most common

and effective treatment for rashes caused by atopic dermatitis. They are used until the rash clears up. Low-strength topical corticosteroids should be used on the face. Over-the-counter hydrocortisone (like Bactine, Cortaid, Dermolate, Aveeno Anti-Itch cream) is a low-strength corticosteroid cream that has been used to treat young children.

Zinc Oxide Creams: Ointments that contain zinc oxide (like Desitin, Diaparene) may help relieve diaper rash in babies. The ointment is applied to affected areas of the skin each time the baby's diaper is changed.

INTEGRATIVE THERAPIES

Strong Scientific Evidence

Vitamin D: A number of different approaches are used to treat psoriasis. Mild approaches include light therapy, stress reduction, moisturizers, or salicylic acid to remove scaly skin areas. For more severe cases, treatments may include ultraviolet A (UVA) light, psoralen plus UVA light (PUVA), retinoids-like isotretinoin (Accutane), corticosteroids, or cyclosporine (Neoral, Sandimmune). The manmade vitamin D_3 analog calcipotriene (Dovonex) appears to control skin cell growth and is used for moderately severe skin plaques, particularly for skin lesions resistant to other therapies or located on the face. Vitamin D_3 (tacalcitol) ointment has been reported as being safe and well tolerated.

Avoid if allergic or hypersensitive to vitamin D or any of its components. Vitamin D is generally well tolerated in recommended doses. Doses higher than recommended may cause toxic effects. Individuals with overactive thyroid, kidney disease, sarcoidosis, tuberculosis, or histoplasmosis are at a higher risk of experiencing toxic effects. Vitamin D is generally considered safe for pregnant women. It may be necessary to give infants vitamin D supplements along with breast milk. The recommended intake of vitamin D for normal infants, children, and adolescents is 200 international units daily.

Good Scientific Evidence

Aloe Vera: Early evidence suggests that extracts from aloe in a hydrophilic cream may be an effective treatment of psoriasis vulgaris. Additional research is needed in this area before a strong recommendation can be made.

Avoid if allergic to aloe or other plants of the Lilaceae family (garlic, onions, tulips). Do not inject aloe into the skin. Do not apply to open surgical wounds or pressure ulcers. Patients should not take aloe by mouth if they have diarrhea, bowel blockage, intestinal diseases, bloody stools, hepatitis, a history of irregular heartbeat (arrhythmia), electrolyte imbalances, diabetes, heart disease, or kidney disease. Avoid taking by mouth if pregnant or breastfeeding.

Evening Primrose Oil: Several small human studies suggest that taking evening primrose oil by mouth may help treat atopic dermatitis (eczema) in adults and children. Large, well-designed studies are needed before a strong recommendation can be made.

Evening primrose oil is approved for atopic dermatitis in several countries outside of the United States. Individuals who are allergic to plants in the Onagraceae family, gamma-linolenic acid, or other ingredients in evening primrose oil should avoid the substance. Individuals with seizure disorders and pregnant or breastfeeding women should also avoid evening primrose oil.

Probiotics: Probiotics show promise for reducing or preventing atopic eczema/dermatitis syndrome in children. Infants benefit when their mothers take probiotics during pregnancy and breastfeeding. Direct supplementation of infants may reduce the incidence of atopic eczema by as much as half. It may also reduce cow's milk allergy and other allergic reactions during weaning. Probiotics may stabilize the intestinal barrier function and decrease gastrointestinal symptoms in children with atopic dermatitis. Children do differ, however, in their responsiveness to specific probiotics.

Probiotics are generally regarded as safe for human consumption. Long-term consumption of probiotics is considered safe and well tolerated.

Unclear or Conflicting Scientific Evidence

Acupuncture: Further research is needed to determine whether acupuncture can effectively treat skin disorders such as hives (itchy, red welts that form on the skin).

Needles must be sterile in order to avoid disease transmission. Avoid with heart valve disease, infections, bleeding disorders or drugs that increase the risk of bleeding (anticoagulants), medical conditions of unknown origin, and neurological disorders. Avoid on areas that have received radiation therapy and during pregnancy. Use cautiously with pulmonary disease (like asthma or emphysema). Use cautiously in elderly or medically compromised patients, diabetics, or history of seizures. Avoid electroacupuncture with arrhythmia (irregular heartbeat) or in patients with pacemakers.

Agrimony: It remains unclear whether agrimony can effectively treat skin disorders and rashes.

Further research is needed to determine if the herb is safe and effective.

Avoid if allergic or hypersensitive to agrimony or its related species. When used as recommended, agrimony is considered to be safe. Avoid with bleeding disorders, kidney or liver disease, or diabetes. Use cautiously with drugs that lower blood pressure.

Avocado: Early scientific research showed promising results using avocado in a cream for psoriasis. Additional studies are needed in this area before a firm recommendation can be made.

Avoid if allergic or hypersensitive to avocado, banana, chestnut, or natural rubber latex. Use cautiously with anticoagulants (like warfarin). Avoid with monoamine oxidase inhibitors. Doses greater than found in a normal diet are not recommended if pregnant or breastfeeding. Some types of avocado may be unsafe when breastfeeding.

Butterbur: There is limited human evidence in this area, although preliminary research suggests that butterbur may not suppress allergic skin reactions when compared to the prescription drug fexofenadine (Allegra), which does suppress these reactions. Additional research is needed.

Use cautiously if allergic or sensitive to *Petasites hybridus* or other plants from the Asteraceae/Compositae family (like ragweed, marigolds, daisies, and chrysanthemums). Raw, unprocessed butterbur plant should not be eaten due to the risk of liver or kidney damage or cancer. Avoid if pregnant or breastfeeding.

Calendula: Limited animal research suggests that calendula extracts may reduce inflammation when applied to the skin. Human studies are lacking in this area.

Avoid if allergic to plants in the Aster/Compositae family like ragweed, chrysanthemums, marigolds, and daisies. Severe allergic reaction (anaphylactic shock) has been reported after gargling with a calendula preparation. Caution is advised while driving or operating machinery. It is not clear if calendula is safe for use during pregnancy or breastfeeding.

Chamomile: Topical chamomile preparations have traditionally been used to soothe skin inflammation. The existing human evidence shows that chamomile may be of little, if any, benefit, while animal studies support its antiinflammatory action. Additional human research is needed in this area.

Avoid if allergic to chamomile or any related plants such as aster, chrysanthemum, mugwort, ragweed, or ragwort. Stop use two weeks before

S

surgery/dental/diagnostic procedures with bleeding risk, and do not use immediately after these procedures. Use cautiously if driving or operating machinery. Avoid if pregnant or breastfeeding.

Chondroitin Sulfate: Early research suggests that chondroitin may help treat psoriasis. Well-designed clinical trials are needed to confirm these results.

Use cautiously if allergic or hypersensitive to chondroitin sulfate products. Use cautiously with bleeding disorders and with blood thinners like warfarin (Coumadin). Avoid if pregnant or breastfeeding.

Dehydroepiandrosterone (DHEA): DHEA is a hormone that is produced by the adrenal glands in the body. Overall, study results suggest that DHEA likely offers no benefit to individuals with psoriasis, but some disagree. Additional research is needed before a firm conclusion can be made.

Avoid if allergic to DHEA. Avoid with a history of seizures. Use with caution in adrenal or thyroid disorders or anticoagulants or drugs, herbs, or supplements for diabetes, heart disease, seizure, or stroke. Stop use two weeks before surgery/dental/diagnostic procedures with bleeding risk, and do not use immediately after these procedures. Avoid if pregnant or breastfeeding.

Euphorbia: Early research of *Euphorbia acaulis* has demonstrated an effect on patients with eczema. More trials are needed to evaluate the effect of *Euphorbia acaulis* for eczema.

Avoid if allergic or hypersensitive to pollen from *Euphorbia fulgens*. Use cautiously with history of Epstein-Barr virus infection or stomach conditions. Avoid if pregnant or breastfeeding.

Gamma-Linolenic Acid (GLA): A number of randomized clinical studies have been conducted to treat atopic dermatitis in adults and children, and in one case a study attempted to prevent atopic dermatitis in infants. Changes in linolenic acid metabolism have been related to eczema where conversion of linolenic acid to GLA is inhibited in persons with atopic dermatitis. However, the studies in the past 20 years reveal minimal therapeutic improvements with GLA as therapy for atopic dermatitis, noted by only marginal to no improvement in inflammation and itching.

GLA is generally considered nontoxic and well tolerated for up to 18 months. Use cautiously with anticoagulants (blood thinners) and avoid if pregnant or breastfeeding.

Gamma-Oryzanol: A few studies have used gamma-oryzanol by mouth or applied on the skin to treat skin conditions. Although these studies seem to indicate that gamma-oryzanol may be useful, additional research is needed to assess gamma-oryzanol's effects.

Avoid if allergic/hypersensitive to gamma-oryzanol, its components, or rice bran oil. Use cautiously if taking anticoagulants (blood thinners), central nervous system suppressants, growth hormone, drugs that alter blood sugar levels, immunomodulators, luteinizing hormone or luteinizing hormone–releasing hormone, prolactin, cholesterol-lowering agents, thyroid drugs, and herbs or supplements with similar effects. Use cautiously with diabetes, hypothyroidism, hypoglycemia, hyperglycemia, or high cholesterol. Avoid if pregnant or breastfeeding.

Grapefruit: There is early but inconclusive evidence to support the use of grapefruit seed extract in the treatment of atopic eczema. Additional research is needed to confirm these findings.

Avoid if allergic to grapefruit. Grapefruit may interact with prescription drugs, herbs, and supplements. Use cautiously if taking cytochrome P450 3A4 substrates such as anticoagulant/antiplatelets (agents that affect blood clotting), antiarrhythmics (medications used to treat abnormal rhythms in the heart), seizure drugs, antidepressants, antihistamines, drugs that affect blood pressure, benzodiazepines (a class of psychotropic drugs that have a hypnotic and sedative action), calcium channel blockers, caffeine, corticosteroids (antiinflammatories), erectile dysfunction drugs, estrogens, immune modulators, 3-hydroxy-3-methylglutaryl coenzyme A reductase inhibitors, macrolide antibiotics, and protease inhibitors. Use cautiously if drinking red wine or tonic water. Use cautiously when smoking and with liver cirrhosis or at risk for kidney stones. Use cautiously in patients who have undergone gastric bypass surgery. Use cautiously if pregnant or breastfeeding.

Hydrotherapy: There is insufficient evidence to determine whether hydrotherapy is an effective treatment for atopic dermatitis (eczema) or psoriasis.

Avoid sudden or prolonged exposure to extreme temperatures in baths, wraps, saunas, or other forms of hydrotherapy, particularly with heart disease, lung disease, or if pregnant. Avoid with implanted medical devices such as pacemakers, defibrillators, or hepatic (liver) infusion pumps. Vigorous use of water jets should be avoided with fractures, known blood clots, bleeding disorders, severe osteoporosis, open wounds, or pregnancy. Use cautiously with Raynaud's disease, chilblains, acrocyanosis, erythrocyanosis, and impaired temperature sensitivity, such as neuropathy. Use cautiously if pregnant or breastfeeding. Hydrotherapy should not delay the time to diagnosis or treatment with more proven techniques or therapies and should not be used as the sole approach to illnesses. Patients with known illnesses should consult their physicians before starting hydrotherapy.

Hypnotherapy: Further research is needed to determine whether hypnotherapy is an effective treatment for skin conditions, including eczema and psoriasis.

Use cautiously with mental illnesses like psychosis/schizophrenia, manic depression, multiple personality disorder, or dissociative disorders. Use cautiously with seizure disorders.

Khella: Preliminary evidence suggests that khellin taken by mouth may be an effective therapy for psoriasis. However, additional study is needed to confirm these results.

Avoid if allergic to members of the Apiaceae family (flowering plants). May cause liver poisoning (hepatotoxicity) in high doses. Use cautiously with liver problems or asthma. Avoid prolonged exposure to sunlight or UV radiation. Avoid if pregnant.

Licorice: Topical licorice extract gel has been shown to be effective in the treatment of atopic dermatitis in preliminary human study. Further research is needed to confirm these results.

Avoid licorice if you have a known allergy to licorice, any component of licorice, or any member of the Fabaceae (Leguminosae) plant family. Avoid licorice with history of congestive heart failure, coronary heart disease, kidney disease, liver disease, fluid retention, high blood pressure, or hormonal abnormalities and/or if taking diuretics. Licorice can cause abnormally low testosterone levels in men or high prolactin or estrogen levels in women. This may make it difficult to become pregnant and may cause menstrual abnormalities.

Marshmallow: Marshmallow extracts have traditionally been used on the skin to treat inflammation. Several laboratory experiments, mostly in the 1960s, reported marshmallow to have antiinflammatory activity, but limited human study is available. Safety, dosing, and effectiveness compared to other antiinflammatories have not been examined.

Historically, marshmallow is generally regarded as being safe in healthy individuals. However, since studies have not evaluated the safety of marshmallow, proper doses and duration in humans are not known. Allergic reactions may occur. There is not enough scientific evidence to support the safe use of marshmallow during pregnancy or breastfeeding.

Neem: Limited human data on the effect of neem on psoriasis are available. Further research is needed before a firm conclusion can be made.

Avoid if allergic or hypersensitive to neem (*Azadirachta indica*) or members of the Meliaceae family. Use cautiously with liver disease. Avoid in children and infants. Avoid if pregnant or breastfeeding.

Omega-3 Fatty Acid: There is insufficient evidence to determine whether omega-3 fatty acid can effective treat skin conditions, including eczema or psoriasis. Further research is warranted.

Avoid if allergic or hypersensitive to fish, omega-3 fatty acid products that come from fish, nuts, linolenic acid, or omega-3 fatty acid products that come from nuts. Avoid during active bleeding. Use cautiously with bleeding disorders, diabetes, or low blood pressure or drugs, herbs, or supplements that treat any such conditions. Use cautiously before surgery. The Environmental Protection Agency recommends that intake be limited in pregnant/nursing women to a single six-ounce meal per week and in young children to less than two ounces per week. For farm-raised, imported, or marine fish, the U.S. Food and Drug Administration recommends that pregnant/breastfeeding women and young children avoid eating types with higher levels of methyl mercury and less than 12 ounces per week of other fish types. Women who might become pregnant are advised to eat seven ounces or less per week of fish with higher levels of methyl mercury or up to 14 ounces per week of fish types with about 0.5 parts per million (such as marlin, orange roughy, red snapper, or fresh tuna).

Polypodium: Laboratory and animal studies report that *Polypodium leucotomos* extract (anapsos) may reduce skin inflammation associated with skin disorders like eczema and psoriasis. However, further research is needed to confirm these results.

Avoid if allergic to ferns (in the family Polypodiaceae) or if pregnant or breastfeeding.

Psychotherapy: Atopic dermatitis is a skin disease associated with an increased anxiety level. Psychotherapy may be helpful for atopic dermatitis patients with high levels of anxiety. However, more research is needed before a recommendation can be made.

Use cautiously with serious mental illness or some medical conditions because some forms of psychotherapy may stir up strong emotional feelings and expression.

Rutin: In one clinical trial O-(beta-hydroxyethyl)-rutoside offered benefit in terms of skin irritation to individuals with breast cancer undergoing radiation treatment. More well-designed clinical trials are required in this field before recommendations can be made.

S

Avoid if allergic/hypersensitive to O-(beta-hydroxyethyl)-rutosides or plants that rutin is commonly found in, such as rue, tobacco, or buckwheat. Use cautiously in elderly patients. Use cautiously with skin conditions. Use cautiously if taking medications for edema, diuretics, or anticoagulation medications. Use cautiously if pregnant or breastfeeding.

Selenium: Further research is necessary to determine whether selenium can be used to effectively treat psoriasis.

Avoid if allergic or sensitive to products containing selenium. Avoid with history of nonmelanoma skin cancer. Selenium is generally regarded as safe for pregnant or breastfeeding women. However, animal research reports that large doses of selenium may lead to birth defects.

Shark Cartilage: Shark cartilage products have been tested by mouth or on the skin in people with psoriasis. However, no clear benefits have been shown. More research is needed before a conclusion can be drawn.

Avoid if allergic to shark cartilage or any of its ingredients (including chondroitin sulfate and glucosamine). Use cautiously with sulfur allergy. Avoid with history of heart attack, vascular disease, heart rhythm abnormalities, or heart disease. Use cautiously with history of liver or kidney disorders, tendency to form kidney stones, breast cancer, prostate cancer, multiple myeloma, breathing disorders (like asthma), cancers that raise calcium levels (like breast, prostate, multiple myeloma, or squamous cell lung cancer), or diabetes. Avoid if pregnant or breastfeeding.

St. John's Wort: Early research of *Hypericum* cream for the topical (applied to the skin) treatment of mild to moderate atopic dermatitis shows positive results. Further studies are needed before a firm conclusion can be made.

Avoid if allergic or hypersensitive to plants in the Hypericaceae family. Rare allergic skin reactions like itchy rash have been reported. Avoid with HIV/AIDS drugs (protease inhibitors) like indinavir (Crixivan) or nonnucleoside reverse transcriptase inhibitors like nevirapine (Viramune). Avoid with immunosuppressant drugs (like cyclosporine, tacrolimus, or myogenic acid). Avoid with organ transplants, suicidal symptoms, or before surgery. Use cautiously with history of thyroid disorders. Use cautiously with drugs that are broken down by the liver, with monoamine oxidase inhibitors or selective serotonin reuptake inhibitors, digoxin, or birth control pills. Use cautiously with diabetes or with history of

mania, hypomania (as in bipolar disorder), or affective illness. Avoid if pregnant or breastfeeding.

Tea Tree Oil: One small study shows that topical tea tree oil may reduce skin inflammation caused by an allergic reaction. Further research is needed to confirm these results.

Thyme: Historically, thyme has been applied to the skin for a number of skin conditions. Results are mixed. Additional research is needed in this area.

Avoid if known allergy/hypersensitivity to members of the Lamiaceae (mint) family or to any component of thyme or to rosemary (*Rosmarinus officinalis*).

Avoid use if allergic to tea tree oil or plants of the Myrtle (Myrtaceae) family, balsam of Peru, or benzoin. Use caution with history of eczema. Avoid taking tea tree oil by mouth because reports of toxicity have been reported. Avoid if pregnant or breastfeeding.

Thymus Extract: It remains unclear whether thymus extract can effectively treat skin conditions such as psoriasis or eczema. Early research results are inconclusive. Further research is needed.

Avoid if allergic or hypersensitive to thymus extracts. Use bovine thymus extract supplements cautiously due to potential for exposure to the virus that causes "mad cow disease." Avoid use with an organ transplant or other forms of allografts or xenografts. Avoid with immunosuppressive therapy, thymic tumors, myasthenia gravis (neuromuscular disorder), untreated hypothyroidism, or hormonal therapy. Avoid if pregnant or breastfeeding; thymic extract increases human sperm motility and progression.

Zinc: Preliminary research on the effectiveness of zinc to treat skin conditions, including diaper rash, psoriasis, and eczema, are inconclusive. Further research is necessary before a firm conclusion can be made.

Zinc is regarded as relatively safe and generally well tolerated when taken at recommended doses, and few studies report side effects. Zinc should only be given to pregnant or breastfeeding women under the supervision of their qualified healthcare providers.

Fair Negative Scientific Evidence

Boron: Preliminary human research of an ointment containing boric acid does not report significant benefits in psoriasis.

Avoid if allergic or sensitive to boron, boric acid, borax, citrate, aspartate, or glycinate. Avoid with history of diabetes, seizure disorder, kidney disease, liver disease, depression, anxiety, high blood pressure, skin rash, anemia, asthma, or chronic obstructive pulmonary disease. Avoid with hormone-sensitive conditions like breast cancer or prostate cancer. Avoid if pregnant or breastfeeding.

Evening Primrose Oil: Initial research does not show a benefit from evening primrose oil in the treatment of psoriasis.

Individuals who are allergic to plants in the Onagraceae family, GLA, or other ingredients in evening primrose oil should avoid the substance. Individuals with seizure disorders and pregnant or breastfeeding women should also avoid evening primrose oil.

Lavender: In a small clinical trial, essential oils were used in combination with massage to treat childhood atopic eczema. It was found that there was deterioration in the patient's eczema, which may have been due to a possible allergic contact dermatitis provoked by the essential oils themselves. Additional research of the effect of lavender essential oil alone is needed before any firm conclusions can be made.

Avoid if allergic or hypersensitive to lavender. Avoid with history of seizures, bleeding disorders, eating disorders (anorexia, bulimia), or anemia (low levels of iron in the blood). Avoid if pregnant or breastfeeding.

PREVENTION

Avoid exposure to known allergens (like pollen, dust mites, animal dander, mold, and certain foods and medications).

Individuals who have experienced anaphylactic reactions should avoid allergy-causing food, medications, or substances. Individuals with a history of anaphylaxis should carry an autoinjectable epinephrine device (known as an EpiPen) with them at all times. A trained family member or friend may help the patient administer the epinephrine if necessary.

Avoid unnecessary exposure to other environmental irritants such as insect sprays, tobacco smoke, air pollution, and fresh tar or paint.

Patients can take precautions to avoid contracting infections that may cause rashes. Patients should thoroughly wash their hands with soap and water. Patients should talk to their healthcare providers about recommended immunizations. Patients should minimize or avoid close contact with individuals who have contagious illnesses.

To help prevent diaper rash, regularly change diapers as soon as they become wet or dirty. Thoroughly dry the baby's bottom before putting a new diaper on.

Wear sun block when outside to help prevent a skin rash. Patients should choose a sun block with a sun protection factor of 15 or higher. The sun block should offer protection against both UVA and UVB rays. Also, patients should look for products that are "PABA free." PABA is a chemical that is found in many sun blocks, and it is known to cause irritation in sensitive patients.

Individuals should learn what poison ivy, poison oak, and poison sumac look like in order to prevent contact with the plants. Individuals who are allergic to poisonous plants should wear long pants and long-sleeved shirts when they are in wooded areas.

Topical creams like bentoquatam (IvyBlock), which are available over the counter, may help prevent or reduce allergic rashes caused by poison plants. The cream is applied to exposed areas of skin before possible exposure to poison ivy, poison oak, or poison sumac. The cream should not be applied to open cuts, sores, or wounds.

S

SLEEP DISORDERS

BACKGROUND

Sleep disorders occur when an individual has problems with his/her sleep cycle. As a result, it may take patients longer to fall asleep; patients may wake up during the night or wake up early; they may fall asleep throughout the day; or they may have severe nightmares (called night terrors), act out their dreams, or stop breathing during sleep. The most common types of sleep disorders include delayed sleep phase syndrome (DSPS), insomnia, narcolepsy, night terrors, rapid eye movement sleep behavior disorder (RBD), and sleep apnea. There are two phases of sleep: non–rapid eye movement (NREM) sleep and rapid eye movement sleep (REM). The first hour or two of sleep is called NREM sleep. During this phase, the brain waves slow down. After one to two hours of NREM sleep, the brain activity increases and REM sleep begins. This is when most dreaming occurs. During REM sleep, the eyes (although closed) move rapidly, breathing becomes irregular, blood pressure rises, and individuals are in a state of temporary sleep paralysis. This temporary immobility prevents individuals from acting out their dreams. Most sleep disorders can be managed with lifestyle changes and/ or medications.

DELAYED SLEEP PHASE SYNDROME (DSPS)

Overview: DSPS—also called circadian rhythm sleep disorder, delayed sleep phase type—occurs when a person's internal clock is not in sync with the normal sleep patterns of most adults. The patient's sleep pattern is delayed by two or more hours, causing later bedtimes and wake times. When patients follow their internal clocks and go to bed when they are tired, they get enough sleep. However, patients with DSPS have abnormal internal clocks, and they typically do not feel tired until 2:00 AM or later. Since this does not match normal school and work schedules, patients feel tired when they try to follow conventional sleeping schedules.

DSPS patients typically find that sleeping aids do not help them fall asleep any earlier.

DSPS is a long-term condition that is most common among adolescents. DSPS can develop suddenly or gradually. Symptoms generally go away spontaneously without treatment.

Causes: DSPS is not caused by jet lag, working late shifts, working irregular shifts, or other external factors. Instead, DSPS is caused by an abnormality in the patient's internal clock (called the circadian rhythm).

Symptoms: Patients with DSPS generally have difficulty falling asleep before 2:00 AM Individuals often feel tired upon waking. Individuals may continue to feel fatigued or drowsy throughout the day.

Diagnosis: If it is suspected that a patient has DSPS, the individual may be asked to keep a sleep log. In the log, patients write what time they fell asleep and woke up each day. In order for DSPS to be diagnosed, symptoms must last at least three months. However, DSPS is often misdiagnosed because symptoms of this disorder are very general and similar to insomnia or some types of mental illness (such as depression).

Treatment: There is currently no cure for DSPS, but symptoms generally go away on their own. Treatment is available to help manage symptoms by reprogramming the patient's internal clock. The goal is to synchronize the patient's sleep patterns with their work and/or school schedules. Treatment often includes light therapy and chronotherapy. Patients may also benefit from melatonin supplements taken 30 minutes to one hour before bed. Melatonin should be used cautiously because high doses may disturb sleep and cause nightmares and uncontrollable yawning the next day. If treatment does not help, patients may need to change their work and social lives to accommodate their internal clocks.

INSOMNIA

Overview: Insomnia occurs when individuals have difficulty falling or staying asleep and they wake up too early in the morning. It is a common health problem that can cause excessive daytime sleepiness and a lack of energy. Long-term insomnia may cause an individual to feel tired, depressed, or irritable. Individuals may also have trouble paying attention, learning, and remembering, which may prevent them from performing fully on the job or at school. Severe insomnia can result in neurochemical (brain chemical) changes that may lead to problems, such as depression and anxiety, further complicating the insomnia.

Causes: There are many potential causes of insomnia. Psychological disorders, such as stress, anxiety, depression, and bipolar disorder, may lead to insomnia. Certain health conditions, including arthritis, overactive thyroid glands, gastrointestinal disorders (such as diarrhea or ulcers), Alzheimer's disease, Parkinson's disease, sleep apnea (discussed in detail below), and restless legs syndrome, may cause insomnia. Other factors, such as taking certain medications (such as stimulants, nasal decongestants, and some antidepressants), consuming caffeine, jet lag, wake-sleep pattern disturbances, excessive sleep during the day, and excessive physical or intellectual stimulation before bed, may cause insomnia.

Symptoms: The main signs and symptoms of insomnia are trouble falling or staying asleep or waking early, followed by a distinct feeling of fatigue (tiredness) the following day. Most often, daytime symptoms will bring people to seek medical attention. Daytime problems caused by insomnia include anxiousness, irritability, fatigue, poor concentration and difficulty focusing, impaired memory, decreased motor coordination, irritability, impaired social interaction, and motor vehicle accidents because of fatigued, sleep-deprived drivers.

Diagnosis: A doctor will ask the individual experiencing insomnia questions to evaluate his/her medical history. Questions investigate mental health problems, medications (prescription and nonprescription drugs, herbs, and supplements), history of pain, leisure habits, work and home situation, and others. The doctor will also inquire about the individual's sleep history. Questions about length and severity of the sleeping problem, routines before sleeping, snoring, and noise levels may also be asked. The doctor will also give the individual a full physical exam, including blood tests for conditions (such as thyroid problems) that may interfere with sleep. A polysomnogram is a recording of the breathing, movements, heart function, and brain activity during sleep. For this study, the individual sleeps overnight at a sleep center or hospital. A sleep study will be recommended if there are signs of sleep apnea or restless legs syndrome.

Treatment: Treatment for insomnia depends on the underlying cause. For instance, if a psychological problem is causing symptoms, a healthcare provider may recommend psychotherapy or cognitive behavioral therapy. If a medication is the suspected cause, a healthcare provider may be able to recommend a different drug or dosage.

There are many sedative-hypnotic medications available to help patients fall asleep and stay asleep throughout the night. Commonly prescribed medications for insomnia include temazepam (Restoril), flurazepam (Dalmane), estazolam (ProSom), triazolam (Halcion), zolpidem (Ambien), zaleplon (Sonata), and eszopiclone (Lunesta).

However, the U.S. Food and Drug Administration (FDA) has issued warnings for all sedative-hypnotic drugs used for sleep because they may cause serious side effects. Anaphylaxis and severe facial angioedema (swelling) can occur the first time a sleep product is taken. Complex sleep-related behaviors may include sleep-driving (driving while not fully awake and with no memory of driving), making phone calls, and preparing and eating food while asleep.

Over-the-counter (OTC) sleep aids may be used short term to treat insomnia. For instance, diphenhydramine (Benadryl) is the most commonly used OTC antihistamine sleep aid. It can be purchased alone (Benadryl, Nytol, Sominex) or in combination with other OTC items such as acetaminophen (Tylenol PM). OTC sleep aids are not intended for long-term use because dependency can develop.

Melatonin agonists, such as ramelteon (Rozerem), have also been used to treat insomnia. Ramelteon promotes the onset of sleep by increasing levels of the natural hormone melatonin, which helps normalize normal circadian rhythm and sleep/wake cycles. These drugs are less likely to cause morning drowsiness than sedative-hypnotics. Side effects are generally mild and may include daytime sleepiness, dizziness, and fatigue.

Sedating antidepressants, including trazodone (Desyrel), amitriptyline (Elavil), and doxepin (Sinequan), have been used to treat insomnia. When used to promote sleep, these medicines are used in lower doses than when used to treat depression. Side effects may include dry mouth, blurred vision, a "hangover" in the morning, constipation, urinary retention, and nausea.

NARCOLEPSY

Overview: Narcolepsy is a sleep disorder that occurs when individuals are overwhelmingly tired and spontaneously fall asleep throughout the day. Patients have a hard time staying awake for extended periods of time regardless of the circumstances or how much sleep they get. The severity of narcolepsy varies among patients. Most patients are diagnosed between the ages of 10 and 25. It is uncommon for patients to be diagnosed with the disorder when they are older than 40 years of age.

Causes: Researchers are still performing studies to fully understand the causes of narcolepsy. Scientists believe that genetics may play a role in the disorder.

However, since only about 2% of narcoleptic patients have family histories of the disorder, other factors besides genetics are probably involved. Narcoleptic patients may have imbalances in the brain chemicals that help control sleep. For instance, one chemical called hypocretin has been shown to help individuals wake from sleep and stay awake. Patients with narcolepsy typically have low levels of this chemical. However, researchers do not know what causes individuals to have low levels of hypocretin. It has been suggested that the body's immune system might attack hypocretin-producing cells by mistake.

Symptoms: Patients with narcolepsy are excessively tired throughout the day. Individuals can fall asleep at any time or any place throughout the day. For instance, they may fall asleep in the middle of conversations with friends. These sleep attacks may last anywhere from a few minutes to a half hour. Individuals also experience decreased alertness and concentration.

About 70% of narcoleptic patients also experience periodic episodes of cataplexy, which is a sudden and temporary loss of muscle tone. This condition, which may last anywhere from a few seconds to a few minutes, may cause symptoms that range from slurred speech and drooling to complete muscle weakness. Laughter or strong emotions, especially excitement and sometimes fear or anger, typically trigger cataplexy. Some patients may only experience cataplexy a few times a year, while others may experience symptoms several times a day.

Sleep paralysis may also occur while the individual is falling asleep or awakening. This temporary inability to move typically lasts anywhere from a few seconds to several minutes. When sleep paralysis occurs, patients may feel scared because they are often aware of what is happening even though they cannot move.

Some patients may experience hallucinations. This occurs if the patient is semiawake when he/she starts dreaming.

Additional symptoms may include restless nighttime sleep or sleepwalking. Some patients may also act out their dreams and talk or move their arms or legs.

Diagnosis: If narcolepsy is suspected, the patient may be required to spend the night at a sleep center. During the night, a team of specialists will observe the patient's sleep patterns and behavior. Electrodes may also be placed on the patient's scalp before he/she falls asleep. This test, called a polysomnogram, measures the electrical activity of the brain and heart as well as the movements of the muscles and

eyes. Patients may also be asked to fill out a sleep questionnaire, called the Epworth Sleepiness Scale. This survey asks the patient to rank how tired they are during certain activities. A multiple sleep latency test may also be performed at a sleep center. The patient will be asked to take several naps that are about two hours apart. Narcoleptic patients will fall asleep quickly and enter REM sleep almost immediately.

Treatment: Because narcolepsy is a neurological disorder, the condition does not improve if the patient gets more sleep. Although there is no cure for narcolepsy, medications can help manage symptoms. Patients typically receive medications called central nervous system stimulants. These drugs help narcoleptic patients stay awake during the day. Modafinil (Provigil), a newer stimulant, is less addictive and better tolerated than other older types of stimulants. However, some patients need treatment with methylphenidate (Ritalin) or other types of amphetamines.

In addition, patients often take antidepressants, such as protriptyline (Vivactil), imipramine (Tofranil), and amitriptyline (Elavil). These medications suppress REM sleep. As a result, they help control symptoms of cataplexy, hallucinations, and sleep paralysis.

Another prescription medication, called sodium oxybate (Xyrem), may also be prescribed to some patients. This medication, which is taken at night, helps reduce symptoms of sleep paralysis, hallucinations, and cataplexy. Even though this medication is taken at night, high doses may also help control daytime sleepiness. Serious side effects, including difficulty breathing during sleep, sleepwalking, and bedwetting, have been reported. Therefore, this medication is only taken when other medications are unsuccessful. Xyrem is not sold in local pharmacies. Instead, a healthcare provider must enroll a patient in a restricted distribution risk-management program that offers the drug from a single centralized pharmacy, the Xyrem Success Program.

NIGHT TERRORS

Overview: Night terrors are similar to nightmares. However, night terrors are scarier and more intense. Night terrors typically cause individuals to scream and thrash about during sleep. Individuals usually do not remember their night terrors when they wake in the morning. Night terrors primarily affect young children, usually between the ages of four and 12. Night terrors during childhood are not usually a cause for concern, and most children outgrow night terrors by adolescence. In rare cases, adults may experience night terrors, usually in response to extreme stress or anxiety. Adults may benefit from medications if they experience frequent night terrors.

Causes: Many factors, including fatigue, stress, illnesses (especially those that cause fevers), and medications that affect the brain or spinal cord (such as stimulants), may cause night terrors.

Symptoms: Night terrors typically occur two to three hours after an individual has fallen asleep. During sleep, the patient may scream or yell, sit up in bed, thrash around, sweat, or breathe rapidly. If a parent or bedmate tries to hold or comfort the patient during a night terror, the patient may unknowingly put up a fight. Adults, who are larger and stronger than children, may even injure their bedmate as they thrash around during night terrors. Most night terrors only last a few minutes. Once the individual wakes up, he/she probably will not remember the episode.

Diagnosis: Night terrors usually do not require a diagnosis. A healthcare provider may perform a physical and/or psychological exam to determine what might be triggering the terrors.

Treatment: Children who experience night terrors generally do not require any treatment. Parents may gently restrain their children to try and calm them down. Speaking softly and calmly is recommended because shouting or shaking the child awake typically worsens the episode. Although rarely used, medications called benzodiazepines, such as clonazepam (Klonopin) may be used short term to reduce symptoms in children. Antidepressants, such as imipramine (Tofranil), may also help if night terrors affect the child's performance at school. Adults may also benefit from these medications if they experience frequent night terrors or if they are harming their bedmates during episodes. If stress or anxiety seems to be causing night terrors, a healthcare provider may recommend psychotherapy. It is also important to ensure that the patient's bedroom is safe. For instance, children who experience night terrors should not sleep on the top of a bunk bed. Consider blocking stairways with a gate. Any sharp or unsafe objects should be out of the patient's reach.

REM Sleep Behavior Disorder

Overview: REM sleep behavior disorder (RBD) occurs when patients do not experience temporary paralysis during REM sleep. As a result, patients act out their dreams, which are often intense, vivid, and violent. The patient may yell, punch, kick, jump up from bed, and punch the air. RBD typically occurs in middle-aged to elderly patients. It is more common in men than women.

Causes: The exact cause of RBD remains unknown. However, the disorder has been linked to many degenerative neurological (brain) disorders, including Parkinson's disease. It is important to note that not all patients with RBD develop neurological disorders. Symptoms of RBD may also occur during withdrawal from alcohol or sedative-hypnotic drugs. However, this form is only temporary and goes away once the person has gone through withdrawal.

Symptoms: Patients with RBD act out their dreams. This may include yelling, screaming, thrashing around, kicking, punching, sitting up in bed, or getting out of bed during sleep. In some cases, RBD may cause self-injury or injury to the bed partner. If the person wakes up in the middle of an attack, he/she is often able to remember the dream in detail.

Diagnosis: A polysomnographic video recording is typically performed to diagnose RBD. During the test, the patient will spend the night at a sleep center. When the patient is asleep, researchers will monitor the electrical activity of the brain and heart, the movement of the muscles, the movements of the eyes, and breathing patterns. A video recording is also made to monitor the physical behavior of the patient during sleep. Patients with RBD will have an increase in muscle movements in association with increased brain activity.

Treatment: Patients with RBD typically take a medication called clonazepam (Klonopin) before bed. This medication has been shown to be effective in 90% of patients. Sleep talking and mild to moderate limb twitching may continue even with treatment. Symptoms generally start to improve within one week of treatment. The treatment is lifelong in order to prevent symptoms from returning.

It is important to ensure the safety of the patient, as well as anyone else who shares a bed with the patient. Any sharp or potentially harmful objects should be removed from the bedroom. Any objects, including furniture, should be removed from the side of the bed in case the patient falls or jumps out of bed. Padded bedrails may also be beneficial. Patients should consider placing the mattress on the floor or placing pillows on the side of the bed. The bedmate should sleep in another bed until the patient's symptoms have been resolved. However, it is recommended that the bedmate is within earshot of the patient. That way, he/she can help the patient in case an injury occurs.

Sleep Apnea

Overview: Sleep apnea is a serious condition that occurs when the individual stops breathing for short periods of time during sleep. Because sleep apnea causes individuals to wake up frequently throughout the night, patients are often drowsy during the day.

Causes: There are two main types of sleep apnea: obstructive sleep apnea and central sleep apnea. Obstructive sleep apnea is the most common form that occurs when the muscles in the throat relax. These muscles support the soft palate, the small piece of tissue that hangs from the soft palate (called the uvula), the tonsils, and the tongue. When these muscles relax, the patient is unable to breathe. The brain senses this inability to breathe and causes the individual to wake up and start breathing again. This process may occur 20 to 30 times or more each hour during sleep. Most patients do not even realize this happens.

Obstructive sleep apnea occurs most often in older adults. It is also twice as likely to occur in men as women. Obese individuals have an increased risk of experiencing obstructive sleep apnea because they have excess fat in their upper airways.

Central sleep apnea occurs when the brain does not send proper signals to the muscles that control breathing during sleep. This is usually caused by heart disease. They are more likely to remember waking up in the middle of sleep than patients with obstructive sleep apnea.

It is possible to have a combination of both types of sleep apnea, which is called complex sleep apnea. Central sleep apnea may develop at any age, and it affects males and females equally. Some evidence suggests that 15% of patients with sleep apnea have complex sleep apnea.

Symptoms: Many of the symptoms of obstructive sleep apnea and central sleep apnea are the same. Common symptoms of both of these disorders include loud snoring, waking from sleep abruptly, difficulty staying asleep, waking up with a dry mouth or sore throat, and drowsiness during the day. In addition, individuals with central sleep apnea often wake up with shortness of breath and headaches. Patients with central sleep apnea may also experience shortness of breath and headaches when they wake up from sleep.

Diagnosis: If sleep apnea is suspected, the patient may be asked to spend a night at a sleep center. At a sleep center, the patient's sleep patterns will be observed and analyzed. Several tests, including a nocturnal polysomnography, oximetry, and portable cardiorespiratory test, may be performed to monitor the patient's conditions.

During a nocturnal polysomnography test, a specialist will monitor the electrical activity of the brain and heart, the movement of the muscles, the movements of the eyes, and breathing patterns of the patient during sleep.

During an oximetry test, a small machine monitors and records the oxygen level of the patient during sleep. A small sleeve is placed over one of the fingers. This test may be performed at a sleep center or at home. Patients with sleep apnea will have low levels of oxygen before each awakening.

A healthcare provider may give the patient a portable cardiorespiratory test to perform at home. These tests involve oximetry, measurement of breathing patterns, and the measurement of airflow.

Treatment: Milder cases of sleep apnea may be treated with lifestyle changes, including weight loss and smoking cessation. More severe cases may be treated with devices to open the airway and/or surgery.

A machine called a continuous positive airway pressure (CPAP) is the most common and effective treatment for patients with moderate to severe sleep apnea. This machine delivers air through a mask that is placed over the nose during sleep. The mask does not breathe for the patient. Instead, it pushes air into the patient's mouth when he/she inhales. This air movement keeps the airways open, preventing sleep apnea and snoring. Patients who use a CPAP should tell their doctors if their weight changes. If the patient loses or gains weight, the pressure settings may need to be changed.

Patients may also wear devices over their mouths to control sleep apnea. Some devices bring the jaw forward in order to open the throat and control symptoms of mild obstructive sleep apnea. Patients should talk to their dentists to determine the best oral appliance for them. Patients should visit their dentists every six months for the first year once they find an oral appliance that works for them. After the first year, patients should visit their dentists and healthcare provider annually to make sure that the device is effectively relieving symptoms of sleep apnea.

In addition to CPAP, patients with central sleep apnea may benefit from bilevel positive airway pressure. This device provides a higher air pressure when the patient inhales and a lower pressure when the patient exhales. The goal of this treatment is to strengthen the weak breathing pattern of central sleep apnea. Some machines can be set to automatically provide oxygen if the device detects a breath has not been taken in a certain amount of seconds.

Another airflow device, called an adaptive servoventilation, may be used to treat central sleep apnea and complex sleep apnea. This device detects the patient's normal breathing pattern and stores it in a built-in computer. When the patient falls asleep, the machine uses the stored information to regulate the patient's breathing pattern and prevent sleep apnea.

Moderate to severe sleep apnea may need to be treated with surgery. During surgery, the extra tissue from the throat or nose that is blocking the airway passage is removed.

INTEGRATIVE THERAPIES
Good Scientific Evidence

Melatonin: Melatonin is a neurohormone produced in the brain. Levels of melatonin in the blood are highest before bedtime. Good evidence suggests that melatonin may help treat symptoms of DSPS. Several human studies report that melatonin taken by mouth before bedtime decreases the amount of time it takes to fall asleep ("sleep latency") in elderly individuals with insomnia. However, most studies have not been high quality in their designs, and some research has found limited or no benefits. The majority of trials have been brief in duration (several days long), and long-term effects are not known. There are multiple trials investigating melatonin use in children with various neuropsychiatric disorders, including mental retardation, autism, psychiatric disorders, visual impairment, or epilepsy. Studies have demonstrated reduced time to fall asleep (sleep latency) and increased sleep duration. Well-designed, controlled trials in select patient populations are needed before a stronger or more specific recommendation can be made. Multiple human studies have measured the effects of melatonin supplements on sleep in healthy individuals. A wide range of doses has been used, often taken by mouth 30 to 60 minutes before bedtime. Most trials have been small, brief in duration, and have not been rigorously designed or reported. However, the weight of scientific evidence does suggest that melatonin decreases the time it takes to fall asleep ("sleep latency"), increases the feeling of sleepiness, and may increase the duration of sleep. Better research is needed in this area.

There are rare reports of allergic skin reactions after taking melatonin by mouth. Avoid with bleeding disorders or blood thinners. Use cautiously with seizure disorders, major depression, psychotic disorders, diabetes, low blood sugar levels, glaucoma, high cholesterol, atherosclerosis, or risk of heart disease. Use cautiously if driving or operating heavy machinery.

Music Therapy: During music therapy, music is used to influence physical, emotional, cognitive, and social well-being. It may involve listening to or performing music, with or without the presence of a music therapist. In older adults, music may result in significantly better sleep quality as well as longer sleep duration, greater sleep efficiency, shorter time needed to fall asleep, less sleep disturbance, and less daytime dysfunction. There is also evidence of benefit in elementary-age children who use music during naptime and bedtime. Music therapy may also be as effective as chloral hydrate in inducing sleep or sedation in children undergoing electroencephalographic testing.

Valerian: Valerian is an herb native to Europe and Asia. Today, the herb grows in most parts of the world. Several studies in adults suggest that valerian improves the quality of sleep and reduces the time to fall asleep (sleep latency) for up to four to six weeks. Ongoing nightly use may be more effective than single-dose use, with increasing effects over four weeks. Better effects have been found in poor sleepers. However, most studies have not used scientific ways of measuring sleep improvements, such as sleep pattern data in a sleep laboratory.

Use cautiously if allergic to valerian or other members of the Valerianaceae family. Use cautiously with liver disorders. Use cautiously before surgery. Avoid if driving or operating heavy machinery, as it may cause drowsiness. Avoid if pregnant or breastfeeding.

Unclear or Conflicting Scientific Evidence

5-Hydroxy-L-Tryptophan (5-HTP): 5-HTP is the precursor for serotonin. Serotonin is the brain chemical associated with sleep, mood, movement, feeding, and nervousness. There is insufficient evidence regarding the use of 5-HTP for sleep disorders. Additional studies are needed before a conclusion can be drawn.

Avoid if allergic to 5-HTP. Avoid with eosinophilia, Down syndrome, or mitochondrial encephalomyopathy. Avoid if taking monoamine oxidase inhibitors. Use cautiously with gastrointestinal disorders. Use cautiously with kidney disorders. Use cautiously if taking antidepressants, carbidopa, phenobarbital, pindolol, reserpine, tramadol, or zolpidem. Avoid if pregnant or breastfeeding.

Acupressure, Shiatsu: During acupressure, finger pressure is applied to specific acupoints on the body. Acupressure is used around the world for relaxation, wellness promotion, and the treatment of many health problems. Early evidence suggests that acupressure may help prevent and treat sleep apnea. Larger, well-designed studies are needed before conclusions can be drawn. Patients with known or suspected sleep apnea should consult with their licensed healthcare professionals. Preliminary research supports the use of acupressure for improving sleep quality in elderly patients and possibly in healthy adults of all ages. Better-designed trials are needed to support these results.

With proper training, acupressure appears to be safe if self-administered or administered by an experienced therapist. No serious long-term complications have been reported, according to scientific data. Hand nerve injury and herpes zoster ("shingles") cases have been reported after shiatsu massage. Forceful acupressure may cause bruising.

Acupuncture: Acupuncture is commonly used throughout the world. According to Chinese medicine theory, the human body contains a network of energy pathways through which vital energy, called "chi," circulates. These pathways contain specific points that function like gates, allowing chi to flow through the body. Needles are inserted into these points to regulate the flow of chi. Traditional Chinese medicine commonly uses acupuncture to treat insomnia. A review of the available studies found reports of benefit, but major weaknesses in the design of the research makes the evidence insufficient to recommend for or against acupuncture for insomnia.

Needles must be sterile in order to avoid disease transmission. Avoid with valvular heart disease, medical conditions of unknown origins, or infections. Acupuncture should not be applied to the chest in patients with lung diseases or on any area that may rely on muscle tone to provide stability. Avoid use in infants, young children, and patients with needle phobias. Use cautiously with bleeding disorders, neurological disorders, seizure disorders, or diabetes. Use cautiously in elderly or medically compromised patients. Use cautiously in patients who will drive or operate heavy machinery after acupuncture. Use cautiously if taking anticoagulants. Avoid if pregnant.

Aromatherapy: Aromatherapy refers to many different therapies that use essential oils. The oils are sprayed in the air, inhaled, or applied to the skin. Essential oils are usually mixed with a carrier oil (usually a vegetable oil) or alcohol. Based on human use, lavender and chamomile aromatherapy are thought to be effective sleep aids. Although preliminary small studies suggest some hypnotic effects, there have been no well-designed human trials. Further research is needed before any recommendation can be made. There is early study

of lavender essential oil inhalation as a sedative for patients following intubation (placement of a breathing tube). Evidence in this area is preliminary, and a firm conclusion cannot be drawn.

Essential oils should be administered in a carrier oil to avoid toxicity. Avoid with a history of allergic dermatitis. Use cautiously if driving or operating heavy machinery. Avoid consuming essential oils. Avoid direct contact of undiluted oils with mucous membranes. Use cautiously if pregnant. Sage, rosemary, and juniper oils should be avoided if pregnant or breastfeeding.

Ayurveda: Ayurveda is a form of natural medicine that originated in ancient India more than 5,000 years ago. Ayurveda is an integrated system of techniques that uses diet, herbs, exercise, meditation, yoga, and massage or bodywork to achieve optimal health on all levels. There is evidence from one well-designed study that a traditional Ayurvedic formula (Blissful Sleep, Maharishi Ayurvedic Products International), containing valerian (*Valeriana wallichi*), rose petals (*Rosa centifolia*), muskroot (*Nardostachys jatamansi*), heart-leaved moonseed (*Tinospora cordifolia*), winter cherry (*Withania somnifera*), pepper (*Piper nigrum*), ginger (*Zingiber officinalis*), aloe weed (*Convolvulus pluricaulis*), and licorice root (*Glycyrrhiza glabra*), may decrease sleep latency (time needed to get to sleep) in people with sleep-onset insomnia, with no side effects. Further research is needed to confirm these results.

Ayurvedic herbs should be used cautiously because they are potent, and some constituents can be potentially toxic if taken in large amounts or for a long time. Some herbs imported from India have been reported to contain high levels of toxic metals. Ayurvedic herbs may interact with other herbs, foods, or drugs. A qualified healthcare professional should be consulted before taking.

Chamomile: Chamomile is an herb that has an applelike smell and taste. It is commonly taken as a tea. Traditionally, chamomile preparations, such as tea and essential oil aromatherapy, have been used to treat insomnia. Better research is needed to determine if chamomile is an effective sedative.

Avoid if allergic to chamomile or any related plants, such as aster, chrysanthemum, mugwort, ragweed, or ragwort. Avoid with heart disease, breathing disorders, hormone-sensitive conditions, or central nervous system disorders. Avoid if taking cardiac depressive agents, central nervous system depressants, respiratory depressive agents, or anticoagulants. Use cautiously if taking benzodiazepines, antiarrhythmic medications, calcium channel blockers, alcohol, sedative agents, anxiolytic medications, spasmolytic drugs, oral medications, or agents that are broken down by the liver. Use cautiously if driving or operating machinery. Avoid if pregnant or breastfeeding.

Creatine: Early evidence suggests that creatine may be an effective treatment for sleep apnea. However, further research is needed in this area.

The FDA has advised consumers to consult their physicians before consuming. Avoid with impaired kidney function or dehydration. Avoid in combination with ephedra. Use cautiously with diabetes, seizure disorders, irregular heartbeat (arrhythmia), deep vein thrombosis, kidney stones, or neuromuscular disorders. Use cautiously in athletes. Use cautiously if taking caffeine, nonsteroidal antiinflammatory drugs, nephrotoxic medications, probenecid, trimethoprim, or cimetidine.

Guided Imagery: Guided imagery may involve a number of techniques, including metaphor, storytelling, fantasy, game playing, dream interpretation, drawing, visualization, active imagination, or direct suggestion. Early research supports the value of combined pharmacotherapy and relaxation training in the treatment of insomnia. Further research is necessary in order to make a firm recommendation.

Guided imagery is usually intended to supplement medical care, not to replace it. Guided imagery should not be relied on as the sole therapy for a medical problem. Contact a qualified healthcare provider if mental or physical health is unstable or fragile. Never use guided imagery techniques while driving or doing any other activity that requires strict attention. Use cautiously with physical symptoms that can be brought about by stress, anxiety, or emotional upset because imagery may trigger these symptoms. Individuals who have a history of trauma or abuse or those who feel unusually anxious while practicing guided imagery should speak with their qualified healthcare providers before practicing this therapy.

Hops: The hop is a climbing plant native to Europe, Asia, and North America. The conelike, fruiting bodies of the plant are most commonly used as a flavoring agent in beer. Animal studies report that hops may have sedative and sleep-enhancing (hypnotic) effects. However, little human research has evaluated the effects of hops on sleep quality. Further study is needed in this area before a recommendation can be made.

Avoid if allergic to hops pollen, peanut, chestnut, or banana. Use cautiously with a history of breast cancer, uterine cancer, cervical cancer, prostate cancer, or endometriosis. Use cautiously while driving or operating heavy machinery. Use cautiously with a history of diabetes, stomach ulcers, seizures, or asthma. Hops may affect hormone levels, including estrogen levels. Dust from hops may contain harmful bacteria. Avoid if pregnant or breastfeeding.

Hypnotherapy, Hypnosis: Hypnosis is a trancelike state in which a person becomes more aware and focused and is more open to suggestion. Hypnotherapy has been used to treat health conditions and to change behaviors. Several early studies report that hypnosis may decrease the amount of time it takes to fall asleep, increase the duration of sleep, and improve sleep quality. However, this research is not well designed or reported and cannot be considered definitive.

Use cautiously with mental illnesses (e.g., psychosis/schizophrenia, manic depression, multiple personality disorder, or dissociative disorders) or seizure disorders.

Kundalini Yoga: Kundalini yoga is one of many traditions of yoga that share common roots in ancient Indian philosophy. Kundalini yoga incorporates multiple modalities, including physical postures, chanting, meditation, breathing exercises, and visualization. One small study suggests improved sleep quality with the help of a regimen of Kundalini yoga practices. However, there is insufficient evidence on which to base recommendations for or against this intervention for insomnia.

Avoid exercises that involve stoppage of breath with heart or lung problems, insomnia, poor memory, or concentration. Avoid certain inverted poses with disk disease of the spine, fragile or atherosclerotic neck arteries, extremely high or low blood pressure, glaucoma, detachment of the retina, ear problems, severe osteoporosis, cervical spondylitis, or risk of blood clots. Use cautiously with mental disorders. Kundalini yoga is considered safe and beneficial for use during pregnancy and breastfeeding when practiced under the guidance of expert instruction. Teachers of yoga are generally not medically qualified and should not be regarded as sources of medical advice for the management of clinical conditions.

Lavender: Oils from lavender flowers are used in aromatherapy, baked goods, candles, cosmetics, detergents, jellies, massage oils, perfumes, powders, shampoo, soaps, and teas. Lavender aromatherapy is often promoted as a sleep aid. Although early evidence suggests possible benefits, more research is needed before a firm conclusion can be drawn.

Avoid if allergic or hypersensitive to lavender. Avoid with a history of seizures, bleeding disorders,

S

eating disorders (such as anorexia, bulimia), or anemia (low levels of iron). Avoid if pregnant or breastfeeding.

Lemon Balm: Lemon balm (*Melissa officinalis*) is a lemon-scented herb that is native to southern Europe. High-quality clinical evidence supporting the use of lemon balm as a sedative/hypnotic is lacking. The available evidence is conflicting. Additional study is required to better support the use of lemon balm as a sedative/hypnotic.

Based on available research, lemon balm taken by mouth has been reported to be relatively well tolerated when taken for up to eight weeks. Evidence for topical administration of cream suggested minimal side effects for up to 10 days of application. Avoid if allergic or hypersensitive to lemon balm. Avoid with Graves disease. Avoid if taking thyroid hormone replacement therapy. Use cautiously with glaucoma. Use cautiously while driving or operating heavy machinery. Lemon balm preparations may contain trace amounts of lead. Avoid if pregnant or breastfeeding.

Melatonin: Melatonin is a neurohormone produced in the brain. Levels of melatonin in the blood are highest before bedtime. Studies and individual cases suggest that melatonin, administered in the evening, may correct circadian rhythm disorders in blind patients. Large, well-designed, controlled trials are needed before a stronger recommendation can be made. Study results have been inconsistent, with some studies reporting benefits on sleep latency and subjective sleep quality and other research finding no benefits. Most studies have been small and not rigorously designed or reported. Better research is needed before a firm conclusion can be drawn. Notably, several studies in elderly individuals with insomnia provide preliminary evidence of benefits on sleep latency (discussed above). Limited case reports describe benefits in patients with RBD who receive melatonin. However, better research is needed before a clear conclusion can be drawn. There are several studies of melatonin used for improving sleep quality in people who work irregular shifts, such as emergency room personnel. Results are mixed. Additional research is necessary before a clear conclusion can be drawn.

There are rare reports of allergic skin reactions after taking melatonin by mouth. Avoid with bleeding disorders or if taking blood thinners. Use cautiously with seizures disorders, major depression, psychotic disorders, diabetes, low blood sugar levels, glaucoma, high cholesterol, atherosclerosis, or risk of heart disease. Use cautiously if driving or operating heavy machinery.

Relaxation Therapy: Relaxation techniques include behavioral therapeutic approaches that differ widely in philosophy, methodology, and practice. The primary goal is usually nondirected relaxation. Several human trials suggest that relaxation techniques may be beneficial in people with insomnia, although effects appear to be short lived. Research suggests that relaxation techniques may produce improvements in some aspects of sleep such as sleep latency and time awake after sleep onset. Cognitive forms of relaxation, such as meditation, are reported as being slightly better than somatic forms of relaxation such as progressive muscle relaxation. However, most studies in this area are not well designed or reported. Better research is necessary before a firm conclusion can be drawn.

Avoid with psychiatric disorders such as schizophrenia/psychosis. Jacobson relaxation (flexing specific muscles, holding that position, and then relaxing the muscles) should be used cautiously with illnesses such as heart disease, high blood pressure, or musculoskeletal injury. Relaxation therapy is not recommended as the sole treatment approach for potentially serious medical conditions, and it should not delay the time to diagnosis or treatment with more proven techniques.

Yoga: Yoga is an ancient system of relaxation, exercise, and healing with origins in Indian philosophy. Preliminary research reports that yoga may benefit sleep efficiency, total sleep time, number of awakenings, and quality of sleep. Well-designed research is necessary before a firm recommendation can be made.

Yoga is generally considered to be safe in healthy individuals when practiced appropriately. Avoid some inverted poses with disk disease of the spine, fragile or atherosclerotic neck arteries, extremely high or low blood pressure, glaucoma, detachment of the retina, ear problems, severe osteoporosis, cervical spondylitis, or risk for blood clots. Certain yoga breathing techniques should be avoided with heart or lung disease. Use cautiously with a history of psychotic disorders. Yoga techniques are believed to be safe during pregnancy and breastfeeding when practiced under the guidance of expert instruction. However, poses that put pressure on the uterus, such as abdominal twists, should be avoided in pregnancy.

Fair Negative Scientific Evidence

Vitamin B$_{12}$: Vitamin B$_{12}$ is a water-soluble vitamin and is commonly found in many foods, including fish, shellfish, meats, and dairy products.

According to available evidence, taking vitamin B_{12} orally, in methylcobalamin form, does not seem to be effective for treating DSPS. Supplemental methylcobalamin, with or without bright light therapy, does not seem to help people with primary circadian rhythm sleep disorders.

Vitamin B_{12} is generally considered safe when taken in amounts that do not exceed the recommended dietary allowance. Avoid vitamin B_{12} supplements if allergic to cobalamin, cobalt, or any other product ingredients. Avoid with coronary stents or Leber's disease. Use cautiously if undergoing angioplasty.

PREVENTION

Avoid consuming caffeine (such as coffee or tea) or using nicotine (such as cigarettes) one to two hours before bedtime. Caffeine is a stimulant that may make it difficult to fall asleep.

Performing quiet and relaxing activities, such as taking a warm bath or reading, may help individuals fall asleep quicker. These activities have also been shown to help prevent night terrors in children.

Night terrors usually occur at the same time each night. Parents or bedmates can wake up individuals a few minutes before a night terror is suspected to occur. However, this should not be performed more than once a night because it will disrupt the individual's sleep and may make the individual feel drowsy the next day.

Children who are overtired are more likely to experience night terrors. If a child is not getting enough sleep, try an earlier bedtime or a more regular sleep schedule.

Avoid large meals and excessive fluids before bedtime, as they can cause trouble falling asleep.

Controlling the environment, such as light, noise, and temperature, may help prevent insomnia. Night shift workers especially must address these factors.

Going to bed at the same time daily helps develop the natural circadian rhythm cycle and the sleep/wake cycle.

Maintaining a healthy body weight helps reduce the risk of developing sleep apnea.

Patients with sleep apnea should avoid sleeping on their backs. This position increases the risk of breathing problems during sleep.

Patients with sleep apnea should avoid alcohol and other sedative medications. These relax the muscles in the back of the throat and may interfere with breathing during sleep.

Patients with narcolepsy should also avoid alcohol or drugs, herbs, or supplements that cause drowsiness. These substances may worsen symptoms of narcolepsy.

S

STROKE

CONDITION: Stroke

BACKGROUND

A stroke (or cerebrovascular accident) is much like what a heart attack is to the heart, but to the brain. A stroke involves the sudden interruption of blood flow and oxygen to areas in the brain and can cause brain damage and loss of function. Stroke develops suddenly, usually in a matter of minutes, and causes symptoms such as paralysis, numbness or weakness often affecting one side of the body, confusion, dizziness, speech problems, and loss of vision. How a stroke patient is affected depends on where the stroke occurs in the brain and how much the brain is damaged. There are two main types of strokes: ischemic and hemorrhagic. Ischemic strokes are by far the more common type and occur when a blood clot or plaque (protein, cholesterol, and material) deposit blocks an artery supplying blood to the brain. A hemorrhagic stroke occurs when an artery in the brain bursts, causing blood to flow into the surrounding tissue. The mortality rate is higher for hemorrhagic stroke than for ischemic stroke, with most deaths occurring within the first 48 hours of the event. A transient ischemic attack (TIA) is a type of stroke that usually lasts only 10-20 minutes. TIAs are sometimes considered to be "mini-strokes." While TIAs cause no long-term damage, having a TIA puts an individual at increased risk of acute stroke. Symptoms of TIAs may go unnoticed and may be confused with other conditions such as epilepsy, migraines, or diabetes. Stroke is a medical emergency. Prompt treatment of a stroke could be the difference between life and death. Early treatment can also minimize damage to the brain and potential disability. In the United States, stroke is a leading cause of adult disability and the third-leading cause of death. Only heart disease and cancer cause more deaths annually. Men are 1.25 times more likely to suffer from strokes than women, yet 60% of deaths from stroke occur in women. Eighty percent of strokes are preventable, which would save approximately 600,000 Americans annually.

TYPES OF STROKE

Ischemic Stroke: About 80% of strokes are ischemic strokes. Blood clots or other particles such as cholesterol may block arteries to the brain and cause severely reduced blood flow (ischemia). This deprives the brain cells of necessary oxygen and nutrients and may lead to cell death within minutes.

The most common ischemic strokes include thrombotic stroke and embolic stroke.

Thrombotic Stroke: This type of stroke occurs when a blood clot (thrombus) forms in one of the arteries that supply blood to the brain. Areas damaged by atherosclerosis (hardening of the arteries) are highly susceptible to developing a blood clot. Arteries in the brain or in the neck (carotid arteries) that carry blood to the brain are susceptible. An ischemic stroke may also be caused by plaque (deposits of fat, protein, and other particles in the blood) that narrows or completely clogs an artery. This narrowing is called stenosis.

Embolic Stroke: An embolic stroke occurs when a blood clot or other particle forms in a blood vessel away from the brain (such as the heart) and travels through the blood to eventually lodge in narrower brain arteries (called an embolus). Emboli may often be caused by irregular beating in the heart's two upper chambers (atrial fibrillation). This abnormal heart rhythm can lead to stagnant (sluggish) blood flow and the formation of blood clots.

Hemorrhagic Stroke: Hemorrhage means bleeding. Hemorrhagic stroke occurs when a blood vessel in the brain leaks or breaks open (ruptures). Hemorrhages can result from a number of conditions that affect the blood vessels, including uncontrolled high blood pressure (hypertension) and weak spots in the blood vessel walls (aneurysms). A less common cause of hemorrhage is the rupture of an arteriovenous malformation (AVM), or a malformed tangle of thin-walled blood vessels present at birth. There are two types of hemorrhagic stroke: intracerebral hemorrhage and subarachnoid hemorrhage.

Intracerebral Hemorrhage: In this type of stroke, a blood vessel in the brain bursts and spills into the surrounding brain tissue, damaging cells. Brain cells beyond the leak are deprived of oxygen and are also damaged. High blood pressure is the most common cause of this type of hemorrhagic stroke, causing small arteries inside the brain to become fragile and susceptible to tearing and rupture.

Subarachnoid Hemorrhage: In this type of stroke, bleeding starts in a large artery on or near the membrane surrounding the brain and spills into the space between the surface of the brain and skull. A subarachnoid hemorrhage is often signaled by a sudden, severe "thunderclap" headache. This type of stroke is commonly caused by the rupture of an aneurysm, which can develop with age or result from a genetic predisposition. After a subarachnoid hemorrhage, vessels may go into vasospasm, in which arteries near the hemorrhage widen and narrow erratically, causing brain cell damage by further restricting or blocking blood flow to portions of the brain.

RISK FACTORS AND CAUSES

Age: A stroke can happen to anyone, but the risk of stroke increases with age. After the age of 55, the risk of stroke doubles every 10 years (decade).

Gender: Stroke is more common in men than women, but more women than men die from stroke. Women tend to be older than men when a stroke occurs and are less likely to recover due to age and fragility. Also, use of hormonal replacement therapy, birth control pills, and pregnancy can increase the risk of stroke in women.

Race: African-American individuals are at an risk of stroke almost double that of Caucasians. Hispanics or Asian/Pacific Islanders also have a higher risk of stroke than Caucasians.

Family History: If a relative in a patient's immediate family, such as a parent or sibling, has had a stroke, a patient's risk of stroke is increased.

Previous Stroke or TIA: A prior stroke or a TIA (mini-stroke) increases the chances of another stroke within five years by approximately 25-40%.

High Blood Pressure (Hypertension): High blood pressure is a risk factor for both ischemic and hemorrhagic strokes. It can weaken and damage blood vessels in and around the brain, leaving them vulnerable to atherosclerosis (hardening of the arteries) and hemorrhage. High blood pressure increases stroke risk four to six times and is the most common cause of stroke.

High Cholesterol: High cholesterol levels, especially low-density lipoprotein (LDL) cholesterol ("bad cholesterol"), may increase the risk of atherosclerosis. In excess, LDL and other materials build up on the lining of artery walls, where they may harden into plaques. The blood must now force its way through tiny openings, if any opening at all. When the blood flow is completely blocked, a lack of oxygen causes cells to die and may cause a stroke in the brain.

Smoking: Cigarette smoking places an individual at a much higher risk of stroke than nonsmokers. Smoking contributes to plaques in arteries. Nicotine makes the heart work harder by increasing heart rate and blood pressure. The carbon monoxide in cigarette smoke replaces oxygen in the blood (called hypoxia), decreasing the amount of oxygen delivered to the brain and the rest of the body.

Diabetes: Diabetes is a major risk factor for stroke. People with diabetes are at increased risk of stroke because diabetes may damage arteries, predisposing them to atherosclerosis (hardening of the arteries). Overall, the risk of cardiovascular disease (including stroke) is two-and-a-half times higher in men and women with diabetes compared to people without diabetes.

Obesity: A high body mass index, or the amount of fat on the body, increases the chances of developing high blood pressure, heart disease, atherosclerosis, and diabetes, all of which increase risk factors associated with stroke.

Cardiovascular Disease: Cardiovascular diseases, or coronary heart disease, can increase the risk of a stroke. Coronary heart diseases include congestive heart failure, a previous heart attack, an infection of a heart valve (endocarditis), a particular type of abnormal heart rhythm (atrial fibrillation [AF]), aortic or mitral valve disease, valve replacement, or a hole in the upper chambers of the heart (patent foramen ovale). AF increases stroke risk up to six times because the abnormal pumping of the heart allows blood to pool within the chamber and form clots, which are then pumped into the bloodstream and travel throughout the body and potentially into the brain. About 15% of all people who have a stroke have AF. Additionally, atherosclerosis in blood vessels around the heart may indicate atherosclerosis in other blood vessels, including those in and around the brain.

Elevated Homocysteine Levels: The amino acid homocysteine occurs naturally in the body. Elevated levels of homocysteine have been linked with a high risk of coronary heart disease and stroke. Homocysteine stimulates the growth of cells that help form plaque (deposits of protein and cholesterol) in blood vessels, encouraging blood clotting and blockages in the vessels.

Birth Control Pills and Hormone Therapy: The risk of stroke is higher among women who take birth control pills (oral contraception), especially among smokers and those older than 35. Lower dosages may help decrease the risk of stroke. Hormone replacement therapy used during menopause also carries an increased risk of stroke.

Sickle Cell Anemia: Sickle cell anemia, which can cause blood cells to clump up and block blood vessels, also increases stroke risk. Stroke is the second leading killer of people under 20 who suffer from sickle cell anemia.

Others: Hypercoagulable (increase in blood clotting) conditions such as factor V Leiden (the most common), prothrombin gene mutation (a hereditary condition), elevated levels of fibrinogen (a protein involved in clotting), deficiencies of natural proteins that prevent clotting (called anticoagulant proteins [such as antithrombin, protein C and protein S]), and "sticky" platelets (easily clump together) increase the risk of stroke. Heavy or binge drinking (drinking more than two drinks per day may increase stroke risk by 50%), the use of illicit drugs such as cocaine and methamphetamine, some prescription stimulant drugs (amphetamines), and uncontrolled stress can also increase the risk of stroke.

SIGNS AND SYMPTOMS

Signs and symptoms of a stroke include sudden numbness or weakness of the face, arm, or leg, especially on one side of the body; sudden confusion; trouble speaking or understanding; sudden trouble seeing in one or both eyes; sudden difficulty walking; dizziness; loss of balance or coordination; and sudden, severe headache with no known cause. For most people, stroke has no warning. One possible indicator of a future stroke is a TIA. A TIA is a temporary interruption of blood flow to some part of the brain. TIA signs and symptoms are similar to stroke but last for a shorter period of time (usually several minutes to 24 hours), and then disappear with no apparent permanent effects. Individuals who have had a TIA are at a very high risk of having a stroke.

DIAGNOSIS

Physical Examination and Tests: Risk factors of stroke are evaluated, including high blood pressure, high cholesterol levels, diabetes, medications, elevated levels of homocysteine, and obesity. Stroke symptoms are documented after the occurrence, often using scoring systems such as the National Institutes of Health Stroke Scale, the Cincinnati Stroke Scale, and the Los Angeles Prehospital Stroke Screen. These tests ask medical history questions and measure left and right paralysis (loss of muscle control and movement). The latter is used by emergency medical technicians to determine whether a patient needs transport to a stroke center (a hospital specializing in stroke).

Carotid Ultrasonography: This procedure evaluates blood flow using a wandlike device (transducer) that sends high-frequency sound waves into the neck. Narrowing or clotting in the carotid arteries can be determined.

Arteriography: Arteriography views arteries in the brain not normally able to be seen in x-rays. During this procedure, a thin, flexible tube (catheter) is inserted through a small incision, usually in the groin

area. The catheter is manipulated through the major arteries and into the carotid or vertebral artery. A dye is then injected through the catheter to provide x-ray images of the arteries.

Computerized Tomographic Angiography (CTA): In CTA, a dye is injected into the blood and x-ray beams create a three-dimensional image of the blood vessels in the neck and brain. CTA is used to look for aneurysms (weakened or ruptured blood vessel) or AVMs (masses of abnormal blood vessels growing in the brain) and to evaluate arteries for narrowing. CT scanning, which is done without dye, can provide images of the brain and show hemorrhages but without as much detailed information about the blood vessels.

Magnetic Resonance Imaging: Magnetic resonance imaging uses a strong magnetic field to generate a three-dimensional view of the brain. This test is sensitive for detecting an area of brain tissue damaged by an ischemic stroke. Magnetic resonance angiography uses this magnetic field and a dye injected into the veins to evaluate arteries in the neck and brain.

COMPLICATIONS

A stroke may cause physical or behavioral changes in an individual. Physical changes are dependent on the side and part of the brain affected by the stroke. Stroke may affect the ability to process language, reading, articulation (ability to enunciate words), or even the ability to swallow. Behavioral changes can include depression and other mental illnesses.

Right Brain: Different sides of the brain control opposite sides of the body. Therefore, a stroke affecting one side will result in neurological (nervous system or nerve) complications on the side of the body if affects. For example, if the stroke occurs in the brain's right side, the left side of the body will be affected. The symptoms include paralysis on the left side of the body, vision problems, quick, inquisitive behavioral style, and memory loss.

Left Brain: If the stroke occurs in the left side of the brain, the right side of the body (and the left side of the face) will be affected, producing effects including paralysis on the right side of the body, speech/language problems, slow, cautious behavioral style, and memory loss.

TREATMENT

The earlier the treatment is received, the higher the chance of survival and recovery. It is imperative to seek medical attention immediately if a stroke is suspected. Helping identify a stroke victim includes asking the individual to smile, to raise both arms and keep them raised, or to speak a simple sentence (coherently). Guidelines for stroke prevention have been developed by the American Heart Association. Primary prevention focuses on preventing a stroke, while secondary prevention focuses on preventing stroke in those with a history of stroke or TIA.

Ischemic Stroke

Emergency treatment for an ischemic stroke depends on the location and cause of the clot. Measures are taken to stabilize vital signs, including intravenous (into the veins) fluids and medications such as clot-dissolving drugs and antiplatelet drugs.

Tissue Plasminogen Activator (t-PA): If the stroke is diagnosed within three hours of the start of symptoms, a clot-dissolving medication called t-PA is usually given, which may increase the chance of survival and recovery. t-PA is not safe for hemorrhagic stroke (bleeding in the brain), as use of t-PA would be life-threatening by increasing bleeding.

Antiplatelet Drugs: Platelets are cells in the blood that initiate clot formation. Antiplatelet drugs make the platelets less sticky and are therefore less likely to clump (aggregate) and form clots. The most frequently used antiplatelet medication is over-the-counter aspirin in doses of 81 to 325 milligrams daily. Aggrenox, a prescription combination product of low-dose aspirin and the antiplatelet agent dipyridamole, may also be used to reduce blood clotting. Other antiplatelet drugs, such as clopidogrel (Plavix) or ticlopidine (Ticlid), may also be utilized. The drugs may be used in combination. However, initiation of these therapies is not recommended within 24 hours of treatment with t-PA due to an increase in serious bleeding problems. Side effects include increased risk of bleeding. There are many possible drug and supplement interactions while taking antiplatelet therapy.

Anticoagulants: Anticoagulation treatments slow the time that it takes for the blood to clot. The drugs used in this class include heparin and warfarin (Coumadin). They affect the mechanism of clotting differently than antiplatelet medications. Heparin, an injection, is a fast-acting agent and is used short term in the hospital, while warfarin, taken by mouth, acts more slowly and is used over a longer term. These drugs have a profound effect on blood clotting and require that patients work closely with their providers to ensure that they are within therapeutic range as well as to reduce the risk of adverse bleeding events. As with the antiplatelet medications, there are many possible drug and supplement interactions while taking anticoagulant therapy.

Biological Therapy: Biologic therapy treats the immune system. The use of abciximab (ReoPro) in acute stroke is being studied. This injectable drug has antiplatelet activity and must be used within six hours of stroke.

Other Medications: Other medications may be given to control blood sugar levels (such as oral blood sugar–lowering drugs), fever (including acetaminophen [Tylenol]), and seizures (such as anticonvulsant drugs). In general, high blood pressure is not treated immediately unless systolic pressure is greater than 220 millimeters of mercury (mm Hg) and diastolic is more than 120 mm Hg (reading as 220/120 mm Hg).

Surgical and Other Procedures: Procedures to open up the artery that has been moderately to severely narrowed by plaque (deposits of cholesterol and protein in the blood) may be necessary. These include carotid endarterectomy and angioplasty.

Carotid Endarterectomy: After a stroke has occurred, an incision in the neck is made to expose the carotid artery. The artery is opened and the plaques are removed, thereby reducing the risk of ischemic stroke. However, in addition to the usual risks associated with any surgery, a carotid endarterectomy itself can also trigger a stroke or heart attack by releasing a blood clot or fatty debris in blood vessels in the brain. As a standard practice, surgeons now place filters at strategic points in the bloodstream to "catch" any material that may break free during the procedure, preventing it from traveling to the heart or brain.

Angioplasty: Angioplasty widens the inside of an artery leading to the brain (usually the carotid artery). During this procedure, a balloon-tipped catheter is maneuvered into the obstructed area of the suspected artery. The balloon is inflated, compressing the plaques against the artery walls. A metallic mesh tube (stent) is usually left inside the artery following the procedure to prevent recurrent narrowing. Stents can stay in for many years but occasionally must be replaced. Anticoagulant drugs such as aspirin and/or clopidogrel (Plavix) are commonly used after stent placement.

Hemorrhagic Stroke

Surgery may be used to treat a hemorrhagic stroke or prevent recurrence. The most common procedures include aneurysm (weakened or ruptured blood vessel) clipping and AVM (masses of abnormal blood vessels growing in the brain) removal; both surgeries carry high risks such as an increase in bleeding and damage to the brain, causing long-term complications such as paralysis (loss of muscle control and use) and behavioral changes.

Surgical AVM Removal: Surgical removal of a smaller AVM from a more accessible portion of the brain can eliminate the risk of rupture, lowering the overall risk of hemorrhagic stroke. Other treatment options for AVMs include radiation or embolization, in which the small arteries supplying the blood to the AVM are blocked with clamps, shrinking the AVM and reducing the chances of rupture.

Aneurysm Clipping: A tiny clamp is placed at the base of the aneurysm, isolating it from the circulation of the artery. The clamp is attached to the vessels to keep it from bursting (rupturing) or bleeding.

Coiling: During coil embolization, tiny, soft platinum coils are placed within a bulging brain aneurysm in order to relieve pressure from circulating blood on the walls of the aneurysm and to prevent rupture. The coils are guided to the aneurysm through the use of a catheter inserted into the femoral artery at the groin. Through the use of precision radiologic monitors and three-dimensional imaging, the coils are advanced to the aneurysm.

Recovery and Rehabilitation: Stroke rehabilitation (for both ischemic and hemorrhagic stroke) is the process by which patients with stroke-induced disabilities undergo treatment to help them regain and relearn the skills necessary for everyday living. It also aims to help the survivor understand and adapt to difficulties such as speech and movement, prevent secondary complications, and educate family members to play a supporting role. Following a stroke, the period of recovery and rehabilitation necessary varies between patients depending on the area of the brain involved and the amount of tissue damaged. Harm to the right side of the brain may impair movement and sensation on the left side of the body. Damage to brain tissue on the left side may affect movement on the right side; this damage may also cause speech and language disorders. In addition, individuals who have experienced a stroke may experience problems with breathing, swallowing, balancing, and hearing and loss of vision, or bladder or bowel function. Recovery may take years. Some may recover in full while others may not progress at all. This depends on each individual and the extent of the stroke damage.

INTEGRATIVE THERAPIES
Unclear or Conflicting Scientific Evidence

Acupuncture: The practice of acupuncture, or the insertion of needles into the body to move energy, or "chi," in a particular area, originated in China 5,000 years ago. Acupuncture has been used traditionally in China for treatment of stroke complications such as paralysis (loss of muscle control and use). Several studies have been conducted in stroke rehabilitation, with positive results. More studies are needed to determine what can be expected in the use of acupuncture with regard to this application.

Aortic Acid: Aortic extract is derived from the hearts of animals, usually sheep, cows, or pigs. There are many substances included in aortic acid. Mesoglycan, a preparation of glycosaminoglycans, is the most studied of these constituents. Mesoglycan has shown activity in anticoagulation (blood thinning) and increasing blood vessel health. Preliminary randomized, controlled studies also indicate that it may be helpful in reducing recurring ischemic cerebral attacks (stroke) and improving quality of life. However, some nonsubjective tests do not show any benefit by mesoglycan. High-quality studies are needed.

Arnica: Arnica (*Arnica montana*) is a widely used herbal supplement. It is also available as a homeopathic drug approved by the U.S. Food and Drug Administration. Homeopathic drugs are very dilute substances and have no apparent side effects or adverse reactions. Homeopathic arnica has been used in stroke recovery. More research is needed.

Betel Nut: Betel nut comes from the betel palm (*Areca catechu*). Several poor-quality studies report the use of betel nut taken by mouth in patients recovering from stroke. In light of the potential toxicities of betel nut, additional evidence is needed in this area. Constituents of areca may be potentially carcinogenic. Long-term use has been associated with oral submucous fibrosis as well as the formation of precancerous oral lesions and squamous cell carcinoma. Acute effects of betel chewing include worsening of asthma, low blood pressure, and rapid heartbeat.

Choline: Choline is an essential nutrient related to the water-soluble B-complex vitamins. The largest dietary source of choline is egg yolk. Though many studies have found promising results, others have not shown statistical significance when assessing choline for the treatment of acute ischemic stroke. Further well-designed trials are needed. Choline supplements are not recommended during pregnancy or breastfeeding unless otherwise advised by a doctor.

Ginkgo: Ginkgo (*Ginkgo biloba*) has been used medicinally for thousands of years. Today, it is one of the top-selling herbs in the United States. Laboratory studies suggest that ginkgo may be helpful immediately following strokes because of possible antioxidant or blood vessel effects. However, initial study of ginkgo in people having strokes found no benefits, and ginkgo has been reported to increase intracranial bleeding. Further research is needed in this area. Caution is advised when taking ginkgo supplements, as numerous adverse effects, including subarachnoid hemorrhage and drug interactions, are possible. Ginkgo supplements are not recommended during pregnancy or breastfeeding unless otherwise advised by a doctor.

L-Carnitine: L-carnitine, or acetyl-L-carnitine, is an amino acid that occurs naturally in the body. We get L-carnitine from foods such as meat and dairy products. There are a limited number of studies showing a positive effect of L-carnitine on cerebral blood flow and metabolism of the brain in patients who have suffered from stroke. Additional study is required.

Melatonin: The natural hormone melatonin aids in the regulation of sleep/wake cycles (circadian rhythm). Theories suggest that the antioxidant properties of melatonin may reduce the amount of neurological damage patients experience after stroke. In addition, melatonin levels may be decreased in people immediately after stroke, and it has thus been suggested that melatonin supplementation may be beneficial, although this has not been shown in humans. A laboratory animal study found that melatonin supplementation decreased the brain tissue damage caused by stroke. At this time, the effects of melatonin supplements given immediately after a stroke are not clear. Caution is advised when taking melatonin supplements, as numerous adverse effects including drug interactions are possible. Melatonin is not recommended during pregnancy or breastfeeding unless otherwise advised by a doctor. Healthcare professionals recommend using melatonin for more than four to six weeks.

Moxibustion: Moxibustion is a healing technique employed across the diverse traditions of acupuncture and oriental medicine for over 2,000 years. Moxibustion uses the principle of heat to stimulate circulation and break up congestion or stagnation of blood and chi. Moxibustion is more closely related to acupuncture, as it is applied to specific acupuncture points. One study suggests that electroacupuncture may reduce spasticity in patients who have experienced stroke, but there was no evidence that moxibustion offered any additive benefit. More studies are needed to determine whether or not moxibustion may contribute to recovery from stroke.

Omega-3 Fatty Acids: Omega-3 fatty acids are essential fatty acids found in some plants and fish. Caution is advised when taking omega-3 supplements, as numerous adverse effects including an increase in bleeding and drug interactions are possible. Omega-3 supplements should not be used if pregnant or breastfeeding unless otherwise directed by a doctor. Several large epidemiological studies have examined the effects of omega-3 fatty acid intake on stroke risk. Some studies suggest benefits, while others do not. Effects are likely on ischemic (lack of blood flow) or thrombotic (blood clots) stroke risk, and very large intakes of omega-3 fatty acids may actually increase the risk of hemorrhagic (bleeding) stroke. At this time, it is unclear if there are benefits in people with or without a history of stroke, or if effects of fish oil are comparable to other treatment strategies. If the individual has an allergy to fish, other sources of omega-3 fatty acids include eggs and walnuts.

Physical Therapy: Physical therapy was first documented in China around 3000 BC with the use of joint manipulation and massage to relieve pain. Physical therapy is a popular choice for patients undergoing stroke rehabilitation. It aims to strengthen weakened muscle groups through repetitive motion, increase overall function including cognitive function, and improve gait and walking. Available studies have used a variety of exercises, which makes it nearly impossible to compare the evidence. Furthermore, physical therapy is often used as a control group in these studies. Higher quality studies are needed.

Psychotherapy: Psychotherapy is an interactive process between a person and a qualified mental health professional (psychiatrist, psychologist, clinical social worker, licensed counselor, or other trained practitioner). Its purpose is the exploration of thoughts, feelings, and behavior for the purpose problem solving or achieving higher levels of functioning. Studies show mixed results about the efficacy of cognitive behavioral psychotherapy for depression following stroke. More research needs to be done in this area.

Relaxation Therapy: Relaxation techniques include behavioral therapeutic approaches that differ widely in philosophy, methodology, and practice. The primary goal is usually nondirected relaxation. Most techniques share the components of repetitive focus (on a word, sound, prayer phrase, body sensation, or muscular activity), adoption of a passive attitude towards intruding thoughts, and return to the focus. Research suggests that relaxation techniques may help stroke victims with facial paralysis recover more rapidly. Better research is necessary before a firm conclusion can be drawn.

S

Transcutaneous Electrical Nerve Stimulation (TENS): TENS is a noninvasive technique in which a low-voltage electrical current is delivered through wires from a small power unit to electrodes located on the skin. Studies of TENS in poststroke rehabilitation report inconsistent findings, and benefits have not consistently been demonstrated. Additional research is necessary before a clear conclusion can be reached.

Vitamin C (Ascorbic Acid): There are variable results of studies that have measured the association of vitamin C intake and risk of stroke. Some studies have reported no benefits, while other research reports that daily low-dose vitamin C may reduce the risk of death from stroke. Vitamin C is an antioxidant; antioxidants help protect the blood vessels from fragility (weakening) and damage. Additional research is necessary before a clear conclusion can be reached.

Yoga: Yoga is an ancient system of relaxation, exercise, and healing with origins in Indian philosophy. Preliminary research reports that yoga may benefit sleep efficiency, total sleep time, number of awakenings, and quality of sleep. Well-designed research is necessary before a firm recommendation can be made.

LIFESTYLE CHANGES AND PREVENTION

Guidelines for stroke prevention have been developed by the American Heart Association. Primary prevention focuses on preventing a stroke, while secondary prevention focuses on preventing stroke in those with a history of stroke or TIA.

High Blood Pressure (Hypertension) Control: One of the most important interventions that can be made in prevention of strokes is the reduction of high blood pressure. Lowering a patient's blood pressure can help prevent a subsequent TIA or stroke. Exercising, managing stress, maintaining a healthy weight, and limiting sodium and alcohol intake are all ways to keep hypertension in check. Medications to treat hypertension, such as diuretics, angiotensin-converting enzyme inhibitors, and angiotensin receptor blockers may also be utilized.

Cholesterol and Saturated Fat Intake Reduction: Eating less cholesterol and fat, especially saturated fat, may help prevent further buildup of plaque in the arteries. Medications from the statin drug-class, which work by inhibiting an enzyme (3-hydroxy-3-methylglutaryl coenzyme A reductase) that is used to make cholesterol in the body may be prescribed to help reduce unhealthy cholesterol levels.

Smoking Cessation: Quitting smoking reduces the risk of stroke. Smoking can double or triple the chances of having a stroke.

Diabetes Control: Managing diabetes with diet, exercise, weight control, and medication is essential. Strict control of blood sugar may reduce damage to the brain in the case of a stroke. Increases in blood sugar levels can damage fragile blood vessels in the body, including the brain, and increase the risk of rupture (breaking open).

Weight Control: Being overweight contributes to other risk factors for stroke, such as high blood pressure, cardiovascular disease, and diabetes. Weight loss of as little as 10 pounds may lower blood pressure and improve cholesterol levels.

Exercise: Exercise can lower blood pressure, increase the level of high-density lipoprotein cholesterol ("good cholesterol"), and improve the overall health of blood vessels and heart. It also helps control weight, control diabetes, and reduce stress. Thirty minutes daily of exercise is normally recommended, but each individual should develop an exercise program for his/her own physical ability. A study reported that men with the highest degree of physical fitness were more than three times less likely than men with the lowest degree of physical fitness to have a stroke.

Stress Management: Stress can cause an increase in blood pressure along with increasing the blood's tendency to clot. Finding ways to decrease stress is important in preventing stroke, especially if an individual has other risk factors.

Alcohol Consumption: Alcohol can be both a risk factor and a preventive measure for stroke. Binge drinking and heavy alcohol consumption increase the risk of high blood pressure and of ischemic and hemorrhagic strokes. However, drinking small to moderate amounts of alcohol (one to two drinks a day) can increase high-density lipoprotein cholesterol and decrease the blood's clotting tendency. Both factors can contribute to a reduced risk of ischemic stroke.

Illicit Drugs Elimination: Street drugs, such as methamphetamine (crystal meth, ice), cocaine, and ecstasy are established risk factors for a TIA or a stroke.

Dietary Modification: Eat healthy foods. A healthy diet should include five or more daily servings of fruits and vegetables, foods rich in soluble fiber (such as oatmeal and beans), foods rich in calcium (dairy products, spinach), soy products (such as tempeh, miso, tofu and soy milk), and foods rich in omega-3 fatty acids, including cold water fish such as salmon, mackerel, and tuna. Pregnant women and women who plan to become pregnant in the next several years should limit their weekly intake of cold water fish because of the potential for mercury contamination, which can cause fetal damage.

AIDSinfo. http://aidsinfo.nih.gov. Accessed November 29, 2007.

AIDS.org. http://www.aids.org. Accessed November 29, 2007.

Alcoholics Anonymous. http://www.alcoholics-anonymous.org. Accessed October 9, 2007.

Allard ML, Jeejeebhoy KN, Sole MJ. The management of conditioned nutritional requirements in heart failure. Heart Fail Rev. 2006;11(1):75-82.

Alzheimer's Association. http://www.alz.org. Accessed May 14, 2007.

American Academy of Allergy Asthma & Immunology. http://www.aaaai.org. Accessed March 11, 2007.

American Academy of Child and Adolescent Psychiatry. http://www.aacap.org.

American Academy of Dermatology. http://www.aad.org. Accessed November 27, 2007.

American Academy of Family Physicians. http://familydoctor.org. Accessed November 15, 2007.

American Academy of Family Physicians. http://www.aafp.org. Accessed March 29, 2007.

American Academy of Family Physicians. Information from your family doctor. Nightmares and night terrors in children. Am Fam Physician. 2005 Oct 1; 72(7):1322.

American Academy of Orthopedic Surgeons. http://www.aaos.org. Accessed May 25, 2007.

American Academy of Pediatrics. http://www.aap.org. Accessed August 28, 2007.

American Academy of Pediatrics Committee on Infectious Diseases. Antiviral therapy and prophylaxis for influenza in children. Pediatrics. 2007 Apr;119(4):852-60.

American Arthritis Society. http://www.americanarthritis.org. Accessed June 20, 2007.

American Association of Neurological Surgeons. http://www.neurosurgerytoday.org. Accessed May 25, 2007.

American Cancer Society. http://www.cancer.org. Accessed December 28, 2007.

American Chiropractic Association. http://www.amerchiro.org. Accessed May 25, 2007.

American Chronic Pain Foundation. http://www.theacpa.org. Accessed July 18, 2007.

American College of Gastroenterology. http://www.gi.org. Accessed July 23, 2007.

American College of Obstetricians and Gynecologists. http://www.acog.org. Accessed September 3, 2007.

American Dermatological Association. http://www.amer-derm-assn.org. Accessed May 10, 2007.

American Diabetes Association. http://www.diabetes.org. Accessed July 27, 2007.

American Foundation for AIDS Research. http://www.amfar.org. Accessed November 29, 2007.

American Gastroenterological Association. http://www.gastro.org. Accessed July 18, 2007.

American Hair Loss Association. http://www.americanhairloss.org. Accessed November 27, 2007.

American Heart Association. http://www.americanheart.org. Accessed August 4, 2007.

American Lung Association. http://www.lungusa.org. Accessed August 28, 2007.

American Lung Association. Epidemiology & Statistics Unit, Research and Program Services. Trends in Asthma Morbidity and Mortality. May 2005. http://www.lungusa.org. Accessed April 23, 2007.

American Pain Foundation. http://www.painfoundation.org. Accessed July 3, 2007.

American Pregnancy Association. http://www.americanpregnancy.org. Accessed September 2, 2007.

American Psychiatric Association. http://www.psych.org.

American Sleep Apnea Association. http://www.sleepapnea.org. Accessed October 7, 2007.

American Social Health Association. http://www.ashastd.org. Accessed July 19, 2007.

American Society for Metabolic and Bariatric Surgery. http://www.asbs.org. Accessed September 4, 2007.

American Society of Addiction Medicine. http://www.asam.org. Accessed October 9, 2007.

American Stroke Association. http://www.strokeassociation.org. Accessed April 25, 2007.

American Urological Association. http://www.auanet.org. Accessed November 15, 2007.

Andersen RE, Crespo CJ, Bartlett SJ, et al. Relationship between body weight gain and significant knee, hip, and back pain in older Americans. Obes Res. 2003;11(10):1159-62.

Anxiety Disorders of America. http://www.adaa.org.

Arkema JM, Paget WJ, Meijer A, et al. Seasonal influenza beginning in Europe: report from EISS. Euro Surveill. 2007 Jan 25;12(1):E070125.3.

Arthritis Foundation Homepage. http://www.arthritis.org. Accessed June 20, 2007.

Assimakopoulos K, Panayiotopoulos S, Iconomou G, et al. Assessing sexual function in obese women preparing for bariatric surgery. Obes Surg. 2006 Aug;16(8):1087-91.

Association for the Advancement of Retired Persons. http://www.aarp.org. Accessed June 21, 2007.

Asthma and Allergy Foundation of America. Asthma. http://www.aafa.org. Accessed April 23, 2007.

Atkinson M, Yanney M, Stephenson T, et al. Effective treatment strategies for paediatric community-acquired pneumonia. Expert Opin Pharmacother. 2007;8(8):1091-101.

Baldwin DS, Hutchinson J, Donaldson K, et al. Selective serotonin re-uptake inhibitor treatment-emergent sexual dysfunction: randomized double-blind placebo-controlled parallel-group fixed-dose study of a potential adjuvant compound, VML-670. J Psychopharmacol. 2008 Jan;22(1):55-63.

Bank AJ, Kelly AS, Kaiser DR, et al. The effects of quinapril and atorvastatin on the responsiveness to sildenafil in men with erectile dysfunction. Vasc Med. 2006 Nov;11(4):251-7.

Barkan AL. Growth hormone as an anti-aging therapy-do the benefits outweigh the risks? Nat Clin Pract Endocrinol Metab. 2007 Jul;3(7):508-9.

Barr KP. Review of upper and lower extremity musculoskeletal pain problems. Phys Med Rehabil Clin N Am. 2007;18(4):747-60.

Becker JM. Surgical therapy for ulcerative colitis and Crohn's disease. Gastroenterol Clin North Am. 1999 Jun;28(2):371-90, viii-ix.

Berner MM, Hagen M, Kriston L. Management of sexual dysfunction due to antipsychotic drug therapy. Cochrane Database Syst Rev. 2007;(1):CD003546.

Bertone-Johnson ER, Hankinson SE, Bendich A, et al. Calcium and vitamin D intake and risk of incident premenstrual syndrome. Arch Intern Med. 2005;165(11):1246-52.

Bianchi C, Penno G, Romero F, et al. Treating the metabolic syndrome. Expert Rev Cardiovasc Ther. 2007;5(3):491-506.

Bijlsma JW, Knahr K. Strategies for the prevention and management of osteoarthritis of the hip and knee. Best Pract Res Clin Rheumatol. 2007 Feb;21(1):59-76.

Blanchard EB, Appelbaum KA, Radnitz CL, et al. Placebo-controlled evaluation of abbreviated progressive muscle relaxation and of relaxation combined with cognitive therapy in the treatment of tension headache. J Consult Clin Psychol. 1990;58(2):210-5.

The Body: The Complete HIV/AIDS Resource. http://www.thebody.com. Accessed November 29, 2007.

Boekholdt SM, Sandhu MS, Day NE, et al. Physical activity, C-reactive protein levels and the risk of future coronary artery disease in apparently healthy men and women: the EPIC-Norfolk prospective population study. Eur J Cardiovasc Prev Rehabil. 2006;13(6):970-6.

Bogart LM, Berry SH, Clemens JQ. Symptoms of interstitial cystitis, painful bladder syndrome and similar diseases in women: a systematic review. J Urol. 2007 Feb;177(2):450-6.

Boney CM, Verma A, Tucker R, et al. Metabolic syndrome in childhood: association with birth weight, maternal obesity, and gestational diabetes mellitus. Pediatrics. 2005;115(3):e290-6.

Brown SA, Guise TA. Drug insight: the use of bisphosphonates for the prevention and treatment of osteoporosis in men. Nat Clin Pract Urol. 2007;4(6):310-20.

Bruno D, Feeney KJ. Management of postmenopausal symptoms in breast cancer survivors. Semin Oncol. 2006;33(6):696-707.

Carrero JJ, Fonolla J, Marti JL, et al. Intake of fish oil, oleic acid, folic acid, and vitamins B6 and E for 1 year decreases plasma C-reactive protein and reduces coronary heart disease risk factors in male patients in a cardiac rehabilitation program. J Nutr. 2007;137(2):384-90.

Catalan V, Gomez-Ambrosi J, Rotellar F, et al. Validation of endogenous control genes in human adipose tissue: relevance to obesity and obesity-associated type 2 diabetes mellitus. Horm Metab Res. 2007;39(7):495-500.

Centers for Disease Control and Prevention. Guidelines for laboratory test result reporting of human immunodeficiency virus type 1 ribonucleic acid determination. Recommendations from a CDC working group. MMWR Recomm Rep. 2001 Nov 16;50 (RR-20):1-12.

Centers for Disease Control and Prevention. http://www.cdc.gov. Accessed November 29, 2007.

Centers for Disease Control. Surveillance for Asthma—United States, 1960-1995, MMWR. 1998; 47(SS-1). http://www.cdc.gov. Accessed April 5, 2007.

Chakrabarty S, Zoorob R. Fibromyalgia. Am Fam Physician. 2007;76(2):247-54.

Chakravorty SS, Rye DB. Narcolepsy in the older adult: epidemiology, diagnosis and management. Drugs Aging. 2003;20(5):361-76.

Chancellor MB, Yoshimura N. Treatment of interstitial cystitis. Urology. 2004 Mar;63(3 Suppl 1):85-92.

Chen H, O'Reilly E, McCullough ML, et al. Consumption of dairy products and risk of Parkinson's disease. Am J Epidemiol. 2007;165(9):998-1006.

Clark KL. Nutritional considerations in joint health. Clin Sports Med. 2007;26(1):101-18.

The Cleveland Clinic Health Information Center. Allergy Overview. http://my.clevelandclinic.org/disorders/allergies/hic_Allergy_Overview.aspx. Accessed March 11, 2007.

Cline JS. Sexually transmitted diseases: will this problem ever go away? N C Med J. 2006 Sep-Oct;67(5):353-8.

Combe B. Early rheumatoid arthritis: strategies for prevention and management. Best Pract Res Clin Rheumatol. 2007 Feb;21(1):27-42.

Compton MT, Weiss PS, West JC, et al. The associations between substance use disorders, schizophrenia-spectrum disorders, and axis IV psychosocial problems. Soc Psychiatry Psychiatr Epidemiol. 2005 Dec;40(12):939-46.

Cossu G, Sampaolesi M. New therapies for Duchenne muscular dystrophy: challenges, prospects and clinical trials. Trends Mol Med. 2007 Dec;13(12):520-6.

A critique of low-carbohydrate ketogenic weight reduction regimens. A review of Dr. Atkins' diet revolution. JAMA. 1973;224(10):1415-1419.

Crohn's and Colitis Foundation of America. http://www.ccfa.org. Accessed April 5, 2007.

Cuschieri A. Non-surgical options for the management of gallstone disease: an overview. Surg Endosc. 1990;4(3):127-31; discussion 136-40.

Dauchet L, Amouyel P, Hercberg S, et al. Fruit and vegetable consumption and risk of coronary heart disease: a meta-analysis of cohort studies. J Nutr. 2006;136(10):2588-93.

Dawber RP. Guidance for the management of hirsutism. Curr Med Res Opin. 2005 Aug;21(8):1227-34.

De la Rosette JJ. Extracorporeal shock wave lithotripsy and the "end of the stone age." Eur Urol. 2006 Sep;50(3):400-1.

DermNet NZ. Dermatitis. http://dermnetnz.org. Accessed May 10, 2007.

Dey AN, Schiller JS, Tai DA. Summary health statistics for U.S. children: National

Health Interview Survey, 2002. Vital Health Stat 10. 2004 Mar;(221):1-78.

DiMeo PJ. Psychosocial and relationship issues in men with erectile dysfunction. Urol Nurs. 2006 Dec;26(6):442-6, 453; quiz 447.

Does eflornithine help women face hirsutism? Drug Ther Bull. 2007 Aug;45(8):62-4.

Douglas S. Premenstrual syndrome. Evidence-based treatment in family practice. Can Fam Physician. 2002 Nov;48:1789-97.

Duffey KJ, Gordon-Larsen P, Jacobs DR Jr, et al. Differential associations of fast food and restaurant food consumption with 3-y change in body mass index: the Coronary Artery Risk Development in Young Adults Study. Am J Clin Nutr. 2007;85(1):201-8.

Eccles R, Pedersen A, Regberg D, et al. Efficacy and safety of topical combinations of ipratropium and xylometazoline for the treatment of symptoms of runny nose and nasal congestion associated with acute upper respiratory tract infection. Am J Rhinol. 2007 Jan-Feb;21(1):40-5.

Elizabeth Glaser Pediatric AIDS Foundation. http://www.pedaids.org. Accessed November 29, 2007.

Enders M, Regnath T, Tewald F, et al. Syphilis. Dtsch Med Wochenschr. 2007 Jan 19;132(3):77-8.

Estevez M, Gardner KL. Update on the genetics of migraine. Hum Genet. 2004;114(3):225-35.

Family Caregiver Alliance. http://www.caregiver.org. Accessed May 14, 2007.

Fehring RJ, Schneider M, Raviele K, et al. Efficacy of cervical mucus observations plus electronic hormonal fertility monitoring as a method of natural family planning. Obstet Gynecol Neonatal Nurs. 2007 Mar-Apr;36(2):152-60.

Femiano F, Gombos F, Scully C. Recurrent herpes labialis: a pilot study of the efficacy of zinc therapy. J Oral Pathol Med. 2005; 34(7):423-5.

Fisher Center For Alzheimer's Research Foundation. http://www.alz.org. Accessed May 14, 2007.

Flipp E, Raczynski P, El Midaoui A, et al. Chlamydia trachomatis infection in sexually active adolescents and young women.

Med Wieku Rozwoj. 2005 Jan-Mar;9(1):57-64.

Flora SJ. Role of free radicals and antioxidants in health and disease. Cell Mol Biol (Noisy-le-grand). 2007 Apr 15;53(1):1-2.

Frank-Herrmann P, Heil J, Gnoth C, et al. The effectiveness of a fertility awareness based method to avoid pregnancy in relation to a couple's sexual behavior during the fertile time: a prospective longitudinal study. Hum Reprod. 2007 May;22(5):1310-9.

Fronczek R, van der Zande WL, van Dijk JG, et al. Narcolepsy: a new perspective on diagnosis and treatment. Article in Dutch. Ned Tijdschr Geneeskd. 2007 Apr 14;151(15):856-61.

Fux CA, Christen A, Zgraggen S, et al. Effect of tenofovir on renal glomerular and tubular function. AIDS. 2007 Jul 11;21(11):1483-5.

Gagnon J. Gallstones: a choice of treatments. Can Nurse. 1992 Oct;88(9):38-40.

Gallstones: advances in treatments. More and better choices in the arsenal against the intense pain of a gallbladder attack. Health News. 2007 May;13(5):9-10.

Gamblers Anonymous. http://www.gamblersanonymous.org. Accessed October 9, 2007.

Giannini C, de Giorgis T, Mohn A, et al. Role of physical exercise in children and adolescents with diabetes mellitus. J Pediatr Endocrinol Metab. 2007;20(2):173-84.

Glick AM. Focal segmental glomerulosclerosis: a case study with review of pathophysiology. Nephrol Nurs J. 2007 Mar-Apr;34(2):176-82.

Gordon-Larsen P. Obesity-related knowledge, attitudes, and behaviors in obese and non-obese urban Philadelphia female adolescents. Obes Res. 2001 Feb;9(2):112-8.

Gorman SK, Slavik RS, Marin J. Corticosteroid treatment of severe community-acquired pneumonia. Ann Pharmacother. 2007;41(7):1233-7.

Green EC, Halperin DT, Nantulya V, et al. Uganda's HIV prevention success: the role of sexual behavior change and the national response. AIDS Behav. 2006 Jul;10(4): 335-46; discussion 347-50.

Guin JD. Treatment of toxicodendron dermatitis (poison ivy and poison oak). Skin Therapy Lett. 2001 Apr;6(7):3-5.

Gynaecological illness after sterilization. Br Med J. 1972 Mar 18;1(5802):748-9.

Hafron J, Kaouk JH. Ablative techniques for the management of kidney cancer. Nat Clin Pract Urol. 2007 May;4(5):261-9.

Hair Loss Information Center. http://www.hairloss.com. Accessed November 27, 2007.

Halperin DT, Steiner MJ, Cassell MM, et al. The time has come for common ground on preventing sexual transmission of HIV. Lancet. 2004 Nov 27-Dec 3;364(9449):1913-5.

Hanna L, Adams M. Prevention of ovarian cancer. Best Pract Res Clin Obstet Gynaecol. 2006;20(2):339-62.

Hardie TL. The genetics of substance abuse. AACN Clin Issues. 2002 Nov;13(4):511-22.

Hargrove JT, Abraham GE. Endocrine profile of patients with post-tubal-ligation syndrome. J Reprod Med. 1981 Jul;26(7):359-62.

Harlap S, Kost K, Forrest JD. Preventing pregnancy, protecting health: a new look at birth control choices in the United States. New York: Alan Guttmacher Institute, 1991.

Harman SM. Estrogen replacement in menopausal women: recent and current prospective studies, the WHI and the KEEPS. Gend Med. 2006;3(4):254-69.

Harris WS, Assaad B, Poston WC. Tissue omega-6/omega-3 fatty acid ratio and risk for coronary artery disease. Am J Cardiol. 2006 Aug 21;98(4A):19i-26i.

Heathcote EJ. Diagnosis and management of cholestatic liver disease. Clin Gastroenterol Hepatol. 2007 Jul;5(7):776-82.

Heid E, Bekkali A, Lazrak B, et al. Neurofibroma, poliosis and vitiligo [in French]. Ann Dermatol Venereol. 1978 Jun-Jul;105 (6–7):645-6.

Heidemann C, Hoffmann K, Klipstein-Grobusch K, et al. Potentially modifiable classic risk factors and their impact on incident myocardial infarction: results from the EPIC-Potsdam study. Eur J Cardiovasc Prev Rehabil. 2007;14(1):65-71.

Hepatitis Foundation International. Caring for Your Liver. http://www.hepfi.org. Accessed March 27, 2007.

Hepatitis Information Network. http://www.hepnet.com. Accessed March 27, 2007.

Herpes.com. http://www.herpes.com. Accessed March 29, 2007.

Hershey AD, Tang Y, Powers SW, et al. Genomic abnormalities in patients with migraine and chronic migraine: preliminary blood gene expression suggests platelet abnormalities. Headache. 2004;44(10):994-1004.

Hoffman R, Monga M, Elliot S, et al. Microwave thermotherapy for benign prostatic hyperplasia. Cochrane Database Syst Rev. 2007;(4):CD004135.

Hofmanova I. Pre-conception care and support for women with diabetes. Br J Nurs. 2006;15(2):90-4.

Hollman D, Alderman E. Substance abuse counseling. Pediatr Rev. 2007 Sep;28(9):355-7.

Holloszy JO, Fontana L. Caloric restriction in humans. Exp Gerontol. 2007 Aug;42(8):709-12.

Hu G, Jousilahti P, Nissinen A, et al. Body mass index and the risk of Parkinson disease. Neurology. 2006;67(11):1955-9.

Human papillomavirus vaccine: new drug. Cervical cancer prevention: high hopes. Prescrire Int. 2007 Jun;16(89):91-4.

IJzelenberg H, Meerding WJ, Burdorf A. Effectiveness of a back pain prevention program: a cluster randomized controlled trial in an occupational setting. Spine. 2007;32(7):711-9.

International Foundation for Functional Gastrointestinal Disorders. http://www.aboutibs.org. Accessed July 18, 2007.

International Osteoporosis Foundation. http://www.iofbonehealth.org. Accessed July 15, 2007.

Irminger-Finger I. Science of cancer and aging. J Clin Oncol. 2007;25(14):1844-51.

Irwin RW, Watson T, Minick RP, et al. Age, body mass index, and gender differences in sacroiliac joint pathology. Am J Phys Med Rehabil. 2007;86(1):37-44.

Isakow W, Morrow LE, Kollef MH. Probiotics for preventing and treating nosocomial infections: review of current evidence and recommendations. Chest. 2007;132(1):286-94.

Janikowski TP, Glover NM. Incest and substance abuse: implications for treatment professionals. J Subst Abuse Treat. 1994 May-Jun;11(3):177-83.

Jiang W, Kuchibhatla M, Clary GL, et al. Relationship between depressive symptoms and long-term mortality in patients with heart failure. Am Heart J. 2007;154(1):102-8.

Jovanovic L. Nutrition and pregnancy: the link between dietary intake and diabetes. Curr Diab Rep. 2004;4(4):266-72.

Kafi R, Kwak HS, Schumacher WE, et al. Improvement of naturally aged skin with vitamin a (retinol). Arch Dermatol. 2007 May;143(5):606-12.

Kallio P, Kolehmainen M, Laaksonen DE, et al. Dietary carbohydrate modification induces alterations in gene expression in abdominal subcutaneous adipose tissue in persons with the metabolic syndrome: the FUNGENUT Study. Am J Clin Nutr. 2007;85(5):1417-27.

Kendrick JM, Wilson C, Elder RF, et al. Reliability of reporting of self-monitoring of blood glucose in pregnant women. J Obstet Gynecol Neonatal Nurs. 2005;34(3):329-34.

Kirchberger S, Majdic O, Stockl J. Modulation of the immune system by human rhinoviruses. Int Arch Allergy Immunol. 2007;142(1):1-10.

Klatte T, Pantuck AJ, Kleid MD, et al. Understanding the natural biology of kidney cancer: implications for targeted cancer therapy. Rev Urol. 2007 Spring;9(2):47-56.

Koh KA, Sesso HD, Paffenbarger RS Jr, et al. Dairy products, calcium and prostate cancer risk. Br J Cancer. 2006;95(11):1582-5.

Koletzko B, Cetin I, Thomas Brenna J, for the Perinatal Lipid Intake Working Group. Dietary fat intakes for pregnant and lactating women. Br J Nutr. 2007 Nov;98(5):873-7.

Kolotkin RL, Binks M, Crosby RD, et al. Obesity and sexual quality of life. Obesity (Silver Spring). 2006 Mar;14(3):472-9.

Kolotkin RL, Head S, Hamilton M, et al. Assessing impact of weight on quality of life. Obes Res. 1995 Jan;3(1):49-56.

Koushik A, Hunter DJ, Spiegelman D, et al. Fruits and vegetables and ovarian cancer risk in a pooled analysis of 12 cohort studies. Cancer Epidemiol Biomarkers Prev. 2005;14(9):2160-7.

Kristal AR, Stanford JL. Cruciferous vegetables and prostate cancer risk: confounding by PSA screening. Cancer Epidemiol Biomarkers Prev. 2004;13(7):1265.

Kwon MA, Shim WS, Kim MH, et al. A correlation between low back pain and associated factors: a study involving 772 patients who had undergone general physical examination. J Korean Med Sci. 2006;21(6):1086-91.

Lang E, Kastner S, Neundorfer B, et al. Effects of recommendations and patient seminars on effectivity of outpatient treatment for headache. Schmerz. 2001;15(4):229-40.

Lata PF, Elliott ME. Patient assessment in the diagnosis, prevention, and treatment of osteoporosis. Nutr Clin Pract. 2007;22(3):261-75.

Leung DY, Bieber T. Atopic dermatitis. Lancet. 2003 Jan 11;361(9352):151-60.

Loutfy MR, Antoniou T, Shen S, et al. Virologic and immunologic impact and durability of enfuvirtide-based antiretroviral therapy in HIV-infected treatment-experienced patients in a clinical setting. HIV Clin Trials. 2007 Jan-Feb;8(1):36-44.

Lupus Foundation of America. http://www.lupus.org. Accessed January 28, 2008.

Madani M, Madani F. The pandemic of obesity and its relationship to sleep apnea. Atlas Oral Maxillofac Surg Clin North Am. 2007 Sep;15(2):81-88.

Malatesta VJ. Sexual problems, women and aging: an overview. J Women Aging. 2007;19(1-2):139-54.

Mantle D, Gok MA, Lennard TW. Adverse and beneficial effects of plant extracts on skin and skin disorders. Adverse Drug React Toxicol Rev. 2001 Jun;20(2):89-103.

Marin Caro MM, Laviano A, Pichard C. Impact of nutrition on quality of life during cancer. Curr Opin Clin Nutr Metab Care. 2007;10(4):480-7.

Marmouz F. Adult celiac disease. Allerg Immunol (Paris). 2007 Jan;39(1):23-5.

MayoClinic.com. Asthma. http://www.mayoclinic.com. Accessed March 28, 2007.

Meade CS, Graff FS, Griffin ML, et al. HIV risk behavior among patients with co-occurring bipolar and substance use disorders: associations with mania and drug abuse. Drug Alcohol Depend. 2008 Jan 1;92(1-3):296-300.

Mental Health America. http://www. nmha.org. Accessed August 11, 2007.

Merikangas KR, Avenevoli S. Implications of genetic epidemiology for the prevention of substance use disorders. Addict Behav. 2000 Nov-Dec;25(6):807-20.

Meston CM, Bradford A. Sexual dysfunctions in women. Annu Rev Clin Psychol. 2007;3:233-56.

Michael J. Fox Foundation for Parkinson's Research. http://www. michaeljfox.org. Accessed May 31, 2007.

Middleton ET, Steel SA. The effects of short-term hormone replacement therapy on long-term bone mineral density. Climacteric. 2007;10(3):257-63.

Miller VA, Palermo TM, Powers SW, et al. Migraine headaches and sleep disturbances in children. Headache. 2003;43(4):362-8.

Modi P. Diabetes beyond insulin: review of new drugs for treatment of diabetes mellitus. Curr Drug Discov Technol. 2007;4(1):39-47.

Moffitt JE, Golden DB, Reisman RE, et al. Stinging insect hypersensitivity: a practice parameter update. J Allergy Clin Immunol. 2004 Oct; 114(4):869-86.

The Movement Disorder Society. http://www.movementdisorders.org. Accessed May 25, 2007.

Nakabeppu Y, Tsuchimoto D, Yamaguchi H, et al. Oxidative damage in nucleic acids and Parkinson's disease. J Neurosci Res. 2007;85(5):919-34.

Napryeyenko O, Borzenko I. GINDEM-NP Study Group. Ginkgo biloba special extract in dementia with neuropsychiatric features. A randomised, placebo-controlled, double-blind clinical trial. Arzneimittelforschung. 2007;57(1):4-11.

Narcotics Anonymous. http://www. na.org. Accessed October 9, 2007.

National Alliance on Mental Illness. http://www.nami.org. Accessed August 11, 2007.

National Association of Neurological Disorders and Stroke. http://www. ninds.nih.gov. Accessed May 31, 2007.

National Cancer Institute. http://www. cancer.gov. Accessed December 28, 2007.

National Clearinghouse for Alcohol & Drug Information. http://ncadi. samhsa.gov. Accessed October 9, 2007.

National Council on Aging. http://www. ncoa.org. Accessed June 21, 2007.

National Diabetes Education Program. http://www.ndep.nih.gov. Accessed July 27, 2007.

National Digestive Diseases Information Clearinghouse. http:// digestive.niddk.nih.gov. Accessed July 18, 2007.

National Digestive Diseases Information Clearinghouse. Viral Hepatitis: A Through E and Beyond. http://digestive.niddk.nih. gov. Accessed March 27, 2007.

National Headache Foundation. http:// www.headaches.org. Accessed April 4, 2007.

National Heart, Lung, and Blood Institute. http://www.nhlbi.nih.gov. Accessed September 4, 2007.

National Institute of Alcohol Abuse and Alcoholism. http://www.niaaa. nih.gov. Accessed October 9, 2007.

National Institute of Allergy and Infectious Diseases. http://www. niaid.nih.gov. Accessed November, 29, 2007.

National Institute of Arthritis and Musculoskeletal and Skin Diseases. http://www.niams.nih.gov. Accessed July 15, 2007.

National Institute of Diabetes and Digestive and Kidney Diseases. http://niddk.nih.gov. Accessed July 27, 2007.

National Institute of Environmental Health Sciences. Asthma and Its Environmental Triggers. http:// www.niehs.nih.gov.

National Institutes of Health. http:// www.nih.gov. Accessed October 7, 2007.

National Institute of Mental Health. http://www.nimh.nih.gov. Accessed May 14, 2007.

National Institute of Neurological Disorders and Stroke. http://www. ninds.nih.gov. Accessed October 7, 2007.

National Institute on Aging. http:// www.nia.nih.gov. Accessed June 21, 2007.

National Kidney and Urologic Diseases Information Clearinghouse. http://kidney.niddk. nih.gov. Accessed July 23, 2007.

National Kidney Foundation. http:// www.kidney.org. Accessed July 23, 2007.

National Migraine Association. http:// www.migraines.org. Accessed April 4, 2007.

National Osteoporosis Foundation. http:// www.nof.org. Accessed July 15, 2007.

National Pain Foundation. http:// www.nationalpainfoundation.org. Accessed June 23, 2007.

National Parkinson Foundation. http:// www.parkinson.org. Accessed May 31, 2007.

National Sleep Foundation. http:// www.sleepfoundation.org. Accessed October 7, 2007.

National Stroke Association. http://www. stroke.org. Accessed April 25, 2007.

National Student Speech Language Hearing Association. http://www. asha.org. Accessed May 31, 2007.

National Women's Health Center. http://womenshealth.gov. Accessed September 3, 2007.

National Women's Health Information Center. http://www.4woman.gov. Accessed April 4, 2007.

Natural Standard: The Authority on Integrative Medicine. 2008. http:// www.naturalstandard.com.

Navarro Silvera SA, Jain M, Howe GR, et al. Dietary folate consumption and risk of ovarian cancer: a prospective cohort study. Eur J Cancer Prev. 2006;15(6):511-5.

Nemours Foundation. http:// kidshealth.org.

Nemours Foundation. Inflammatory Bowel Disease. http://www.nemours. org. Accessed March 28, 2007.

Neugut AI, Ghatak AT, Miller RL. Anaphylaxis in the United States: an investigation into its epidemiology. Arch Intern Med. 2001 Jan 8;161(1):15-21.

Nguyen-Michel ST, Unger JB, Spruijt-Metz D. Dietary correlates of emotional eating in adolescence. Appetite. 2007 Sep;49(2):494-9.

NIH Consensus Development Conference on celiac disease. NIH Consens State Sci Statements. 2004 Jun 28-30;21(1):1-23.

North American Menopause Society. http://www.menopause.org. Accessed August 31, 2007.

Oliver G, Wardle J, Gibson EL. Stress and food choice: a laboratory study. Psychosom Med. 2000 Nov-Dec;62(6):853-65.

Pacheco RC, Oliveira LC. Lipase/amylase ratio in biliary acute pancreatitis and alcoholic acute/acutized chronic pancreatitis.

Arq Gastroenterol. 2007 Mar;44(1):35-38.

Palacios S. Androgens and female sexual function. Maturitas. 2007;57(1):61-5.

Pandemic Flu Guide. http://www. pandemicflu.gov. Accessed March 29, 2007.

Park S. Medical management of urinary stone disease. Expert Opin Pharmacother. 2007 Jun;8(8):1117-25.

Parkinson's Disease Foundation. http://www.nlm.nih.gov. Accessed May 31, 2007.

Penninx BW, Messier SP, Rejeski WJ, et al. Physical exercise and the prevention of disability in activities of daily living in older persons with osteoarthritis. Arch Intern Med. 2001 Oct 22;161(19):2309-16.

Peters U, Foster CB, Chatterjee N, et al. Serum selenium and risk of prostate cancer—a nested case-control study. Am J Clin Nutr. 2007 Jan;85(1):209-17.

Phatak S, Foster HE. The management of interstitial cystitis: an update. Nat Clin Pract Urol. 2006 Jan;3(1):45-53.

Pines A. Postmenopausal hormone therapy: The way ahead. Maturitas. 2007 May 20;57(1):3-5.

Polizzi S, Pira E, Ferrara M, et al. Neurotoxic effects of aluminium among foundry workers and Alzheimer's disease. Neurotoxicology. 2002;23(6): 761-74.

Porst H, Behre HM, Jungwirth A, et al. Comparative trial of treatment satisfaction, efficacy and tolerability of sildenafil versus apomorphine in erectile dysfunction—an open, randomized cross-over study with flexible dosing. Eur J Med Res. 2007 Feb 26;12(2):61-7.

Porter SE, Hanley EN Jr. The musculoskeletal effects of smoking. J Am Acad Orthop Surg. 2001;9(1):9-17.

Prostate Cancer Foundation. http:// www.prostatecancerfoundation.org. Accessed November 15, 2007.

Raiford DS. Pruritus of chronic cholestasis. QJM. 1995 Sep;88(9):603-7.

Resnick SM, Coker LH, Maki PM, et al. The Women's Health Initiative Study of Cognitive Aging (WHISCA): a randomized

clinical trial of the effects of hormone therapy on age-associated cognitive decline. Clin Trials. 2004;1(5):440-50.

Rieck G, Fiander A. The effect of lifestyle factors on gynaecological cancer. Best Pract Res Clin Obstet Gynaecol. 2006;20(2):227-51.

Riegel B, Moser DK, Powell M, et al. Nonpharmacologic care by heart failure experts. J Card Fail. 2006;12(2):149-53.

Rigopoulos D, Gregoriou S, Paparizos V, et al. AIDS in pregnancy, part II: treatment in the era of highly active antiretroviral therapy and management of obstetric, anesthetic, and pediatric issues. Skinmed. 2007 Mar-Apr;6(2):79-84.

Rosano GM, Vitale C, Marazzi G, et al. Menopause and cardiovascular disease: the evidence. Climacteric. 2007;10 Suppl 1:19-24.

Rosenberg M, Parsons CL, Page S. Interstitial cystitis: a primary care perspective. Cleve Clin J Med. 2005 Aug;72(8):698-704.

Rousseau JC, Delmas PD. Biological markers in osteoarthritis. Nat Clin Pract Rheumatol. 2007 Jun;3(6):346-56.

Rupp RE, Stanberry LR, Rosenthal SL. Vaccines for sexually transmitted infections. Pediatr Ann. 2005 Oct;34(10):818-20, 822-4.

Schulze MB, Schulz M, Heidemann C, et al. Fiber and magnesium intake and incidence of type 2 diabetes: a prospective study and meta-analysis. Arch Intern Med. 2007;167(9):956-65.

Segraves RT, Lee J, Stevenson R, et al. Tadalafil for treatment of erectile dysfunction in men on antidepressants. J Clin Psychopharmacol. 2007 Feb;27(1):62-6.

Seksik P, Daniel F, Marteau P, et al. Refractory proctitis [in French]. Gastroenterol Clin Biol. 2007 Apr;31(4):393-7.

Shadiack AM, Sharma SD, Earle DC, et al. Melanocortins in the treatment of male and female sexual dysfunction. Curr Top Med Chem. 2007;7(12):1137-44.

Shapiro J, Lui H. Treatments for unwanted facial hair. Skin Therapy Lett. 2005 Dec-2006 Jan;10(10):1-4.

Shen M, Kim Y. Osteoporotic vertebral compression fractures: a review of current surgical

management techniques. Am J Orthop. 2007;36(5):241-8.

Shoelson SE, Herrero L, Naaz A. Obesity, inflammation, and insulin resistance. Gastroenterology. 2007;132(6):2169-80.

Shrestha S, Pradhan G, Bhoomi K, et al. Review of laparoscopic cholecystectomy in Nepal Medical College Teaching Hospital. Nepal Med Coll J. 2007 Mar;9(1): 32-5.

Siddiqui MA, Perry CM. Human papillomavirus quadrivalent (types 6, 11, 16, 18) recombinant vaccine (Gardasil). Drugs. 2006;66(9): 1263-71; discussion 1272-3.

Simasek M, Blandino DA. Treatment of the common cold. Am Fam Physician. 2007 Feb 15;75(4):515-20.

Singh BB, Udani J, Vinjamury SP, et al. Safety and effectiveness of an L-lysine, zinc, and herbal-based product on the treatment of facial and circumoral herpes. Altern Med Rev. 2005;10(2):123-7.

Smith CA, Collins CT, Cyna AM, et al. Complementary and alternative therapies for pain management in labour. Cochrane Database Syst Rev. 2006;(4): CD003521.

Smith SD. Oral appliances in the treatment of obstructive sleep apnea. Atlas Oral Maxillofac Surg Clin North Am. 2007 Sep;15(2):193-211.

Society for Interventional Radiology. http://www.sirweb.org. Accessed August 16, 2007.

Sohen S. Adverse effects of corticosteroids in treatment of rheumatoid arthritis [in Japanese]. Nippon Rinsho. 2005 Jan;63 Suppl 1:556-9.

Sperling LC. Hair and systemic disease. Dermatol Clin. 2001 Oct;19(4):711-26, ix.

Stander H, Traupe H. Hair loss: a review of possible causes [in German]. Med Monatsschr Pharm. 2000 Oct;23(10):316-22.

Staud R. Treatment of fibromyalgia and its symptoms. Expert Opin Pharmacother. 2007;8(11): 1629-42.

Steele AC, McLennan MT. The painful bladder: urinary tract infection and interstitial cystitis in women. Mo Med. 2007 Mar-Apr;104(2):160-5.

Stein RT, Marostica PJ. Community acquired pneumonia: a review and recent advances. Pediatr Pulmonol. 2007 Dec;42(12): 1095-103.

Steinmaus CM, Nunez S, Smith AH. Diet and bladder cancer: a meta-analysis of six dietary variables. Am J Epidemiol. 2000;151(7):693-702.

Storch A, Jost WH, Vieregge P, et al. Randomized, double-blind, placebo-controlled trial on symptomatic effects of coenzyme Q10 in Parkinson disease. Arch Neurol. 2007 Jul;64(7):938-44.

Straub DA. Calcium supplementation in clinical practice: a review of forms, doses, and indications. Nutr Clin Pract. 2007 Jun;22(3):286-96.

Sun Y, Yang J. Experimental study of the effect of Astragalus membranaceus against herpes simplex virus type 1. Di Yi Jun Yi Da Xue Xue Bao. 2004;24(1):57-8.

Swanenburg J, de Bruin ED, Stauffacher M, et al. Effects of exercise and nutrition on postural balance and risk of falling in elderly people with decreased bone mineral density: randomized controlled trial pilot study. Clin Rehabil. 2007;21(6):523-34.

Tamlcr R, Mechanick JI. Dietary supplements and nutraceuticals in the management of andrologic disorders. Endocrinol Metab Clin North Am. 2007;36(2):533-52.

Targonski PV, Poland GA. Pneumococcal vaccination in adults: recommendations, trends, and prospects. Cleve Clin J Med. 2007;74(6):401-6, 408-10, 413-4.

Tham LM, Lee HP, Lu C. Enhanced kidney stone fragmentation by short delay tandem conventional and modified lithotriptor shock waves: a numerical analysis. J Urol. 2007 Jul;178(1):314-9.

Thomas SL, Wheeler JG, Hall AJ. Micronutrient intake and the risk of herpes zoster: a case-control study. Int J Epidemiol. 2006;35(2): 307-14.

Thompson R, Bandera E, Burley V, et al. Reproducibility of systematic literature reviews on food, nutrition, physical activity and endometrial cancer. Public Health Nutr. 2008 Oct;11(10):1006-14.

Thorpy M. Therapeutic advances in narcolepsy. Sleep Med. 2007 Jun;8(4):427-40.

Tikkanen MJ, Jackson G, Tammela T, et al. Erectile dysfunction as a risk factor for coronary heart disease: implications for prevention. Int J Clin Pract. 2007 Feb;61(2): 265-8.

Tsiodras S, Mooney JD, Hatzakis A. Role of combination antiviral therapy in pandemic influenza and stockpiling implications. BMJ. 2007 Feb 10;334(7588):293-4.

U.S. Food and Drug Administration. http://www.fda.gov. Accessed November 29, 2007.

Ueki A, Otsuka M. Life style risks of Parkinson's disease: association between decreased water intake and constipation. J Neurol. 2004;251 Suppl 7:vII18-23.

United States Administration on Aging. http://www.aoa.gov. Acccssed May 14, 2007.

United States Department of Health and Human Services. http://www. hhs.gov. Accessed March 29, 2007.

Vas J, Perea-Milla E, Mendez C, ct al. Efficacy and safety of acupuncture for chronic uncomplicated neck pain: a randomised controlled study. Pain. 2006;126(1-3): 245-55.

Vina J, Borras C, Miquel J. Theories of ageing. UBMB Life. 2007 Apr;59(4):249-54.

Viner RM, Haines MM, Taylor SJ, et al. Body mass, weight control behaviours, weight perception and emotional well being in a multiethnic sample of early adolescents. Int J Obes (Lond). 2006 Oct;30(10):1514-21.

Vogt TM, Ziegler RG, Patterson BH, et al. Racial differences in serum selenium concentration: analysis of US population data from the third National Health and Nutrition Examination Survey. Am J Epidemiol. 2007 Aug 1;166(3):280-8.

von Haehling S, Doehner W, Anker SD. Nutrition, metabolism, and the complex pathophysiology of cachexia in chronic heart failure. Cardiovasc Res. 2007;73(2): 298-309.

Vrouenraets SM, Wit FW, van Tongeren J, et al. Efavirenz: a review. Expert Opin Pharmacother. 2007 Apr;8(6):851-71.

VZV Research Foundation. http:// www.vzvfoundation.org. Accessed March 29, 2007.

Wager TD, Scott DJ, Zubieta JK. Placebo effects on human micro-opioid activity during pain. Proc Natl Acad Sci U S A. 2007;104(26):11056-61.

Wanga QM, Chen SH. Human rhinovirus 3C protease as a potential target for the development of antiviral agents. Curr Protein Pept Sci. 2007 Feb;8(1):19-27.

Weaver BA. Epidemiology and natural history of genital human papillomavirus infection. J Am Osteopath Assoc. 2006 Mar;106(3 Suppl 1):S2-8.

White A, Foster NE, Cummings M, et al. Acupuncture treatment for chronic knee pain: a systematic review. Rheumatology (Oxford). 2007;46(3):384-90.

Wilson LF. Adolescents' attitudes about obesity and what they want in obesity prevention programs. J Sch Nurs. 2007 Aug;23(4): 229-38.

Women's Health America. http:// www.womenshealth.com. Accessed September 2, 2007.

World Health Organization. http:// www.who.int. Accessed March 29, 2007.

Worldwide Education and Awareness for Movement Disorders. http:// www.wemove.org. Accessed May 31, 2007.

Wu T, Zhang J, Qiu Y, et al. Chinese medicinal herbs for the common cold. Cochrane Database Syst Rev. 2007 Jan 24;(1):CD004782.

Zhang J, Villar J, Sun W, et al. Blood pressure dynamics during pregnancy and spontaneous preterm birth. Am J Obstet Gynecol. 2007;197(2):162.e1-6.

Zhou P, Qian Y, Xu J, et al. Occurrence of congenital syphilis after maternal treatment with azithromycin during pregnancy. Sex Transm Dis. 2007 Jul;34(7):472-74.